D0857973

MIND AND BRAIN

MIND AND BRAIN
The Many-Faceted Problems

Selected Readings from the
Proceedings of the International Conferences
on the Unity of the Sciences

Edited by Sir John Eccles

PARAGON HOUSE

Washington

Printed in the United States of America

International Standard Book Number: 0-89226-016-5

Library of Congress Catalogue Card Number: 82-083242

The International Cultural Foundation, Inc. (ICF, Inc.)

International Headquarters:
G.P.O. Box 1311, New York, NY 10116

Tokyo Office:
Rm. 1006, TBR Bldg., 2-10-1 Nagata-cho
Chiyoda-ku, Tokyo, Japan

London Office:
44 Lancaster Gate,
London W23NA, England

— CONTENTS —

About the Authors

Karl H. Pribram is Professor of Neuroscience, Stanford University, Stanford, California

Henry J. Jerison is Professor of Psychiatry, University of California, Los Angeles, California

Diane McGuinness is Lecturer in Psychology, Stanford University, Stanford, California

Roger W. Wescott is Professor of Anthropology, Drew University, Madison, New Jersey

Ragnar A. Granit is a Professor of Neurophsiology, The Medical Nobel Institute, Stockholm, Sweden

Benjamin Libet is Professor of Physiology, University of California Medical School, San Francisco, California

Holger Hyden is Professor and Director of The Institute of Neurobiology, University of Goteborg, Goteborg, Sweden

Robert J. White is Professor and Co-Chairman of Neurosurgery, Case Western Reserve University, Cleveland, Ohio

Gunther S. Stent is Professor of Molecular Biology, University of California, Berkeley, California

Marius Jeuken is Professor of Theoretical Biology, State University, Leiden, Netherlands

Daniel N. Robinson is Professor of Psychology, Georgetown University, Washington, DC

Juan Antonio Gomez is Director of the Institute for Scientific Investigation, University of Bogota, Bogota, Columbia

J.W.N. Watkins is Professor of Philosophy, London School of Economics, London, England

Grover Maxwell is Professor of Philosophy, University of Minnesota, Minneapoplis, Minnesota

Roger Sperry is Hixon Professor of Psychobiology, California Institute of Technology, Pasadena, California

J.W.S. Pringle is Linacre Professor of Zoology, Oxford University, Oxford, England

Brian D. Josephson is Professor of Physics, University of Cambridge, Cambridge, England

W.H. Thorpe is Professor of Zoology, Jesus College, Cambridge, England

H.D. Lewis is Professor of History and Philosophy of Religion, King's College, London, England

Mary Carman Rose is Professor of Philosophy, Goucher College, Towson, Maryland

Bradley T. Scheer is Professor of Biology, Westmont College, Santa Barbara, California

Kai Nielsen is Professor of Philosophy, University of Calgary, Alberta, Canada

W. Norris Clarke is Professor of Philosophy, Fordham University, New York, New York

Ravi Ravindra is Associate Professor of Physics and Religion, Dalhousie University, Halifax, Nova Scotia

Sir John Eccles is Distinguished Emeritus Professor, State University of New York-Buffalo, USA/Switzerland and Past Chairman of the International Conference on the Unity of the Sciences V and VI

*H.B. Jones, Professor of Medical Physics and Physiology, University of California, Berkeley, California

*Duke L.V.P.R. de Broglie, Secretary of the Academy of Science, *Academie Francaise*, Paris, France

---

*deceased

Preface

The annual International Conferences on the Unity of the Sciences (ICUS) have been the occasion for the exploration of a wide range of topics covering a large part of human culture—from the natural sciences to the social sciences and to the humanities as exemplified in art, philosophy and religion. The proceedings of seven of these conferences (1972 to 1978) have been published, and it is from these published records that I have compiled this book, selecting those contributions that could be considered as relating to a theme of discourse and argument that rightly has now become a topic of great interest, namely the body-mind or mind-brain problem.

I have chosen to interpret this theme very broadly on the grounds that this problem has a quite unique relationship to the human quest for a meaning and value for life. In fact the question is that of ultimate concern especially when this mysteriously wonderful conscious life is viewed as ending in death. There is a termination of our consciously experiencing selves and our memories with the death of the brain.

The topics assembled in this book extend in a spectrum from evolutionary biology through to the philosophy of life and death. I have organized them into four main sections: A.) The biology of consciousness; B.) Cerebral correlates of consciousness; C.) Philosophical contributions to the mind-brain problem; and D.) Meaning of life and death in the context of the mind-brain problem. In these sections there are contributions from some of the foremost thinkers of the world, who do in fact present widely different beliefs. Thus it is hoped that this book provides an excellent educational opportunity for the reader to view a wide variety of beliefs. Since the papers necessarily are limited to a brief text for presentation in 30 minutes or less, references to more extensive works by the authors are appended to each paper. Unfortunately there has been no recording of many of the interesting discussions aroused by the presented papers and the associated commentaries.

Sir John Eccles
Locarno, Switzerland

Sir John Eccles

Introduction

A. The Biology of Consciousness

The papers of this section of the mind-brain problem are grouped around biological ideas, particularly evolution and purposiveness. The chairman's introduction by *Karl H. Pribram* helps to orientate our thinking to evolution and to consciousness in its many states.

Henry J. Jerison gives an excellent account of the factors probably concerned in that most wonderful of all evolutionary achievements, the creation of Homo Sapiens. Necessarily attention is concentrated on brain performance with the superposition of consciousness and language.

Diane McGuinness develops the provocative idea that the role of females in the evolution of Homo Sapiens has been overlooked because of the preoccupation of evolutionists, particularly Darwin, with natural selection by prowess in hunting and warfare. She makes a most convincing case for the dominant female influence in important aspects of human evolution, such as food-gathering, food-sharing and language. In his discussion paper *Roger W. Wescott* in part agrees, but outlines a balanced position.

Ragnar A. Granit approaches evolutionary theory from the standpoint of a neurophysiologist, and stresses the importance of concepts of purposiveness and adaptability, even speaking of immanent teleology with which I approve.

Sir John Eccles uses the three-world philosophy of Popper to illuminate the process of cultural evolution, which is exclusively human. Homo Sapiens has created culture, and each human being (Nature) has to be created as a person by the culture he is immersed in (Nurture).

B. Cerebral Correlates of Consciousness

This section embraces papers that are concerned in one way or another with the responses of the brain and their relationships to conscious experiences.

1

The first paper of this section was a plenary lecture by *Sir John Eccles*, there being no discussion. The theme embraces the intimate association of the human person with its brain and follows on thematically from the last paper of the preceding section (A 6). In particular there is an account of the modular structure and operation of the neocortex with conjectures about the way in which mind can relate to the enormous complexity of the spatio-temporal modular patterns, so giving the unity of conscious experience.

Empirical evidence on the mind-brain interaction is presented by *Benajim Libet*. The temporal discrepancy between brain events and the related conscious experiences provides a difficulty for any variety of identity theory (cf. C4, C5, C6).

Robert J. White describes remarkable surgical interventions on primates whereby brains or heads (cephalons) are transplanted and remain viable, as shown by electroencephalograms and reactions. The vexed question of human head transplants arises as a menacing spectre.

W. Horsley Gantt's contribution is of particular interest for its rich historical material. He is one of Pavlov's most famous pupils, but developed scientifically and philosophically away from Pavlov. It is remarkable for its wisdom and deep insight into the mind-brain problem.

Holger Hyden presents the outcome of many years of neuro-chemical investigations on the brain, particularly in respect to learning. He has always stressed the important role of messenger ribonucleic acid and the subsequent protein synthesis. As the discussant, *Robert J. White*, indicates, it is important to synthesize these concepts with the neurophysiological mechanisms of the brain—with synaptic actions, impulse discharges, modular patterns, etc.

Sir John Eccles discusses the philosophical problem of the freedom of the will in the light of the hypothesis of dualist- interactionism (cf. C7). Suggestions are given as to how the mind influences could provide information modifying the spatio-temporal modular patterns of the neocortex.

C. Philosophical Contributions to the Mind-Brain Problem

I am particularly happy with the contributions collected into this section, as they present a wide range of speculative thought by scientists who have pondered deeply on a great variety of problems oriented around the mind-brain problem.

In his philosophical essay *Gunther S. Stent* views the failure of positivism in relation to its successors, particularly structuralism. He attempts to relate the structure and functioning of the neural machinery of the brain to the subconscious and the conscious, as exhibited particularly in language in Chomsky's structuralist linguistic theory. *Marius Jeuken* follows up with penetrating comments and criticisms, but unfortunately Stent's reply was not recorded.

Daniel N. Robinson presents an historical and critical appraisal of the mind-body problem. It is regarded as a bona fide issue for science and central to the attempt to understand homo cogitans. No solution is offered, but the way to a solution is indicated.

In his analysis of the mind-brain problem *Juan Antonio Gomez* uses his neurological expertise in giving an account of the linguistic performance of the brain at all levels of its activity.

By a masterly logical analysis *J.W.N. Watkins* develops a seemingly insuperable objection to the Identity-hypothesis, particularly as defined by Moritz Schlick. He concludes that "if physiology were ever to show that the above-mentioned properties of consciousness are *also* properties of the brain, then the brain would be utterly different from the brain as described by contemporary physiology and, indeed, from *any* physical system so far known to us." I would fully agree.

On the same theme *Grover Maxwell* contemplates the possibility that the neural machinery of the brain may have completely different properties from anything yet discovered, having mental attributes *per se*, and so there could be a strict identity of mind and brain.

Sir John Eccles critically evaluates all materialist theories of the brain-mind problem and discounts the suggestion that the neurosciences will eventually provide a complete explanation of all mental phenomena, which is labelled as promissory materialism. The alternative hypothesis of a strong dualist-interactionism is outlined. Further consideration of this hypothesis is provided in Section B 1.

Karl H. Pribram gives a general and critical survey of the mind-brain problem in which he favors a structuralist basis for a solution (cf. C 1).

Philosophical implications of the brain-mind problem are discussed at length by *Roger Sperry*. He states that his aim is to show that the traditional separation of science and values and the related limitations it has implied for science as a discipline are no longer valid in the context of the current mind-brain theory. He develops a wholistic concept of the mind-brain relationship that is opposed to reductionism and materialism on the one hand and to dualism on the other. This closely reasoned paper deserves critical attention. He concludes that "Science deals with values as well as with facts".

JW.S. Pringle presents a rich field of speculative thought. He regards the human brain as being central to *all* problems. There is an initial section on temporal patterns of oscillators which are presented as a possible model of brain action in contrast to the customary spatial relations. Then the treatment becomes more general with valuable sections on the evolution of consciousness and the emotions. In his commentary *Brian D. Josephson* raised important points with respect to the blocks produced by the conditioning of scientists to consider only material happenings. He instanced the understanding of such phenomena as ESP and even of the possible intervention of God in the natural world. I would further suggest the mind-brain problem as being in this category.

D. Meaning of Life and Death in the Context of the Mind-Brain Problem

There can be no doubt but that the mind-brain problem must be of paramount concern because of the key position it necessarily occupies in the human quest for meaning, not only of life, but also of death. I am happy to present a series of papers that give widely differing and even antagonistic viewpoints.

In his plenary [ICUS] lecture *W.H. Thorpe* concentrates on the human search for meaning that has been threatened by "the monistic views of so many scientists and humans of the present day". He counteracts these threats firstly by reference to the recent revolution that suggests a deep relationship between ourselves and the whole cosmological story from the Big Bang onwards. Secondly he postulates a real disposition of the world for the evolution of mental awareness. He concludes that "the human mind and soul which operates in liaison with it, has latent possibilities and capacities for further emergence and transcendence — capacities to which we can set no limit."

The late *Duc de Broglie* presents the quest for meaning, as it appears to a great physicist, immersed in the materialist philosophy of science, though spiritual overtones are lightly sketched in.

H.D. Lewis gives a very well argued account of the philosophical concept of persons. An historical account of the idealism-materialism controversies leads him to develop his own critical attack on materialism. He then presents his philosophy of dualism and the human person, which is similar to what I have given in sections B 1 and C 6. He insists on the "notion of the distinct and ultimate identity of persons", which he suggests continues after death. *Mary Carman Rose* comments in a well reasoned, wise and deeply thoughtful paper on the philosophy of the human person as conceived in the great religions. *Bradley T. Scheer* also comments on the Lewis paper. He develops a good synthesis of biology and personhood. He stresses particularly that the person represents a history of expression, reception, creation and transmission of information. Finally he considers the person as having "the property of eternity" in conformance with the "Will of the Creator".

Kai Nielsen develops a philosophical position diametrically opposed to that of Lewis and his commentators. He presents a clever atheistic argument which is essentially that of the majority of scientists and humanists of this day. He attempts to show that for an atheist life can have meaning and moral commitment, and even hope.

W. Norris Clarke's paper is in great contrast to Nielsen's. He presents a very clear and authoritative account of the traditional Christian position on death and the meaning of life. With the

coming of the Christian message death "becomes no longer the
ultimate darkness, the end without issue, but rather the gateway
to a new and indestructible fullness of life." He finishes with
reference to "the mystery of the total meaning of human life, as
seen in the partly revealing, partly concealing light of death."

Ravi Ravindra presents the Hindu response to death and the
meaning of life, which is in great contrast to the views expressed
in sections D 5 and D6. There is a relativity of life and death, of
death and rebirth. The meaning of life consists in the opportunity
it affords for liberation from this endless repetition of life and
death and rebirth.

Sir John Eccles attempts to bring to a conclusion this extraordinary variety of contributions. He outlines a position that can be
developed from the principles of Natural Theology, but which is
not in conflict with the Christian tradition.

Karl H. Pribram

A1 Evolution of Consciousness

Today's topic is "The Evolution of Consciousness". Before we
hear the speakers we should make some definitions so that we
will better understand what they are talking about. Yesterday we
were exposed to many statements regarding consciousness. But
one of the problems was that people were often not communicating because terms remained undefined. So I would like to first
recall to you a definition of evolution. Dr. Wescott yesterday talked about evolution, and suggested that evolution means change,
and that the change must be in essence either gradual or come in
stages. There may be some discontinuities but the discontinuities
have to be related to each other in some fashion. The difference
between evolution and revolution is that in evolution the stages
can be related to each other, and that there is not some major discontinuity in the change. Empirically the problem is to find the
missing links that relate stages.

Consciousness is perhaps more difficult to define. But we can
start with the difference between states of consciousness which
we have all experienced. We have one state of consciousness when
we are asleep and dreaming, another state of consciousness when
we are awake (hopefully) attending a conference such as this.
There are discontinuities between states, and we cannot as Sir
Eccles said last night, remember in one state what occurred in the
other. This state specificity of memory and thus of the articula-
tion that defines consciousness applies to many more states of
consciousness than just dreaming on the one hand and being
awake on the other. Sometimes even different scientific disciplines
appear to provide different stages of consciousness in this sense.
One of the problems of a transdisciplinary conference such as this
is that the articulated consciousness which one discipline gives to
an individual limits him, and he cannot somehow get to the other
state of consciousness within which someone else is speaking.
States of consciousness mutually exclude each other: A salmon
spawning does not eat. A salmon eating does not spawn. A

behaviorist in psychology does not speak about consciousness at all. He has no consciousness.

There is much talk about altered states of consciousness these days. I don't think there is such a thing; rather, there are alternate states of consciousness. And (although we can't go into detail this morning) the bio-chemistry and electro-physiology of the brain seems to have a great deal to do with establishing these states. The idea that a conceptual discipline can determine a state of consciousness may seem a little farfetched when brain bio-chemistry is concerned to be the root of a conscious state. But in our own work, we've established the fact that the areas of the brain involved in cognitive operations, the so-called association areas, modulate the activities of the biochemical mechanisms. At least the anatomy of the connection has been worked out and the electro-physiology, so whatever becomes organized cognitively can then change the chemistry of the brain.

These brain mechanisms help define the states of consciousness, but they do not define the contents of consciousness. The contents of consciousness are our perceptions and feelings. What relates the states of consciousness to their contents are what we call attentional processes. We'll hear a great deal about these processes today.

But this is not the total range of ways in which consciousness is talked about. One way compatible with the above definitions is the manner the neurosurgeon, e.g. Bob White, will be talking about consciousness this morning. The neurosurgeon is interested in whether the patient is conscious or not conscious. Remember I noted that dreaming is a state of consciousness. Well how do we know that? We poke a person who's asleep and dreaming and he wakes up. He's not in coma, he's not in a stupor. And so we make useful distinction between consciousness and unconsciousness in that fashion. Freud used the term in a similar fashion: when we have ready access to the determinants of behavior (that we know why we did something) we call it consciously determined. If on the other hand, access is difficult or eludes us then we call its determination unconscious. This is one set of definitions.

Another set of definitions became evident yesterday in the session on religion and philosophy. The problem of self-consciousness, the problem of awareness of the self, what philosophers call intentionality. The difference between being able at one and the same time to be aware of the contents of consciousness and of the process of being aware—i.e. simultaneously aware of one's self and one's environment. That is a second way in which consciousness is defined: people don't always use the term self-consciousness—they simply use the word consciousness to cover this intentional aspect of consciousness.

And finally, there is a way of talking about consciousness which is still different. Sir John Eccles has been talking to us in these terms for a number of years, and often we have not understood him. I'm beginning to understand him now and will label this form of consciousness 'transcendental'. This definition holds that consciousness extends beyond, is not just the product of, the interaction through this brain and senses of an organism and his environment. This is the mystic's way of conceiving consciousness. We must not confuse this transcendental consciousness with either the content definition of self-consciousness nor with the state definition of consciousness.

I now ask the speaker to let us know which definition of consciousness he is addressing: whether he is speaking to the problems of states or contents or transcendence of consciousness. This should help us understand each other.

Harry J. Jerison

A2 The Evolution of Consciousness

The evolutionary biology of consciousness cannot be studied directly for several obvious reasons. First, we know consciousness as an essentially private experience. It cannot be analyzed directly in a group of people, a human population. There is, therefore, no direct information on variations in human consciousness. Variation is the stuff of evolution, and without information about it an evolutionary analysis is impossible. The second source of difficulty follows from the first. If we are to analyze the evolution of a trait we must have some sense of its nature in different species. If we cannot have direct access to the consciousness of another human how much less likely is it that we will ever have direct access to the consciousness of individuals of nonhuman species of animals.

But in making these points I am belaboring the obvious. Their value is primarily in emphasizing the requirement for indirect assessments of consciousness and, thus, of definitions of consciousness that are both acceptable and useful in suggesting indirect measures. I will not plunge into measures and data, and the necessary definitions at this time can be much more vague and yet retain some utility.

To begin with, let us recognize that all aspects of life can be viewed as adaptions, that is, as characters or traits that evolved as a way of making animals work more successfully in their normal environments. The consciousness that we know individually is as much a biological adaptation as the hand or eye. I think that I can characterize this consciousness in a way that will help us appreciate its biological role, which I believe is an inevitable one for animals more complex than simple invertebrate species to cope with the challenge of an environment. I would start with the place of the nervous system in coping with information about the environment.

The biological problem raised by the existence of nervous systems that contain more than a few thousand neurons is how to control the responses of a whole animal. Even if the animal worked as a piece of clockwork, with each bit of information from the environment triggering fixed sensory and motor responses and movements of muscles, it would be impossible for the system to work accurately without further organization. The chain of events, which we should call reflexes, would never complete an appropriate response to stimuli if more than a few dozen elements were involved. The difficulty is due to the fact that neurons are built with some uncertainty inherent in their operation. And the uncertainty is such that the system would produce impossibly many errors unless the chain of nerve cells in the reflex arc had no more than a dozen or so elements in it.

The solution to the biological problem was undoubtedly by chunking or clumping the information-processing procedure, analogously to the way computer programmers write their programs by putting "instructions" together into subroutines and then calling up subroutines when a complex instruction is needed, rather than attempting to rewrite a complete detailed instruction on every occasion that it is needed. An even better analogy from computers is in the way user-languages, such as FORTRAN, have evolved in which the simplest element in the language is already a complex set of electrical yes-no events as described in "machine-language."

Consider the information-processing problems faced by an "average" mammal such as a cat as it stalks a mouse, and let us restrict ourselves to visual information even though this may be one of the less important channels of information. The visual image of the mouse could be captured without difficulty on photographic film placed at the cat's retina. But at the living retina the physical image becomes a remarkably complex, elaborate, and almost innumerable set of events. Literally millions of sensory cells are excited to different degrees and at different times, and the bleaching of pigments in those actually excited at a given time is the source of nerve impulses in addition millions of nerve cells in the cat's eye. Not in what we conventionally recognize as its brain. The neural retina is technically brain tissue, but since it lies outside the cranial cavity it is usually treated as non-brain. A complex pattern of exitation and inhibition is transmitted by several hundred thousand nerve cells in the retina upward into the brain. The "information" in this pattern consists of perhaps 10 events or so per second, on the average, with some neurons passing more than 100 events per second into the first stage of analysis in the brain.

I am not about to treat you to a lesson in elementary neuroanatomy, so let me sum up this issue by noting that before the instantaneous information about the mouse in space is fully analyzed by the cat's brain, before the half second or so of analysis is complete, it is likely that more than 100,000,000 neurons will have been involved (I am probably an order of magnitude too low in this estimate). It is inconceivable that a system adapted to process information, the brain in this instance, could work directly on so much information. It would have to be chunked, and there would have to be hierarchies of chunks.

Now let us consider the same cat but other modalities. If the mouse moved it might produce some sound. That would reach some 70,000 sense cells in the cat's ears, and the signals would eventually be processed in millions of neurons in the brain. A comparably complex or even more complex situation exists for smell, and it is likely that we misread the role of this modality. As primates, we are severely crippled in our ability to use olfactory information. Our sense organ is, in a real sense, atrophied at least when compared to that of other orders of land mammals. (The weak olfactory system of primates will be a central element in later analysis here; it certainly keeps us from understanding intuitively the experience of most other species of mammals.) We must assume comparable chunking and hierarchies of chunks for auditory and olfactory brain and for visual brain.

As a thought problem, let us try to imagine the nature of the chunks produced by the brain as it processes information. Within each modality these can be arbitrarily constrained. The essential requirement would be to have the highest level of chunking produce chunks that would be reasonably stable labels for the source, the environmental source, of stimulation. The whole animal might be thought of as an object that has to move through physical space (with the option of remaining stationary, or freezing in position, a zero-movement among the "movements".) As the animal moves the pattern of neural stimulation must change dramatically even if the environment is entirely stable. The highest-level-chunks must represent the stability of the environment and, where appropriate, the fact of the animal's motion through a stable environment. Now a further problem: the highest-level olfactory chunk, representing stalked mouse against environmental background, and the highest level visual chunk and auditory chunk for the same information-complex are very likely in different parts of the brain. Furthermore, with respect to the neural constraints on processing information there is no necessary relationship among these modality-specific chunks. It is only in the ultimate use of the information, perhaps in guiding a leap by the cat as it catches the mouse, that a unity is or must be developed.

It is obvious what that unity must be. The mass of information, the changes-of-state of many nerve cells, has to be converted into a useful entity, namely a "mouse" that exists in a "world out there." The chunk must represent an object in space. And the olfactory and visual and auditory chunks, though perhaps distinct as smells and sights and sounds, must all refer to the object: the smell of the mouse, its appearance, and the effects of its movements and squeaks.

This constructive act by a complex nervous system is more complex than I have indicated here. The mouse is known against some environmental background. It is in some position in space. In the visual system, space of a sort is inherent in the structure of the system. There are labeled spatial coordinates, essentially x, y, z labels for the points of space, and one assumes that this system (x, y *coordinates given by the retina of the eye; z-coordinate* added in some analytic fashion from stereopsis and from the many other cues for the third dimension of visual space) is also represented by appropriate higher-order chunks.

The fact of time, of the organization of events in time, which appears so natural and elementary to us, is not a simple phenomenon from a neural point of view. Simultaneity is as much of a problem for the psychologist and for the sensory physiologist as it is for the physicist. Certain departures from physical simultaneity — temporal disparaties among neural events — may yet be experienced as simultaneity with added character. I have a specific example in mind. If the cat's mouse happened to squeak, and certain neurons in the cat's medulla were activated within 5 millionths of a second of one another, the information would be chunked (or put into a super-chunk higher in the hierarchy) as indicating that the mouse was directly in front of the cat. If the physical temporal disparity between the events in the medulla were, let us say, 1/10,000th of a second, the mouse's squeak (and the mouse) would be experienced as off to one side or other, but not in line with the cat's midline. The squeak would still be a unitary event in time, but it would be displaced in space. The time-difference in the brain would be structured as a spatial deviation — a localization of sound in space.

The reason for developing as much detail as I have is to make a central point for the analysis of consciousness as a biological phenomenon. The point is that reality as we ordinarily understand and experience it is not a phenomenon of the outside physical world. Rather it is a construction of the brain, a phenomenon of what we might correctly consider as the inside physical world of the brain. This is not to be solipsistic on the matter. Our naively experienced phenomenal reality bears a close relationship to physical reality (as understood from sophisticated analysis of the nature of the physical world). But phenomenal reality is very much a construction of the brain, as can be shown by the tricks and failures of experience in illusions, dreams, and hallucinations.

My approach to the evolution of consciousness takes the idea of a constructed reality as its basis. To be conscious is first to experience a real world. It is as simple as that. Certain "events" are constructed by the brain as part of experience. These include space, time, and a variety of objects. The puzzle and confusion in the analysis of consciousness is certainly on the role of the self as one of the objects in one's world. I doubt that many would argue that relatively complexly organized animals, such as mammals, do not experience a reality that is at least comparable to the one that we experience. And all but a few odd philosophers would agree that my reality is essentially the same as yours in its basic structure, though the events that we experience at any given moment will differ, of course, depending on where we are and what we happen to be doing.

The evolution of consciousness can then be analyzed from at least two perspectives. How do the basic structures of consciousness differ in different species of animals to reflect specific adaptions and unique environmental niches? Second, can we find some hierarchy with respect to the level of organization of consciousness in different species, to characterize some as higher and others as lower? These two questions will occupy the rest of this analysis. The answer to the first is entirely in the context of environmental niche and the available neural apparatus for adaption to the niche. The answer to the second question also concerns the environmental niche and its pressures, but also concerns encephalization—the evolution of more neural tissue and of a more important role for the brain (especially its "higher centers") in more advanced species. The concept "more advanced" can be tricky, and I will try not to trap you in the illogic of the idea of directed progressive evolution.

Consciousness as a Biological Adaption

It may be unfortunate that the word "consciousness" appears here, because the basic adaptation is the construction of a real world within which to behave. That this construction differs in different species has been appreciated for generations. Popularized as *Umwelt* by the neoKantian biologist, Jacob von Uexhull, the concept is well illustrated in pictures of the same environment as it might be experienced by animals of different species. Obvious examples include the visual world of carnivores, such as dogs, which are relatively insensitive to color and the comparison of this world with the color-rich world of man and other primates. But there are more dramatic and radical examples that may be beyond our ability at representation. The visual world of the horse and rabbit and of most birds is not the proscenium stage that we experience. Rather it is a complete hemisphere or sphere (depending on whether the earth forms a platform or, as a bird in flight, the animal is in the center of an almost complete sphere). We are reasonably certain that these are the visual "real" worlds from reconstructions of the visual field represented on the retina of the eye. The two retinas of these species are at the sides of the head, more or less parallel to one another, and a reconstruction of the visual field covered by the two retinas turns out to involve more than 360 degrees, both in front of and behind the head. Can you imagine living in such a 360-degree physical universe experienced at each instant of time? You probably can, because even in our natural proscenium-stage world, the limited 120-degree extent of visual space is recognized as a limited experience that could easily be extended by turning our heads about. I would ask you to stretch your imaginations here, however, to guess at the world of the horse in which the instantaneously visible includes the world behind the head as well as the one in front of it.

The picture of reality, of conscious experience, is really more complex than these examples suggest. Our world is the peculiarly visual world of a species of primate. It is also richly auditory, especially in the human world of heard speech. But it is an under-privileged world of odors and the olfactory sense. You need only watch your dog as it moves about sniffing at objects and dropping a few drops of urine (if it is male) and thus marking its world. The marks are intelligible to other dogs, so much so that present views are that they give information about specific individuals. The world of knowledge conveyed by scent-marks and scents, so rich for dogs and other canids (wolves, foxes, etc.) is unknown to us except when analyzed with sophisticated scientific procedures. Even then we can be reasonably sure that the gap between our understanding of the message of the dog's urine and the place of the message in the dog's world is as great as the gap between the representation of speech in sophisticated sound-pictures, a sonogram or an oscilloscopic trace, and the place of its message in our lives.

The adaptation involved in the creation of a real world is one that enables an animal to make sense of an otherwise overwhelming load of neural information. The workings of this adaptation can be illustrated by pictures of what the world of experience "looks like". The best illustration of this adaptation may be at the other end of its operation, but the way movements are controlled.

As I write these words, I sit at the typewriter (since that is my habitual way) and my thoughts are eventually converted into marks on a piece of paper. The observable end of this conversion as a biological process is in the movement of my fingers striking keys. Note how complex that analysis has to be. There is the microscopic level, analogous to machine-language or the operation of yes-no devices in a computer, in which millions of neural and muscular events are recordable every second in the fibers running to the musculature of fingers, arm, shoulders and elsewhere. It is obviously impossible to handle instructions to this system by working at this machine-language level. But it would be as serious a mistake to imagine the operation at any of several higher, chunked, levels, such as the movements of individual fingers or even sequences of movements. I can control the motions by ordering: "Move index finger from coordinate position x_1, y_1, z_1, to position x_2, y_2, z_2." Further reduced, I might rephrase the order as a sequence of commands: flex index finger, extend ring finger, etc. Neither of these make much sense and neither is a true picture of the activity or of the instructions. Yet even these false overly reductionist pictures are highly chunked organized versions of commands in the form: 1_1, t_1, i_2, t_2, . . . where i refers to a nerve impulse and t to a time and the subscripts are summary statements to identify the position and order of the events. The last is the measurable biological output of the system, but the controls are at a much higher level. If I were typing single letters without further semantic content the instruction would very likely take the form: "type k," the same as the intent to have the letter k typed. The resultant action would involve the ballistic movement of one finger oriented in space with respect to the key on the typewriter for the letter k, and the execution would be through the reduction of "error" in the relative positions of finger and key, coupled with "subroutines" specifying force etc. That is a still higher order chunking than noted before, and here it is important to recognize that "finger" and "key" will have been constructed by a brain as elements of a reality in which "events" can take place — all chunks of a higher order. The actual performance, as I sit and type, is one which only I can report with even approximate clarity. I type not as motions of my fingers on the typewriter, unless I attend to these motions. Rather I "speak" to an imaginary listener, and my speech is not through my voice box but through my fingers. If I took time to think of each movement of each finger I would give this up as a bad job. My chunks are larger units, syntactic and lexical units, and I have evidence for that in my errors. A common one for me is: *I no what I'm saying* in place of *I know what* . . . . Clearly my fingers take an acoustic message and can confuse homonyms.

To summarize the biological adaptation, it is one that determines a way to chunk neural information into useable units. The elements of my reality are similar to the elements in yours, and the experience of these elements is similar. Hence we know similar worlds. It is impossible to imagine a radically different world in other animals, even if we imagine intriguing species-typical adaptations. This naive awareness, phenomenal experience, or consciousness is a necessary aspect of information processing, and we are only vaguely aware of it as being special or unusual or a problem.

Human Consciousness and Speech and Language

Just as the reality of a species, as a construction of its brain, must to some extent be unique to the species, so must consciousness be unique to a species. I have tried to suggest the way in which reality is structured as being part of the adaptation of brain as a bodily organ, and I will carry this analysis forward to consider the special adaptations of *Homo sapiens* and their implications for our reality. It is in the uniqueness of our reality that we will appreciate the uniqueness of human consciousness.

Note first that I have argued for consciousness as a general adaptation, an aspect of the chunking of information in (moderately) large brains. I have reported elsewhere a detailed analysis of the evolution of encephalization in mammals as a 200-million year old adaptation that enabled our ancestors at that remove to cope with an unusual environmental niche, and I will summarize that analysis now. It is prologue to the analysis of the evolution of human consciousness.

The problem was to account for the appearance of enlarged brains in the earliest mammals which distinguished them from their immediate ancestors among the reptiles. The "larger" brain was about one gram; the smaller, ancestral brain about ¼ gram. My solution involved the often (and I believe, correctly) assumed adaptations of early mammals as nocturnal animals. Add to this the fact that reptiles of that period were almost certainly diurnal, with highly developed visual systems (and associated chunking of visual information), it was natural to consider the hypothesis that the earliest mammals were "reptiles" that had invaded a new environmental niche, that of life on land at nightfall and through the night.

Without detailing the full analysis, it is sufficient to note that the visual system is much less useful to a nocturnal animal than to a diurnal one. If the species invading the new niche were to conserve as many adaptations as possible it would have to evolve new distance-sensing machinery analogous to the visual sense of reptiles. I considered the likelihood that hearing and smell were elaborated for this purpose in the earliest mammals. I could then show, easily, that to pack a number of neurons into the auditory and olfactory systems that would be comparable in number to those packed into the retina of reptiles would require a significant enlargement of the brain. Thus the enlarged brain of early mammals, the encephalization of these species, could be accounted for as the solution of a packing problem: where to put the information-processing neurons for auditory and olfactory information that would function analogously to those relatively useless neurons of the neural retina.

The full argument acknowledged the persistent role for the retina at twilight (including the evolution of the rod-system of the retina that functions primarily in a dark-adapted eye and is presently a typical mammalian adaptation). Night vision, coupled with audition and olfaction in the early mammals would then be providing information from the same points in space. Organizing that information with code-representations or chunks as "objects" in space and time were clearly useful adaptions that would provide a selective advantage for animals dependent on information about the distant environment. It was possible to argue, further, that the construction of "space" was natural for a visual system structurally organized with spatial coordinates in at least two dimensions. The category, "space," would be supplemented in the early mammals by comparable constructions based on the unique elements of the other neural systems — audition and olfaction. The auditory system, with its intrinsically temporal organization (witness the conversion of microsecond differences between physical neural events into spatial displacement for the localization of sound, as described earlier), would in its normal operation chunk events into a construction that we would know as "time." The picture for the olfactory system is more obscure, since, as noted earlier, our intuitions about an olfactory world are necessarily poor.

The essence of the analysis was to account for a novel development in evolution, the enlargement of the brain while other organs of the body remained at an appropriate size, by seeing in the novelty nothing more than a conventional adaptation to an understood environmental requirement. The major point was that the earliest mammals were "reptiles" trying to make a living as animals on land at night. The nocturnal niche was new for reptiles and there was the novelty. The adaptive response was conventional: add neuronal material to process environmental information that can be handled by existing sensory systems. In this "addition" there was a new adaptation: encephalization. I will presently develop the same kind of analysis for human encephalization, a unique phenomenon as far as we know at present for the past 3 million years or so in the history of life on earth.

The facts of the history of encephalization can be stated fairly simply. During the 500 million years or so of known vertebrate life most vertebrate species have had brains that were fairly similar in encephalization, that is, in relative size with respect to their body-sizes. This means that most species were comparable in their ability to process neural information; because encephalization is a measure of general information-processing capacity. This majority of species includes almost all fish, amphibians and reptiles. Birds and mammals have been more encephalized throughout the past 150-200 million years, and I have analyzed the history of early encephalization in mammals with you in the preceding paragraphs. After the great extinctions about 65 million years ago, there was a major evolution of encephalization in mammalian species, correlated with the reinvasion diurnal niches. A new evolution of the visual system would have been required for corticalized vision to interact with the auditory and olfactory system at the level of higher brain centers in the neocortex and cerebellum. The primates formed an unusual order of mammals in this respect, much more encephalized than other orders (about twice as much brain per unit body size, on the average) throughout their known history of over 50 million years. The primates probably were encephalized to this extent because of their highly visual behavior, which involved color vision, fancy stereopsis, and perhaps other adaptations of the system. But the primates also were peculiar in their underdeveloped peripheral olfactory systems. The key element now is derived from the anatomy of the latter systems so I have to go through a bit of neurology with you.

The olfactory system of the brain is a highly elaborate one, scarcely olfactory in the simple-minded sense, but nevertheless treated so by classical neurology because it is connected to the olfactory bulbs. The olfactory bulbs are essentially that, "bulbs" of nerve tissue attached to stalks that are nerve fiber tracts, known as the olfactory tracts. These can be tracked into the inside of the brain.

Once inside the brain these tracts connect to enormous systems of cells named collectively as "rhinencephalon" (smell brain), limbic system, or paleocortex. Primates have very small olfactory bulbs compared to the bulbs of other mammals of similar body size. But they are perfectly normal mammals with respect to the rest of the "olfactory" system. In fact, that system is notorious in modern neurobiology as the neural system involved in emotions, motivation, and even in some types of memory, everything except "smell," hence the discarding of the old term, rhinecephalon.

To skip now from neurology to behavior, I want to reconstruct the niche invaded by that group of primates that included our immediate ancestors, family Hominidae which branched away from the manlike apes perhaps 15 million years ago. This family is rather well known as of about 3 or 4 million years ago as the australopithecines, whose environment can be reconstructed with some confidence. More, their way of life can also be constructed. They were likely social predators living in relatively open country (rather than forests). It is in that niche or adaptive zone that I have sought to understand the evolution of many of the peculiarly human features of our brain and behavior.

Let us recall, before lunging into this analysis, that we must deal with adaptations to existing environments, not *preadaptations* appropriate for environments that might be entered later. The model social predator is the wolf, and we should imagine the ecology and neurobiology of the australopithecines (and their predecessors) in terms of species of primates trying to make a living doing what comes naturally to wolves. The missing element for primates is as easy to think about as the missing visual world for early mammals as "reptiles" in a nocturnal niche. That element is the olfactory sense associated with environmental markers. To appreciate the importance of this lack of effective olfaction, let us see its place in the wolves' niche. In its normal life, a wolf pack may number a half dozen individuals. The pack ranges over a territory that is hundreds of kilometers in extent. Its members can mark the territory with urine, know their friends of the pack, and members of adjacent packs, and navigate the territory with daily treks of tens of kilometers. There is little doubt that an individual wolf retains an excellent mental map of its territory, and the problem faced by a primate attempting a comparable life would very likely begin with the methods for constructing a useful cognitive map to navigate its extended range. I would argue that primates accomplished this without the olfactory and scent-making skills by adaptations of their auditory and vocal systems for analogous functions. The internal portions of the olfactory system, the existing smell-brain or rhinencephalon, would also participate in the neural adaptation.

In short, I imagine the early primates as "marking" their territory with sounds, recording the auditory label of the sounds, talking to themselves, as it were, about where they were in space and where their positions were relative to other marked positions in space. This speech would be elementary, of course, prelinguistic or protolanguage at best. But it is in this kind of adaptation that I would seek the eventual adaptation that we know as language.

Many puzzles fall into place if we adopt this view. Living languages are tools for communication, but peculiar tools for living

animals. For one thing, they are severely hampered by the requirement that they be learned through an elaborate cultural ritual.
Strangely (in terms of newer developments in the neurosciences),
the learning of language is more like the learning of sensory-
perceptual abilities than of communicational abilities, at least in
the perspective of general biology. Most animals communicate
fairly instinctively with one another with only rare instances of
major contraints imposed by early environments. But they must
be exposed to normal environments for their sensory systems to
develop normally. Another feature of human language is its function as a kind of representation of reality rather than as a method
of commanding or eliciting actions from others. It is a cognitive
rather communicational domain. Further, human language is controlled by extensive neocortical networks in the brain, as opposed
to the paleocortical and subcortical systems that appear to be
most relevant for the analysis of the control of communication in
other species. Finally, there are important cognitive functions for
paleocortical systems, including the involvement of the limbic
system in language and of the hippocampus in memory.

The peculiar element in the human construction of reality is
the place of language in that construction. Recognizing consciousness as the labelling of reality, the important place of language in
our reality must have immediate consequences. Linguistic labels
are themselves representations of things, hence their use as a
part of reality makes the representational activity, the second-
order "object" a part of our reality. To see a table and the word,
"table", and to recognize the differences and associations of these
"events" in our reality makes our reality representational as well
as a world of immediate experience with object. Words (their
sounds, appearances, etc.) are as real as the things they represent, and to encompass both realities in our reality certain reflexive features are inevitable. The words about our selves, our
bodies, and perhaps most important, our thoughts and memories,
are also elements of the reality. (We may not require actual words
—brain processes of a comparable sort in the deaf or blind must
still occur and contribute to the chunks that become objects and
things in our individual real worlds.)

It is evident to me that the evolution of human consciousness must be related first to the evolution of hierarchical structures in the brain's analytic machinery. That aspect of consciousness must be shared with many other species of animals that have even moderately large brains. As processing capacity increased, either through encephalization or the increases in body size, more and different kinds of chunking must have occurred. The peculiar features of human consciousness: self-consciousness, reflexive events or knowing that we know and that others know, must be related to special constructions, special kinds of chunks, in human brains. Given the representational activity of language systems of the brain it seems evident that all of these "higher order" conscious activities would have to follow. They are not so much higher order as specialized and different orders of conscious activity, but like other adaptations of essentially familiar systems (chunking and hierarchically organized systems in this case) their ultimate effects may be difficult to predict or understand. The dominant place of *Homo sapiens* in the present world of nature is an outcome of this adaptation, applied in new ways and thus creating a new environmental niche within which we live our lives.

Diane McGuinness

A3 Was Darwin Conscious Of His Mother?

Darwin and His Descendants

In the *Descent of Man* Darwin sets out the major distinctions between ape and man.[1] For the majority of these distinctions, bipedalism, development of tools, increased intelligence, and social behavior, etc., Darwin attributes the selection process solely to hunting and warfare, going so far as to conclude that benevolence and empathy are a direct result of male cooperation during war.

Continued speculation about factors leading to human evolution has not changed since Darwin. Washburn derives his theory on sharing from the hunt.[2] Shepher, writing in 1978 in *The Journal of Social and Biological Structures*, concludes after reviewing many theories that the evolution of pair-bonding derived from the transition to hunting.[3] This in turn led to larger brains because of tool-making, causing larger skulls, earlier parturition, wider hips and long lactation, sexual specialization, and less muscular, more cuddly females!

Apart from one or two authors, such as Lancaster and Morgan,[3] evolutionary theorists seem convinced that male specific behavior provides the only relevant clues to man's evolutionary descent. Because of this onesidedness the theories are remarkably contrived and unconvincing. To remedy this state of affairs I wish to explore the possibility of developing a model based largely on female-specific behaviors.

The truth is no doubt somewhere in between, but as will be seen, natural selection based upon female aptitudes gets us considerably further from the apes than selection based exclusively on male aptitudes. This approach also has merit from a genetic point of view. Females have two X chromosomes. Genetic information from *either* chromosome can be passed on to offspring of both sexes. Information from the male Y chromosome, however, can only go to one sex. No information about Y chromosomes is ever passed on to females. Thus, females maintain the dominant gene pool, sharing their *female* characteristics with both sons and daughters. As will be seen, this genetic arrangement is a direct parallel of behavioral distinctions.

The Puzzle of the Enlarging Brain

The major dilemma in the attempt to understand man's origins is related to *why* and *how* the brain began to change in size so dramatically. Man's nearest genetic relative, the chimpanzee, has a body weight of 45 kilograms and a brain size of approximately 400cm³. This is a ratio of 1kg to 8.75 cm³. Homo sapiens' body weight/brain size ratio is 1 kg to 22 cm³ (57 kg to 1230 cm³). The most important clues to the nature of this transition lie not only in the difference in mass of tissue, but in specific areas of development. The most prominent distinction is found in the four-fold increase in the size of the cerebral mantle. Both posterior and frontal cortical areas are grossly enlarged, and in humans the left hemisphere is larger than the right. This difference between the hemispheres is not found in the apes.

Bipedalism and use of tools, long considered to be fundamental antecedents of the changing brain, have largely been ruled out as salient contributors to man's evolution. Bipedalism and tool use occurred long before the radical change in brain size. Observations from Darwin's period to current studies by Goodall show that apes frequently use tools for a number of purposes.[5] The discovery of a "home-base" for primitive man prompted a theory which suggested that we evolved *because* of discovering how to stay in one place and share food instead of foraging. However, the establishment of home bases has been shown to precede the change in the size of the brain. Bones, stone artifacts and crude tools have been found in small contained sites estimated as well over two and one-half million years old.

Nor is hunting the answer. Apes occasionally "go hunting" if they accidentally come across game while foraging. They will grab whatever weapons are available in the form of branches, stones, etc., and attack the animal and consume it on the spot with enormous excitement, agitation and vocalizations. A number of lower mammals hunt successfully without the need for large brains.

Despite the legend of man-the-hunter handing down his genes to his sons and thus passing on skill in aimed throwing, there is simply no evidence to support this notion as a model for evolution. Hunting was and is a sporadic endeavor. Apes throw quite well. Wolves hunt in packs, cooperatively, without the need for language that some have proposed derived from hunting expeditions. In fact, studies have shown that *silence*, not speech, is essential to the successful hunt.

Washburn, in an intriguing hypothesis, proposed the theory that *sharing* became important because of geographical and climatic factors. He interpreted this insight, however, in a straight Darwinian tradition. Sharing is presumed to be derived from *hunting*;[2] though there is little logic in this assumption. In most hunter-gatherer societies the majority of food is obtained through gathering. Another problem with Washburn's theory is that severe climatic conditions such as those during the Pliocene drought, actually drive out game. In modern day desert dwelling tribes, gathering is the primary source of food. The gatherers, Bushman women, living in harsh desert conditions will walk up to 10-15 miles a day in search of small plants and insects, carrying them back to the home base. Because of the difficulties with Washburn's hypothesis, Lancaster proposed that *gathering, carrying* and *sharing* are the critical factors in our evolution.[4] She suggests that sharing began as a cooperative endeavor by females. One of the most primary distinctions between apes and men is not the proclivity for hunting, but the fact that apes are hairy and we are not. Young apes are transported by clinging to their mother's fur. Human mothers, being hairless, have to *carry* their infants. Whatever clues may be found to solve the riddle of our hairlessness, the fact remains that human beings carry their children, and this has a multitude of consequences. The propensity for carrying is available even in monkeys through ventral-ventral contact between mother and infant. In studies on Rhesus macaques carried out by Gary Mitchell at the University of California at Davis, they found that pairing infants with males produced bonding largely through play behavior.[6] There was an almost total absence of ventral-ventral contact between infants and their male "mothers".

Here is the hint then, that one of the more radical shifts in evolution may have had something to do with the female: her need to carry her child, the reliance of the tribe or troupe on her skills in gathering food, and her ability to share both the gathering and in the distribution of food. The bones of a theory proposing that evolutionary changes leading to Homo sapiens were produced somehow through selection of female specific behaviors is given more flesh when considering the differences between apes and men.

Differences That Make a Difference

There are four primary differences between humans and the apes all of which combine to produce the elements and artifacts of human culture. As will be seen subsequently all of these differences are female-specific apptitudes. Three of these differences are psychological. The first is language, the second a vastly superior memory and the third, self-awareness, or context dependent behavior. The final difference is a vast superiority in sequencing fine-motor behavior. In almost all other respects involving the sensitivities of sensory systems, strength, agility and so forth, apes and men are remarkably similar. As each of these differences reflects a refinement of an aptitude, not merely the possession of that aptitude, they rely on changes in *cortical* tissue.

Apes, of course, do share all of these abilities but to an exceedingly lower degree. The pioneering studies of the Gardners and those of David Premack have illustrated that chimpanzees are able to master certain aspects of language using signs or tokens, specifically nominalization and a rudimentary form of sequencing signs and symbols.[7] The Gardner's chimp, Washoe, has subsequently invented "words" by combining two signs into a novel relationship. There is considerable debate, however, that the ape's capacity for language contains an ability to master syntax and any grammar with semantic connotations. No ape has ever been taught to utter human sounds beyond a few words, suggesting that the brain region governing the fine motor control for the vocal apparatus is undeveloped. Fine-motor control of all types is noticeably lacking.

Apes must remember in order to master language, but their memory span is short. Immediate memory involving the processing of a number of items at one time is directly related to span of attention. Maintaining items in awareness, or paying attention involves the ability to remain undistracted by irrelevant information. The outcome of processing efficiency is a more stable and functional use of coding strategies and hence retrieval from a permanent memory store. As noted above, apes use objects as tools, but generally discard them when they have obtained their goal. Remembering specific objects and noting their permanence is essential to the development of an understanding of object relationships in the physical world. It leads ultimately to a sense of time and place. A highly developed memory for time and place is essential to a species who searches for specific foods at specific seasons and can bring food back from remote locations to a home base.

The remaining psychological distinction and perhaps the most significant to this conference is the human's capacity for self-awareness or the ability to view the self in the context of others. Self-awareness or self-consciousness therefore leads to context-sensitive behavior, specifically to the ability to imagine oneself in situations or states observed in others. This is the beginning of empathetic understanding, the beginning of rule governed behavior, and of values. It is the preliminary requirement for *sharing*. The complications of this form of consciousness will be considered later in this paper.

Female Influence on Evolution

Current data reveal that almost all of the abilities outlined above are female specific aptitudes.[8] One, female ability in language skills of all types is well documented. Females speak earlier, use longer words and more words per utterance than males, and this facility continues into adulthood. Two, females also have superior memories for both visual and auditory information. Three, females are context sensitive. They analyze information *in the context* of each specific situation (one of the reasons, perhaps, that women

are always accused of changing their minds). This is particularly
relevant in social settings where female empathy has been documented at all ages. Four, females are fine-motor specialists particularly for rapid sequencing of movement and show fewer deficiencies than males in all forms of speech production, less stutter-
ing or inability to pronounce certain combinations of sounds.

Not only are these sex differences found in humans, but the
seeds of these differences exist in all non-human primate species.
It may not only be because of female apes having a more docile
nature that all the "talking" apes are female. Patterson reports
that by age 5½ Koko had acquired 450 signs. Her playmate
Michael at the same age, signs only 35.[9] Female non-human primates are more socially oriented, more empathetic and emit
vocalizations that are more often used to signal contact or to
calm other troupe members. Male vocalizations are almost all
antagonistic, accompanying gestures of threat. Females in most
non-human primate species do the major portion of grooming,
and in some species are the only groomers. Primatologists have
suggested that the presence of grooming is the major indicator
that a socially cohesive group exists.[10]

In hard times the non-human primate female preserves and
protects her young; the male preserves himself. The skill needed
to care for others and maintain life becomes essential to a social
unit. Foraging for oneself does not support a social system. In
terrestrial primate colonies, once the males are old enough, they
are pushed out by their mothers and find themselves on the periphery of the colony. It is only through the long experience of rough
and tumble play that they can then adapt and fit into a dominance
order. Females and their daughters remain on the inside of the
colony. This arrangement works well when all that is required is a
loose arrangement to protect a large territorial domain. In a situation where sharing becomes the means of survival and cooperative behavior is essential, the food supply would inevitably be
controlled by the females. The female would thus determine who
survived and who did not. Infants of clever females adept at cooperative endeavors, aided by some form of gesture, or rudimentary
speech, with excellent memories for place (the source of the food
supply) and time (knowledge of seasons) would be the successful

mothers. Sons of these mothers would survive. Sons of mothers who were inept, uncooperative and lazy would, along with their mothers, be driven out or starve.

Ultimately a type of cooperative interaction between the sexes would arise, with males maintaining and patrolling the territory, attempting to bring in food from hunting, and females providing the major sustenance within it. It is possible that the initial cooperation between the sexes came about through mother-son interactions, and only subsequently through unrelated male-female pairs. Though the division of labor with specialist functions for each sex is already present in non-human primate colonies (even pair bonding is observed in species like the gorilla), what is lacking is sharing the food supply. Those primitive peoples more able to share and cooperate, more able to value skills which could maintain a troupe, more able to specialize in order not to waste energy, would become the most effective species.

A New Male: A Conflict of Empathy and Territoriality

Cooperation, awareness of self in the context of others, extended memory, and the evolution of language to establish an effective means of organizing work parties, monitoring the young, sharing out food by learning to count, all have implications for male behavior. The genes that effective mothers pass on to their sons cause behaviors that become integrated with male-specific activities. Two of these male activities are rituals of dominance and the manipulation and construction of tools and weapons. In some ways these are related. Darwin was the first to propose that the drastic change in the shape of the adult human skull with its small jaw and teeth came about through the invention of weaponry. Weaponry obviates the need for what Washburn has described as the "anatomy of bluff." Washburn, like Darwin, was puzzled by the presence of huge teeth in male but not female apes.[2] Apes are largely vegetarian, and females are as well nourished as males. Large incisors appeared to have no function.

The anatomy of bluff involves muscle mass and size as well as a number of specific muscle groups around the face and skull, permitting certain facial gestures of threat that function to promote dominance. Although intra-species aggression is exclusively male (Moyer calls this inter-male aggression),[11] females do have a function in establishing male dominance positions. Evidence from observations of a colony of Rhesus macaques in Oregon, shows that dominant males tend to be the sons of dominant females. The form dominance takes in the females is the observed ability to stand up for her young against threat from other mothers and juveniles. Confidence, it appears, is part of the dominance game.

With the discovery that weapons can function to promote dominance, males skilled in the manufacture and wielding of weapons would predominate and contribute to the gene pool. In times of hardship and danger, a cooperative use of weapons becomes useful and necessary. Weapons are used in hunting and in fending off invaders. Cooperative hunting with weapons and cooperative warfare or defense against attack requires *planning*. Skill in strategic warfare involves the same brain system, namely the frontal lobes, that cooperative, context-sensitive behavior involves. Thus the female capacity for cooperation and planning, passed on to her sons, combines with strength, agility, dominance, manufacture of weapons, all male specific aptitudes.

In advanced civilizations these skills and abilities have increased enormously. Yet we still find a continual shift between the female principle and the male principle. Communal life, respect for other's needs and empathy, vie with territoriality, dominance and power and an emphasis on the individual emerging from the ranks through competition. How then does this interplay emerge in human consciousness?

The Evolution of Self-Consciousness

Consciousness, the ability to pay attention, to be aware of one's surroundings, is a characteristic of all mammals. What is open to debate is whether or not other species besides the great apes and man have achieved self-consciousness. The classic test of self-consciousness has been the ability to recognize one's self in a mirror. Dogs and cats do not appear to do this. Yet social animals like dogs and wolves work cooperatively and appear to distinguish self from other. Domesticated dogs respond to human demands by signalling what appears to be similar to a sense of guilt following a misdemeanor. A dog is aware that *he* and not another has produced an unacceptable act. Thus it seems that all social animals may possess some rudimentary form of self-consciousness.

What then is unique to man? And how seriously should one consider the assumption raised by Julian Jaynes that self-consciousness only arose when man could distinguish his thoughts from the voices of Gods?[12]

It is my contention that human self-consciousness has taken two forms. One form has its roots in cooperative endeavors characteristic of all social mammals. It goes beyond this in the heightened awareness of context dependent behavior. Situational factors govern what is appropriate and what is not. Context-dependent sensitivity predicated on social systems, leads to an ever increasing refinement in the ability to read social signals, to interpret acts, to assist another and to exhibit empathy. As noted above, the ability to share, to take turns, determining what is *fair*, stem from female-specific aptitudes. The rudiments of these skills are found in all non-human primates in the act of grooming.

Once language is achieved, self-consciousness becomes a dominating force. First, it allows one to distinguish verbally between self and other. Secondly, language provides a new domain for thought, the domain of pragmatics. Whereas semantics and syntax involve cues and rules for establishing the meaning of objects and events, pragmatics enable one to determine *intent*. In recent research on mother-infant interactions, Bruner and his colleagues have discovered that a primary focus for training an infant's speech is forcing the child to specify intent. The mother responds to a request by an attempt to determine its sincerity.[13]

> Requesting requires an indication that you want *something* and *what* it is you want. In the earliest procedures used by children it is difficult to separate the two. First the child vocalizes with a characteristic intonation pattern while reaching eagerly for the desired nearby object—which is most often held by the mother. As in virtually all early exchanges, it is the mother's task to interpret, and she works at it in a surprisingly subtle way. During our analysis of Richard when he was from 10 to 24 months old and Jonathan when he was 11 to 18 months old, we noticed that their mothers frequently seemed to be teasing them or withholding obviously

desired objects. Closer inspection indicated that it was not teasing at all. They were trying to establish whether the infants really wanted what they were reaching for, urging them to make their intentions clearer.

When the two children requested nearby objects, the mothers were more likely to ask "Do you really want it?" than "Do you want the X?" The mother's first step is pragmatic, to establish the sincerity of the child's request.

J.S. Bruner, *Human Nature*, 1978, *1* (9). p. 46.

Note that this joint activity is carried out between *mothers* and their children, not by fathers. In fact, McGlaughlin has shown in studies on game playing, employing mother-child and father-child interactions, that only mothers attempt to determine the exact level of understanding of their child.[14] This tuning process by the mother shows clearly her empathetic aptitude and her insistence that the child become aware of the nature of his/her endeavors and goals. The child becomes self-aware, *self- conscious*, through the verbal interchange of specifying intent in the context of the situation. Context sensitivity arises from a female specific ability to force linguistic competence and precision on her offspring.

The second form of consciousness is referred to by Jaynes in *The Origin of Consciousness in the Breakdown of the Bicameral Mind.* Whether or not one accepts Jaynes' view that early man was able to distinguish his own ideas and thoughts from the "voices" of the Gods, Jaynes has documented a radical shift in consciousness during the period of the early Greeks. This shift is a shift towards individualization, and I contend that it is a shift toward a male self-consciousness. It is no accident that this period saw the beginning of monotheistic religions and the birth of a new belief in the power of the individual. The concept of self *against* the others, self as unique, apart from nature and capable of controlling nature, is the beginning of man's conquest of his environment. Man *against* the world, *against* the universe, is an extension of the principle of dominance and it marks a crucial turning point in our cultural evolution. Primitive tribes consider they are part of the natural world, brothers of the animals and trees. Once one recognizes that one can take charge of nature, determine its structure and change its face, one begins the long road to scientific discovery, technology and mastery of the secrets of the universe. Consciousness of the self as *unique*, rather than merely as other, is a male consciousness and is a powerful force for change. The ultimate question then is what *value* do we put on male and female forms of consciousness and how can these forms be brought into harmony?

REFERENCES

1. Darwin, C. *The Descent of Man,* London: John Murray, 1871.
2. Washburn, S.L. and Lancaster, C.S. The evolution of hunting. In: R.B. Lee and I. DeVors (Eds.) *Man the Hunter.* Chicago: Aldine, 1968.
——————— The evolution of man. *Scientific American, 1978,* 239, September, pg. 194.
3. Shepher, J. Reflections on the origin of the human pair-bond. *J. of Social and Biological Structures,* 1978, *1,* 253-264.
4. Lancaster, J.B. *Primate Behavior and the Emergence of Human Culture.* New York: Holt, Rinehart and Winston, 1975.
——————— Carrying the sharing in human evolution. *Human Nature,* 1978, *1,* February.
Morgan, E. *The Descent of Woman.* New York: Stein and Day, 1972.
5. Goodall, J. Continuities between chimpanzees and human behavior. In: G. Isaac, E. McCown (Eds.) *Human Origins: Louis Leakey and the East African Experience.* W.A. Benjamin, Inc. 1976, pp. 483.
6. Mitchell, G. Parental behavior in non-human primates. In: J. Money and H. Musaph (Eds.) *Handbook of Sexology.* Amsterdam: Elsevier, 1977.
7. Gardner, R.A. and Gardner, B.T. Early signs of language in child and chimpanzee. *Science,* 1975, *187* (4178), 752-753.
Premack, D. The education of Sarah: A chimp learns the language. *Psychology Today,* 1970, *4,* 55-58.
8. McGuinness, D. Sex differences in perception and cognition. In: B. Lloyd and J. Archer (Eds.) *Exploring Sex Differences.* New York: Academic Press, 1976.
——————— and Pribram, K.H. The origins of sensory bias in the development of gender differences in perception and cognition. In: M. Bortner (Ed.), *Cognitive Growth and Development: Essays in Memory of Herbert G. Birch.* New York: Brunner/Mazel, 1978.
9. Patterson F. Conversations with a gorilla. *National Geographic,* 1978, *154,* October, p. 438.
10. Missakian, E.A. The timing of fission among free-ranging rhesus monkeys, *Amer. J. of Physical Anthropology,* 1973, *38,* 621-624.
11. Moyer, K.E. *The Psychobiology of Aggression,* New York: Harper & Row, 1976.
12. Jaynes, J. *The Origin of Consciousness in the Breakdown of the Bicameral Mind.* Boston: Houghton Mifflin, 1977.
13. Brunner, J.S. Learning the mother tongue. *Human Nature,* 1978, *1,* Sept. 42-49.
14. McGlaughlin B. Report in preparation.

R. W. Wescott

A4 Human Evolution: His and Hers

Before dealing with the broader question raised by Dr. McGuinness—that of the male and female components in our developing human consciousness—I should like to deal first with the narrower one: that of Charles Darwin's awareness of his mother, Josiah Wedgwood's daughter Susannah, who died when Darwin was 8 years old. Darwin had, in fact, so little memory of her that he did not even mention her in his autobiography.[1] For some years before her death, Susannah Darwin had been an invalid. Her son's mental avoidance of her may have represented an effort on his part to reject illness as a lifestyle. If so, the effort clearly backfired, since he spent much of his adult life housebound by ill health of obscure origin. A Freudian would no doubt label Darwin's chronic indisposition psychogenic and attribute it to the unconscious guilt he felt over his unfilial behavior.

In a larger sense, Darwin may have been representative of the attitude of scientists toward women. Since most scientists were—and still are—men, a predictable element of androcentricity has crept into their thinking about most subjects susceptible to sexual bias. Certainly human evolution is one such subject. Because men have historically been the leaders in the conversion of horticultural society into urban society, our behavioral scientists too readily assume that males have guided females into each new phase of their joint evolution. We know, however, that male initiative has not inevitably characterized our simian cousins in times of collective behavioral reorientation. Among Japanese macaque monkeys, for example, it is juvenile females who have recently pioneered in the introduction of both food-washing and hot-spring bathing to the behavioral repertory of their troops.[2]

It may be, then, that some of the puzzles of human evolution can be better solved by positing female leadership at certain stages in our collective development than by clinging to the habitual assumption that males introduced every major change which our lineage has undergone. A case in point is what Dr. McGuinness calls "the riddle of our hairlessness," which the conventional wisdom, as represented by Sherwood Washburn, explains as an adaptation to the male hominid's new Pleistocene career as a pack-hunter.[3] Washburn's reasoning is that we lost our ape-fur because it impeded rapid heat-dissipation in the long-distance chase. The difficulty with this argument is that it is directly contravened by another anatomical conundrum—the fact that we, alone among the primates, have a substantial deposit of subcutaneous fat, which acts to retain body heat rather than to facilitate its dissipation!

The resolution of this paradox which was suggested by Sir Alister Hardy is that the Pliocene hominids, between 3 and 12 million years ago, went through an aquatic stage, in which they lost their fur (as had the dugongs and dolphins) in a way that facilitated swimming, but gained an underskin fat layer (like that of most marine mammals) which protected them from chilling.[4] Elaine Morgan adopted Hardy's thesis and expanded it, explaining our large noses, busts, and buttocks as adaptations to life in shallow water, along with bipedality, a preference for pebble tools, and the practice of ventral coitus.[5]

What Morgan never states explicity but seems (quite clearly, to me) to imply is that women not only "took the Pliocene plunge" before men but embraced the aquatic life more fully than men, with the result that women even today remain smoother and more streamlined in bodily contours than do their male counterparts.

Well before the Hardy/Morgan Hypothesis was advanced, various theorists, taking note of our exceptionally large brains and gracile bone-structure, had, in effect, defined human beings as fetalized and domesticated apes. If we accept the view of Hardy and Morgan, we may have to expand this definition to describe ourselves, additionally, as aquaticized and feminized apes.

The degree to which wide-spread myths and legends can or should be correlated with known and inferred paleontological facts remains a question. But, were I to attempt such correlations, I would associate the Garden of Eden tradition with the Miocene Epoch, about 12 to 25 million years ago, when our dryopithecian forebears enjoyed a richly frugivorous forest diet; the matriarchal tradition with the Pliocene Epoch described above, when drought shrank the forests but carnivores made the savannas dangerous, inducing our ramapithecian ancestors to undergo collective baptism; and the Nimrod tradition with the Pleistocene epoch, about 3 million to 10,000 years ago, when glacial and pluvial conditions spawned the large herds of ungulates and proboscideans which made big-game hunting and trapping easy.

There are few of Dr. McGuinness' arguments to which I respond in a sex-stereotyped way. Yet one such is her contention that women are more social than men. I can accept this only if I am permitted to substitute the compound "micro-social," meaning familially social, for the word "social." For I would say that, although women tend to be more empathetic toward members of their immediate kin-groups then men do, men tend to be more responsive toward members of the external community than women do. In this sense, men are, I would say, more "macro-social" than women. Putting the matter differently, we might state that the interpersonal attention which women are inclined to direct toward a small number of close associates, men are inclined to direct toward a larger number of more distant associates. The overall sociability of each sex, though comparable in quantity, would then differ only in focus.

I am inclined, however, to agree wholly with Dr. McGuinness' assertion that "consciousness of the self as unique, rather than merely as other, is a male consciousness and is a powerful force for change." The non-hominid primate precondition for such consciousness may well be the strong tendency for juvenile males, expelled from the troop upon reaching adolescence, to live either in solitude or in "bachelor bands" for a time before finding other troops to attach themselves to at a more adult level. A sense of unique selfhood, on the other hand, is probably not only distinctively human but comparatively recent, dependent on the abandonment, by adherents of the doctrinal religions of the last three millennia, of the totemic view of man as embedded in nature.[6]

Dr. McGuinness' last question—"What value do we put on male and female forms of consciousness, and how can these forms be brought into harmony?"—is crucial. During the past five millennia, our agricultural, urban, and industrial civilization has evaded this question by taking it for granted that, where male cultural initiative is paramount, male consciousness must also be paramount. Under these circumstances, female consciousness tends to be regarded as constituting, at best, an imperfect approximation of male consciousness. Today, however, when miniaturization and computerization are rendering masculine muscle increasingly superfluous, patriarchal presumptions are increasingly unconvincing. Broadly construed, that "unity of the sciences" to which all of us, as ICUS conferees, are committed seems to me to require not only that we relate disparate disciplines to one another but also that we seek to integrate male with female ways of knowing. To do less would be to settle for a monocular view of a world for which we are coming to realize that we need, at the very least, fully stereoscopic vision.

REFERENCES

1. Sir Francis Darwin, *Charles Darwin's Autobiography*, Schumann, New York, 1950.
2. Atsuo Tsumori, "Newly Acquired Behavior and Social Interaction of Japanese Monkeys," in *Social Communication Among Primates*, Stuart A. Altmann, Editor, University of Chicago Press, Chicago, Illinois, 1967.
3. Sherwood L. Washburn, *Ape into Man*, Little Brown, Boston, Massachusetts, 1974.
4. Alister C. Hardy, "Was Man More Aquatic in the Past?", *The New Scientist*, Volume 7, 1960, pp. 642-5.
5. Elaine Morgan, *The Descent of Woman*, Stein and Day, New York, 1972.
6. Roger Wescott, "Language, Taboo, and Human Uniqueness," *The Bucknell Review*, Lewisburg, Pennsylvania, December, 1969, pp. 28-30.

Ragnar A. Granit

A5 Adaptability of the Nervous System and Its Relation to Chance, Purposiveness, and Causality

To the biologists themselves biology nowadays is either organismic, physico-chemical or molecular but if you ask a layman what biology might be he would almost certainly think of the evolution of animals, genetics, chromosomes, hybridization, new species of plants, breeding of horses or dogs. Behind this is — I suspect—a flood of popular conceptualization based on slogans such as the survival of the fittest, the struggle for life, our origin from apes and perhaps also the tough resistance of anti- Darwinism in some well-known trials in a certain state within the United States. To many of these topics people feel an irresistible urge to add their own contribution.

In the science of neurophysiology experimenters are cautious, unwilling also to popularize and hesitant to discuss general principles for fear of exposing themselves to disparaging remarks from their colleagues. As a consequence their science stands isolated from contact with the rest of the biological sciences in which a running discussion of first principles is being maintained. I thought of giving our science a push in what I hope is the right direction to show in what way we can add a note of our own to the concert of voices explaining concepts such as purposiveness, adaptation, causality and chance. How do we look upon them in our field?

The best background is evolutionary theory in which purposiveness is given a definite role in the disguise of 'directiveness'. While physiologists may speak about teleological explanations, the evolutionary biologist speaks about 'teleonomic directiveness' or 'teleonomic purposiveness' (Mayr). Pantin maintains that it is impossible to use 'purposiveness' because purpose implies "striving after a future goal retained as some kind of image or idea". The neurophysiologist can immediately mention any number of highly purposive reactions which are wholly automatic, be they inherited or acquired. Thus he has no reason to discard the classical term: teleological explanations—without or with an image of the goal. When in evolutionary theory 'purposiveness' has to be toned down by the attribute 'teleonomic', the reason for this is that the consensus of opinion in this field holds 'purpose' to be apparent only and the direction of evolution to be fundamentally explainable on the basis of mutations and recombinations. Their viability is tested by natural selection. The testing itself takes place in the phenotype and the whole operation in a population. It is thus statistical.

If one asks how the effect of the testing ultimately leads to fixation of the mutant in a population, the answer may be illustrated in the following experiment by Waddington: a strain of *Drosophila melanogaster* produced flies with a break in the posterior crossvein of the wing only when pupae aged 21-23 hours were subjected to 40° for four hours. They did not do so at 25°. After 14 generations of selection with the heat treatment some flies were found to show the effect without being exposed to the heat shock. Thus this typical acquired character had entered the genetic make-up by selection which so increased the frequency of the salient gene that it became stabilized for some generations. The evolutionary progress is postulated to have taken place by small changes over millions of years of exposure to natural selection. These have ultimately been fixed in the coded genome.

Mayr (1963) points out that evolutionary biology deals with two questions, "how come" and "what for". I take it that the synthetic theory of evolution, as briefly outlined above, deals with both of them simultaneously in their explanations. This field is distinguished from "functional biology"—says Mayr—which deals with questions of "how" in a manner inseparable in principle from that of physics and chemistry. I shall come in a moment to the fact that no one can think of understanding the central nervous system without encountering any number of why-questions.

In the meantime let us realize that the coded instructions of evolutionary theory cannot easily be translated into characters paired with genes. Characters are polygenetic and an additional complication is polymorphism, an important variability reflected in the process of natural selection. The programmed codes, for these and many other reasons, cannot be rigid. The genetic instructions are within limits open. An outsider would like to understand why this sometimes is obviously true, while at other times it is equally obvious that great rigidity has prevailed, for instance, in species which have been constant for 500 million years.

Perhaps I should also add an instance of open instructions. We can take it from Lucretius, *De rerum natura*, Chapter IV, where he pointed out that the tongue existed before speech became possible. Everybody knows that the dog also uses the tongue for heat regulation. This is what one might call the serendipitous trait in evolution. Something is begun somewhere in the phylum and after millions of years is found to be useful for something else. Because the coded instructions are open and tested by the environment in the phenotype, such strokes of inspired magic are possible.

The leading workers in evolutionary biology realize that the explanation of evolution by the synthetic theory is a postulate, also that it is non-predictive. Nevertheless it is the best explanation we have. It embodies deep insight, a great deal of real creative knowledge, and it will live with us into the future.

Approaching this theory from the point of view of the neurosciences, I believe that a significant contribution might be a discussion of the act of testing of the phenotype, as it is seen from the physiological end. It seems to me essential that if we can understand the role of 'purpose' in neurophysiology and thereby its role in the elaboration of the phenotype, we have in a way given teleological purposiveness a place also in evolution.

It is of course not difficult to show that teleological explanations play a decisive role in practical neurobiology. We ask *why* an observed event takes place and by this means arrive at an essential element of understanding. A very good example is the work of Karl von Frisch on the communication and orientation of the bee. The two questions of 'how' and 'why' are clearly outlined. *How* is it that the bee can orientate itself over long distances of flight? The answer was, as is well known, that it differs from us in having retinal units with eight radially placed detectors of light polarized in different planes. Sunlight is naturally polarized as it is reflected from the blue sky and, thus, as long as part of the sky is visible, the bee has at its disposal a map by which to adjust its angle of flight.

Why is it that bees returning to the hive from distant sources of honey execute a curious dance on the glass wall of the observation hive? Von Frisch called it "Schwanzeltanz". To many scientists this would just have been an oddity, a curio to be placed on the roomy shelf of other innumerable curios in the biological world. It could in fact be understood merely by asking for its purpose and then von Frisch proved that its purpose was communicative. The bee danced in a circle divided into two semicircles by a diagonal which showed the direction of the flight while the number of tours in the dance indicated the distance from the hive. In the observation-hive the bee danced on a vertical plane so that its companions in addition had to project it on a horizontal plane — rather an intricate piece of geodetic geometry on the part of such a relatively small mass of neurons.

So far my questioning merely has concerned the practical use of why-questions. They make it possible to detect biological adaptions and the evolutionary biologist would agree and maintain — as to the bee — that this is a typical instance of *telenomic* purposiveness laid down in the genetic instructions.

But then true *teleological* purposiveness is what evolution has produced in developing our brain. Let me quote Sherrington: "The dog not only walks but it walks to greet its master. In a word the component from the roof-brain alters the character of the motor act from one of generality of purpose to one of narrowed and specific purpose fitting a special occasion. The change is just as if the motor act had suddenly become correlated with the finite mind of the moment". This is meant to emphasize that the conscious purposive brain represents the final hierarchic stage in the development of our capacity to adjust ourselves to the environment. An adaptation — the dog walks — has become *adaptable* by being subjected to cerebral control—it walks to greet its master. In the neurosciences the great and fascinating problem is what to do with *adaptability*. From the genetic point of view evolution has led to diverse adaptations. Animals are adapted to swim, to fly, to feed on grass etc. But purposive adaptability deals with the range and pliability of such genetically fixed adaptations.

To begin analyzing such problems with 'the dog walking to greet its master', is to begin from the end, the top level of dog performance. Pavlov did this when he trained dogs to salivate to a tone by the simple expedient of letting a reward of food in repeated trials succeed the tone. In order to appreciate the role of purposiveness in creating such 'conditioned reflexes' one need but imagine the 'reward' (today called 'reinforcement') to be given *before* sounding the tone instead of *afterwards*. Purpose, meaning motivation, are terms that in different ways show what made sense of this undertaking.

We have to begin with simpler questions and the one I propose is as follows: can we change a normal response of a single cortical cell or a number of them by impressing upon them properties which are at crosspurpose with an ingrained purposive adaptation? This question is particularly interesting from the evolutionary and developmental points of view.

My first example is Sperry's experiment (1951) in which the optic nerve of a frog was cut, the eye bulb turned round in its socket by 180° and regeneration allowed to take place. It was found that by some kind of chemically determined specificity the nerve fibers grew into their original sites in the optic tectum. The frog never adapted itself to this reversal of the optical image. A fly in the upper field of vision excited the animal to catch it in the lower field. Once established the ingrained adaptation was too resistant to allow any adaptability.

In this experiment inherently open genetic instructions have been closed but it can be shown that originally they had been open at an early stage of amphibian ontogenetic development. If at the time rotation took place normal purposive (fly-catching) reflexes developed. Jacobson and Hunt's analysis showed that the critical period for the operative rotation in *Xenopus,* another

amphibian, was between 32 and 40 hours of amphibian life. Its
retinal ganglion cells were born at about 34 hours and their nerve
fibres reached the optic tectum 15 hours later. The empirically established new correlations between the retinal and the cortical
maps closed the genetical instructions, possibly aided by functional sanction of synaptic chemical 'markers'.

It is easy enough to enumerate cases of developmental plasticity which are lost later in life, even in man. The language areas in
the brain are well known to be in the parietal and temporal lobes
of the left hemisphere. Destruction of them leads to permanent
aphasia. But, if this region is lost before the age of about twelve,
the right hemisphere takes over and develops new language
areas.

On the other hand, there are also functions of the roof-brain or
cortex in which re-purposing against an ingrained purpose succeeds. In this respect man is supreme. Long ago it was shown by
Sperry (1947) that operative exchange of flexors and extensors
even in the monkey was not perfectly compensated. But if one
looks up "Bunnell's Surgery of the Hand" (Boyes 1964) one finds
it stated explicitly that in the hand and the forearm any muscle
and tendon, when transferred to a new site, can carry out any
desired motion. "A wrist extensor can act as a digital extensor, a
digital flexor, a wrist flexor or a motor for opposition and adduc-
tion of the thumb" (p. 444). These movements have then been re-
programmed in the brain under the guidance of feedback from the
eye, the muscles, and, oddly enough, from the skin which has
been found to be very important for programming a prosthesis
(Moberg). In Sperry's experiments training for e.g., one flexor
movement was not transferable to flexion in another situation:
the measure of re-adaption achieved required months, even two
years.

However, I would like to return to vision and make some comparisons between cat and man with respect to adaptability tested
by 'repurposing' an afferent response of the brain. This concerns
the perception of orientation of lines appearing in the receptive
field of a cortical cell in the primary visual projection area 17. It
presupposes knowledge of the discovery of Hubel and Wiesel that
the cells of the type called 'simple' are sensitive to the orientation

of oblongs or lines and yield optimal responses for correct orientations. In the visual cortex of the cat an assembly of such cells represents all orientations of visual stimuli in a non-preferential manner. But if young kittens are reared in a vertically or horizontally striped environment the cortical cells begin to respond preferentially to these directions. Blakemore who did this work, following Hirsch and Spinelli, found that no more than an hour's exposure to such visual experiences sufficed to modify the preferred orientation of most units, provided that this experiment was followed by a minimum of two weeks in the dark. But if the kittens had more than 5 hours of such abnormal experience the effect became virtually ineradicable by other visual stimuli. Nothing else distinguished these cortical units from normal ones.

What about ourselves? There is now a large number of experiments in which people have been wearing inversion lenses or prismatic goggles or even colored filters to create a visual world at cross-purposes with ingrained experience. The first ones, by Stratton in 1897, showed that on the fifth day of wearing a monocular inversion lens with the other eye covered, Stratton had adapted so well to the originally inverted world that "there was no anticipatory drawing in of the chin and chest when a solid object passed through the visual field in the direction which in normal vision would have meant a blow". Both the perceived world and the reflexes were adapted to the new experience.

From work on monkeys we are entitled to conclude that directionally sensitive cells exist also in our visual cortex. An average response of such cells can actually be studied objectively by measuring on the scalp the amplitude of electrical potentials evoked in response to visual stimuli of variable orientation. It is known that vertical and horizontal targets are better resolved by human observers than oblique patterns, also that evoked potentials by their amplitude indicate these preferential sensitivities.

In Pisa Fiorentini, Ghez and Maffei proceeded to investigate what happens when seven adult subjects wore tilting prisms continually for seven days. The prisms produced a tilt of the target of 30^0 or 40^0 from the vertical, and the angle between the apparent vertical and the real vertical was measured and compared with the amplitudes of their evoked potentials. These served to indicate the degree of perceptual compensation. In all subjects perceptual 're-purposing' to the tilt occurred already in the first hours, and compensation was virtually complete on the second day. The adaptive effects were accompanied by a decrease of the mean difference between the amplitudes of evoked potentials for the vertical and oblique patterns. And this is now the final experiment that I shall mention in support of the fact that man has carried a high degree of plastic adaptability with him into maturity. I would now like to discuss the facts rather than multiply them.

There are many things we would like to understand in these observations, (i) the mechanism of compensation, (ii) why man is superior to cat and (iii) their general significance in relation to purposiveness, chance and causality.

(i) <u>Verticality</u>, like most percepts, <u>is a complex affair</u>. If we tilt our head, a vertical oblong remains vertical in spite of the tilted retinal image and the new receptors concerned. Verticality has a kind of relative constancy, like size, velocity of movement and object color. The size of our hands alters continually, regarded as a retinal image, but is constant as a percept. There are clearly definite frameworks of reference, some external, but probably most of them internal. The percept of verticality has important components other than visual ones. There is first and foremost an internal world of reference based on feedback from the balance organs in the head, on sense organs in the neck muscles, along the spine, in muscles of the leg, and skin sensations from the soles. The perennial necessity of compensating for gravity sees to it, that the experience of verticality is solidly anchored by those feedback impulses in a cellular organization capable of error detection. This is based on the information returning to it.

A permanent distortion of the visual input by prismatic goggles is a non-plausible illusion which goes against the grain of all the other sources of information, in particular against those most directly concerned with the position of the head in relation to gravity. Error detection leads by feedback to error correction in this highly purposeful, or let us say, sensible brain of ours. These events produce alterations in the wiring diagram which is wired up with a redundancy, very likely exceeding that of all other mammals. We do not know which particular processes are responsible for the error correction but there is no lack of possible alternatives, judged by experimental results from adjacent neurophysiological fields. The axoplasmic flow of chemical material in nerve fibres is well known and intensely studied today. It may serve to cement new connections, the old ones may withdraw in a mechanical sense because of dis-use while new ones may expand by use. A synaptic cleft, after all, is no more than a few hundred Angstrom (2 nm), or there may be active inhibition involved in the error correction. Even if we do not know what is the explanation, it is one that does not seem to be wholly beyond reach by experimentation. From Cragg's work we are also quite familiar with electronmicroscopically recordable synaptic alterations by use and disuse. And, as to error correction by feedback, it is well known from the experiments on maintaining constant length and tension of a muscle in the face of load variations. We have the wiring diagram of this circuit and the whole process is essentially spinal though the sensitivity of the error detectors (muscular sense organs) is adjustable from the brain. The new element introduced by the experiments on perceived verticality reviewed here is the durable effect of error detection, the permanent nature of the compensation. This may be maintained by use.

(ii) In considering a likely explanation of why man is superior to the cat, the enormous expansion of our cortex and the high degree of encephalization, that is, of the shift of final control to this cortex, suggest themselves as the basic elements in any workable hypothesis.

Beginning with the question of why in early development the genetic instructions are open, later on to become closed, I feel much attracted by the hypothesis of Jacobson which is well-founded and capable of an experimental expansion. Jacobson, a developmental physiologist, uses the terms specification and speaks of non-specified cells: "Some neurons are highly specified and all their connections are fully determined, but there are also some incompletely specified neurons with indeterminate connections. During ontogeny there is a tendecy for neuronal specificity to increase and for connections to become more highly determined, but the developmental stage at which these changes occur, as well as their extent and duration, varies for different neurons ... Neurons of class I are those that originate early in embryonic development. They are mainly macroneurons, that is, large neurons with long axons. They form the primary afferent and efferent neurons of the central nervous system of vertebrates, and their central connections usually have a topographical arrangement. Their connections are specified during early embryonic development, and are invariant and unmodifiable thereafter. Sensory stimulation is not required for their development and there are few, if any, lasting changes following electrical activity of class I neurons. By contrast, class II neurons are interneurons of various kinds, and especially the small neurons with short axons, the Golgi II type. They originate later than class I neurons in any particular part of the nervous system, and the production of class II neurons continues into postnatal life in some parts of the brain. The connectivity of these neurons is more variable than that of class I neurons. Specific kinds of sensory stimulation are required for the full development and maintenance of class II neurons or of their connections. Electrical activity in these neurons may result in changes of long duration. Specification of class II neurons occurs slowly and is contingent on specific kinds on sensory stimulation" (Jacobson, 1970 p. 333).

The talent for re-purposing against an ingrained purpose is thus not a universal property of all brain cells. It is based on the variable connectivity of the interneurons of the Golgi II type of cell which are the large majority of all cells in the cortex. According to Ramon y Cajal their number increases upwards in the phylum. One of the directive purposes of evolution in creating such an organ for encephalization of control may well be to give the new instrument the adaptability of which I have spoken. The ultimate controls are drawn into the sphere of action of the small internuncial cells at a site where their number is great enough to be decisive in responding purposively to experience beyond the stage of ontogenetic development.

From this point of view it seems to follow that man should be the most adaptable adult organism in existence. His brain is the relatively largest one. Relative to what? It is with its 1350 cc in the averages smaller than, for instance, that of the blue whale which is 2800 cc. But phylogenetically brain volumes are related to body surface, the formula relating brain size to weight being the same as the one relating weight to surface. We are apparently more significantly related to the environment by our surface than by our weight. But in the formula there is also a constant that determines the degree of encephalization and this is wherein man excels.

(iii) I wish I could do better on degrees of connectivity in this cellular organization that is our cortex. Such figures are very difficult to come by, because there is no good technique for measuring what Cragg's average figure of 30,000 synapses per cell or 60,000 synapses for the large cells really means. Is it an enormous branching of a few fibres of contact or does it represent a very large number of projecting axons and thus a high degree of connectivity. Following Cragg (1967) there would, at a conservative estimate, by 56 neurons interconnected with each neuron in the monkey visual cortex, 600 in its motor cortex where the neurons are larger. In another paper dealing with the rat visual cortex his estimate is 300 for each neuron. Man tends to have more large neurons than other animals of the same size. For the cat Scholl found each stellate neuron to branch around 4000 other neurons. For man Cragg gives the average figure of 50 million cells per cc in the visual area. Others give values of 78 and 97 millions, as collected and tabulated by Cragg. But then, of course, the absolute number of neurons also would be relevant and there the estimates for the whole cortex of man range from 2.6 x 10^9 to 14 x 10^9.

Despite all these variations I think we move on certain ground when we state that no man-made computer has a connectivity anywhere near this order of magnitude. It simply is fabulous and adds an element of futility to the hope of ever solving the riddle of brain function merely by wiring diagrams.

What it does show, however, is that the numerous small cells of Group II with their adaptability or plasticity relative to environmental changes are numerous enough to give chance a chance. At this stage we have to turn to biological analogies to realize that we are up against a trick that Nature has used elsewhere. There are plants producing an enormous number of seeds, and in one ejaculation of the rabbit there is said to be an average of

700,000,000 sperms. Behind all this is, of course, a basic stability of the genetic code, just as in the brain there are fixed connections by cells of Type I and variable ones by cells of Type II, capable of being influenced by environmental challenges.

The best analogy there is to brain function is a comparison with the immuno-system (Jerne, 1973). The small B-lymphocytes, rather than specializing on certain common diseases, generate an extraordinary number of antibodies. Specialization would have led to a fixed rather than to an adaptable adaptation. Adaptability is achieved by the existence of random chemical specificities for pattern recognition, their number being large enough for matching antibodies to most of the inimical epitopes that are likely to occur. These fits are remembered by the system and we know them as immunities for the agents that provoked them, at least when the immunity refers to a diagnosed disease with a name fixed to it. In this manner the immuno-system responds adequately to an enormous variety of signals, it learns from experience and remembers the lessons it has been taught by foreign agents. The chemical markers concerned in this activity are the immunoglobulins.

The analogy implies that in both cases there are systems making use of chemical specificities and relying on chance for adaptability to environmental challenges. Chance comes in as a multiplication of alternatives. Both systems have other cells for fixed tasks. In brain physiology and anatomy the fixed organizations and the various adaptations that they represent have obviously been in the center of neurophysiological research. To quote Brodal: "we may consider the brain as consisting of a multitude of small units each with its particular morphological (and presumably functional) features. These units collaborate by way of an immensely rich, complicated and different network of connections, which are very precisely and specifically organized. The anatomical possibilities for (more or less direct) cooperations between various parts of the brain must be almost unlimited".

Finally, having seen now how purposiveness and adaptability are, so to speak, partners in an indissoluble marriage between the organism and its environment, what about casusality? It is perfectly clear that teleological explanations do not imply that we are casting adrift from causality. The aim of a purposive response is predictive; it assumes that the environment behaves in a predictable manner, and adjusts itself to correct for deviations from the predictable. Thus, inasmuch as the external world is concerned, purposiveness relates to definite causes. The experimenter can relate different purposes to the responses he is engaged in studying. We can never escape from the purposive causal relation to the environmental challenge. The teleological explanation may be put aside while we try to study the mechanisms by which it is realized in the organism, but it is nevertheless there clamoring for an answer.

The limitations we encounter in discussing casual teleology are on the inside of the organism. We don't know the inside causes residing in memory, motivation and in as yet unknown properties of the nervous system. To these unknown quantities we can add mind or consciousness which, of course, is the supreme instrument for dealing with purposiveness in all its aspects. I have left consciousness outside my talk because I have been interested in seeing to what an extent it is possible to get at the 'hardware' of purposive responses in relation to definite environmental factors. In other words, I have wanted to find out how far we can go with things accessible to physiological and anatomical approaches. There is no denying that it would have been an easy choice to go for experiments that emphasize the complexity of internal causes, as, for instance, those referring to numerous illusions.

If I may return for a brief moment to evolutionary theory on the notion that lectures should end where they began, I would like to point out that my reasoning amounts to a study of the act of testing of the phenotype and this process is an essential component of the synthetic theory. I think my analysis has shown that adaptability is a teleological concept, with or without awareness of goal. I would not hesitate one moment to speak of an *immanent teleology*. People are afraid of this because they think it implies accepting a vitalism, which in my opinion has been dead for half a century. I would just as happily speak about immanent gravity or immanent magnetism. In all three cases no knowledge about ultimate causes is assumed. On the contrary, the term 'immanent' means that we have no idea about the nature of the gravitational force and therefore have to accept it as a fact, inherent in our world of observations and for this reason as an essential element in our scientific superstructure. Similarly immanent teleology belongs to the scientific structure dealing with the living organism in its relation to the environment and we should try to make sense of it. My view has been that trying to understand adaptability, in the present phase of physiological work, is a step in the right direction.

REFERENCES

Blakemore, C. and Cooper, G.F. (1970). Development of the brain depends on the visual environment, *Nature (Lond.) 228*, 447-478.

Blakemore, C. and Mitchell, D.E. (1973). Environmental modification of the visual cortex and the neural basis of learning and memory. *Nature (Lond.) 241*, 467-468.

Boyes, J.H. (Ed.) (1964). *Bunnell's Surgery of the Hand.* 4th ed. Lippincott, Philadelphia.

Brodal, A. (1974). M.I.T. Conference. To be published.

Cragg, B.G. (1967). The density of synapses and neurons in the motor and visual areas of the cerebral cortex, *J. Anat., 101,* 639-654.

Fiorentini, A., Ghez, C. and Maffei, L. (1972). Physiological correlates of adaptation to a rotated visual field, *J. Physiol. (Lond.) 227,* 313-322.

Frisch, K. von (1953). *Aus dem Leben der Bienen.* Springer Verlag, Gottingen, Heidelberg.

Hirsch, H.V.B. and Spinelli, D.N. (1970). Visual experience modifies distribution of horizontally and vertically oriented receptive fields in the cat. *Science 168,* 869-871.

Hubel, D.H. and Wiesel, T.N. (1959). Receptive fields of single neurons in the cat's striate cortex. *J. Physiol. (Lond.) 148,* 574-591.

Jacobson, M. (1970). *Developmental Neurobiology.* Holt, Rinehart and Winston Inc., New York.

Jacobson, M. and Hunt, R.K. (1973). The origins of nerve-cell specificity. *Sci. Amer., 228,* 26-35.

Jerne, N.K. (1973). The immune system. *Sci. Amer., 229,* 52-60.

Mayr, E. (1963). Cause and effect in biology. *Science 134,* 1501-1506.

Moberg, E. (1972). Fingers were made before forks. In *The Hand, 4,* 201-206.

Pantin, C.F.A. (1968). *The Relations between the Sciences.* Cambridge Univ. Press.

Ramon y Cajal, S. (1952). *Histologie du Systeme Nerveux de Phomme et des Vertebres.* Instituto Ramon y Cajal, Madrid.

Sherrington, C.S. (1941). *Man on his Nature.* The Gifford Lectures, Edinburgh 1937-38. Macmillan, New York and Cambridge Univ. Press.

Sholl, D.A. (1956). *The Organization of the Cerbral Cortex.* Methuen, London.

Sperry, R.W. (1947). Effect of crossing nerves to antagonistic limb muscles in the monkey. *Arch. Neurol. Psychiat. (Chicago) 58*, 452-473.

Sperry, R.W. (1951). Mechanisms of neural maturation. In *Handbook of Experimental Psychology*, S.S. Steven (Editor). Wiley, New York, pp. 236-280.

Stratton, G.M. (1897). Vision without inversion of the retinal image. *Psychol. Rev. 4*, 341-360; 463-481.

Waddington, C.H. (1953). Genetic assimilation of an acquired character. *Evolution 7*, 118-126.

Discussion

Stephen Prickett: I was fascinated by the Kantian possibilities that seem to be illustrated there, where it became clear that so many of the attributes we push into the external world can in fact be seen as qualities within the mind. Could Professor Granit comment further?

Granit: As a matter of fact there is a secret undercurrent in all this work, that we are trying to discover clues for the mind. The physiology of the special senses is in many cases a physiology designed to discover the clues for any kind of mental processes. We have gone rather far now in this direction in present day physiology. We are now at single cells in the cortex of animals and I think even sometimes in man—they can be obtained in surgical operations on man since the brain doesn't feel any pain and so people allow such experiments to be done. Some clues are very direct like that of horizontality and verticality. There are many other clues that are not so directly translatable now. For example, we can locate distances acoustically—it is the difference in time between the two ears that is decisive, but it doesn't give any indication of the location of the source; whereas these experiments on horizontality and verticality have a more precise connection with the mind, if I may say so.

Erick Jantsch: I wonder whether the concept of immanent teleology is not convergent with the aims and the concepts of general systems theory?

Granit: Well many people do like to think of cybernetics as a teleological science, but I am a little hesitant on that. I think that if you have say a Kreb's cycle and push a good reaction into a Kreb's cycle you have done something important—you have put a new reaction into an old structural process. In the same way we have these cybernetical restrictions and many things can be put into this concept, but personally, I think it isn't so very different from pushing a reaction into the Kreb's cycle, or pushing a reaction process into the cybernetic machinery or constraints which can be of course handled mathematically.

Nand Keswani: Professor Granit, you spoke of the adaptability of the nervous system to the needs of the human body. How about the relationship of the brain to the adaptability of the human being to a community and to the society. We know that the brain, in experimental animals as well as in man, has centers controlling feeding and also the sex urge. The herding mentality is also closely associated with these urges. Some chromosome aberrations have also been blamed for criminal tendencies and antisocial behavior in these individuals. What is your comment?

Granit: Well you are asking me to go far beyond my limits of competence. I am a neurophysiologist and I therefore have thought very little about the application of these ideas into society. I think that I shall leave it to you.

R.V. Jones: Could you tell us anything about the 'moon illusion' and how it arises. You have explained about the vertical perception.

Granit: When I was a child I was riding on a horse and saw the moon jumping along the treetops at the speed at which the horse moved. The explanation is that the image on the retina is a constant, but as you are moving, the trees are being left behind you, and then you have an illusion — a sensible movement — because something which goes ahead with the trees must be moving in order to remain in the background. These fall into internal frameworks of reference for which we have very little physiological knowledge but we have to accept them, since we have created such frameworks.

Tor Ragnar Gerholm: In the 18th century a physicist named Mobertius advanced the theory that every action for every natural phenomenon occurs according to a principle of least action. This was clearly a teleological idea which was very much detested by the Newtonian physicists. The Principle of Least Action has been formulated into a mathematical language finally arriving in a pure logical mathematical way at a formula, which is exactly the same one as one obtained by Newtonian Mechanics. It followed that the distinction between the teleological explanation and a causal one is actually a matter of how you speak about it, rather than accounting for a difference in principle in nature. I don't know if this has any relation to what Professor Granit was speaking about today. It seems to me that there is really no difference in principle between teleological explanations and causal explanations, but that depends on a particular situation which you are dealing with as to which one of the two modes make more sense. Certainly in physiology, it makes more sense to have a teleological explanation. Would Professor Granit please comment?

Granit: This is very much in line with what I wanted to say. I agree that causal explanations are teleological explanations, but the only difficulty is, within us, internal forces have become master. With respect to the environment we can very often do very well with teleological explanations because they are causal and essentially the same. We can't help doing it, but when dealing with organisms which have to eat, have to reproduce, have to defend themselves, so they are related to the environment in a causal way and that's what I wanted to do, merely to show you how far we can go experimentally in this field these days.

Earl of Halsbury: When I refer to the blackboard, I take a piece of chalk and draw a curved line across and I record the results as a graphical fact. Now, given that graphical fact, I can invent various alternative analytic descriptions. One can set up a co- ordinate system and express it as an equation between the dependent and independent variables. Alternatively I can set up a differential equation and provided I know one point on this curve and the tangent at that point as a first order differential equation, I can describe it exactly in the same way, but by an alternative means. Now, if instead I choose to take a point at the beginning of the curve and a point at the end of the curve, and to say that the curve goes through those two points subject to an external condition such that there is some constraint on the action, there is a third analytic description of a graphical fact. Now it is only when we introduce an anthropomorphic rejection into these alternate descriptions of graphical facts that we begin to talk of:

Description for the first;
Natural Law for the second;
Teleology for the third.

We imagine that we human beings are the tip of that piece of chalk. That, in the first sense we are doing what we are doing. In the second sense we are obedient to a law, and in the third sense that we are trying to accomplish something.

Now, goal-seeking mechanisms were rather mysterious creatures to the biologists of the last century who drew from Aristotle the concept of teleology as a means of explaining the rather unfamiliar properties of living organisms. But even then, Clark Maxwell at about the time that he was inventing the electromagnetic theory of light gave the first analytic description of the centrifugal governor of the steam engine which we would now call a linear control device. Goal-seeking mechanisms are now the commonplace of the control engineer's laboratory. You can have mechanisms like those that are at Edinburgh University where they take a child's toy in pieces and by trial and error find out how to put it together. Then when they feel a little tired, they plug themselves into a source of electricity in order to have a meal and be able to carry on. These are really almost the trivia of control engineering and the great question is: Have the teleological descriptions of anthropomorphic character which we project into them really got anything in common with human purpose, which is self-conceived. Because the one thing that no computer, I can imagine functioning, can do for itself is to decide the next problem which to work on. This has got to be done by human beings and so long as that is true, then all mechanical analogies of human purposes will, I believe, fail.

Granit: I agree completely with you, and have nothing against your point of view. We can't go too far with such things as cybernetics and so on, but I think there are some concepts in Information Theory which are very useful for us. After all, the engineer cannot design any machines that his brain cannot design for him. But, nevertheless there are some things different in the whole machinery that we don't understand.

I have been thinking always in hierarchic terms. You can't explain by the potential of the individual cell, you can't explain the whole operation that is performing. But, when you come to a higher level of hierarchy you cannot explain it by going down and down. There is a limit to that.

Sir John Eccles

A6 Culture: The Creation of Man and the Creator of Man

Philosophical Introduction —The Three Worlds

Before discussing the brain-mind problem it is essential to give an account of the philosophical position which forms the basis of my discussion. I have written at length on this philosophy in my book *Facing Reality*. It is developed from the fundamental contributions of Sir Karl Popper in defining the three worlds which subsume the whole of reality, in developing their philosophical status and in describing their interaction (K.R. Popper, *Objective Knowledge*, 1972, Chapters 3 and 4). Both Sir Karl and I are thus trialists and trialist interactionists. My lecture will give many examples of the explanatory power of these new concepts.

The scope of the three worlds can be seen in the tabular classification of Fig. 1 (p. 76), which indicates that Worlds 1, 2 and 3 take care of everything in existence and in experience.

In Fig. 1, World 1 is the world of physical objects and states. It comprises the whole cosmos of matter and energy, all of biology including human brains, and all artifacts that man has made for coding information, as for example the paper and ink of books or the material base of works of art. World 1 is the total world of the monist materialists. They recognize nothing else. All else is fantasy.

World 2 is the world of states of consciousness and subjective knowledge of all kinds. The totality of our perceptions comes in this world. But there are several levels. In agreement with Polten (1973), I tend to recognize three kinds of levels of World 2, as indicated in Fig. 2 (pg. 77), but it may be more correct to think of it as a spectrum.

The first level (*outer sense*) would be the ordinary perceptions provided by all our sense organs, hearing and touch and sight and smell and pain. All of these perceptions are in World 2, of course: vision with light and color; sound with music and harmony; touch with all its qualities and vibration; the range of odors and tastes, and so on. These qualities do not exist in World 1, where correspondingly there are but electromagnetic waves, pressure waves in the atmosphere, material objects, and chemical substances.

In addition there is a level of *inner sense*, which is the world of more subtle perceptions. It is the world of emotions, of feelings of joy and sadness and fear and anger and so on. It includes all memory, and all imaginings and planning into the future. In fact there is a whole range of levels which could be described at length. All the subtle experiences of the human person are in this inner sensory world. It is all private to you but you can reveal it in linguistic expression, and by gestures of all levels of subtlety.

Finally, at the core of World 2 there is the *self* or *pure ego*, which is the basis of our unity as an experiencing being throughout our whole lifetime.

This World 2 is our *primary reality*. Our conscious experiences are the basis of our knowledge of World 1, which is thus a world of *secondary reality*, a derivative world. Whenever I am doing a scientific experiment, for example, I have to plan it cognitively, all in my thoughts, and then consciously carry out my plan of action in the experiment. Finally I have to look at the results and evaluate them in thought. For example, I have to see the traces on the oscilloscope and their photographic records or hear the signals on the loudspeaker. The various signals from the recording equipment have to be received by my sense organs, transmitted to my brain, and so to my consciousness, then appropriately measured and compared before I can begin to think about the significance of the experimental results. We are all the time, in every action we do, incessantly playing backwards and forwards between World 1 and World 2.

And what is World 3? As shown in Fig. 1 it is the whole world of culture. It is the theme of this lecture that World 3 was created by man and that reciprocally made man. The whole of language is here. All our means of communication, all our intellectual efforts coded in books, coded in the artistic and technological treasures in the museums, coded in every artifact left by man from primitive times — this is World 3 right up to the present time. It is the world of civilization and culture. Education is the means whereby each human being is brought into relation with World 3. In this manner he becomes immersed in it throughout life, participating in the heritage of mankind and so becoming fully human. World 3 is the world that uniquely relates to man. It is completely unknown to animals.

Following the thought of Popper we can say that the self or ego is the result of achieving a view of ourselves from the outside, as we emerge from the solipsism of babyhood. In that way we each place ourselves in our bodies in the spatial domain and with a time sequence dependent on memories that bridge the diurnal gaps that sleep gives to the stream of consciousness of each of us. The concept each of us has of our own ego is dependent on our intuitive acceptance of the World 3 in which we are immersed in all our cognitive life, which would include all perceiving, thinking and communication.

Sir Charles Sherrington (1947) has written in his own exquisite style on the ego or self.

> "Each waking day is a stage dominated for good or ill, in comedy, farce or tragedy, by a *dramatis persona*, the 'self.' And so it will be until the curtain drops. This self is a unity. The continuity of its presence in time, sometimes hardly broken by sleep, its inalienable 'interiority' in (sensual) space, its consistency of view-point, the privacy of its experience, combine to give it status as a unique existence."

A frequent objection to the concept of the ego or self is that its perception involves an infinite regress. This criticism arises from a misunderstanding. Reference to Fig. 2 shows that the conscious experiences listed under the categories outer sense and inner sense are perceived by the ego or self. In contrast, the ego or self is experienced, not perceived. Following Kant, we can make the distinction by saying that the self or ego is apperceived. As Polten (1973) states:

> "The ontological basis for the difference between apperception and perception is that the pure ego is a mental thing in itself, whereas the mental phenomena of inner and outer sense are appearances. For that reason, too, subject and object merge in the act of the pure ego's self-observation, while inner and outer data are the pure ego's objects."

Sherrington (1940) develops a comparable theme in relation to a voluntary motor act.

> "This 'I' which when I move my hand I experience as 'I-doing', how do I perceive it? I do not perceive it. If perception means awareness through sense I do not perceive the 'I'. My awareness and myself are one. I experi-

ence it. The 'I-doing' is my awareness of myself in the motor act . . . This
'I' belongs more immediately to our awareness than does even the spatial
world about us, for it is directly experienced. It *is* the 'self'."

The Evolution of Culture

As we survey the cultural story of mankind the most remarkable discovery is that there were eons of incredibly slow development (cf. Dobzhansky, 1962; Hawkes, 1965). There was an immense
time lag between man's development of a large brain and his significant progress in cultural evolution, *i.e.* in the creation of
World 3. For the greater part of the immensely long Paleolithic
age, some 500,000 years, all we know is the slow development of
stone tools — from flaked pebbles to the very gradualy improved
hand-axe. It is generally believed that this almost unimaginable
slowness demonstrates that man was greatly handicapped by not
having yet an effective communication by speech.

Evidently, as recognized by Dobzhansky (1967) and Popper
(1972), immense and fundamental problems are involved in the
evolution of the brain that occurred as man was gradually developing his means of communication in speech. One can imagine
that speech and brain development went on together in the evolving process and that from these two emerged the cultural performance of man. Over hundreds of millenia there must have been
a progressive development of language from its primitive form as
expressive cries to a language that became gradually a more and
more effective means of description and argument. In this way,
by forging linguistic communciation of ever increasing precision
and subtlety, man must gradually have become a self-conscious
being aware of his own identity or selfhood. As a consequence he
also became aware of death, as witnessed so frequently and vividly
in other members of the tribal group that he recognized as beings
like himself. We do not know how early in the story of man this
tragic and poignant realization of death-awareness came to him,
but it was at least a hundred thousand years ago, as evidenced by
the ceremonial burial customs with the dead laid in graves with
antlers, weapons, ornaments, etc.

It was not until the Upper Paleolithic era that man seemed to
have achieved a new awareness and sense of purpose — as witness

the remarkable progress in a few thousand years, relative to the virtual stagnation for the previous hundreds of thousands of years. As one can readily imagine, by a language that gave clear identifications of objects and descriptions of actions and even more importantly the opportunity of discussing and arguing, man was lifted to a new level of creativity. We can presume that because of this linguistic communication man was enabled to progress in the development of the large variety of stone tools with greatly improved design, which is the most important characteristic of the upper Paleolithic age.

But the most fascinating insight into the artistic creativity of Upper Paleolithic man is given by the cave paintings of southern France and northern Spain. When I saw the marvellous paintings of Lascaux, I was overwhelmed by the feeling that these artists had highly developed imagination and memory as well as a refined aesthetic sense. Undoubtedly they had a fully developed language so that they could discuss the techniques they employed and the ideas that inspired them. One has the impression that, at this period of about 15,000 BC, man was very richly contributing to the world of culture. At the same time there were carvings and modellings of animals and of archetypal female figures that probably are representative of Mother Goddesses. Many would achieve distinction in modern sculpture exhibitions!

In the subsequent Mesolithic age man developed and perfected hunting methods and also clothing and housing, but artistically it was disappointing after the great achievements of the later Paleolithic. This technological Mesolithic period beginning at 10,000 to 8,000 BC was relatively brief.

The Neolithic age of settled farming communities began as early as 7,000 BC in Jericho and at 6,500 BC at Jarmo in Mesopotamia. The settled towns and villages of the Mesopotamian region soon became remarkable for their substantial houses and for the fine pottery and weaving. These developments were possible because of the prosperous farming with crops of barley and wheat and with domesticated animals, sheep, ox, goat, pig and dog. In addition the stone tools were finely made with polished surfaces. The pottery clearly reveals that Mesopotamian man was guided by an aesthetic sense. The decorative patterns of Hasuma and

Jarmo were in part abstract, but also, as with the Samarra pottery of the 5th millenium BC, there was a very sophisticated stylization of animal forms to give designs that display a high artistic sense. This Mesopotamian pottery is remarkable for the combination of utility and elegance. Already they had invented the potter's wheel. Cultural evolution was well advanced and the ceramics of Susa represent their highest artistic performance in this field.

About 1000 years after its development in Mesopotamia, Neolithic culture had spread from there to Egypt, so seeding the great periods of Egyptian civilization. Later there was a wide dispersal to Europe and to Asia (first to the Indus valley and later to China) of this central feature of the Neolithic culture, namely farming with settled communities of villages and towns. Meanwhile great developments continued in Mesopotamia, which undoubtedly led the world during the magnificent periods of Sumerian civilization from 3,500 BC for more than a millenium. The Neolithic age gave place to the Bronze age at about 4,000 BC and, during the third millenium BC, gold, silver and bronze workmanship was of a high order.

The greatest of all contributions of the Sumerians to culture was the development of a written language. The beginnings were about 3,300 BC, but for some hundreds of years it was still in the form of ideograms that had been developed from pictograms. The Sumerians progressively simplified the forms so that eventually it was completely abstract, consisting of various arrangements of tapered signs inscribed in soft clay tablets by a stylus made like a wedge, hence the name "Cuneiform" for the first written language that was fully developed by about 2,800 BC.

A written language must rank as one of the greatest discoveries in human history, for by means of it man could live beyond time. Thoughts, imaginings, ideas, understandings and explanations experienced and developed by men living in one age can be written down for distribution in that age and also for recovery in later ages. A man's creative insights need no longer die with him, but, when encoded in written language, can be re-experienced by later men who have the ability to decode. And so we enter into the historical epochs where the different civilizations have left records of their economic and political activities, their myths and legends, their drama, poetry, history, philosophy and religion.

Culture Exclusively Human

It must be recognized that each human individual has to be educated from babyhood to be able to participate even at the simplest level in the Culture he has been born into, though of course he carries genetically the potentiality for this participation. This generalization applies to babies from all races. Their cultural development from that of the stone age culture of primitive men of today in which they may be born to that of the advanced technological cultures is dependent on their opportunities to learn. A very young child from a stone age culture can be assimilated readily to our culture, its achievement being of course dependent on what we may call "brain potentiality;" and, conversely, a very young child of our culture if immersed in a stone age culture would carry no genetic memory whatsoever of our culture, and merely be assimilated to the primitive culture of his society. Completely different propositions obtain for all of the instinctive behaviors of animals. This behavior is largely if not entirely inborn, but it is of course modified by environmental influences. Animals brought up in isolation exhibit a remarkable ability to develop the behavior patterns of the normal adult, for example nest-building or bird-song, but with birds and mammals the finesse of the performance is dependent on having examples on display, i.e. the details of the performance have an imitative basis (Tinbergen, 1951; Thorpe, 1956).

It can be concluded that animal behavior in constructions on the one hand and human purpose and design at all levels of doing and making on the other hand are quite distinct. The one belongs to the biological evolution, the other to the cultural evolution. Animals are innocent of culture and civilization, which are distinctively human. There is no trace of them in the whole of animal evolution, which is governed by trial and error acting blindly, but of course being guided by instinctive and learning behavior. I use the world "blind" because there is no evidence that animal behavior pattern is based on the understanding of a situation, in the way that we use the word "understanding" in respect of human behavior.

Culture and Man

Popper (1970) has expressed very well the specific relationship of World 3 (the world of objective knowledge or culture) to World 2 (the self of ego).

"My central thesis . . . is that the self or the ego is anchored in the third world, and that it cannot exist without the third world. Before discussing this thesis more fully it may be necessary to remove the following difficulty. As I have here so often said, the third world is, roughly, the universe of the products of our minds. How can this be if, on the other hand, our minds or our selves cannot exist without the third world? The answer to this apparent difficulty is very simple. Our selves, the higher functions of language, and the third world have evolved and emerged together, in constant interaction; thus there is no special difficulty here. To be more specific, I deny that animals have states of full consciousness or that they have a conscious self. The self evolves together with the higher functions of language, the descriptive and the argumentative functions."

In summary we can state that World 3 is a world of storage, for the whole of human creativity through the prehistory and the history of the cultures and civilizations. What we call in old-fashioned terminology a cultured man is a man able to retrieve from this storage and to enter into an understanding of it. But of course this retrieval is also right up to the contemporary scene, where critical evaluation is concerned in elimination of error or banality and in the setting of standards.

I believe that central to each human being is the primary reality of conscious experience in all the richness and diversity that characterizes World 2 existence. Furthermore this experience is self-reflective in the sense that we know that we can know. Our ultimate efforts are to understand this primary reality in relation to the secondary realities of the matter-energy world (World 1) and of the world of objective thought that embraces the whole of civilization and culture (World 3). We as experiencing beings must be central to the explanations, because all the experiences derived from Worlds 1 and 3 are recognizably dependent on the manner in which we obtain information by means of the transductions effected by sense organs and the coded transmission to our brains.

The story of man's thoughts on the meaning of life and on the ultimate human destiny in death provide a poignant testimony. Myths and religions and philosophies have been concerned with this tragic enigma of "ultimate concern" that faces each one of us. Is human destiny but an episode between two oblivions? Or can we have hope that there is meaning and transcendent significance in the wonderful, rich and vivid conscious experience that is our birthright?

And that brings me to assert that any fundamental question in philosophy must be considered in the full context of related questions, and never in some arbitrary isolation. The question of death-awareness and self-annihilation must not be discussed except in relation to the question of birth and the subsequent self-actualization, which has been expressed by Plato in the Phaedo. As I have argued previously (Eccles, 1970), I believe that my experiencing self is only in part explained by the evolutionary origin of my body and brain, that is of my World 1 component. It is a necessary but not a sufficient condition. About the origin of our world of conscious experience (World 2) we know only that it can be described as having an emergent relation to the evolutionary development of the human brain. The uniqueness of individuality that I experience myself to have cannot be attributed to the uniqueness of my genetic inheritance, as I have already argued (Eccles, 1970, Chapt. V). Our coming-to-be is as mysterious as our ceasing-to-be at death. Can we therefore not derive hope because our ignorance about our origin matches our ignorance about our destiny? Cannot life be lived as a challenging and wonderful adventure that has meaning to be discovered?

Let us look now at the future for cultural evolution. It is my thesis that this will provide man with virtually unlimited opportunities in the many rich fields of World 3. Even before the great and pioneering cultural achievements of Sumerian civilization, we can assume that the cerebral potentiality of man had evolved to the level of modern man. It seems that in this respect there has been no signficant evolutionary advance in the last tens of millenia — perhaps from the latter part of the upper Paleolithic age. From then on biological evolution had given place to cultural evolution. And if we survey the recent history of man, century by century, we can see that there have been tremendous achievements in one or other aspect of culture. Not all aspects advance continuously. Great creative discoveries and inspiring leadership by men of genius have led to a flourishing of now one great cultural discipline, now another. At one time it is in literature, at another in philosophy or in the plastic arts or in music or in science and technology. For example the classical age of Greece was remarkable for architecture, sculpture, literature and philosophy. In the Renaissance there were great developments in architecture, painting, sculpture and literature; later came music, philosophy, cosmology and science. It would be generally agreed that for more than a century the greatest cultural achievements of man have been in science and technology.

I will now recapitulate my thesis. It has been argued that man differs *radically in kind* from other animals. As a transcendence in the evolutionary process there appeared an animal differing fundamentally from other animals because he had attained to propositional speech, abstract thought and self-consciousness, which are all signs that a being of transcendent novelty had appeared in the world—creatures existing not only in World 1 but realizing their existence in the world of self-awareness (World 2) and so having in the religious concept, souls. And simultaneously these human beings began utilizing their World 2 experiences to create another world, the third World of the objective spirit. This World 3 provides the means whereby man's creative efforts live on as a heritage for all future men, so building the magnificent cultures and civilizations recorded in human history. Do not the mystery and the wonder of this story of our origin and nature surpass the myths whereby man in the past has attempted to explain his origin and destiny?

We can have hope as we recognize and appreciate the wonder and mystery of our existence as experiencing selves. Mankind would be cured of his alienation if that message could be expressed with all the authority of scientists and philosophers as well as with the imaginative insights of artists. In my recent book (Eccles, 1970) I expressed my efforts to understand a human person, namely myself, as an experiencing being. I offered it in the hope that it may help man to discover a way out of his alienation and

to face up to the terrible and wonderful reality of his existence —
with courage and faith and hope. Because of the mystery of our
being as unique self-conscious existences, we can have hope as we
set our own soft, sensitive and fleeting personal experience against
the terror and immensity of illimitable space and time. Are we not
participants in the meaning, where there is else no meaning? Do
we not experience and delight in fellowship, joy, harmony, truth,
love and beauty, where there else is only the mindless universe?

REFERENCES

Dobzhansky, T. (1962). Mankind evolving: *The evolution of the human spe-cies*. Yale University Press, New Haven.

Dobzhansky, T. (1967). *The Biology of Ultimate Concern*. New York: New American Library.

Eccles, J.C. (1970). *Facing Reality*. Springer-Verlag New York, Heidelberg, Berlin. 210 pp.

Hawkes, J. (1965). Prehistory in History of Mankind. Cultural and Scientific development. Vol. 1, Part 1. UNESCO. London, New English Library Limited.

Polten, E.P. (1973). *A critique of the psycho-physical identity theory*. Mouton Publishers, The Hague.

Popper, K.R. (1970). Personal communication.

Popper, K.R. (1972). Objective knowledge: an evolutionary approach. Clarendon Press: Oxford.

Sherrington, C.S. (1940). Man on His Nature. London: Cambridge University Press. 413 pp.

Sherrington, C.S. (1947). Foreword to 1947 edition. The integrative action of the nervous system. Cambridge University Press.

Thorpe, W.H. (1956). Learning and Instruct in Animals. Methuen London.

Tinbergen, N. (1951). The Study of Instinct. Clarendon Press, Oxford. 228 pp.

WORLD 1

PHYSICAL OBJECTS AND STATES

1. INORGANIC
   - Matter and energy of cosmos
2. BIOLOGY
   - Structure and actions of all living beings
     - human brains
3. ARTEFACTS
   - Material substrates
     - of human creativity
     - of tools
     - of machines
     - of books
     - of works of art
     - of music

⇄

WORLD 2

STATES OF CONSCIOUSNESS

Subjective knowledge

Experience of
- perception
- thinking
- emotions
- dispositional intentions
- memories
- dreams
- creative imagination

⇄

WORLD 3

KNOWLEDGE IN OBJECTIVE SENSE

Records of intellectual efforts
- philosophical
- theological
- scientific
- historical
- literary
- artistic
- technological

Theoretical systems
- scientific problems
- critical arguments

Fig. 1. Tabular representation of the three worlds that comprise all existents and all experiences as defined by Popper (1970).

WORLD OF CONSCIOUSNESS

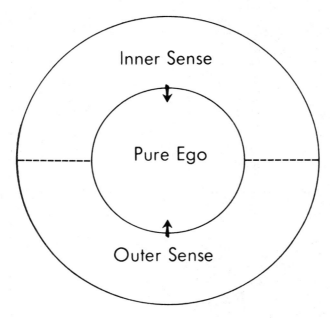

Outer Sense	Inner Sense	Pure Ego
Light	Thoughts	The self
Color	Feelings	The soul
Sound	Memories	
Smell	Dreams	
Taste	Imaginings	
Pain	Intentions	
Touch		

Fig. 2. World of consciousness. The three postulated components in the world of consciousness together with a tabulated list of their components.

Section B:
Cerebral Correlates
of Consciousness

— B1 —
The Human Brain and the Human Person
Sir John Eccles

— B2 —
Subjective and Neuronal Time Factors in Conscious Sensory Experience, Studied in Man, and Their Implications for the Mind Brain Relationship
Benjamin Libet

Commentary:
K.B. Madsen

— B3 —
Experimental Transference of Consciousness
Robert J. White

— B4 —
The Science of Behavior and the Internal Universe
W. Horsley Grantt

— B5 —
The Brain, Learning and Values
Holger Hyden

Commentary:
Robert J. White

— B6 —
Cerebral Activity and the Freedom of the Will
Sir John C. Eccles

Sir John Eccles

B1 The Human Brain and the Human Person

The theme of my talk relates to this mysterious experience that each of us continually has of being a person with a self-consciousness — not just conscious, but knowing that you know. In defining "person" I will quote two admirable statements by Immanuel Kant: "A person is a subject who is responsible for his actions;" and "A person is something that is conscious at different times of the numerical identity of its self." These statements are minimal and basic, and they could be enormously expanded. For example, Popper and I have just published a 600-page book on *The Self and Its Brain*.

We are now able to go much further than Kant in defining the relation of the person to its brain. We are apt to regard the person as identical with the ensemble of face, body, limbs, etc., that constitutes each of us. It is easy to show that this is a mistake. Amputation of limbs and losses of eyes, for example, though crippling, leave the human person with its essential identity. This is also the case with removal of internal organs. Many can be excised in the whole or in part. The human person survives unchanged after kidney transplants or even heart transplants. You may ask what happens with brain transplants. Mercifully, this is not feasible surgically, but even now it would be possible to successfully accomplish a head transplant. Who can doubt that the person "owning" the transplanted head would now "own" the acquired body and not vice versa!? We can hope that with human persons this will remain a Gedanken experiment, but it has already been successfully done in mammals by Professor White (B3). We can recognize that all structures of the head extraneous to the brain are not involved in this transplanted ownership. For example, eyes, nose, jaws, scalp, etc. are no more concerned with ownership than are other parts of the body. So we can conclude that it is the brain and the brain alone that provides the material basis of our personhood.

But when we come to consider the brain as the seat of the conscious personhood, we can also recognize that large parts of the brain are not essential. For example, removal of the cerebellum gravely incapacitates movement, but the person is not otherwise affected. It is quite different with the main part of the brain, the cerebral hemispheres. They are very intimately related to the consciousness of the person, but not equally. In more then 95% of persons there is dominance of the left hemisphere, which is the speaking hemisphere (Fig. 1). Except in infants its removal results in a most severe destruction of the human person, but not annihilation. On the other hand, removal of the minor hemisphere (usually the right) is attended with loss of movement on the left side (hemiplegia) and blindness on the left side (hemianopia), but the person is otherwise not gravely disturbed. Damage to other parts of the brain can also greatly disturb the human personhood, possibly by the removal of the neural inputs that normally generate the necessary background activity of the cerebral hemispheres. A tragic example of this is shown by the vigil coma that often follows severe head injury in accidents. The subject remains in deep unconsciousness even though the cerebral hemispheres themselves have not been damaged. Damage at lower levels of the brain, for example of the reticular activating system, has caused the cerebral hemispheres to be inactive and so to be functionally dead. This terrible state can go on for months. Sometimes there is a slow and often imperfect awakening some weeks after the accident, but often this never occurs. The electroencephalograms show an almost complete silence, which indicates little or no activity in the cerebral cortex. In other cases the cerebral cortex may be so severely damaged that the diagnosis of brain death can be sustained, as for example following a long interruption of the heart beat. The person is literally dead though the rest of the body and its organs can function indefinitely when respiration is provided by an iron lung.

So to sum up the evidence, we can say that the human person is intimately associated with its brain, probably exclusively with the cerebral hemispheres, and is not at all directly associated with all the remainder of its body. The association that you experience of limbs, face, eyes, etc., is dependent on the communication by nerve pathways to the brain, where the experience is generated.

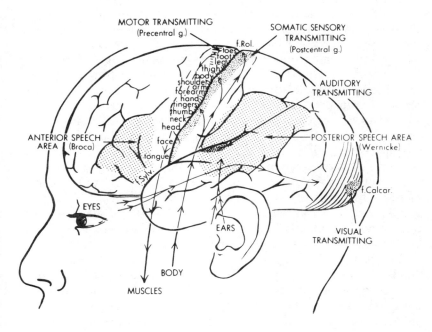

Fig.1. Motor and sensory transmitting areas of the cerebral cortex. The approximate map of the motor transmitting areas is shown in the precentral gyrus, while the somatic sensory receiving areas are in a similar map in the postcenral gyrus. Other primary sensory areas shown are the visual and auditory, but they are largely in areas screened from this lateral view. The frontal, parietal, occipital and temporal lobes are indicated. Also shown are the speech areas of Broca and Wernicke.

Let us now briefly consider how a human embryo and baby eventually become a human person. It is a route that all of us have traversed, but much is unremembered. A baby is born with a brain that is very fully formed in all its detailed structure, but of course it has yet to grow to the full adult size of about 1.4 kg. The nerve cells and the unitary components of the brain have almost all been made. All the major lines of communication from the periphery and from one part of the brain to another have been grown ready for use. Much before birth the brain has been causing the movements sensed by the mother. And even before birth the child can respond to sounds. Its hearing system is already functioning well by birth, which is far earlier than the vision system. It is remarkable that by seven days after birth a baby has learned to distinguish its mother's voice from other voices, just as happens with lambs. Then follows a long period of learning to see and to move in a controlled manner.

As we all know, even in the first months of life a baby is continually practicing its vocal organs and so is beginning to learn this most complex of all motor coordinations. Movements of larynx, palate, tongue and lips have to be coordinated and blended with respiratory movements. It is another variety of motor learning, but now the feedback is from hearing and is at first imitative of sounds heard. This leads on to the simplest types of words like "dada", "papa", and "mama" that are produced at about one year. It is important to realize that speech is dependent on feedback from hearing the spoken words. The deaf are mute. In linguistic development recognition outstrips expression. The child has a veritable word hunger, asking for names and practicing incessantly even when alone. It dares to make mistakes evolving from its own rules, as for example with the irregular plural of nouns. Language does not come about by simple imitation. The child abstracts regularities and relations from what it hears and applies these principles in building up its linguistic expressions.

To be able to speak given even minimal exposure to speech is part of our biological heritage. This endowment has a genetic foundation, but one cannot speak of genes for language. On the other hand the genes do provide the instructions for the building of the special areas of the cerebral cortex concerned with language

(Fig. 1), as well as all the subsidiary structures concerned in vocalization.

The 3 World philosophy of Popper (c.f. A5) forms the basis of my further exploration of the way in which a human baby becomes a human person. All the material world including even human brains is in the matter-energy World 1. World 2 is the world of all conscious experiences (c.f. Fig. 2) and World 3 is the world of culture including especially language. At birth the human baby, has a human brain, but its World 2 experiences are very rudimentary and World 3 is unknown to it. It, and even a human embryo must be regarded as a human being, but not as a human person.

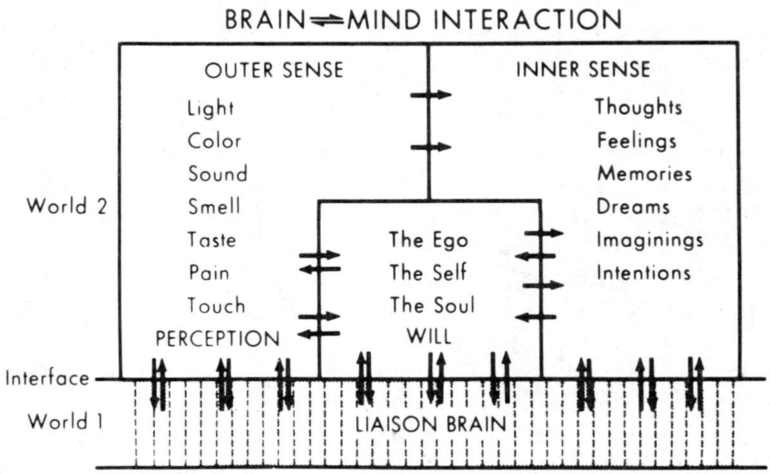

Fig. 2. Information flow diagram for brain-mind interaction. The three components of World 2: outer sense, inner sense and the ego or self are diagrammed with their connectivities. Also shown are the lines of communication across the interface between World 1 and World 2, that is from the liaison brain to and from these World 2 components. The liaison brain has the columnar arrangement indicated (cf. Fig. 6). It must be imagined that the area of the liaison brain is enormous with open modules (cf. Fig. 7) probably numbering up to 1 million and not just the 40 here depicted.

The emergence and development of self-consciousness (World 2) by continued interaction with World 3 is an utterly mysterious process (c.f. Eccles, 1979). It can be likened to a double structure

(Fig. 3) that ascends and grows by the effective cross-linkage. The vertical arrow shows the passage of time from the earliest experiences of the child up to the full human development. From each World 2 position an arrow leads through the World 3 at that level up to a higher, larger level which illustrates symbolically a growth in the culture of that individual. Reciprocally the World 3 resources of the shelf act back to give a higher, expanded level of consciousness of that self (World 2). And so each of us has developed progressively in self-creation. The more the World 3 resources of the individual, the more does it gain in the self-consciousness of World 2. What we are is dependent on the World 3 that we have been immersed in and how effectively we have utilized our opportunities to make the most of our brain potentialities. The brain is necessary but not sufficient for World 2 existence and experience, as is indicated in Fig. 2, which is a dualist-interactionist diagram showing by arrows the flow of information across the interface between the brain in World 1 and the conscious self in World 2.

There is a recent tragic case illustrative of Fig. 3 (Curtiss, 1978). A child, Genie, was deprived of all World 3 influences by her psychotic father. She was penned in isolation in a small room, never spoken to and minimally serviced from the age of 20 months up to 13 years and 8 months. On release from this terrible deprivation she was of course a human being, but not a human person. She was at the bottom rung of the ladder in Fig. 3. Since then with the dedicated help by Dr. Susan Curtiss she has been slowly climbing up that ladder of personhood for the last 8 years. The linguistic deprivation seriously damaged her left hemisphere, but the right hemisphere stands in for a much depleted language performance. Yet, despite this terribly delayed immersion in World 3, Genie has become a human person with selfconsciousness, emotions, and excellent performance in manual dexterity and in visual recognition. We can recognize the necessity of World 3 for the development of the human person. The brain is built by genetic instructions (that is Nature), but development to human personhood is dependent on the World 3 environment (that is Nurture). With Genie there was a gap of over 13 years between Nature and Nurture.

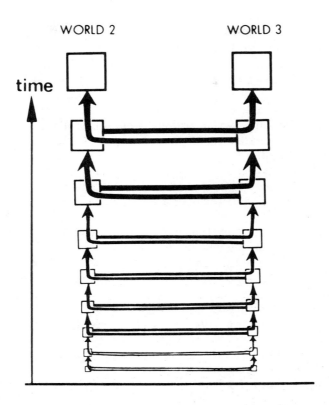

Fig. 3. Diagramatic representation of the postulated interrelationship of the developments of self consciousness (World 2) and of culture (World 3) in time as shown by the arrows. Full description in text.

It may seem that a complete explanation of the development of the human person can be given in terms of the human brain. It is built anatomically by genetic instructions and subsequently developed functionally by learning from the environmental influences. A purely materialist explanation would seem to suffice with the conscious experiences as a derivative from brain functioning. However, it is a mistake to think that the brain does everything and that our conscious experiences are simply a reflection of brain activities, which is a common philosophical view. If that were so, our conscious selves would be no more than passive spectators of the performances carried out by the neuronal machinery of the brain. Our beliefs that we can really make decisions and that we have some control over our actions would be nothing but illusions. There are of course all sorts of subtle cover-ups by philosophers from such a stark exposition, but they do not face up to the issue. In fact all people, even materialist philosophers, behave as if they had at least some responsibility for their own actions. It seems that their philosophy is for "the other people, not for themselves," as Schopenhauer wittily stated.

These considerations lead me to the alternative hypothesis of dualist-interactionism (c.f. C6), that has been expanded at length in the recent book, (Popper and Eccles, 1977). It is really the commonsense view, namely that we are a combination of two things or entities: our brains on the one hand; and our conscious selves on the other. The self is central to the totality of our conscious experiences as persons through our whole waking life. We link it in memory from our earliest conscious experiences. It lapses during sleep, except for dreams, and it recovers for the next day by the continuity of memory. But for memory we as experiencing persons would not exist. Thus we have the extraordinary problem that was first recognized by Descartes: how can the conscious mind and the brain interact?

Let us look at this question by considering what is involved in vision. When we sense an object visually, the upside down retinal image is conveyed to the brain by the Morse code-like signals of nerve impulses, dots only, in the million lines of each optic nerve and in the brain there is an enormous expansion (Fig. 4). In the initial stage hundreds of millions of cortical nerve cells are involved, and even more in the further stages of brain response to the image of the retina. But never in the brain is the retinal image reconstituted. What we have is the immense and complicated coded information about lines and angles and location, which is all that the machinery of the brain can do. The fully evolved coded response of the brain is read out by the mind to give the visual experience from moment to moment with all the qualities of light and color and form and contour. More wonderfully this experience gives meaning—the perceived world that we recognize with ob-

jects and distances and movements. The mind is not passive in
this transaction, but is selecting and interpreting the immense
mass of information that is provided by the brain in coded form.
We are of course far from understanding how this miraculous
transformation can occur. It is important to realize that in the
world that we sense with vision there are none of the properties
that we experience, even light and color. All that the world has for
our sensing are patterns of electromagnetic radiation of various
frequencies and intensities. The vivid pictures of the world that
we experience are actually created in the mind.

This generalization is also true of our other senses, hearing,
touch, smell and taste, which all have counterparts in the material world. It is otherwise with the sense of pain for which there is
no physical or chemical counterpart. It is signalled to the brain
by very simple sense organs that are sensitive to injury. Again
after much complication by the neural machinery of the brain, the
messages come to the cerebral cortex where eventually they are
transmitted to the experience of pain. This is a unique creation by
the mind with the extreme range from unpleasantness to agony.

Other ranges of conscious experiences are independent of
signalling by sense organs and are listed in Fig. 2 under Inner
Sense. They are more subtle and even more uniquely private to us
and so are denoted by rather vague descriptive words such as
feelings, thoughts, imaginings, intentions, dreams, memories.
Yet they have counterparts in brain actions. Changes in the electrical potentials in the brain accompany dreams and mental tasks
such as mental arithmetic or the attempt to recall a memory.
Also, the willing of a simple movement such as the bending of a
finger generates electrical potentials that begin in the brain almost one second before the movement occurs.

It is useful to think of the brain as an instrument, our instrument, that has been our lifelong servant and companion. It provides us, as conscious persons, with the lines of communication
from and to the material world (World 1) which comprises both
our bodies and the external world. It does this by receiving information by the immense sensory system of millions of nerve fibres
that fire impulses into the brain where it is processed into the
coded patterns of information that we read out from moment to

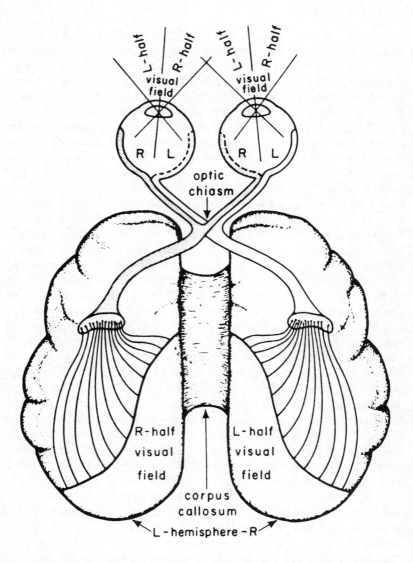

Fig. 4. Diagram of visual pathways showing the L-half and R-half visual fields with the retinal images and the partial crossing in the optic chiasma so that the right-half of the visual field of each eye goes to left visual cortex, after relay in the lateral geniculate body (LGB), and correspondingly for left visual field to right visual cortex.

moment in deriving all our experiences — our percepts, thoughts, ideas, memories. But we as experiencing persons do not slavishly accept all that is provided for us by our instrument, the neuronal machine of our sensory system and of our brain. We select from all that is given according to interest and attention, and we modify the actions of the neuronal machinery, for example, to initiate some willed movement or in order to recall a memory or to concentrate our attention (c.f. Eccles, 1980).

How then can we develop ideas with respect to the mode of operation of the brain? How can it provide the immense range of coded information that can be selected from by the mind in its activity of reading out conscious experiences? It is now possible to give much more informative answers because of very recent work on the essential mode of operation of the neocortex. By the use of radiotracer techniques (Goldman and Nauta, 1977) it has been shown that the great brain mantle, the neocortex, is built up of units or modules (Szentagothai, 1978). The total human neocortex has an area of about 2500 cm.^{2} and is about 3 mm. thick. It contains about ten thousand million nerve cells. These are arranged in small ensembles in the form of a column or module, that runs through the whole thickness of the cortex, three millimeters across. It is a functional unit because of its selective communication with other modules of the neocortex (Fig. 5). The projection is seen to be in a completely overlapping manner and not diffusely.

This modular organization has provided most valuable simplification of the enterprise of trying to understand how this tremendously complex structure worked. The potential performance of ten thousand million individual units is beyond all comprehension. The arrangement in modules of about 2500 nerve cells reduces the number of functional units of the neocortex to about 4 million. These modules have a complex internal operation that is still very little understood, but the structural arrangements have been now fairly well defined by Szentagothai (1978; Fig. 6). The remarkable new discovery is that the modules act as communication units. Each one gives out at least 500 nerve fibres to other modules, but this output is strictly channelled to a few (Fig. 5), perhaps 20 other modules. On the basis of this communi-

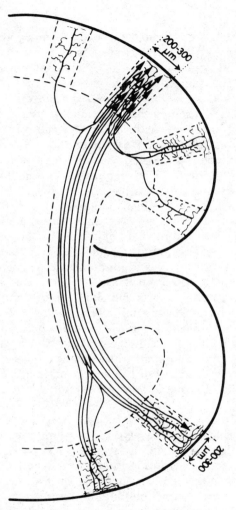

Fig. 5. The general principle of cortico-cortical connectivity is shown diagrammatically in the two hemispheres of the brain. The connections are established in highly specific patterns between vertical columns of 200-300 um diameter in both hemispheres. Ipsilateral connections are derived mainly from cells located in layer III (cells shown at left in outlines), while contralateral connections (cells shown in full black) derive from all layers II-VI. The diagram does not try to show the convergence from afferents originating from different parts of the cortex to the same columns.

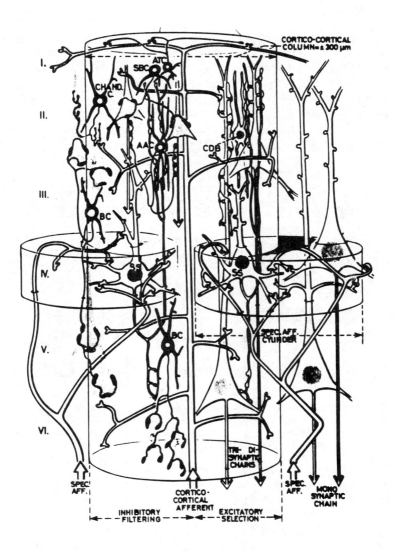

Fig. 6. Diagram illustrating a single cortico-cortical column and two specific subcortical afferent arborization cylinders. Lamination is indicated on the left margin. The right half of the diagram indicates impulse processing over excitatory neurone chains, while the left half shows various types of inhibitory interneurones (in full black). Further explanation in the text.

cation system of each module receiving from 20 and giving to 20, it can be imagined how a sensory input, visual for example, could be rapidly (in a fraction of a second) evolved to a spatio-temporal pattern of active modules that will uniquely encode the information provided by that sensory input, as is shown for one instant in the greatly simplified diagram of Fig. 7. It is postulated that such scintillating spatio-temporal patterns are read out by the mind in its performance of providing a unique perceptual experience.

Pattern of open and closed modules

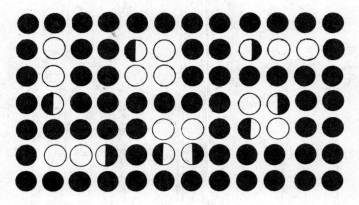

Fig. 7. Diagrammatic plan of cortical modules as seen from the surface. As described in the text the modules are shown as circles of three kinds, open, closed (solid black) and half open. Further description in text. For the human brain this pattern has to be extended about 200 times in each direction.

It can, however, be questioned if the four million modules of the neocortex are adequate to generate the spatio-temporal patterns which encode the total cognitive performance of the human brain — all the sensing, all memories, all linguistic expression, all creativities, all aesthetic experiences — and for our whole life time. The only answer I can give is to refer to the immense potentialities of the 88 keys of a piano. Think of the creative performances of the great composers, Beethoven and Chopin for example. They could utilize only four paramaters in their creation of

music with the 88 keys, each of which has invariant pitch and to-
nal quality. And a comparable four parameters are utilized in
creating the spatio-temporal patterns of activity in the four million modules of the human brain. I will consider these four parameters in turn, pointing out the comparable features.

Firstly, there is intensity. In music this is the loudness of the
note, whereas with the module it is the integral of the impulse firing in the output lines from the module. It has to be recognized
that in the analogy the keys of the piano have a pitch differentiation, whereas in the brain, the modules or keys have location
which is the basis of coded properties that give the kind of perception read out from them, e.g., light or color or sound. *Secondly,*
there is the duration of the note or of the impulse firing from a
module. *Thirdly,* there is the sequence of the notes which gives a
melody with piano music and the temporal pattern of modular activities in the brain. One can imagine that this modular pattern is
dispersed over the surface of the brain. (c.f. Fig. 7). *Fourthly,*
there is the simultaneous activation of several notes, a chord, or
of several modules in the brain. With the chord the maximum
number is ten. With the modules it may be thousands.

I think it will be recognized that the enormous generation of
musical patterns using the 88 keys of a piano points to a virtually
infinite capacity of the four million modules to generate unique
spatio-temporal patterns. Moreover it must be realized that, just
as with piano keys, these patterns giving the conscious experiences are dependent on the four parameters listed above. We can
imagine that the intensities of activation are signalled symbolically by the lighting up of modules. So if we could see the surface
of the neocortex, it would present an illuminated pattern of 50
cm. by 50 cm. composed at any moment of modules $\frac{1}{4}$ mm. across
that have all ranges from dark to dim to lighter to brilliant. And
this pattern would be changing in a scintillating manner from
moment to moment, giving a sparkling spatio-temporal pattern
of the four million modules, appearing exactly as on a TV screen.
This symbolism gives some idea of the immense task confronting
the mind in generating conscious experiences. The dark or dim
modules would be neglected. Moreover it is an important feature
of the hypothesis of mind-brain interaction that neither the mind

nor the brain is passive in the transaction. There must be an active interchange of information across the frontier (Fig. 2) between the material brain and the non-material mind. The mind is not in the matter-energy world so there is no energy exchange in the transaction, merely a flow of information. Yet the mind must be able to change the pattern of energy operations in the modules of the brain, else it would be forever impotent.

It is difficult to understand how the self-conscious mind can relate to such an enormous complexity of spatio-temporal modular patterns. This difficulty is mitigated by three considerations. Firstly, we must realize that our self-conscious mind has been learning to accomplish such tasks from our babyhood onwards, a process that is colloquially called "learning to use one's brains." Secondly, by the process of attention the self-conscious mind selects from the total ensemble of modular patterns those features that are in accord with its present interests. Thirdly, the self-conscious mind is engaged in extracting "meaning" from all that it reads out. This is well illustrated by the many ambiguous figures, for example, a drawing that can be seen either as a staircase or an overhanging cornice (Fig. 8). The switch from one interpretation to the other is instantaneous and holistic. There is

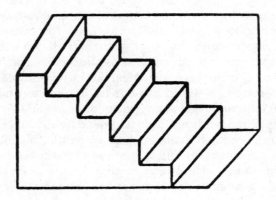

Fig. 8. Ambiguous figure that can be interpreted either as an ascending staircase or an overhanging cornice.

never any transitional phase in the reading out by the mind of the modular pattern in the brain.

A key component of the hypothesis of brain-mind interaction is that the unity of conscious experience is provided by the self-conscious mind and not by the neuronal machinery of the neocortex. Hitherto, it has been impossible to develop any theory of brain function that would explain how a diversity of brain events comes to be synthesized so that there is a unity of conscious experience. The brain events remain disparate, being essentially the individual actions of countless modules.

I have endeavoured to keep the story of mind-brain interaction as simple as possible. How should we expect to have an easy solution of the greatest problem confronting us? I do not claim to have offered a solution, but rather to have indicated in general outline the way the solution may come. In some mysterious way the human brain evolved with properties of a quite other order from anything else in nature. At the summit of these brain properties I would place initially the interaction with another, non-material world (World 2). The coming-to-be of self-consciousness is a mystery that concerns each person with its conscious and unique selfhood. And our self-conscious forebears with their creative imagination built the world of culture and civilization that has played a key role in enriching the formation of each of us as human persons with our culture and our values. The coming-to-be of each unique selfhood lies beyond scientific enquiry, as I have argued elsewhere (c.f. Eccles, 1980). It is my thesis that we have to recognize that the unique selfhood is the result of a supernatural creation of what in the religious sense is called a soul.

I hope that I have shed some light on the great and mysterious problem of the human brain and the human person. Each person must be primarily considered as a unique self-conscious being that interacts with its environment — especially with other persons — by means of the neuronal machinery of the brain. Beyond the scope of this lecture there is the realm of the human person with all the human values that has been the theme of so much of this conference. I have concentrated on the dualist-interactionist view of this mind-brain transaction, because, as Popper and I have argued, all monist-materialist explanations are mistaken simplifications. I offer no final solution of this age-old problem, but hope that I have indicated the way that deeper understanding may be won. Certainly there will be no cheap solutions of a doctrinaire kind.

REFERENCES

Curtiss, S.: Genie: A psycholinguistic study of a modern-day "Wild Child". New York: Academic Press (1977)

Eccles, J.C.: The Human Mystery. Berlin, Heidelberg, New York: Springer International (1979)

Eccles, J.C.: The Human Psyche. Berlin, Heidelberg, New York: Springer Verlag (1980)

Goldman, P.S., Nauta, W.J.H.: Columnar distribution of cortico-cortical fibres in the frontal association, limbic and motor ortex of the developing rhesus monkey. Brain Res. 122: 393-413 (1977)

Popper, K.R., Eccles, J.C.: The Self and its Brain. Berlin, Heidelberg, New York: Springer International (1977)

Szentagothai, J.: The neuron network of the cerebral cortex: A functional interpretation. Proc. Roy. Soc. B 201: 219-248 (1978)

Benjamin Libet

B2 Subjective and Neuronal Time Factors in Conscious Sensory Experience, Studied in Man, and Their Implications For the Mind-Brain Relationship

I propose to confront you with a rather recent experimental discovery of ours that we think has an important bearing on the mind-brain problem. It was made with neurosurgical patients in whom electrodes were implanted for therapeutic purposes. That gave us the opportunity to try to investigate what kinds of neuronal activities might be required at cerebral levels for producing a conscious sensory experience. The particular experimental finding I want briefly to get across to you deals with time factors in the relationship between the neuronal and the subjective events. There were two experimental questions involved. Firstly, when are the neuronal activities adequate to produce the conscious sensory experience after a sensory stimulus is delivered? There is a second, less obvious question that we found had to be addressed, namely, is the timing of the subjective experience the same or different from the time of the neuronal adequacy that is necessary for occurrence of the experience. The answer to the second question appears to bear on the issue at least of psychophysiological parallelism, and in that sense perhaps on identity theory.

We attempt to place an electrode on the lateral surface of the cerebral hemisphere, in particular on the postcentral gyrus, which receives sensory representation of various parts of the body on it. When we electrically stimulate an appropriate site here in the awake human subject, he reports a sensation in the hand or finger area of the opposite side of the body. Now you will notice that the subject does not experience the sensation in his brain where we are stimulating; he experiences it as being referred to a peripheral part of his body. This immediately tells us that there is not an identity between the actual neuronal-spatial configurations that being activated and the spatial locations of the subjective experience that results from it, because the latter is in an entirely different place altogether. Now we consider the time factors involved. We found that one single electrical pulse was completely inadequate to produce a conscious sensory experience; it requires repetition of stimulation pulses. More surprisingly, the repetition, at least near the threshold levels, had to go on for around a half a second, 500 milliseconds, before the subject would report anything. Using different frequencies of pulses makes no difference to this requirement. If we stopped the stimulus train just short of a half a second, the subject would report he felt absolutely nothing. Additional evidence indicated that there seemed to be a corresponding delay of about 0.5 sec in the subjective experience for this cortical stimulus.

When we stimulated the skin, however, the situation became even more interesting. At the skin one single electrical pulse, as many of you may know, is sufficient to give rise to a sensory experience, even when it's very weak. So the question there becomes, first of all, is there also an actual delay at cerebral levels of up to about 500 msec, before the neuronal responses to that single pulse become adequate? Evidence was developed from two lines of experiments. In one, it was found that a conditioning stimulus, delivered to the cerebral cortex up to 200-500 msec *after* a skin stimulus, could retroactively affect the conscious experience elicited by the prior skin stimulus; this indicated that cerebral process going on for some time after the skin stimulus could still be altered before actual production of the sensory experience. In another line, it was shown that the early electrophysiological indicators of the cerebral cortex responses to a skin stimulus were clearly insufficient to elicit a sensory experience; later components of this electrophysiological complex were necessary. This evidence led to the conclusion that even though a single pulse to the skin is adequate to elicit a sensation, it is in fact followed by a series of events at cortical levels before the neuronal system becomes adequate for the production of conscious experience.

The *subjective* experience for the skin stimulus, on the other hand, seemed to appear with no appreciable delay! I cannot give the details of the evidence for this in the time available. In brief, the evidence was based on the order of the subjective timing of experience for a skin stimulus relative to that for a cortical stimulus (the latter known to require at least 500 msec before it could produce any experience).

Let us summarize the situation. When you stimulate the skin with one single pulse, there are initiated, after a brief delay of 10 to 20 milliseconds, a series of electrophysiological changes recordable at the cortex; these in fact go on for about a half a second or more. The early or primary portion of this is by itself not adequate to produce any conscious experience. In fact, you can produce conscious experience without having the primary response there at all. The apparent delay of up to about a half a second before there is neuronal adequacy for the production of the conscious sensation, is thus paradoxically coupled with the apparent absence of any delay for appearance or timing of the subjective experience that is "produced" by the neuronal acitivity. To explain this we proposed (a) that the initial primary response of the cortex to the fast message which arrives via a specific projection system, acts as a "time market"; and (b) that, after neuronal adequacy for the production of the sensation is achieved, the experience is somehow referred back automatically to this initial time marker. As far as the subject is concerned, therefore, there would be no delay whatsoever. With different sensory inputs delivered synchronously to different parts of the body, including also visual or auditory, you know you have no jitter or asynchrony in your experiences. They are all, in our thesis, referred back to the initial fast signals for each input case, and thereby appear to be subjectively synchronous.

So we have the proposition, then, that there is a discrepancy between the time of neuronal adequacy, delayed for up to about a half a second before in fact a conscious sensory experience can be produced, and the time of the subjective experience "produced" by this neuronal activity. I'm going to touch briefly on one or two points that relate this discrepancy to the mind-brain relationship. A substantial delay for neuronal adequacy would mean that if you make a quick response to a stimulus, it would have to be made unconsciously. If quick responses are unconscious, that puts a time constraint on what you can refer to as being an act of free will, since free will could presumably be exercised consciously. If by experimental observation, not theory, the subjective experience of an event seems to have a different time base from the neuronal activity that produced it, the concept of psychophysiological parallelism would have to be stretched to encompass this discrepancy. One could argue that this discrepancy is not different in principle from the discrepancy between a subjective referral of an image in space and the neuronal spatial configuration that is responsible for it. But somehow the discrepancy in time bases seems more disturbing. One cannot conclude that it supplies a rigorous disproof of identify theory, which requires a strict psychoplysiological parallelism. However, it introduces an experimentally based factor that may affect the relative attractiveness of alternative philosophical views of mind-brain interaction.

K.B. Madsen

Commentary

Fortunately, I have had the opportunity to read Sir John's and Sir Karl Popper's book. I got it just before I went on the airplane from Copenhagen and read it, and there were two pages in that book where Sir John tried to put Libet's experimental results in. What I will do now, as Sir John has not already himself done it, is to try to expose that part of his theory which explains these experimental results. First I must say that I think the mind-body problem is the most important philosophical problem, at least for psychologists, and I think from this conference it is one of the most important problems. But I think there had not appeared real new original theories of philosophers about this problem for many years until Sir Karl Popper's theory appeared. I think it was in 1968 that he first exposed his theory about the three worlds, and this theory is already exposed by Sir John, so I can refer to that. And then I will say that even if it was a new philosophical theory, it was after all a philosophy after Sir Karl Popper's own requirement for a scientific theory. It was not a scientific theory because a scientific theory according to his principles had to be a testable theory, a theory which can be falsified. And I don't think his own formulation of it is so that it can be falsified. So we must call it a philosophical theory in the exposition which he gas given. But then Sir John Eccles has in his part of the book transformed this philosophical theory to a real and scientific theory which can be falsified, and I think what you have heard here is one of the things which is testing this theory, and I shall mention another thing.

First I must repeat the three most important hypotheses in the version of the theory which Sir John presents in the latest book. First, what you have already heard, the interaction between mind and brain is going on in the liaison-brain, which is the cortex or the dominant hemisphere of the cortex. That we have already heard.

Second, integration of information in perception is the function of the mind, not of the brain. And this explains the delay of the half second which Libet has found, because it's the function of the mind and not of the brain. I cannot avoid referring to a very old experimental fact in psychology, one of the most well-testing areas, classical conditioning. Pavlov and many of his followers have found that a half-second is the optimal time interval between presenting the unconditioned stimulus and the conditioned stimulus. So it seems to be as if there has been already there the requirement of some kind of, what shall we say, conscousness in the dog or whatever animal it is which they experiment with, because it was just the same time interval. That was the second hypothesis.

The third hypothesis could be framed in this way, or formulated in this way: The decision and plan of action is of the mind and not of the brain. And this is demonstrated, or it is tested by the experiment which Kornhuber has made, in which he found that the delay between the decision, the act of will, and the performance of the movement was 0.8 seconds. That is a parallel to what we have heard here. Now it is the other side of the interaction, and there is a time lag of almost a second, 0.8, and I think that's an interesting thing that the time lag is not the same on the input side as on the output side. The input side and the output side between the interaction of the mind and brain is perhaps not the same, and I should like to hear some comments from Libet and Sir John about this difference in time in these two experiments.

Of course I cannot here repeat all of the experiments which are set forth and exposed in the book as data which is evidence for the theory as a scientific theory. So here you see the results have an important place in a theoretical frame of reference, which again has place in philosophy.

In the ending, I have one critical remark, and it's half terminology and half real criticism. I think that the mysteriousness of the interaction between these two worlds, as they are called in Sir Karl Popper's theory, will be reduced by two things: first, instead of calling them two worlds or three worlds, you should call them three levels of the same world. I think many people here would

accept the theory if you framed it another way. I can't see it would
hurt the sense of the theory if you called it three levels of the world
instead of three worlds. It will reduce the mysteriousness a little,
I believe. These three levels you can conceive of as only *method-
logical* levels or, if you prefer, *onotological* levels. You need not
take both steps. The first step is enough to deal with the scientific theory, at least.

In addition to these three levels which can be conceived meth-
odologically and onotologically, you could add more levels because
I think that the same problems are coming up in many other places
where sciences are working on borderlines. We have already heard
today that even inside one science, physics, there is a kind of leap
from one level to another, from classical mechanism to the electromagnetic theory. Then of course we leaped from the level of
physics to chemistry and from chemistry to biochemistry: and if
you go on in the line which Pribram has done from *"The Languages of the Brain"* (from 1971), you could say that some psychologists at least, work on the levels from neurochemistry, neurophysiology, brain physiology (where the brain is dealt with as a
whole) and to psychology in the traditional way (where the person is dealt with as a whole). Then on to the social-psychological
level, to the sociological level, to the cultural level where the third
world in Popper's theory is placed, so I think that there are many
such levels in the world but we can think upon it as one world leveled by our sciences, by our methods, by our conceptual frame of
references.

If you like, especially if you like to have a philosophy about
your scientific theory you can think upon these levels as levels in
the reality, and many of you will recognize this as the systems
theorists' approach to the world.

Robert J. White

B3 Experimental Transference of Consciousness: The Human Equivalent

Part I

In recent years we have been able to construct a series of brain models which have permitted us to literally transfer the entire brain of the experimental animal intact and still capable of high performance at all levels. The majority of these experiments utilized the subhuman primate, but, more recently, both the canine and the rodent have been employed in the surgical engineering design of these isolated brain preparations.

The initial experimental protocols involved first, the design of a unique surgical procedure permitting isolation of the complete brain, both vascularly and neurogenetically; and, second, the construction of a support system to insure viability of the brain outside of its own body. This was accomplished by reestablishing cerebral circulation and by employing a hematologically compatible donor or a miniaturized extracorporeal perfusion system. With both of these extracerebral vascular support systems, the brain was in a truly isolated state and the performance of the organ is continuously monitored using ongoing neurochemical and neurophysiological criteria. While, particularly in the donor supported model, data retrieved from these tracking techniques approached normality in character and value, we were unable to assume that the preparation was, in the final analysis, conscious or aware of its existence.

By definition, to isolate the brain required neurogenic separation and, therefore, not only the spinal cord, but all of the cranial nerves must be severed; as a consequence, the inner organizational matrix of the brain is no longer receiving an inrush of information from the peripheral nervous system. It is exclusively dependent on hormonal secretion via the circulation. Obviously the brain is also unable to "express itself" through nerve pathways and, thus, can only remain in contact via the release of neurohormones into the vascular system.

In recent experiments, in which a single cranial nerve complex was purposefully preserved, for example, the auditory or optic nerve, it was demonstrated that with either sound or light stimulation, the appropriate neuroanatomical connections in the isolated brain remained intact and, when the appropriate areas of cerebral cortex (auditory or visual cortex) were instrumented with surface electrodes appropriate responses were recorded, strongly suggesting the preservation and functioning of these intimate and delicate neural fiber tracts and connections subserving these modalities of sensation. Once again, however, this did not provide evidence that the preparation in the isolated state was capable of processing or appreciating this information.

Detailed neurophysiological investigation utilizing stereotaxically oriented depth electrodes in brain stem demonstrated preservation of functioning in the reticular activating relay systems. The accumulation of data strongly supported the concept that, under these experimental conditions, the isolated brain, vascularly supported outside of its body, existed in a recreated environment that provided adequacy of substrate delivery. It was therefore very reminiscent of the in situ situation. Furthermore, neurophysiological sampling at a cortical or subcortical level, particularly in the donor supported isolated brain, appeared to meet the criteria of electroencephalogic normality in hundreds of samplings when compared with similar tracings from awake and intact central nervous system animals. Thus, while we have no objective criteria that the isolated brain model, even in the subhuman primate, was conscious, it did appear that its biochemical and neuroelectrical state would be appropriate for the maintenance of an alert condition.

In more recent years, it has been possible to actually transplant the isolated brain into the body (anatomically either in the neck or in abdominal cavity) by interposing the organ between the arterial and venous system. Under these circumstances, a significant increase in longevity was, and is, possible. In general, these periods have been of the order of three to seven days. Originally the technology required the use of specially designed vascular cannulae to achieve artery to artery and vein to vein anastomosis, necessitating the continuous use of an anticoagulant state. This often required termination of the experiment because of gradually increasing hemorrhage in the preparation. More recently, with the employment of micro-surgical techniques, the vascular anastomosis has been achieved without the use of cannulae and without the requirement of chronic heparinization. Isolated brain models in the transplanted state are equipped with a survey module permitting continuous recording of cerebral blood flow, arterial-venous chemical analysis, cortical and subcortical neuroelectrical recording and temperature sampling. Again, and with great frequency, brain performances in the transplanted subhuman have approached cerebral performance in the intact animal.

There is, of course, no way that we can argue, in spite of the high level of functioning of the brain in the transplanted model, that consciousness or appreciation of environment change is attained or maintained. In order to achieve evidence of responsivity of the brain in isolation, it appeared to us that it would be necessary to retain cranial nerve function. Toward that end, an entirely new generation of brain models had to be developed. This would require the operative transplanting of the entire cephalon of the body of another animal from which the animal's own cephalon had been removed. This has necessitated the development of unique technology where none existed previously, not only in terms of anesthesia and surgery, but, equally important, the construction of advanced engineering suspension and fixation units. In the initial experiments the employment of vascular cannulae were required to make the vascular connections between cervical vessels (arterial and venous). As in the isolated brain transplantation experiments, continuous heparinization was necessitated to prevent clotting of the connecting tubing and, as a result, the experiments frequently were terminated after a day or two.

More recently, using direct microsurgical anastomosis of the arterial and venous vessels, the transplanted cephalon could be surgically connected with only short phase heparinization (during the actual operation.) Under the design of these experiments, it was now possible to examine the brain within the head with the cranial nerves intact and, at long last, to answer the question as to whether or not, when the brain is transplanted, it retains the capability of consciousness and for appropriate response to external stimuli. While this question has now been answered in a more chronic sequence in the preparations that were vascularly associated through microsurgical anastomosis, even in the early models of cephalic transplantation where cannular connection was employed, that with the emergence from anesthesia it was immediately obvious that *the brain had regained a state of consciousness!*

In the ensuing hours following surgery, a completely awake state supervened and, through the available cranial nerve function, the preparation did respond appropriately to external stimulation! It was obvious that the animals could see and did appreciate movement and, indeed, would track with their eyes objects of interest placed in their visual fields. Responsivity to ordinary stimulation was obvious in that, if a loud sound was produced, the cephalon responded by a facial expression of discomfort. Light pin prick of the facial tissues, likewise, gave evidence of discomfort on the part of the animal.

These preparations could and did masticate and swallow food, as well as appropriately handling fluids employing the expected muscle movements of tongue and oral cavity. Indeed, one had the impression that the animals were "hungry and thirsty" and understood the oral processing of food and liquid with alacrity.

While these behaviorial observations might be considered gross, there was no disagreement amongst the examiners that the isolated brain in the cephalon transplantation had achieved consciousness and that its preservation, as reflected in the proper responses of the animal to appropriate cranial nerve stimulation was dependent solely on the maintenance of an adequate circulation and substrate delivery to brain. The sustaining of viability in the unique cephalic transplantation model required a highly sophisticated intensive care unit with detailed programs of management. Maintenance of pulmonary function necessitated continuous mechanical respiratory support and to maintain appropriate levels of blood pressure, exogenous catecholamine infusion techniques required development.

The most advanced transplant model yet devised requires the preservation of the brain stem at a mid-brain level in the body that is to receive the cephalon. Thus, when the cephalon is vascularly connected with the body, the new preparation is able to initiate its own respiratory activity and provide for self-maintenance of blood pressure.

To date the obvious problem of tissue rejection has not been addressed although neuropathological examination of the transplanted brain has not revealed any light microscopy evidence of hyper-rejection of tissue. In actuality, the brain tissue stained with hematoxylin and eosin looked quite normal!

Part II

While the investigations described in Part I deal exclusively with the transference of cerebral function including consciousness in the experimental animal there is every reason to believe that with additional advances in surgical and instrumentation technology, similar operations could be performed in the human. In some ways, the accomplishments presented in Part I enabling the scientist to perform cerebral transplantation in the subhuman primate actually present a more difficult undertaking surgically than would be the case in the human sphere. Thus, because of the extremely small size of the blood vessels in these animal preparations, as opposed to those available in man, the increase in vascular dimensions would markedly increase the ease of constructing the blood vessel anastomosis. Additionally, considerable anatomical and operative information is available on a human level that would permit solution of the problem of designing a surgical technique for cephalic transplantation in man.

Be that as it may, the methodology, as yet, is not available, nor have we undertaken an attempt at preparing such an operative technique. Obviously, if such an operation were to be considered in man, a great deal of work would have to be undertaken in the area of tissue rejection, not only in terms of the brain itself, but as it would relate to other tissues of the cephalon. (It would be interesting to contemplate the construction of a series of subhuman primate cephalic transplantation experiments in which immunological suppressive drugs were utilized much as in renal transplantation to further extend the longevity of these preparations.)

Additionally, and over and above the operative technique itself, a great deal of research would have to directed toward designing support systems to provide viability of the human model, for surely these patients would require an incredible array of monitoring and maintenance equipment, as well as specially trained physician and nursing personnel. Granting the justification of funding and undertaking the necessary research, there is little doubt that, even at the present time, cephalic transplantation in man is a technical reality. Whether we can justify this socially, philosophically, or theologically, there is no question that it can be done. More importantly, there is no question that such a preparation should and would demonstrate a level of consciousness and cerebral performance that we have come to expect in the sub-human primate model nor is there any reason we should not expect that the intrinsic individuality, personality, emotional structure, intelligence, and memory would not continue to function under these experimental circumstances.

Thus, it is already possible to transfer human consciousness provided the organ that subtends such functioning is retained. It could be argued that all of the other body systems and organs have been primarily developed for and, in a sense, subserviant to the concept that brain function must be sustained and that their very existence and design is based on this principle. In other words, the body and its systems are nothing more than a "power pack" for the brain for, in the final analysis, the brain is the tissue substrate for the mind and possibly that which we call the spirit or soul of man.

Science has reached the threshold where *human consciousness can be transferred* provided the organ which supervenes this characteristic is maintained. Whether research directed toward human cephalic transplanation should be undertaken requires extensive review by such fields as philosophy, theology, sociology, and medicine.

W. Horsley Gantt

B4 The Science of Behavior and The Internal Universe

I.

Introduction

At the fourscore year mark my curiosity about the universe having increased rather than diminished, I have the advantage of using the perspective of many years in the background to look forward.

Science began with unity, e.g., Aristotle was not only one of the three great Greek philosophers who dominated thinking down to the Middle Ages, but he was as well an astronomer, a physicist, an anatomist and a biologist.

The Middle Ages saw the foundation of a science with a new outlook, a perspective based upon the experimental method and observation combined with an elaboration of concepts. This foundation was laid especially by Galileo and Newton, with an emphasis on the conceptual side by Francis Bacon and Descartes.

Our interest, however, is centered around John Locke, born in 1723, on account of his emphasis on the relation of the individual to the external environment, his *tabula rasa* upon which experience writes. From him has developed the materialistic point of view in behavior. Hence began the emphasis upon the data brought to us by the sense organs, later greatly amplified by instrumentation. What occurred in the body was likened to what was seen with machines, e.g., the pumping of the blood by the heart and the discovery of the circulation by Harvey to hydrodynamics. Thus, it was apparent that many of the functions of the body obeyed the laws of mechanics.

Behaviorism as we know it today obtained a great stimulus from the discovery of sensory and motor nerves by Bell and Majendie, about the beginning of the 19th century. The Russian physiologist Sechenov in 1863 wrote his "Reflexes of the Brain."

This was a bold step to include thinking and mind on a purely reflex basis, denying the reality of a separate subjective life. This was emphasized by Thomas Huxley in his statement, "No psychosis without neurosis," meaning that all thinking was underlayed by detectable neural processes. Thus the 19th century began to think of mind as equivalent to complex physical and chemical changes in matter.

The study of the nervous system as a vehicle for total behavior was founded around the turn of the 20th century. This development diverged along two paths, the study of gross movement, and the quantitative measurement of secretions to a food stimulus, the former being developed by Bekhterev, Thorndike, Watson, and Skinner, the latter by Pavlov. On this divergence there have been built up two schools called the Operant and the latter the Classical-Pavlovian. Operant conditioning has been greatly expanded in America; its emphasis is chiefly on how the external behavior can be "shaped" according to the wishes of the experimenter. This at first made use only of the skeletal movements, but later has included the autonomic nervous system.

An entirely different elaboration was centered around Pavlov, who had received the Nobel Prize in 1903 for his work on the physiology of digestion. His contributions involved chiefly the use of the dog over its life span, viz., the chronic experiment, the use of quantitative measures (units of saliva), the emphasis on the individual rather than on statistical surveys and the recognition of individual differences by his four "temperaments".

The evaluation of the Pavlovian school, including that of his successors, such as Skinner, the electrophysiologists, and others, fluctuates from the extreme optimism that "the behaviorists are the people who have got to save the world; they may win the race with total destruction" to the more cautious statement of Grey Walter: "At the present time there is still not one single principle of mental physiology that can claim the status of a natural law, in the sense that it receives universal acceptance and permits deductive prediction or extrapolation."

Though they may espouse monism, most scientists will recognize that for the subjective phenomena of our life there are no objective representations. A simple test is to try to communicate to anyone the sensation of the color "blue." No matter what you say about its wave length or other measurable physical properties, these do not even approach the subjective feeling. They are of a different order—and never the twain shall meet.

Pavlov said science must be satisfied with its practical achievements—its ability to give us the measurable relationships in physical, objective items. Perhaps the monist should heed the counsel of Planck, not to ask of science questions it cannot answer.

Finally, Pavlov, as well as every student of the nervous system, owes much to Descartes' concept of reflex. Pavlov and Sherrington adhered to this concept either implicitly or explicitly in their epochal researches. The difference between them is that whereas Sherrington did not think that his laboratory methods could give him the ultimate answers to the riddle of our mental life, Pavlov had the adolescent hope that at some future time "the omnipotent scientific method will deliver man from his present gloom, and will purge him from his contemporary shame in the sphere of interhuman relations."

II.

Many other responses and reactions in the organism have been brought within the conditional reflex (CR) methodology since Pavlov. In the Pavlovian Laboratories, we have extended this field to include vestibular reactions of equilibration, respiratory and cardiovascular responses including heart rate and blood pressure as well as responses to stimuli placed within the central nervous system (interoceptors). In the human being we have added to these the psychogalvanic.

To epitomize, four decades of work from my laboratory on the cardiac reactions: (the cardiac component of the CRs are in general parallel to the secretory and motor) there is a quantitative relationship to the intensity of the excitatory CR, a marked difference between the cardiac component of the excitatory and inhibitory CRs, a precise cardiac time reflex, etc. The inhibitory CR is characterized by a slight rise in heart rate with a marked subsequent decrease below normal. Here we have in the cardiac response a measure of inhibition which gives an explanation to the quiescent phase and sleep which Pavlov found resulting from inhibitions.

George Burch and some others in the USA have contributed to this field through a study of vasomotor responses. Burch in the course of his detailed and painstaking research on the heart and vascular reactions, has shown that the latter are definitely modified through experiences of the individual, i.e., they are capable of being conditional reflexes.

III.

The preceding description of the ability of many systems to form CRs involves many stimuli from the external environment. The relative role of the periphery and the center, the external sense organs and the central nervous system, concerned us. To solve this, we considered the elements of the reflex arc, both the conditional reflex arc and the unconditional reflex arc. We successively eliminated the different parts of the conditional reflex arc—the external sense organs, the peripheral nerves, the spinal pathways to the motor area of the brain, finally the executor organ, viz., the motor movement or the salivary secretion with the result that the only essential part for conditional reflex function is the central nervous system.

This then puts the importance of the adaptation *within* the central nervous system, diminishing the function of the external environment in the healthy subject. This, of course, does not negate the influence of the external environment in such items as nutrition, etc. It means that many adaptations can be found within the central nervous system.

In directing our attention to the inner universe, we must acknowledge the debt we owe to Claude Bernard for his study of the inner world through which study he was led to the realization of the fact that the body maintains a constant chemical composition for its life within. This idea was taken up later by Cannon and made the principle of his "homeostasis". Thus arose an over-emphasis of the ability of the organism—beyond its powers—to regulate its economy and to maintain its equilibrium in an unfavorable environment. In psychiatry it took the form of believing that whatever the individual tended to do represented a healthy, balancing action. The counterpart of this idea was expressed by Pavlov, viz., that the CR was a means of preserving an equilibrium between the individual and its environment. This idea of equilibrium will be discussed later.

In the formation of the conditional reflex we can eliminate the external sense organs (eye, ear, skin) by placing electrodes within the nerves to produce the conditional stimulus. To supplant the unconditional stimulus an electrode may be placed 1) on the posterior nerve root, 2) on the posterior columns of the spinal cord, 3) within the cerebellum, 4) in the motor area of the cortex. In all these regions the movements produced can be conditioned as easily as if the stimulus were applied to the skin receptors. Also for the conditional stimulus may be substituted an electric stimulus in the silent areas of the cortex. In these instances the unconditional stimulus or the conditional stimulus or both are entirely within the central nervous systems. Also the efferent end may be eliminated by crushing of the anterior nerve roots within the spinal canal to a limb, training the animal during the period of paralysis and testing him after recovery; the motor reflex appears on the first trial after several months interval required for regeneration of the nerve.

Thus the conditional reflex can be formed and can exist internally without involvement of the external environment! If the nervous system can form conditional reflexes from a stimulus applied within, albeit an artificial one, it is reasonable to assume that it can elaborate conditional reflexes from stimuli arising from origins peculiar to itself.

IV.

From the consideration of many approaches to the adaptability of the organism during its life experiences we see that its various functions do not make parallel adaptations; some functions readily become CRs, others are absolutely unconditionable. From this we arrive at the law of *fractional conditioning*. Besides this absolute difference, there are differences of degree relative to the speed of formation of a CR and the durability once formed. To this marked difference, first seen with the cardiac conditional reflex, we get the name of *schizokinesis*.

In the study of the cardiac components of the conditional reflex to food or to pain we saw that the cardiac conditional reflex formed rapidly, usually before the motor or the salivary and often after one reinforcement by the unconditional stimulus. Not only did it form first, as a rule, but it generally was much more resistant to extinction. Often the cardiac conditional reflex might continue for several years after the motor or the salivary component had been extinguished by active efforts for extinction. The respiratory conditional reflex behaves in this respect more like the cardiac conditional reflex than like the specific salivary or motor components.

The fact that the cardiac conditional reflex may continue while the other components are absent led to the concept of schizokinesis, a split between the more general functions as the respiratory and the cardiovascular and the specific ones. Such a split—a persistence of one activity in the absence of the other—would seem to represent a maladaptation, a kind of built-in lack of integration of the physiological systems.

The existence of the conditional reflex may at times seem to be a liability and a lack of equilibrium with the environment, and even the opposite, viz., dysfunction. Thus, as shown by Bykov, more oxygen is consumed in performing a given task when the performance is preceded by a conditional stimulus, i.e., the oxygen consumed by the conditional reflex plus the amount consumed by the unconditonal reflex alone not preceded by the conditional stimulus. We have shown a similar thing for the salivary secretion; more saliva is required for the same amount of food when the eating of the food is preceded by the conditional stimulus. The organism must pay in efficiency, i.e., in the amount of energy required, for its function of being ready for emergencies.

The fact that conditional reflexes are so often difficult to eradicate once formed makes the individual a museum of antiquities as he grows older, as I have pointed out previously. He is encumbered with many reactions no longer useful or even those detrimental life. This is especially true for the cardiovascular function, and it is these conditional reflexes that are the most enduring. A person may be reacting to some old injury or situation with his cardiovascular system which no longer exists, and he is usually unconscious of what it is that is causing an increase in heart rate or blood pressure. The result may be chronic hypertension. This may be the explanation of many cardiac deaths.

The persistence of the cardiac conditional reflex and of other general components in the absence of the more specific parts, e.g., the salvation and the movement, should lead to a revision of the idea of *inhibition*. Formerly we considered that the dog was in a state of complete inhibition in regard to a specific stimulus when he no longer gave the salivary secretion and the motor component, but now we see that inhibition can be and probably is, partial, incomplete fractional. The animal may be quiet externally but violently agitated internally. This seems to me a usual and therefore normal occurrence instead of an exceptional and abnormal one.

Autokineses

By means of the chronic experiment, studying the subjective for a long period of its life, we can see important changes within the organism, changes which indicate that interactions among foci of excitations stored in the central nervous system. To this function we give the name of autokinesis.

A familiar example is acquired immunity to disease. Having once had certain diseases — measles, mumps, chicken pox, whooping cough, typhoid fever— the person does not contract them a second time. But what remains? Certainly not the antigen, certainly not the same antibodies. It is the pattern of activity that is present, the ability to react when the stimulus has long since passed. There is some trace left in the living tissue somewhere. There are many other examples, occurring in biology or as a result of individual experience. One is the spontaneous restoration of the conditional reflex. Pavlov, as well as I and others, showed that generally a conditional reflex could be extinguished in one day but that it would reappear the next day, and that sometimes many separate days of repetitions were necessary for complete extinction. As he did not measure all components, this view would have to be modified somewhat at present in the light of the cardiac responses, but essentially the fact of spontaneous restoration remains.

I have noted that sometimes *one* injection of a drug will permanently, or at least for a long time, change the level of reactivity of the dog, the size of his conditional reflexes, though the drug is not repeated. Wiener, recognizing the development of pathologic reactions to formerly innocuous stimuli, explained it by saying that the *level* of feedback had been altered.

Every physician knows that a patient may steadily improve after one visit and consultation, and we all know how one experience in life may change our whole future. When the development is in the direction of making better adaptations this I call positive autokinesis, when the direction is downward, negative autokinesis.

There is growing anatomical evidence that new connections can be made in the nervous system through emerging nervous processes or perhaps even through the origin of new nerve cells. Thus Jerzy Rose has shown that if one of the cortical layers are destroyed by radiation, the axons of the two layers adjacent, on either side of the destroyed layer will grow through the degenerate layer to make new connections with each other. At the XXIII Physiological Congress in Tokyo in 1965, Drs. M. Adal, D. Barker, and M.C. Ip, University of Durham, England, reported the growth of entirely new motor endings of nerves to muscles.

Organ System Responsibility

For the last few years we have been concerned with the comparative study of the renal and cardiac functions in the dog. It had been previously reported that the kidney was susceptible to conditioning to the same extent that the gastrointestinal functions were. However, after a number of years of trying to form renal CRs in the dog we have not found it possible.

When we begin to analyze renal function we come to an explanation of why this difficulty in forming a diuretic CR. The usual way of considering conditioning was a stereotyped one: you select an inborn type of reactivity, an unconditional reflex, you give the adequate stimulus to produce this UR, and then you precede this stimulation with any signal, the conditional stimulus, and *ipso facto* you get a CR. This has been the usual method for obtaining all CRs. There has been little question that the application of this stereotyped method will produce a stereotyped result, viz., the CR.

Recently I have looked for an explanation of why the kidney did not respond the way the salivary and the gastric secretions do, the way the motor system does. The function of the motor system is to adjust in a useful way to the coming events in the external environment, and the cardiovascular and respiratory systems prepare the organism for this action. In a like manner the salivary secretion, the gastric secretions prepare for the ingestion of food. When the signal for one reason or another does not signalize the events that it once did for the CR to occur is no great loss except a slight loss in physical energy. This is because the secretions, salivary and gastric, etc., are poured into the gastrointestinal canal and promptly reabsorbed; there is no loss of either fluids or solutes. Several gallons of saliva, gastric, pancreatic and intestinal secretions and bile are poured into the gut, reabsorbed and reused. It is as if a city continually reused all its sewage, for this happens with the aqueous solutions of the body, except those lost through the skin, lungs and kidney, and a small portion through the feces.

However, if the kidney were to function according to the same stereotyped paradigm, there would occur in the conditioning process a discharge of water and electrolytes which are unrecoverable. This would mean that a thirsty animal responding to the signals for water and also for foods could be depleting itself of these very essential items, leading to the death of the individual. For what the kidney discharges into its pelvis and into the bladder cannot be reabsorbed into the body system and it is therefore lost irrevocably.

The principle of organ responsibility means that the formation of a conditional reflex in greater or lesser degree is in relation to the physiologic function of the system upon which it is operating; a conditional reflex appears impossible to form if it would violate radically the function performed by this system in the body economy, thus opposing the principle of homeostasis.

Organ-system responsibility and the principle of teleology do not mean that we can always make a prediction according to logic, according to teleology; we do not know precisely the teleology of the organ or of the individual. We only know a little about it. So we cannot, as the great physicists—Einstein and Planck have done—sit down with a few figures and, without performing an experiment, make predictions and come out with great laws. You cannot do that with a biological organism because of the tremendous number of factors which are at work. So you have to go to the dog and do the experiment to find out what happens; you cannot bypass the experiment simply by the principle of organ-system responsibility. This leads me to the conclusion, however, that I, as well as other people, can be very wrong by adhering to a stereotyped paradigm without looking at the underlying function of the physiology of that system with which you are working. And although it seems very popular and very alluring to say that everything can become conditioned, that you can cure heart disease, and that you can regulate every autonomic function of the body by the simple bell-and-food paradigm, I think that we have to exercise wisdom, look more at the physiology, and understand what are the organs doing—what are they for—and, thus, get rid of stereotyped thinking.

V.

Pragmatism, the production of Charles Peirce, was developed and applied by William James and John Dewey. It is not reality that we are concerned with (and cannot know) but with only the part accessible to us can we interact.

The laws of the external universe result in pragmatic control. We assume that the external sense organs record accurately the phenomena of the external world, and we work pragmatically with these laws.

Nerves from the internal universe give us a vague sense of the degree of well-being. Furthermore, we know when we are conscious, but these states are not recognizable in any scientific quantitative measurements. For the whole internal universe, we are unaware what goes on, except under pathological conditions.

The significance of the part of the information brought by the nerves of pain is subjective. The electrical impulses conducted over the nerves are of no significance to us, unless they are represented by the subjective feelings of pain.

The *content* of the states of consciousness cannot be communicated—first, these states are not quantitativiely *recordable*, in the terms of which they are significant. Secondly, they are not communicable in their essence. There are objective correlates—e.g., heart rate, motor movements.

In regards to communication, who knows what a baby is thinking when he looks at red?

Therefore, the science that we have and use for the internal universe is a foreign science built on external data.

We are lacking a science for what goes on inside.

In all of this, an important, if not the central role is played by the information brought to the brain by the external sense organs, viz., the visual, auditory, olfactory, gustatory, tactile, temperature functions. All these organs turn outward. They register what goes on in the external universe. Normally they cannot sense even their own existence—the eye does not see itself, the ear hear itself, the tongue taste itself, the olfactory organ smell itself, the skin feel itself. We are concerned here with the *conscious* experiences, not what may be conveyed to the subconscious, nor with the electrical potentials or chemical perceptions since it is the conscious perceptions that are the basis of our science. What the external sense organs bring into consciousness, as far as is obvious and demonstrable, is the *sine qua non* of the science that we know.

Thus our science is constructed from the building blocks of the external sense organs arranged and cemented into place by the inner master architect, the brain.

Furthermore, science is a human product and practically all of this science depends on (involves?) the function of vision. The eye is not only the sense organ at the basis of our human science, but it is the most sensitive instrument that we know, either in nature or man-made. This is true both as regards the amount of energy it can detect—viz., several quanta, nearly at the theoretical physical limit of energy—but the simplicity of its construction to perform its function. And as Sherrington points out, it is constructed mainly from water plus a little of the substance of egg white, entirely in darkness.

Although we do not know of a science devoid of the facts and involvement of vision, it is conceiveable that, given our human brain, we could build a rudimentary science from other external sense organ data. Thus Helen Keller without the sense of vision could understand visual science, because the facts were supplied by other eyes which could see for her. If we had the auditory and tactile sense organs of a bat, or the olfactory sense organs of a dog, or of some worms, we could construct a certain kind of science, but it would include only things which could be heard or smelled and very circumscribed as to distance. Space would have to be estimated as with a bat by resonance of reflected sound waves emitted from the vibration of its own voice, or by the muscular sense of spanning the distance with arms or legs. We would know of the existence of the sun but not of the moon or stars, nor anything of its distance.

Because some animals are guided by delicate sense perceptors, e.g., insects to their goals perhaps by heat radiations, salmon, eels, seals, etc., into streams by a chemical or pressure sense, this is a long way from a science.

So far we have discussed the science that has been erected on the sense organ data of the external universe. But there is an internal universe bounded by our skin plus a few small areas of sensitive mucous membrane and modified visual epithelium, the boundary that prevents any unscheduled interchange of substance between the two universes. This internal universe of which we are a part is immeasurably more complex, infinitely less comprehensible than the external universe of which we are not a part. By the standards of external science it is mainly an unstable aqueous solution comprising at any one instant vitriolic and toxic substances, perhaps many thousands of compounds and to exact proportions, immersed together in a common medium, often strictly limited to one small area (e.g., HCl) or everywhere abundant (hemoglobin), confined rigidly to certain places, but under great pressure, by a watery membrane not visible to the naked eye and thinner than the finest tissue paper, yet strong enough to withstand a constant fluid pressure greater than that of the most powerful suction pump (the epithelial cells of the renal tubules).

Without any known centrally and uniquely controlled mechanism, this living organism of thousands of simultaneous reactions, compositions, functions, structures, infinitely varied and separate, yet with a common goal, maintains itself and contributes its prescribed allotment for the survival of the whole.

But what of the science for this complex internal universe? How does it compare with the science of the infinite external universe, relatively speaking? Have we evolved such an adequate science?

Let us compare the science for the external universe and that for the internal universe. As pointed out, the science of the external universe has been constructed on the data brought to the integrating organism, the brain, by the external sense organs. It has been a science which, though it may reveal only a very minute part of the external universe, of reality, it provides us a pragmatic basis for working with that part of the external universe to which the external sense organs are sensitive.

Now if science for the external universe is dependent upon what the sense organs tell us of the external universe, how can we escape the conclusion that an adequate science of the internal universe must depend upon sense organ data from that internal universe?

But what are the sense organs for this internal universe? Sense organ data for the basis of science must bring information from the universe with which it deals, even though we admit the data is of a relatively small part of the whole. For example, the ear records only vibrations within the range of 16 to perhaps 30,000, the eye between the wave lengths of red and blue, one octave.

The sense organ data from the internal universe that reach consciousness, and these are the only ones that science so far can deal with, are nil under normal conditions. All these myriad interactions work silently and to our sight, blindly. None of us are conscious of the function of the liver, kidney, spleen, adrenals, stomach, vestibular apparatus. We have a proprioceptive sense, but it is doubtful to what degree it normally enters consciousness.

It is true that under conditions of malfunctioning, or pathology, we sometimes feel discomfort or pain, but even this sense is not always present. Thus one can be dying of cancer, silent tumors, unconscious of their presence or location. The surgeon Blalock was not conscious of the cancer of the liver from which he died until it had spread throughout his body. Such facts are too commonplace in medicine to require elaboration.

Even when one had information from the internal universe it is usually vague and imprecise, comparable to what it would be to view an object through a ground glass window, a heavily smoked glass, or to listen for a specific sound in the roar of Niagara. We do often have a sense of well-being or the opposite, but it would be very difficult to measure or to record euphoria objectively.

VI.

On the same basis as we assess the science of the external universe, we have no adequate science for the internal universe.

But as we well know the science that we have evoked for the external universe has produced remarkable results in biology. We have the cure for many diseases, e.g., diabetes, pellagra, scurvy, to say nothing of the drugs for combatting infections, the analgesics, anesthetics, stimulants, etc.

But this science of the external universe applied to the internal universe, though it is useful and often alters profoundly biological processes, we are still lacking in a science that adequately explains life. The science that we have is foreign to life, borrowed from the science of the dead universe.

Even our language when applied to the subjective, the most conscious part of the internal universe, is descriptive of spatial, auditory, visual relations. The terms for this idea, as well as the idea itself come from conversation with my friend John Lamb, who said:

> Our language is replete with words brought from objective descriptions of the external universe. For example: we turn now to the *sub*conscious from which ideas come to the *surface* in the form of mental *images* during a *flash* of insight. The *rate* at which this happens is taken to be a *function* of a person's psychic *energy. Deeply* felt emotions, though, are likely to *color* our ideas and *becloud* our thinking. Those who are deemed the *sharpest* thinkers seem to be most *adept* at *circumventing* these distractions in order to *penetrate* to the *core* of a *tangled mass* of abstractions.

It is perhaps for this inadequate science of the internal universe corresponding to our science of the external universe that we have practically no science of the most important part of the life as we estimate it for ourselves, viz., our subjective life. This we cannot even record scientifically, as we do the elements of the external universe. When we record the change in heart rate, blood pressure, respiration, muscular contraction in pain, we have an objective correlate, but a corelate of a zero function except when we experience it in ourselves. What we record is something of another category, the existence of which is known to ourselves but only inferred in others, animal or human. The science of the external universe does not touch this subjective.

Furthermore some subjective processes — thinking, feeling, perception, etc. — may be below quantum level and therefore theoretically never recordable by any instrument other than mind. This view is especially reinforced by the purest scientists, the modern physicists, Planck and Schroedinger, but also by the philosopher-physiologist Sherrington. Planck states that science cannot deal with our subjective life.

"Science thus fixes for itself its own inviolable boundaries. But man, with his unlimited impulses, cannot be satisfied with this limitation. He must overstep it, since he needs an answer to the most important, and constantly-repeated question of his life: What am I to do? — And a complete answer to this question is not furnished by determinism, not by causality, especially not by pure science, but only by his moral sense, by his character, by his outlook on the world."

And Schroedinger says that our phychical life does not involve energy.

"One can say in a few words why our perceiving and thinking self is nowhere to be found within the world picture, because it itself is this world picture."

And Sherrington:

"Mind, for anything perception can compass, . . . remains without sensual confirmation, and remains without it forever."

The failure by Kety to measure any increased blood supply to the brain during consciousness or thinking, though still not conclusive, may be relevant.

Is it because of the lack of a specific science for the internal universe and the probable inadequacy of the science of the external universe when applied to the internal universe, that there is so much unknown about biology and life? Here the imponderables remain as stubbornly incomprehensible as they were in the dawn of recorded human history. Most of the eminent scientists sense that the existence of mind, love; individual free will, a world with a beginning or a world without a beginning, limited or unlimited space, time, God, are equally difficult. Even with our advanced and advancing science of the external universe, for each one of us what we value most highly are the emotions and the subjective. The objective science of the external universe has no meaning of its own—only as it can affect our subjective. This becomes apparent when we look at how the human values the idea of an after-life; it is not the body that he aspires to preserve, but the spirit, i.e., the subjective part. When there is the lack of interest in an after-life it is not because of the uncertainty of the objective body, but because of the doubt of such a subjective persistence. Thus:

Why if the soul can fling the dust aside,
And naked on the air in Heaven ride,
Were it not a shame, were it not a shame
In this clay house imprisoned to abide.

The situation then is that when a science of the world of the subjective and perhaps of life is not only woefully behind the science of the external universe, but perhaps theoretically it will always remain inadequate.

We could erect a similar though very limited science to the one we have now by using auditory sense data or a system of radar as used by bats. Thus we could form a science of music—pitch and the length of strings—but such a science would be limited only to what could be transmitted through actual matter, or perhaps through the thermal sense and heat rays.

But let us reverse the process of applying the science of the external sense organs to the internal universe, viz., using the internal sense organ data applied to the science of the external universe. The most definite and continually acting internal sense organs are proprioceptive, vestibular, which are mainly below consciousness and therefore, because they are below consciousness, inadequate by the criteria (sense organ data reaching consciousness) for our science of the external universe. The sense organ which preeminently brings us data from within and enters consciousness is the pain sense.

To reverse the process, to found a science of the external universe on the sense organ data from the internal universe: the science, the relationships developed from the perception of pain would be applied to the scientific understanding of the external universe. This would be a poet's world of images rather than a scientific world; the external universe would be explained by subjective terms such as groaning, suffering, etc. Such an idea is evidently preposterous, but I raise the question whether it is not equally absurd to look for an adequate science of the subjective world and of the whole internal universe from the sense organs which bring data from the external universe.

Without doubt it is true that we can produce certain results by studying the living organism as if it were a part of the dead external universe.

When we measure the effect of meditation and other mental states in objective physiological terms—heart rate, blood pressure, oxygen metabolism, etc.—we are doing no more than Pavlov did seventy-five years ago when he converted the state of hunger to a quantitative record, drops of saliva.

What is to be done?

Given the structure of the nervous system and the lack of a basis for a science of the internal universe comparable to the science of the external universe, it is hardly likely that we can ever develop such a science. We then must make what pragmatic use we can of the science that we have.

But if one chief goal of science is to comprehend the nature of the biology of our subjective life we should understand the differences in the study of the external universe compared with the internal universe. Such a point of view will not blind us to the pragmatic value of science, of the wonders revealed by science, of the adventures ahead into the Unknown, of what is knowable and what is unknowable.

In conclusion, we must assess the inadequacy of our present science of the external universe for the complete study of the internal universe, of consciousness and our various subjective states. And despite our misgivings, we shall face all the universe, the external and the internal, with an open mind and the spirit not of despair but of adventure.

Discussion

Sir John Eccles: I am, of course, in general agreement with Dr. Gantt on his external and internal universes, but I would like to point out that I have some differences also. We do have far more sense organs within the skin, shall we say, than pain. And some of these have recently been investigated quantitatively and shown to be very important. Of course, we have known for a long time about proprioception and, for example, the position of a limb is known accurately from joint sensing and from muscle and tension sensing in fascia. But more than the muscle contraction can actually be now sensed and Gantt has shown that this sensing gives rise to many kinds of illusion. We have knowledge of more and more sensing that comes from within the body and which is quantifiable. It has not been recognized until recently because it isn't so overt as other sensing. It is rather like the sense from your vestibular system. You don't normally notice it, but if you are put on a turntable, you get vertigo. Vertigo is a sense derived from your vestibular mechanism. There are many internal senses which can be quantified. That is the first point I want to make.

Secondly, about the subjective states. There is a science of subjective states, in fact it is a very extensive science. One part is called psychophysics, where all kinds of measurements of stimulations are made and compared to the resulting subjective experiences, for example in vision and in hearing with matching a sense with the signals. In fact, Stevens has erected a power law according to which the experienced sense intensity is proportional to the stimulus intensity raised to some specific power. The exponential of this power law has been found for many senses, but has very different values for the kinds of sensing—vision, pressure, vibration and sound. So what I am trying to say is that we do have, in fact, a way of evaluating our internal senses, not perhaps as accurately as the external. Even our scientific observations in the way of measuring and assessing necessitate an internal evaluation of what comes through our senses. We would all agree that we build up the whole of science on sensory impressions. There is no other way, but many of these senses come from the inside and are strictly speaking internal.

Gantt: Well, I am very privileged to have Sir John Eccles' comments, because this is the highest authority and there is nowhere else I would want to go to get this information. But I would just make the comment that although this does throw light on whether we have nerves for internal states, the other part of what I am saying is that the subjective remains forever beyond measurement, in any degree and with any measurement that is essential to itself. You can get measurements of correlates, but they are not the essence of the subjective, and I am sure Sir John would agree with me in that. It is said many times in Sherrington's book; here is just one sentence from Sherrington. "Mind, for anything perception can compass . . . remains without sensual confirmation, and remains without it forever." Now, of course, you can always say that new things will be discovered, but this statement throws light on some possibilities of nerves that come from inside. If you compare these with the precision of the external sense organs, there is no comparison if you talk about what comes into consciousness. These things are probably acting all the time in some subconscious way.

Eccles: Yes, I agree with that, but lest Sherrington be misunderstood in your little quotation, I would like to read your other quotation from Schroedinger here if I may. It reads, "One can say in a few words why our perceiving and thinking self is nowhere to be found within the world picture, because it itself is this world picture". That, I would agree with completely, and that was, of course, the essence of my lecture the other day. I think it is a very good quotation.

Holger Hyden

B5 The Brain, Learning and Values

Thoughts on the Problem

The problem of higher brain functions is very much involved in the question of the unity of sciences, if the ultimate aim is that brain should understand brain. All statements about learning and memory should attach quantitative values to definite positions in a space-time of coordinates, provided the different systems within the brain could be defined by qualitative criteria.

There is a big gap between the psychological experience of a "memory," its expression as complex behavior of an animal or homo and the knowledge of the structure, biochemistry and physiology of brain. An understanding of e.g. insight learning should imply that physical laws suffice to explain biological phenomena. Given mathematical methods to solve nonlinear, partial differential equations, a general systems theory such as proposed by von Bertalanffy could in time express such higher brain functions by isomorphic concepts, at both biological and physical levels for the different hierarchies of the brain. When this will be realized then also the unity of sciences is granted.

When we revisit a summerplace from our childhood and take in the smell of wet grass and jasmin, look out on the familiar sight of the sea and feel the rough surface of the old firtree, we experience these sensory modalities as a whole; the brain is a whole with interacting hierarchies. We look at one instant at a butterfly on a flower — and we discover a moment later that the butterfly is gone. We do not consciously scan the area and subtract the picture minus the butterfly from the picture in our memory in order to make the discovery of the missing butterfly. We take in the sight as a whole.

If we reduce the brain unit to subunits, a simple account of the combinatorial explosion says that one nerve impulse travels to the synapses and triggers the activity in let us say 10 cells by means of synaptic chemical mechanisms. Each of the 10 cells triggers 10 more interactions. The combinations increase from 100 to 10,000. Since each of 10 billion nerve cells may have 100 to

10,000 connections there will be an enormous input from the activated cells. The activation of neurons is very selective!

The activities through the brain are channelled in certain systems, deviated to millions of certain neurons which may be dispersed in several areas. Electrical and chemical activities take
their course determined by phylogenetically developed systems
and hierarchies in the brain. The detailed processing will, however, be determined by the way in which most of the brain cells
have been modified or labelled by experience. We assume that
this process goes on for most of the life cycle. This paper will discuss mechanisms by which a protein differentiation of nerve cells
can serve all brain systems in establishing long-term memories.

Leaving psychological approaches and applying the approach
of molecular biology, a direct question is: does by learning process imply that brain cells—their structure, molecules and
metabolism—undergo remaining changes?

On the basis of present experimental knowledge I would like to
present a theory *in principle* of learning and memory which implies that both shortlasting, reversible , and longlasting, remaining, cell protein changes are biochemical correlates. When an animal begins to learn a suitable and sufficiently difficult task of an
"image-driven" type, a shortlasting production of protein starts
within minutes. The increased synthesis involves at least two
proteins which are specific for the brain—one is called the S100
protein. This production starts in the hippocampus, a phylogenetically old part of the brain. Non-learning controls do not show
this activity. The same type of brain cell production follows in
brain cortical areas after a certain delay. During learning at least
two other protein fractions are synthesized in the membranes of
synapses, the contacts between neurons. This shortlasting protein production (around 24 hours) is redundant and increases the
statistical probability for the remaining nerve cell changes to be
made.

The longlasting nerve cell changes involve protein molecular
changes which become inscribed in a certain pattern into the
membrane of millions of neurons. This brain specific protein interacts with another, contractile protein by mediation of calcium.
On the same stimulus, all neurons with the same membrane pro-

tein pattern and synapse differentiation are assumed to become activated. The renewed, same stimulus makes all those neurons active which share most of the same molecular membrane pattern. This is experienced as a memory.

Between the shortlasting protein synthesis in nerve cells during learning and the longlasting, membrane changes occurs an increased production in the whole brain of a certain protein with a molecular weight around 60,000. We assume that this protein mediates the consolidation of the long-term memory.

When learning starts, there occurs (only in learning animals, not in controls) a new synthesis of messenger RNA (8S and 16S hn RNA and 25S polyadenylate-associated RNA) in nerve cells which will induce the production of certain proteins and molecular patterns as described above. Calcium is the element which helps to translate electrical field changes during learning into longlasting molecular changes in brain cell membranes. The stimulus to learn can thus penetrate to the genome of brain cells and the learning mechanism has its root in the same molecular mechanism as has "instinct behavior," although experiential learning operates only for a life cycle.

Brain and the Critical Period

The present paper will mostly discuss the S100 protein inside and outside the cell membrane, and also a contractile network of protein filaments close to the inside of the nerve cell membrane and attached to the knob-like synapses on the membrane, the contacts between neurons bridged by the thin nerve cell processes. Both S100 and the contractile network interact with calcium. By this reaction we have reason to believe that they interact also with each other. In doing so, the synapse function is affected within that area of the nerve cell surface which has incorporated S100. The effect is in the nature of inhibition.

Observations on man and animals show that the visional, auditory and sensory-somatic modalities converge to a part of the temporal cortex, called the entorhinal cortex, and from there to the hippocampus. An intact and correctly functioning hippocampus is a prerequisite for formation of the long-term memory (if the task is sufficiently difficult and not only a conditioning reflex). From the hippocampus the activities spread out over cortical areas via subcortical centers and one part goes back to the hippocampus.

The hippocampus and surrounding areas belong to the so- called limbic system, deeply hidden by the hem of the temporal lobe, and are parts of the evolutionary old brain.

Around 10 million different pathways are built up in the brain during the embryonic period in the form of systems between collections of nerve cells surrounded by the other type of brain cells, the glial cells. This occurs by a genetical and chemical labelling method. When the outer shape of the brain is sculptured by firm rules, the visual, auditory and sensory-somatic pathways are laid down together with association paths and the still mysterious small and short neurons intermixed with glia in the outer part of the brain cortex. All activity is specific for the pathway proper. The nerve cells are highly differentiated cells. Like all other somatic cells each nerve cell has in its nucleus all genes necessary to produce a complete individual. The genes direct the synthesis of the cell's special products for the daily activity via different types of RNA molecules and proteins in the form of enzymes. The differentiation into specialized cells means that only a certain number and combination of the genes are active. The rest is inactive or blocked but some can be activated by proper stimulation. For neurons in general and for the whole brain there exists a critical period in the beginning of the life cycle during which the proper stimuli seem most important for the development of brain functions, structures and biochemistry in the whole brain. One such period for man is the first two years. When the critical period is over — and there are different periods correlated with different abilities — the possibility to undergo further plastic changes seems to be blocked.

Several types of behavior are present at birth through the bank of information in the genes of the brain cells. More than 99% of all nerve cells are present in the brain at birth. During the first year in homo, the branching processes of the nerve cell body, called dendrites, grow extensively in number and length. The points of contact between neurons, the synapses, will be structured and grow. A number of already formed synapses disappear. Intricate relationships are set up between neurons via neighboring small neurons. During this first postnatal period genetically programmed activities are started by triggering stimuli. Learning by experience begins. For all species the first part of the life cycle is the concentrated period of learning in all its aspects. Expressed in another way, a whole spectrum of stimuli is necessary to realize the genetical potentialities of the brain in an individual. In man, a warm contact between the small child before the age of 2 and an adult is necessary for the development of its emotional life and higher brain functions. This has been amply shown by Skeels and Goldfarb. In animals, brain analyses have been performed during the corresponding critical period. Young rats or mice living in a normal hierarchical group and with a detailed environment to investigate get a thicker brain cortex with a more intensive chemical metabolism and bigger synapses than animals living isolated in a single cage during this critical period. The animals in the "enriched" environment also do better in behavioral tests. What has been lost by lack of proper stimuli during the critical period cannot be regained later on. Results from animal experiments cannot, however, be directly translated to the conditions of man.

It has been convincingly shown that skills learnt during one generation cannot be inherited by the next. There is no Lamarckian mechanism in learning.

A pertinent question is whether learning and memory by experience utilize the same mechanism which operates during embryonic life to build up instinct behavior. Certain results indicate that this is the case, and I would like to return to this problem later on.

The Behavioral Test

How shall an animal learning experiment best be arranged to elicit the same response of the brain as a similar learning demand produces in the animal's natural environment and living conditions? This question has been vastly ignored by many neurobiologists working on behavior. Mostly rats have been used. The rat is a highly intelligent animal, inquisitive and ecologically and socially successful. Briefly put, the rat learning test should be of the type image-driven behavior, rather difficult to solve and modelled on behavior in the natural environment. Conditioning tests with jumping onto a shelf to escape electric shock, or, pressing of a lever to get a food pill, are poor choices. Why is that so? One way to answer this question is the following. That part of the old areas of the brain called the hippocampus must function correctly if learning shall occur and memories be formed. This has been found for man, monkeys and also for the rat. The hippocampus is a paired structure, deeply hidden by the overlaying brain cortex. If the hippocampus is damaged in the rat, it cannot learn to solve a task of medium difficulty, within the capacity of the species. But—and this is significant—the rat without correctly functioning hippocampus will learn conditioning tasks and even better than normal rats! The hippocampus has also another function in the rat. It informs the rat about space-time relations and helps the animal to make three-dimensional maps. In our rat learning experiments we have for twelve years used a transfer of handedness task in retrieving food pills one by one by grasping it by inserting the paw in a narrow glass tube. The control to the learning animal is a rat which uses the preferred paw to get the same number of pills in the same arrangement. The control is under the same conditions as the learning rat. The control can improve its performance but does not learn anything new.

Remaining Protein Changes During a Learning Period

As was mentioned above, during the first part of the postnatal period the neurons develop their intricate processes, the synapses grow and become structured. Contacts are being established with other neurons. The insulating material around the main nerve cell process becomes finished. Genetically programmed activities become activated according to their built-in time schedules. For all species it is a concentrated period of learning. To mention a striking example, between 2 and 4 years a child learns to speak its language, including meaning, grammar, syntax!

To go back to the molecular and structural studies: parts of the

neuronal membrane from adult mammals contain the brain specific S100 protein, firmly bound. The S100 protein is incorporated
into the nerve cell outer membrane during the first part of life.
The membrane S100 constitutes around 10% of the total S100
which in turn is 0.1% of the total brain cell proteins. The S100 is
an acidic protein with a molecular weight of 21,000. It is produced by glial cells but is localized also to the nerve cell outer
membrane and nuclear membrane. Characteristically, S100 binds
calcium and undergoes with this process "conformational" changes. The molecule partly opens up and certain groups are exposed. This enables the protein to react with membranes which
then acquire the ability to regulate the in- and outflux of ions.

Species differences with respect to the formation of mem-
brane-bound S100 are striking and interesting. As examples, the
rat and the rabbit are poorly developed at birth; they are like embryos. At two weeks after birth they first get the young animal's
metabolism and then begin to show the alert behavior of the
young. Rats and rabbits lack membrane S100 in their nerve cells.
At the end of the first fortnight, S100 begins to be incorporated
into the nerve cell membrane. It becomes redistributed in a dramatic way during that period of intensive learning. S100 changes
its main localization from the top of the cell to the basal part of
the cell body from which the impulse carrying process emerges.
During the first month in rats the membrane S100 widens into a
pattern of the cell surface. Eventually it will take up 30-50% of
the surface including the receiving part of the synapses within
that area. As you know, the newborn guinea pig is well developed,
alert and lively at birth and begins almost at once to explore the
environment. It is interesting that already at birth membrane
S100 is present in the nerve cells of the guinea pig. This differentiation of the nerve cell surface including the synapses into one
area which is rich in S100 and another area which lacks S100,
may be of great importance for learning. The reason is the following. Close to the inner side of the nerve cell membrane and attached to the synapses lies a continuous network consisting of
two intercoiled protein filaments. These filaments contain the
contractile protein actin. Both the coiled filaments of the network
and the membrane S100 bind calcium, S100 most avidly. When

the network binds calcium the filaments uncoil. From a physico-chemical point of view, this is a cooperative process. S100 has at least 8 different binding sites for calcium and undergoes a conformational change at binding; the molecule partly unfolds. If one looks at the arrangement of the two proteins in question on the nerve cell, a mechanism reveals itself which seems to affect both synapses and membrane.

An important observation has been that during learning calcium increases in the hippocampus. This is a specific reaction since sodium, potassium and water do not change, so it cannot be increased circulation which is the cause of calcium increase. When calcium is taken up by the S100 that molecule undergoes conformational changes. Inside the cell the concentration of calcium is low, 10^{7} M, and the network remains coiled and exerts a tension on the synapses and that part of the membrane which contains S100. Outside that area there is no competition by S100 for calcium. Therefore, the filaments can bind calcium and uncoil, which may result in a relaxation of synapses and membrane in areas lacking S100. Thus, there exists *a functional linkage between the membrane S100 and the network of contractile protein, and the relation between the cooperative processes is regulated by calcium.*

What may be the function of such an arrangement of two proteins in the nerve cell membrane? The working hypothesis is that the protein differentiation, caused by experience and learning, will secure the concomitant activation of all neurons which have undergone a similar differentiation and on the same stimulus. It does not matter where in the brain the neurons are located.

Shortlasting Synthesis of Brain Cell Protein as an Inducing Phase at Learning

The observations on the nerve cell membrane and theory discussed in previous paragraphs depict a mechanism which introduces cooperative phenomena and functional linkage between brain cell proteins. It could add a further combinatorial level to the already known mechanism of the nerve cell membrane.

The shortlasting, reversible protein production starts within minutes after the training to learn has begun. In general terms it can be stated that at learning neurons become highly active. I would like to contrast *active* against *re-active*. The data available indicate that the learning mechanism of the brain in the first hand is *active*, not *re-active* like a reflex in a conditioning system.

The amount of S100 in the hippocampus increases by 15-20% and the incorporation of radioactive amino acids into cell protein by 300%. A similar increase is shown by another brain specific protein which is localized to the neurons and called 14-3-2. There thus occurs an increased synthesis of defined proteins in the hippocampus when the animals learn a new complicated pattern of behavior. The calcium increase in the hippocampus during learning causes part of S100 to undergo conformational changes. As a sign of the stability of this molecular change S100 has a higher mobility on electrophoresis. The active controls do not display such a response. An increased synthesis of brain specific proteins is observed in cortical areas with a time delay in comparison to that in hippocampus. This series of observation demonstrates that a wave of protein synthesis pervades the brain at learning and starts in the hippocampus. In other words, *system changes occur in brain cell protein during learning*. The leading role of the hippocampus during learning does not seem to be dependent upon the type of learning task. It occurs during the change of handedness in a complicated sensory-motor task as well as during maze learning.

Is the observed synthesis and alterations in brain proteins specific for learning *per se* or is the phenomenon only a sign of increased activity? The specificity of the response has been demonstrated by injecting a monospecific antiserum against the S100 during the training into the lateral ventricles of the brain. By the technique used, it was shown that the antiserum reaches and precipates on the S100 of brain cells in the hippocampal and related regions which are situated closely to the ventricles.

The effect of the antiserum to S100 is seen in the deviation of the learning curve towards zero on further training. Careful controls with antiserum from which antibodies against S100 had been removed did not show any impairing effect. Nor did the injection of other gamma globulins.

Rapport and collaborators, (1976), observed that besides antiserum against S100 also antiserum directed against synaptic protein had such an impairing effect on learning. No other motor or sensory symptoms were observed in the animals treated with antisera.

If one considers the dominating role of the hippocampus in the protein response during learning, it is not surprising that if the membrane mechanism involving S100 is blocked by antiserum, functional disturbances will ensue. The blocking of further learning is clearly observed. It is interesting that the reaction between a membrane antigen of nerve cells and the corresponding antiserum gives rise to an increse of the antigen, the S100 protein. Within half an hour the production of soluble S100 increases significantly in the hippocampus, from 350 g/g wet weight to 450.

A conclusion from these experiments on S100 and behavior is that S100 has an inhibiting effect on neurons.

Several hours after finished training when the animals are back in their cages, a protein fraction with a molecular weight of 60,000 is synthesized in the cortex and other parts of the brain. It may emerge at 8 hours after finished training and reaches a considerable peak after 24 hours. The response has disappeared after 48 hours. As a working hypothesis, this protein fraction may consolidate the long-term memory.

The S100 was localized to the outer cell membrane. The synaptic membrane protein is likewise an object of great interest since synapses are the functional contacts between neurons (Hyden et al. 1974). We have therefore analyzed membrane bound protein in synapses in the hippocampus and cortical areas during learning in rats. The training was followed by an increase of protein around 30,000 and 80,000 molecular weights, beginning in the hippocampus. Later on similar proteins increase in cortical areas. Thus, the distinctive activity of the hippocampus at learning is also observable in the synaptic membrane protein and the synthesis in the cortex follows with a delay.

Shashoua (1975) has found an increased synthesis of three different protein fractions from nerve cells in goldfish trained to acquire a new behavior.

Gene Activation During Learning

It is indeed a puzzling observation that an animal engaged in learning for which it is motivated starts a synthesis of specific brain proteins in its nerve cells which cannot be observed in the corresponding nerve cells of the active control. The latter performs all the movements, is in the same environment and gets the same amount of food as the learning animal. But the control does not learn. Stress has been excluded as a possible cause of such protein changes granted that certain amount of stress is always involved in all learning experiments. Several years ago we took up the question whether the stimulus involved in the acquisition of a new behavior can penetrate to the nucleus of brain cells and activate part of the genome. A positive answer would demand that learning experiments could be shown to lead to a production of messenger RNA (mRNA). Attempts in various laboratories including our own could to begin with only show indirect evidence for mRNA production in brain cells in learning animals. Recently, we have, however, succeeded in demonstrating that hippocampal nerve cells in a learning rat show in increased synthesis compared to active controls of 8S and 16-18S heterogeneous RNA and a synthesis of polyadenylic-associated mRNA of 25S. Both these species of RNA belong to mRNA (Cupello and Hyden, 1976). This means that cognitive stimuli can penetrate to the nucleus of nerve cells and activate genes which results in specific protein synthesis. This phenomenon does not exclude that mRNA which is already present in the cell body can be utilized for protein synthesis before the new mRNA has been assembled, transported to the cytoplasm and organized for protein synthesis. Learning and formation of long-term memories seem therefore to have their roots in the same molecular mechanism as genetically programmed activities.

A Hypothesis

A hypothesis *in principle* of learning and formation of long-term memory can be based on available data with certain assumptions. Perception may take less than a second. Formation of a short-term memory seconds to minutes. Processing and consolidation of a long-term memory may take seconds to many hours, depending on the characteristics of the new information and the level of emotion.

An unknown factor is the stimulus to learning and its nature. It initiates via messenger RNAs a specific protein synthesis in learning animals which synthesis is absent in control animals subjected to the same experimental procedure but without learning.

When learning begins, we assume that outer and inner stimuli cause electrical field changes which induce the shortlasting synthesis of at least two brain specific proteins. Calcium effects and calcium binding proteins have amply shown the important role of that divalent ion for cell processes. Calcium increases at learning and acts as a translator of electrical phenomena to remaining molecular changes. Calcium causes the membrane S100 to undergo conformational changes whereby hydrophobic groups are exposed. This enables S100 to interact with the membrane and to change its behavior towards ions. It is assumed that during acquisition of a new behavior the pattern of the membrane S100 on neurons enlarges successively with more learning. The shortlasting synthesis of S100 which begins in the hippocampus and spreads to cortical areas is a redundancy phenomenon securing that the nerve cells achieve a metabolic state which favours the process of membrane differentiation.

Eight to twenty four hours after finished training to learn, a soluble protein, molecular weight around 60,000, is synthesized in several brain areas. This protein disappears in some hours. We assume that this protein helps to consolidate the new information into a long-term memory.

The shortlasting protein production which is observed in the hippocampus and cortical areas with a time phase shift suggests that small molecules, like peptides, may act as triggering substances. The increased synthesis remains for hours and a steering of the activity by electrical impulses seems unlikely. A diffusion of smaller molecules from area to area is a more likely proposition.

Perception from the outer environment or stimuli from the inner environment activate during learning many millions of neurons belonging to different modalities. Each activation seems at the beginning to be kept within its own system but will soon spread by association mechanisms to other parts. The further paths of the activities lead to the entorhinal and related areas in the cortex and pass on to the hippocampus. The new information processed does not seem to be stored in the hippocampus. Instead, the hippocampus activates its cellular mechanisms, electrical and molecular. The biochemical activity inducing protein differentiation of nerve cell membranes and synapses via subcortical areas to different parts of the cortex. According to this view learning means protein differentiation of brain cells governed by the genetic mechanism. The experiential learning is superimposed upon the structures and mechanisms for genetically programmed activities but belong to the same categories. At retrieval, it is supposed that the same stimuli which induced a growth of brain cell differentiation can activate all brain cells wherever they are located provided only that they share the same pattern of protein differentiation. These brain cells have the same qualitative and quantitative values in the space-time of coordinates. The sum of differentiated activation in the three-dimensional brain is experienced as "memory." Viewed in this way the engram is a process.

REFERENCES

Bertalanffy, L.V., *General System Theory,* George Braziller, New York 1968.

Cupello, A. and Hyden, H., Alterations of the pattern of hippocampal nerve cell RNA labelling during training in rats, *Brain Res.* 1976, 114, 453.

Haglid, K., Hamberger, A., Hansson, H.A., Hyden, H., Persson, P. and Ronnback, L., S-100 protein in synapses of the central nervous system, *Nature,* 1974, 251, 532.

Hyden, H., Changes in brain protein during learning. Nerve cell and their glia: relationship and differences. RNA changes in brain cells during changes in behaviour and function. In *Macromolecules and Behavior,* ed. by G. Ansell and P. B. Bradley, MacMillan, London, 1973, p. 3.

Hyden, H., A calcium-dependent mechanism for synapse and nerve cell membrane modulation, *Proc. Nat. Acad. Sci.,* 1974, 71, 2965.

Hyden, H., and Cupello, A., A comparison of poly(A)-associated RNA from synaptosomes and cytoplasmic subcellular fraction of rat brain,

Brain Res. in press.

Hyden, H. and Lange, P.W., Protein synthesis in hippocampal nerve cells during re-reversal of handedness, *Brain Res.,* 1972, 45, 314.

Hyden, H. and Lange, P.W., Protein changes in different brain areas as a function of intermittent training, *Proc. Nat. Acad. Sci.* 1972, 69, 1980.

Hyden, H. and Lange, P.W., Brain proteins in undernourished rats during learning, *Neurobiology* 1975, 5, 84.

Hyden, H., Lange, P.W., Mihailovic, L. and Petrovic-Minic, B., Changes of RNA base composition in nerve cells of monkeys subjected to visual discrimination and delayed alternation performance, *Brain Res.* 1974. 65, 215.

Hyden, H., Lange, P.W. and Seyfried, C., Biochemical brain protein changes produced by selective breeding for learning in rats, *Brain Res.* 1973, 61, 446.

Karpiak, S.E., Serokoz, M. and Rapport, M.M., Effect of antisera to S-100 and to synaptic membrane fraction to maze performance and EEG, *Brain Res.* 1976, 102, 313.

Pickel, V. M., Reis, D.J., Marangos, P.J. and Zomzely-Neurath, C., Immunocytochemical localization of nervous system specific protein in rat brain, *Brain Res.* 1976, 105, 184.

Shashoua, V.E., Brain metabolism and the acquisition of new behaviors. I Evidence for specific changes in pattern of protein synthesis, *Brain Res.* 1976, 111, 347.

Zilliken, F. and Abdallah, K. Molekularbiologische Grundlagen des Kurz- und Langzeitgedachtnisses, F.K. Schattauer, Stuttgart 1973.

Zomzely-Neurath, C., Marangos, P.J., Hymowitz, N., Parl, W., Ritter, A., Zayas V., Cua, W. and York, C., The effect of a behavioral task on neuronal and glial specific proteins. In press.

Robert J. White

Commentary

Professor Hyden has reviewed for us his unique contributions to the neurochemical understanding of memory and learning necessarily heavily based on his extensive studies of the protein alterations of nerve cells and their membranes associated with the acquisition, storage, and expression of information in the rodent brain. Happily he has gone further, for in his efforts to unravel the intricate properties of the short and long term memory traces and their intimate relationship to each other, he has provided us with a multidimensional general system theory incorporating genetic mechanism and ionic participation to explain learning memory. Without question, his approach is controversial and to some degree conjectural. It will certainly not satisfy the molecular or mathematically oriented neurophysiologist who characterizes such brain functions as memory and learning in terms of nerve nets, steady state ionic equilibrium and fluxes, computer analogies and high ordered mathematical formulations—to name only a few. Nor would many experimental psychologists be pleased with these conclusions and theories for they would question and emphasize the lack of exactness in anatomical localization, appropriateness of the testing design and interpretation, and finally relevance to these neurochemical findings to memory and learning in general. Be that as it may, Professor Hyden's exquisite analytical chemical techniques have repeatedly demonstrated statistical changes in the protein composition of the appropriate loci of the hippocampus and somato-sensory cortex of the rat during and following the learning of a specifically designed difficult task; however, his personal attempt to provide a total conceptualization of memory and learning transgressing both genetics and phylogeny and based on his own experimental work is, of course, open to serious challenge not only neurophysiologically and biophysically (as stated previously) but philosophically.

Before considering this aspect of the problem, let's briefly review several interesting experiments conducted in the sub-human primate which add new dimensions to the stability of the memory trace in this highly encephalized animal. Monkeys trained in the Wisconsin testing device on six separate cognitive tests were subjected to localized cooling of the brain (to 15^0C or lower) employing a simplified extracorporal circuit and at these lower temperatures the brain was rendered totally ischemic for thirty minutes. Upon recovery the animals were retested demonstrating no diminution of intellectual or memory performance: additionally the Rhesus monkey's cephalon has recently been successfully transplanted for short periods of time to the isolated body of another Rhesus, and with the regaining of the conscious state, gives every evidence of preservation of behavior and intellectual performance (cf. Section B4). In addition, the subhuman primate brain has been completely isolated, removed from the cephalon and maintained in a high performance state utilizing a completely mechanical extracorporal perfusion circuit. Studies employing evolved potentials (visual and auditory) indicate preservation ("normalization") of the circuitry subservient to these high ordered functions. This is also true of the neuroelectrical recordings at both a cortical and subcortical level. Thus the memory and intellectual functioning of the subhuman brain demonstrates remarkable stability in spite of drastic physical (cooling and ischemia) and/or surgical (transplantation) dislocation. Perhaps a further subtle argument in favor of Professor Hyden's tenet regarding the memory trace representation in the protein permanency of the cell body and membrane.

Experiments on monkey and rodents are fine, but in the final analysis can we extrapolate these findings to man? For it is man and his values that we are primarily concerned with at this conference.

The human brain is the most complex, most superbly designed biological system known. Before it all human achievements in science and engineering is humbled. Truly the elements and their relationships that compose the "inner space" of the brain-mind continuum are as awesome and challenging as the galaxies and their solar systems in "outer space." Yet it is the human mind utilizing the tissue substrate of the brain which must solve the mysteries not only of the universe, but of itself. As Professor Hyden has stated it: "That the brain should understand brain." Surely one would hope as the intricacies of the central nervous system are unraveled, and human performance and action are explained, scientific unity will be born of the diversities and inconsistencies which presently characterize intellectual endeavor.

Thus the exciting and though provoking experiments and theories of Professor Hyden, dealing with memory and learning in the rodent require re-examination of the uniqueness of the mind-brain relationship, which must characterize all human relationships and acquisition of all knowledge. Wilder Penfield, in the volume entitled: *The Mystery of the Mind*, published just prior to his death, concluded: "That it is easier to rationalize man's being on the basis of two elements than on the basis of one." This famous brain surgeon, however, further adds: "But I believe one should not pretend to draw a final scientific conclusion, in man's study of man, until the nature of the energy responsible for mind-action is discovered as, in my own opinion, it will be."

Thus this world authority in his concluding literary effort is on one hand forced to accept "scientific dualism" as an explanation of the mind-brain continuum, yet even he after years of work on the problem was hopeful of eventually solving the relationship based on a unitary hypothesis. One wonders if neuroscience may eventually be reaching limits in this area which will require the defining of a new "Heisenberg Indetermancy Principle" operant in expressing the intimate association between the mind and its tissue substrate. Our chairman, Professor J.C. Eccles, has likewise expressed himself on this vexing problem and has found it appropriate to employ the "three world" concept of Popper, stating: "But realizing their existence in the world of self-awareness (World 2) and so having in the religious concept, souls." He further recalls a conversation with the great neurophysiologist, Sherrington, who stated: "For me now the only reality is the human soul." Thus many of our most distinguished neuroscientists, after decades of investigation, acknowledge the impossibility of explaining the human mind in terms of computer science, neurochemistry, or neurophysiology. Acknowledging these weighty opinions as well as contemporary theology, the question remains to plague us as to whether the mind-brain problem (including human learning and memory) will ever be completely understood regardless of the expected advances in experimental science. Nevertheless, one must hope and persevere that as the nature of brain, in its biochemical and neuroelectronic dimensions, is slowly unraveled, this will enable mankind to better appreciate and understand human motivations and values permitting a better design of life and living for all.

REFERENCES

Penfield, W.: *The Mystery of the Mind.* Princeton University Press, Princeton and London, 1975.

Eccles, J.C.: *Facing Reality.* Springer-Verlag, New York/Heidelberg/Berlin, 1970.

Wolin, L.R., Massopust, L.C., Jr., White, R.J.: "Behavioral Effects of Autocerebral Perfusion, Hypothermia and Arrest of Cerebral Blood Flow in the Rhesus Monkey." *Exper. Neurol.* 39:336-341, 1973.

White, R.J., Massopust, L.C., Jr., Wolin, L.R., Taslitz, N., and Yashon, D.: "Profound Selective Cooling and Ischemic of Primate brain without Pump or Oxygenator." *Surgery* 66: 224-232, 1969.

White, R.J.: "Experimental Transplantation of the Brain," Chapter 45 in *Human Transplantation,* F.T. Rapaport and J. Dausset (eds.), 1968, Grune & Stratton, Inc., New York.

White, R.J., Wolin, L.R., Massopust, L.C., Jr., Taslitz, N., and Verdura, J.: "Cephalic Exchange Transplantation in the Monkey." *Surgery* 70: 135-138, 1971.

White, R.J., Albin, M.S., Verdura, Jr., and Locke, G.E.: "The Isolated Monkey Brain: I-Operative Preparation and Design of Support Systems." *J. Neurosurg.* 27: 216-225, 1967.

Popper, K.R.: "On the Theory of the Objective Mind." *Akten des XIV. Internationalen Kongresses fur Philosophie,* vol. 1, Wien (1968b). 152, 164, 169, 176.

Sir John Eccles

B6 Cerebral Activity and the Freedom of the Will

Introduction

I have in my lecture (A6) given an account of the philosophical position which will form the basis of my discussion. I refer to the trialist philosophy of Sir Karl Popper in which everything in existence or experience is subsumed in one of the three worlds: World 1, the world of physical objects and states; World 2, the world of states of consciousness and subjective knowledge of all kinds; World 3, the world of man-made culture, comprising the whole of objective knowledge.

Fig. 1 indicates the three levels of World 2, outer sense, inner sense and central to these, the self of pure ego which for each of us is the basis of our unity as an experiencing being throughout out whole lifetime.

The Ego and the Freedom of the Will

"An action to be free must be conscious, purposive, follow open alternative choices; and it by no means follows, as empiricist philosophers always maintain, that because it could be otherwise it need be arbitrary or because it is not mechanically caused, it is not caused at all." (Polten, 1973).

That we have free will is a fact of experience. Furthermore I state emphatically that to deny free will is neither a rational nor a logical act. This denial either presupposes free will for the deliberately chosen response in making that denial, which is a contradiction, or else it is merely the automatic response of a nervous system built by genetic coding and moulded by conditioning. One does not conduct a rational argument with a being who makes the claim that all its responses are reflexes, no matter how complex and subtle the conditioning. For example, one should not argue with a Skinnerian, and moreover a Skinnerian should not engage in argument. Discourse becomes degraded into an exercise that is no more than conditioning and counterconditioning — what we may characterize as Skinnerian games! Nevertheless, despite these logical problems, it is widely held that free will must be rejected on logical grounds. The question can be raised: can free will be accommodated in a deterministic universe?

The diagram of Fig. 1 (p. 162) gives the basis for defining the postulated mode of operation of free will, which is represented symbolically by the arrows stemming from the pure ego or self. Polten (1973) states:

> "The pure ego is the necessary ingredient which changes determination to *self*-determination or libertarianism. If we did not have such an 'unmoved mover' (and it must be the *core* of that which makes up the self!) then we could not master our environment with science and technology, as we undeniably do. Far less would it be possible to give ourselves autonomously the moral law, and act with freedom of choice and responsibility. Both technologist and practical moralist can interfere with natural causal chains only because they themselves (i.e., their pure egos) are not pushed along these inexorable sequences; the pure ego rather impinges its own intentions upon the course of nature, and thus utilizes the laws of nature for its own ends . . . . Those who uphold free will need a pure ego, and the meaning and existence of free will has been so notoriously unclear and vexing largely because the meaning and existence of the pure ego has so far been so unclear. Thus human reflex actions, such as a knee jerk, are unfree because the pure ego is not involved; but conscious thoughts and purposive actions are free because the pure ego directs them."

When discussing causality, Max Planck (1936) made a statement that is relevant in this context.

> "The question of free will is one for the individual consciousness to answer: it can be determined only by the ego. The notion of human free will can mean only that the individual feels himself to be free, and whether he does so in fact can be known only to himself."

The Neurological Problems Arising from the Postulate of Free Will

My position is that I have the indubitable experience that by thinking and willing I can control my actions if I so wish, *although in normal waking life this prerogative is exercised but seldom.* I am not able to give a scientific account of how thought can lead to action, but this failure serves to emphasize the fact that our present physics and physiology are too primitive for this most challenging task of resolving the antimony between our experiences and the present primitive level of our understanding of brain function. When thought leads to action, I am constrained, as a neuroscientist, to postulate that in some way, completely beyond my understanding, my thinking changes the operative patterns of neuronal activities in my brain. Thinking thus comes to control the discharges of impulses from the pyramidal cells of my motor cortex and so eventually the contractions of my muscles and the behavioural patterns stemming therefrom. A fundamental neurological problem is: how can willing of a muscular movement set in train neural events that lead to the discharge of pyramidal cells of the motor cortex and so to activation of the neural pathway that lead to the muscle contraction?

If we have not this ability to exercise a willed or voluntary control over our actions, if we are illuded in this belief, the logical consequences lead to a denial of all personal responsibility for actions no matter how clever the philosophical discussion. Praise or blame become but meaningless noises because all people would be trapped in an inexorable web of cause and effect. To claim freedom of will does not mean that actions are uncaused. — It means that some are not caused or controlled solely by purely physical events in the neuronal machinery of the brain, but that the events in this neuronal machinery are to some extent modulated by the self or ego in the mental act of willing. It is postulated that there is a true interaction of the mental and the physical, and that mental events actually are causal agents in their modulating influence on the patterns of neuronal events that lead to the expression of willed movements.

I will not discuss the many philosophical theories (c.f. Section C6; Popper and Eccles, 1977; Eccles, 1980) that have been developed in order to evade the crucial and fundamental problems raised by the postulate of interaction — that mental events can effectively interact with brain events both in giving and receiving. The existence of mental states is not denied in these various philosophies, but it is regarded as being ineffective — a kind of spin-off from the neural events as in parallelism, epiphenomenalism and even in the more sophisticated version of the psyconeural identity hypothesis (Feigl, 1967). This philosophy is reducible to a materialist monism, but it accepts fully all varieties of conscious experience and explains them as being necessary components or aspects of brain states, there being strictly a psychoneural identity. It is postulated that every brain state has its counterpart in a conscious experience, the analogy being that the brain state can be recognized by external observation, and consciousness is the inner experience of that same state. Unfortunately the philosophical formulation is naive with respect to brain states.

I will not embark on a philosophical disputation, but recently there has been a most critical appraisal of the psycho-physical identity hypothesis by Polten (1973) who has demonstrated that it leads to paradoxes and contradictions and so stands refuted. My attack on the hypothesis is based on a consideration of the brain events and of the manner in which the identity hypothesis relates them to consciousness.

We are now in a position to consider the experiments of Kornhuber and associates (Deecke, Scheid and Kornhuber, 1969; Kornhuber, 1973) on the electrical potential generated in the cerebral cortex prior to the carrying out of a willed action. The problem is to have an elementally simple movement executed by the subject entirely on his own volition, and yet to have accurate timing in order to average the very small potentials recorded from the surface of the skull. This has been solved by Kornhuber and his associates who use the onset of the movement to trigger a reverse computation of the potentials up to 2 sec before the onset of the movement. The movement illustrated was a rapid flexion of the right index finger. The subject initiates these movements "at will" at irregular intervals of many seconds. In this way it was possible to average 250 records of the potentials evoked at various sites over the surface of the skull, as shown in Fig. 2 (p. 163) for the three upper traces. The slowly rising negative potential, called the *readiness potential,* was observed as a negative wave with unipolar recording over a wide area of the cerebral surface, but there were small positive potentials of similar time course over the most anterior and basal regions of the cerebrum. Usually the readiness potential began almost as long as 800 ms (0.8 sec.) before the onset of the movement, and led on to sharper potentials, positive then negative, beginning about 90 ms before the movement. Finally, as shown in the lowest trace, at 50 ms a sharp negativity developed over the area of the motor cortex concerned in the movement, the left precentral hand area in this case. We can assume that the readiness potential is generated by complex patterns of neuronal discharges that eventually project to the appropriate pyramidal cells of the motor cortex and synaptically excite them to discharge, so generating this localized negative wave just preceding the movement.

These experiments at least provide a partial answer to the question: What is happening in my brain at a time when a willed action is in process of being carried out? It can be presumed that during the readiness potential there is a developing specificity of the patterned impulse discharges in neurons so that eventually there are activated the correct motor cortical areas for bringing about the required movement. It can be regarded as the neuronal counterpart of the voluntary command. The surprising feature of the readiness potential is its wide extent and gradual build up. Apparently, at the stage of willing a movement, there is very wide influence on the patterns of neuronal operation, or as we will consider below, on the patterns of module operation. Eventually this immense neuronal activity concentrates on to the pyramidal cells in the proper zones of the motor cortex (Fig. 3) (p. 164) for carrying out the required movement. I will later continue with the neurological problems arising from these remarkable experiments.

The Unique Areas of the Cerebral Cortex

The evolution of man's brain from primitive hominids was associated with an amazingly rapid increase in size, from 550g to 1400g in two million years. But much more important was the creation of special areas associated with speech (Fig. 3). We can well imagine the great evolutionary success attending not only the growth of intelligence that accompanied brain size in some exponential relationship, but also the development of language for communication and discussion. In this manner primitive man doubtless achieved great successes in communal hunting and food gathering, and in adapting to the exigencies of life in linguistically planned operations of the community. We now know that special areas of the neocortex were developed for this emerging linguistic performance, which in about 98% are in the left cerebral hemisphere (Penfield and Roberts, 1959). Usually (in 80% of brains) there is a considerable enlargement of the planum temporale in the left temporal lobe and in the areas bordering the sulcus in the inferior frontal convolution; and this enlargement is developed by the 28th week of intrauterine life in preparation for usage some months after birth. Its development represents a very important and unique construction by the genetic instructions provided for building the human brain.

Sperry's investigations on commissurotomy patients have shown that the dominant linguistic hemisphere is uniquely concerned in giving conscious experiences to the subject and in mediating his willed actions. It is not denied that some other consciousness may be associated with the intelligent and learned behavior of the minor hemisphere, but the absence of linguistic or symbolic communication at an adequate level limits the extent to which it can be discovered. The situation is equivalent to the problem of animal consciousness.

Fig. 4 (p. 165) shows in diagrammatic form the association of linguistic and ideational areas of the dominant hemisphere with the world of conscious experience. Arrows lead from the linguistic and ideational areas of the dominant hemisphere to the conscious self (World 2) (cf. Fig. 1) that is represented by the circular area above. It must be recognized that Fig. 4 is an information flow diagram and that the superior location adopted for the conscious self is for diagrammatic convenience. It is of course not meant to imply that the conscious self is hovering in space above the dominant hemisphere! It is postulated that in normal subjects activities in the minor hemisphere reach consciousness mostly after transmission to the dominant hemisphere, which very effectively occurs via the immense impulse traffic in the corpus callosum, as is illustrated in Fig. 4 by the numerous arrows. Complementarily, as will be discussed in full later, it is postulated that the neural activities responsible for voluntary actions mediated by the pyramidal tracts normally are generated in the dominant hemisphere by some willed action of the conscious self (see downward arrows in Figs. 1 and 4).

It must be recognized that this transmission in the corpus callosum is not a simple one-way transmission. The 200 million fibers must carry a fantastic wealth of impulse traffic in both directions. In the normal operation of the cerebral hemisphere, activity of any part of a hemisphere is as effectively and rapidly transmitted to the other hemisphere as to another lobe of the same hemisphere. The whole cerebrum thus achieves a most effective unity. It will be appreciated from Fig. 4 that section of the corpus callosum gives a unique and complete cleavage of this unity. the neural activities of the minor hemisphere are isolated from those cerebral areas that give and receive from the conscious self. The conscious subject is recognizably the same subject or person that existed before the brain-splitting operation and retains the unity of self-consciousness or the mental singleness that he experienced before the operation. However, this unity is at the expense of unconsciousness of all the happenings in the minor (right) hemisphere.

Structural and Functional Concepts of the Cerebral Cortex
The Modular Concept*

The excitatory level built up in a module is communicated from moment to moment by the impulse discharge along the association fibers formed by the axons of pyramidal cells (Szentagothai, 1978). In this way powerful excitation of a module will spread widely and effectively to other modules. There is as yet no quantitative data on module operation. However the number of neurones in a module is surprisingly large — some thousands of which there would be many hundreds of pyramidal cells and many hundreds of each of the other species of neurones. The operation of a module can be imagined as a complex of circuits in parallel with summation by convergence of hundreds of convergent lines onto neurones and in addition a mesh of feed-forward and feed-back excitatory and inhibitory lines overpassing the

* In Section B1 there has been an account of the modular structure of the cerebral neocortex, and of the communication patterns from module to module (for a more comprehensive treatment see Eccles, 1980, Lecture 2).

simple neuronal circuitry expressed in Fig. 6 of Section B1. Thus
we have to envisage levels of complexity in the operation of a
module far beyond anything yet conceived and of a totally different order from any integrated microcircuits of electronics, the
analogous systems mentioned earlier. Moreover there will be an
enormous range in the output from a module — from high frequency discharges in the hundreds of constituent pyramidal cells to
the irregular low level discharges characteristic of cerebral cortex
in the resting state. The range of projection of the pyramidal cells
is enormous — some go only to nearby modules, others are remote
association fibers, and yet other are commissural fibers traver-
sing the corpus callosum to areas of the other side, which tend to
be in mirror-image relationship.

The Patterns of Module Interaction

Fig. 5 (p. 166) is a diagrammatic attempt to illustrate in the
limited time span of a fraction of a second the on-going module to
module transmission. It attempts to show the manner in which
association fibers from the pyramidal cells in a module can activate other modules by projections of many pyramidal axons in
parallel. These other modules in turn project effectively to further modules. In this assumed plan of a small zone of the neocortex, the pyramidal cells of the modules are represented as circles,
solid or open, according as they participate in one or another
class of modality operation, e.g. to one type of sensory input for
A and to another for B. Main lines of communication between
successive modules are shown by arrows, and there is one example of a return circuit giving a loop for sustained operation in the
manner of the closed self-reexciting chains of Lorente de No. In
addition convergence of the modules for A and B modalities gives
activation of modules by both A and B inputs with a corresponding symbolism — dense-core circles. The diagram is greatly simplified because in it one module at the most projects to two other
modules, whereas we may suppose it to be to tens or hundreds.
There are 3 examples where excitation of modules was inadequate for onward propagation. Thus in the diagram two inputs A
and B give only two outputs A and AB. Fig. 5 represents the kind

of patterning of neuronal activation in the cerebral cortex that was imagined by Sherrington (1940). He likened it to "an enchanted loom, weaving a dissolving pattern, always a meaningful pattern, though never an abiding one, a shifting harmony of subpatterns."

The diagram of Fig. 5 is particularly inadequate in that there is no representation of the irregular background discharge of all types of cortical neurones. The modular activation and transmission must be imagined as being superimposed upon this on-going background noise. Effective neuronal activity is ensured when there is inparallel activity of many neurones with approximately similar connections. Signals are in this way lifted out of noise. Thus instead of the simplicity indicated in Fig. 5, we have to envisage an irregular seething activity of the whole assemblages of neurones, the signals being superimposed on this background by phases of collusive activity of neurones in parallel either within modules or between modules.

One can surmise that from the extreme complexity and refinement of its modular organization there must be an unimagined richness of properties in the active cerebral cortex. It is postulated that in a situation where the pure ego is operative, there will be changed patterns of modular interaction leading eventually to a change in the spatio-temporal pattern of influence playing upon the pyramidal cells in the motor cortex. The "readiness potential" (Fig. 2) bears witness to this cortical activity preceeding the pyramidal tract discharge.

Evidently we have here a fundamental problem that transcends our present neurophysiological concepts. Some tentative suggestions have been made (Popper and Eccles, 1977; Eccles, 1979, 1980). It is necessary to take into account the evidence that the conscious self can act on cortical modules only when the cerebral cortex is at a relatively high level of excitation. If the neuronal activity of the cerebral cortex is at too low a level, then liaison between the mind and the brain ceases. The subject is unconscious as in sleep, anaesthesia, coma. Perception and willed action are no longer possible. Furthermore, if a large part of the cerebral cortex is in the state of the rigorous driven activity of a convulsive seizure, there is a similar failure of brain-mind liaison.

Originally it was suggested that the liaison between mind and brain depended on the "mind influences" being able to modify the discharge of neurons that were critically poised at firing level. In the light of the modular concept a more attractive hypothesis would be that the modules themselves are the detector units for causal input from the pure ego. We may give them a function analogous to radio-receiving units.

Thus, the neurophysiological hypothesis is that the causal action of the conscious self modifies the spatio-temporal activity in the modules of the liaison zone of the dominant hemisphere. It will be noted that this hypothesis assumes that the mind has itself some spatio-temporal patterned character in order to allow it this operative effectiveness.

This concept is closely related to those recently developed by Sperry (1969) who states:

> In the present scheme the author postulates that the conscious pheno-
> mena of subjective experience do interact on the brain processes exerting
> an active causal influence. In this view consciousness is conceived to have
> a directive role in determining the flow pattern of cerebral excitation."
>
> "Conscious phenomena in this scheme are conceived to interact with
> and to largely govern the physiochemical and physiological aspects of the
> brain process. It obviously works the other way round as well, and thus a
> mutual interaction is conceived between the physiological and the mental
> properties. Even so, the present interpretation would tend to restore mind
> to its old prestigious position over matter, in the sense that the mental
> phenomena are seen to transcend the phenomena of physiology and bio-
> chemistry.

Just because World 2 is drawn located above the brain in Figs. 1 and 4, I do not wish to imply that World 2 is floating above the brain and has an autonomous existence and performance independent of the liaison area of the brain! On the contrary it is, so far as we can discover, tightly linked with neuronal activity there. If that stops, unconsciousness supervenes. As shown by the arrows in both directions in Fig. 4, there is an incessant interplay in the interaction between World 2 and the liaison brain, but we know nothing about its nature. This interaction is a tremendous challenge for the future. In this respect we can think of the whole range of psychiatry with such problems as those of the unconscious self, of sleep and dreams, of obsession. Despite our present ignorance of the precise neurological basis of all these problems of the psyche, we can have hope for some clearer understanding because it is now possible to define the liaison areas of the brain, and postulate that only in certain areas and in certain states of the brain does this relationship occur. This insight, limited as it is, provides hope for more understanding in this most fundamental problem.

REFERENCES

Deeke, L., Scheid, P. and Kornhuber, H.H.: Distribution of readiness potential, pre-motion positivity, and motor potential of the human cerebral cortex preceding voluntary finger movements. Exp. Brain Res. 7: 158-168 (1969)

Eccles, J.C.: The neurophysiological basis of mind: The principles of neurophysiology. Oxford: Clarendon Press (1953)

——————— : Facing Reality. Berlin, Heidelberg, New York: Springer (1970)

——————— : The Human Mystery. Berlin, Heidelberg, New York: Springer International (1979)

——————— : The Human Psyche. Berlin, Heidelberg, New York: Springer International (1980)

Feigl, H.: The 'mental' and the 'physical'. Minneapolis, Minn.: University of Minnesota Press (1967)

Kornhuber, H.H.: Cerebral cortex, cerebellum and basal ganglia: An introduction to their motor functions. In: The Neurosciences: Third Study Program. Schmitt, F.O. (ed.) New York: The Rockefeller University Press (1973)

Penfield, W. and Roberts, L.: Speech and Brain Mechanisms. Princeton, New Jersey: Princeton University Press (1959)

Planck, M.: The Philosophy of Physics. London: G. Allen & Unwin, (1936)

Polten, E.P.: A Critique of the Psycho-physical Identity Theory. The Hague: Mouton Publishers (1973)

Popper, K.R.: Objective knowledge: an evolutionary approach. Oxford: Clarendon Press (1972)

Popper, K.R. and Eccles, J.C.: The Self and its Brain. Berlin, Heidelberg, New York: Springer International (1977)

Sperry, R.W.: A modified concept of consciousness. Psychol. Rev. 76: 532-536 (1969)

Szentagothai, J.: The neuron network of the cerebral cortex: A functional interpretation. Proc. Roy. Soc. B 201: 219-248 (1978)

WORLD OF CONSCIOUSNESS

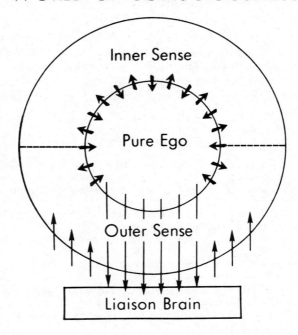

Outer Sense	Inner Sense	Pure Ego
Light	Thoughts	The self
Color	Feelings	The soul
Sound	Memories	
Smell	Dreams	
Taste	Imaginings	
Pain	Intentions	
Touch		

Fig. 1. World of consciousness. The three postulated components in the world of consciousness toghether with a tabulated list of their components.

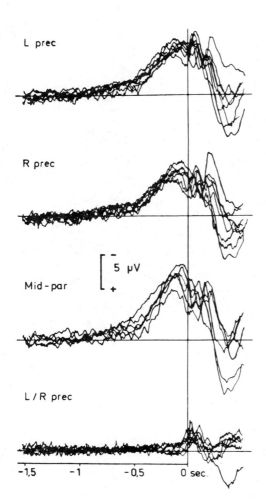

Fig. 2. Cerebral potentials, recorded from the human scalp, preceding voluntary rapid flexion movements of the right index finger. The potentials are obtained by the method of reverse analysis (Kornhuber and Deecke). Eight experiments on different days with the same subject; about 1000 movements per experiment. Upper three rows: monopolar recording, with both ears as reference; the lowermost trace is a bipolar record, left versus right precentral hand area. The readiness potential starts about 0.8 sec prior to onset of movement; it is bilateral and widespread over precentral (L. prec, R. prec) and parietal (Mid-par) areas. The premotion positivity, bilateral and widespread too, starts about 90 msec before onset of movement. The motor potential appears only in the bipolar record (L/R prec), it is unilateral over the left precentral hand area, starting 50 msec prior to onset of movement in the electromyogram. (Experiment of W. Becker, L. Deecke, B. Grozinger, and H.H. Kornhuber, presented at the German Physiological Society Meeting 1969, Pflugers Arch Physiol. 312:108).

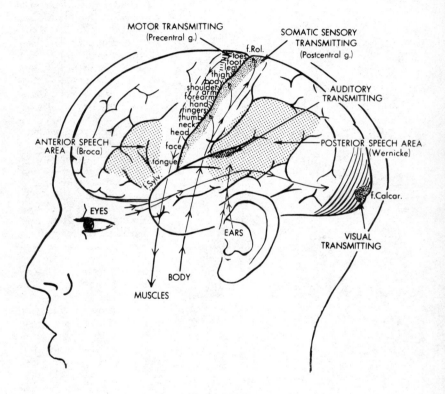

Fig. 3. The motor and sensory transmitting areas of the cerebral cortex. The approximate map of the motor transmitting areas is shown in the precentral gyrus, while the somatic sensory receiving areas are in a similar map in the precentral gyrus. Other primary sensory areas shown are the visual and auditory, but they are largely in areas screened from this lateral view.

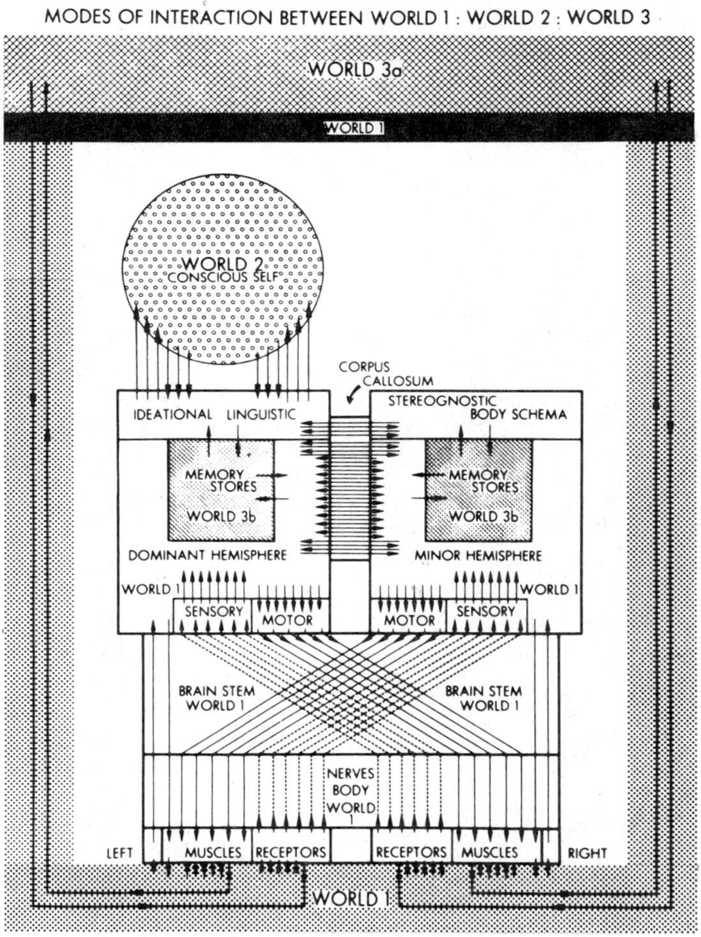

Fig. 4. Communications to and from the brain and within the brain. Diagram to show the principal lines of communication from peripheral receptors to the sensory corices and so to the cerebral hemispheres. Similarly, the diagram shows the output from the cerebral hemispheres via the motor cortex and so to muscles. Both these systems of pathways are largely crossed as illustrated, but minor uncrossed pathways are also shown. The dominant left hemisphere and minor right hemisphere are labeled, together with some of the properties of these hemispheres. The corpus callosum is shown as a powerful cross-linking of the two hemispheres and, in addition, the diagram displays the modes of interaction between Worlds 1, 2, and 3, as described in the text.

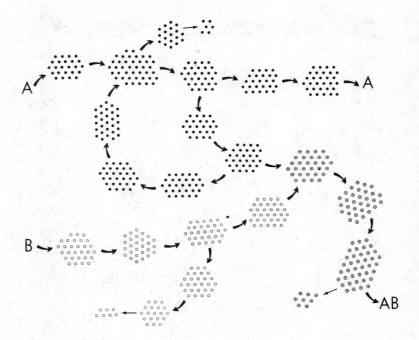

Fig. 5. In this schema of the cerebral cortex looked at from above, the large pyramidal cells are represented as circles, solid or open, that are arranged in clusters, each cluster corresponding to a column or module as diagrammed in Figs. 1, 2, where only a few large projecting pyramidal cells are shown of the hundreds that would be in the column. The large arrows symbolize impulse discharges along hundreds of axons in parallel, which are the mode of excitatory communication from column to column. Two inputs, A and B, and two outputs, A and AB, are shown. Further description in text.

Discussion

Long: Sir John, I have always been troubled by the kind of discussion which you gave us on the mind/brain interaction, because of an inability to understand it fully and perhaps you can help. My problem is that I see the brain as something which is a physical fact, a phenomenon, a biological component of animals, which is itself subject to precisely the kind of studies which you tell us about. It is clearly an inordinately complicated piece of biology, but still it is obviously revealing itself to further and further studies.

In contrast I cannot avoid a feeling that when I deal with something called the mind or something called the ego, I am dealing with a construct which is a useful, important way of thinking of human behavior, but which differs in a somewhat fundamental way from this biological entity. I would appreciate more of your thoughts on this. Am I right? Are we dealing with constructs and physical facts, and secondly, how does one resolve it?

Eccles: Thank you very much for this very searching question. Yes, it is of course terribly hard to come to terms with this complex problem. But if we don't, we are, for example, denying our ability to bring about conscious actions, to be responsible for our actions. If everything is simply neural events operating in the neuronal circuits from input to output in the genetically coded structures of our brains together with the changes brought about conditioning, then that is it! We are no more responsible than an animal is responsible.

I am like Karl Popper. I am a common sense philosopher. I believe that the very earliest knowledge we have is from our experiences. On the one hand there is light and color and sound, which we eventually can transmute into meaning and describe in language and so on, and on the other hand there is an immense neural performance in the cerebral cortex that I did not go into. Again, if we so wish, we can deliberately take action into the external world to bring about events. This happens in the way I was trying to show you. Now, more and more we are defining this mind-brain liaison down to special areas of the brain. It isn't just a general brain action. I think it is going to be an action of very specialized regions of the brain.

The next point I want to make is to warn against the idea that the brain is just a bit of ordinary machinery. Some parts of the brain such as the cerebellum can be regarded as neural machinery, but there is the immense and very different structure, the cerebral cortex. As we go up to the cerebral cortex, we are gradually understanding the kind of structure it is. The immensely complicated patterns of neural activity are still far beyond our understanding being what Sherrington called the enchanted loom, weaving patterns in space and time. I like to think with Szentagothai that there are modular structures in the cerebral cortex each with their own incredible dynamical life. They resemble integrated micro-circuits of electronics but are ever so much more so, within each module up to ten thousand cells linked up synaptically in patterns of activity which we don't yet understand. But gradually we begin to realize that in the brain there evolved a structure with dynamic performances of a different order from anything else in nature, from anything else that physics has ever looked at. And we even may imagine that these structures, when in the right dynamical state, could be functioning, if you will pardon the analogy, like antennae out into the mind world, receiving and giving to it.

I think this is a fundamental problem concerning what happened somewhere along this evolutionary story, at least a hundred thousand years ago. Then man attained to self-consciousness—knew that he knew. Something had happened, mysteriously, wonderfully, in the evolution of the human brain, to give it these potentialities, which as you are quite right in saying, we still are shocked by. We cannot accept that such a thing happened because we are so immersed in the material world, the physical world, the world of science. But let me tell you, that the whole of science itself is a mental construct. The whole of our understanding of nature is in fact mental. It is World 3. The imaginative, creative, scientific efforts of mankind have given us a philosophy that makes it difficult to understand how minds can work on matter. It has given us the laws as you might say, of matter, and left mind out. This was of course due to Descartes, and it was very good up to a point. I am a reductionist, in my work on science, I am a reductionist just as everyone else is. I want to admit that; but metaphysically I am an anti-reductionist.

Jantsch: I am a bit troubled by the internal system which you pointed out and you trace back to Popper, because it does not link World 1 and World 3 although in a later diagram you did link those two. Here in the first diagram, you just had World 1 interacting with World 2 and World 2 interacting with World 3. And I think that the basic trouble with it is that you have reality on one side and you have what you then describe as objective knowledge on the other side. I think if you conceive it as I do it and I arrived at a very similar ternary structure but in a toroidal form you know, with feed-back links centering the whole thing constantly. Then also you have no trouble of admitting that what is going on between World 2 and World 3 may be subjective, or is really subjective from some level, and is objective from some other level.

I have a paper on which I will go into a little bit into the subjectivity and objectivity question and I think that both are just aspects of the same kind of process. I think that if you just call it objective knowledge like that, it means that you believe, or that you infer that there is one absolute truth, which is eventually to be revealed by science; not like what I think is a much more fruitful idea, a continuous process of putting models into the world, into our cultural world which act as myth, and guide our lives for a certain period, but being flexible and having a whole type of cultural evolution which goes to ever new models, and goes to ever new mind regimes, so to say, and keeps our own action within this cultural world alive. So that as someone, I think John Calhoun has put it, man is constantly a "crisis provoker". But what I would also say then is perhaps this view of seeing this at one end of the spectrum as a final objective knowledge, that this comes out maybe also in the view and I did not understand whether you have let us say, very final proof or whether this was a hypothesis that only the linguistic, analytic type of brain function is linked to consciousness. It goes very much against much of the experience which more and more people seek also today that the holistic experience should not directly be linked to consciousness. I think that in a certain way, we are, at least this is my tentative conclusion, we are, we have a holistic way of relating and we have an analytical way of relating. And there is a whole tradition, very much also in the Far Eastern culture which Dr. Sibatani, for example, has pointed out in his paper. Emptying ourselves of the linguistic and analytical ability gives us the possibility of becoming conscious — you may call it sub-consciously conscious, but conscious in a way that it works and acts on our consciousness — of the holistic view which I think, just as an idea, would tie in then very much also with the notions that the mind is not, as you in your last sentence said, let us say, the universe is not as you say it, mindless; but that we all share, as Aldous Huxley has put it, that we all are mind at large in some way. So that we share in some mind and I think I cannot elaborate this more here, but I think there are certain new results coming out, even in physics, which seem to indicate that there is something like a process of evolution which is not mindless but which goes on from the physical, what we call the inanimate world all the way to the social-cultural world.

Eccles: Thank you very much. I am going to get a bit lost, you know, in all the detailed answering. I think I agree with you almost completely. I think that we should start to communicate more, you will be in Committee I, I think, will you not?

Jantsch: Unfortunately I am in Committee II.

Eccles: That is a great pity because I was hoping that we could communicate much more about this. In my first diagram (Section A6, Fig. 1) you have pointed out that I had World 2 and World 3 communicating to each other. That is Popper's suggestion. However for the most part the interaction between these two worlds has to be mediated by sense organs, with all the complexities of coding. So there I agree completely with you. Thank you for pointing that out.

As regards the other main query you made: am I putting consciousness only in the left hemisphere and not in the right? I am putting the ultimate experience of consciousness only in the left hemisphere. However all of the processing, all of the development of the neuronal operations that eventually become associated with conscious experiences goes on in both hemispheres everywhere. The holistic performance goes on in my minor hemisphere. Otherwise, how could I appreciate music? The physical substrate of music comes into my cochlea and is coded in the auditory nerve fiber discharges and eventually in a most sophisticated manner by neuronal machinery of my cerebral cortex to give me an experience of delight in the analysis of the musical patterns of remembrances and associations. Most of that analysis and synthesis comes about in the minor hemisphere and then it is shot through the corpus callosum to be experienced in the liaison areas of the dominant hemisphere, where it comes through to consciousness. In general I think we agree. I don't believe that consciousness is only linguistic. I believe that we have direct consciousness of pictures, of music, of odors and tactile experiences of all kinds of pain without having to talk about them. I think that is a bad fallacy that some people are expressing today, that you never know about anything until you talk about it. We are supposed to spend all our waking time in talking to ourselves. I disagree with this completely. This is only for primitive people.

Now, what is the other point you made? The mindless universe. I am strongly against pan-psychism. I don't believe that it tells us anything. I think it is based upon a fallacious idea that nothing new can come to exist. Even Sherrington thought this, as also Teihard de Chardin and Julian Huxley — that there is an element of mind in all organized matter and gradually it has become perfected in the evolutionary process, eventually to achieve its great flowering in the human brain. I see no evidence for that. My evidence on the contrary is that of my self-consciousness. For each of us that is the only mind we know. If we did not have self-consciousness, we would not start putting mind into anything. It is only because we find mind in ourselves related to our own brains, that we begin to think about minds in other people. Then of course, if you are un-sophisticated, you put minds into animals; and, as in the myths of the past, you can put minds into the various other manifestations of nature. But this is unscientific. We only know of mind as it is in each one of us, and then by subtle communications we recognize mind in others. That is as far as I am going to go!

Jantsh: Just one point. What about plant communication?

Eccles: Communication doesn't involve mind at all, the whole of biochemistry, the whole of physiology, the whole of biophysics is involved in communication, but it operates simply by physical principles. I am a complete reductionist in all these matters. I come out of reductionism not even for the working of my own brain — there I am still a reductionist — but only in the respect of the relationship of the liaison brain to the mind world. There I am, as I said, metaphysically an anti-reductionist.

About all the other questions, I am, of course, not putting up proofs of problems except in some cases which I gave you. Rather I am putting up hypothesis in the Popperian manner hoping to be challenged as you challenged them. That is what we do it for. If we don't define our ideas sharply with diagrams and models, if we only give fuzzy talking expressions, then I don't believe we can ever make progress. We have to dare to make statements which challenge refutation.

Haskell: You mention something to the effect of what is called PSI — telepathy, clairvoyance, perhaps even precognition, there are various forms of it. There have been many books published on it, and some experiments actually done with it. Would you please expand your views on that subject?

Eccles: Yes, I have in fact been to Duke to see experiments of Rhine and have read widely in the literature. I don't see anything definitive against telepathy. We don't know how brain actions communicate to our own spiritual World 2. We don't know how the World 1 to World 2 communication goes on in our brain. It is conceiveable that World 2 could receive from other World 2's but I don't think the experiments have been adequate to prove this extraordinary idea. I would on the other hand keep my options open on it. I don't want to say that it cannot exist because the world has so many incredible events happening in it. For example from our own experiences, we know the creativity and the imagination of man. What are we in fact as human beings? We are indescribably wonderful, beyond our understanding. Therefore, I would say that I would keep my options open on telepathy and I would recommend that if people want to work on it that they should be free to work on it and supported for it. We have many examples in the past where attempts to investigate problems of an esoteric kind were frowned upon. All kinds of pioneers had to fight for their existence. Not that they have always been right, most of them have been wrong, as for example the astrologers or the vitalists. But I would say that the cost is quite small, and we should be prepared to have freedom for people to investigate even extremely unorthodox problems.

Bar-Hillel: Leaving more basic questions such as the explanatory power of your trialist model for Committee I, hopefully at least, let me just use my half a minute to ask you two perhaps minor questions. First, how would you go about corroborating or refuting your conjecture that non-human animals have no awareness of death. Question number one. This primariness of personal experiences and the secondariness of physicalist modes of view, has been an old philosophical tenet, of which you are of course fully aware. It has been called various names, Phenomenalist views, etc., Eigenphysischer by Carnap in 1928 and has as often been shown to be inadequate as it has been proposed and re-proposed. So the question is, do you have any new conceptions to vindicate to the view that in some interesting sense the Eigenphysischer and Lebens are primary relative to the other points of view which have been claimed by other people to be primary? Or relative to the views say of the later Carnap in which this whole problem has become a pseudoproblem so that this talk about primariness and secondariness didn't make much sense any more to him.

Eccles: Thank you very much. The first question is one of observation. When you are studying animals, please remember you have to study them in the wild. Do not study domestic pets. In this case even Joan Goodall's chimpanzees have become her domestic pets. But even then when you watch animals and let us say, I will give you an example, Professor Washburn of Berkeley has studied monkey colonies in the wild. He has observed that, as animals get old and injured, they are rejected by the colony. No monkey takes any notice of an injured or dead animal. The point I would make is that you should observe the behavior of animals in the wild state.

There are occasional reports on elephants which could be used to refute my statement, but elephants are domestic animals. You know where this behavior of caring for the sick or dead is reported the elephants are associated intimately with people and they are very intelligent. It is reported that elephants just cover the dead elephants with leaves. But the chimpanzees in Joan Goodall's experiences take no notice in the end of dead chimpanzees and this is certainly true of Washburn's monkeys in the wild. Therefore, I think that you can say that animals are not aware of death. As soon as an animal is dying they reject it. It is no more interesting to them. They do not recognize it. They never recognize that this too could happen to me. This poignant insight happened to man at least one hundred thousand years ago. When he saw the other members of the tribe dying, he must have got the sense that, they are like me. They die. I too can die. I will look after the dead body to the best of my ability in the hope that when I die, it will be done to me too.

The second question was about the primary and the secondary. I just think that this is simple neurophysiology. Perceptual physiology wasn't well known by Carnap and his colleagues. They did not study the physiological processes concerned in perception. That is the trouble with so many philosophers who have talked and written books on perception. They do not know about the neural events involved in perception—the coding by the sense organs and the successive analysis and synthesis that goes on in the sensory pathways to the brain and the further integration there. I think this would be my answer, that it is just the inadequacy of scientific understanding that leads to these philosophical problems. If philosophers were much better informed upon the basic physiological events involved in perception, I think they would be quite different in their interpretation about primary and secondary reality. And I should mention that the distinguished physicist Eugene Wigner has made this very same statement, and I am following his concept in talking about primary reality and secondary reality.

Anderson: This is by way of comment to Dr. Eccles to see if you would concur in my observation. It seems to me that your unique use of language as the base of culture is of great importance to us, particularly vis-a-vis the term, "communication", as was brought up by one of our other speakers. In the plant world and more so in the lower animal world communication is on a one-to-one kind of non-transformational basis, where in fact a signal for aggression is automatically met by aggression; whereas in man, language is transformational, that a cue for aggression can by way of our higher brain centers, be transformed into a cue for, if you will, non-aggression, non-conflict, but rather, if anything, to amicability. Therefore, I think it calls for a clear distinction between communication and language to allow for this transformation and greater enhancement of culture as your model seems to imply. Would you agree with that?

Eccles: Thank you Dr. Anderson. Of course I would. That is a very nice expression that you have given to the ideas that I was trying to convey. We are in fact, speaking animals. It is through the subtleties of communication in a linguistic mode that I think man came to become human. I was trying to give you these instances of "Genie" and others, to show you that but for this developed communication, we stay animals. Each human child has to be created anew as a human being, a sophisticated human being, through linguistic communication and other methods too of course. I don't want to exclude artistic form, and sound, as with music. These are all part of human language if we think in a wider mode that includes all of the cultural means of communication. This is the wonderful thing that we have been born to. How grateful we should be to be born now into this marvellous cultural world of ours, rather than to have been born, what should we say six thousand years ago in this area, in Japan, or in Europe, or in America. What a difference! No, we are the lucky inheritors of this rich human culture, and this makes it all the more important for us, as responsible beings, to see that this heritage goes on enriched further for subsequent generations. This thought relates to the motto of this conference.

Gunther S. Stent

c1 Culturalism and Biology

For the past two centuries, scientists, particularly in English-speaking countries, have generally viewed their attempt to understand nature from the epistemological vantage of positivism. All the while, positivism had been under attack from philosophers, but it is only since the 1950's that its powerful hold on the students of nature finally seems to be on the wane. There is as yet no generally accepted designation for the philosophical alternatives that are presently replacing positivism, but the view of man known as "structuralism", which has informed certain schools of psychologists and social scientists, appears to be central to the latter-day epistemological scene. As I shall try to show here, in addition to the philosophical and psychological arguments that have been advanced in its behalf, structuralism can draw support also from biological insights into the evolutionary origins and manner of function of the brain. The principal tenet of positivism, as formulated in the 18th century mainly by David Hume and the French Encyclopaedists, is that sensory experience is the source of true knowledge about the world. According to this view the mind at birth is a clean slate on which there is gradually sketched a representation of reality built on cumulative experience. This representation is orderly, or structured, because, thanks to the principle of inductive reasoning, we can recognize regular features of our experience and infer causal connections between events that habitually occur together. The possibility of innate, or *a priori*, true knowledge of the world is rejected as a logical absurdity.

It is unlikely that the widespread acceptance of a positivism had a significant effect on the development of the physical sciences, since physicists have little need to look to philosophers for justification of their research objectives or working methods. Moreover, once a physicist *has* managed to find an explanation for some phenomenon, he can be reasonably confident of the empirical test of its verity. Thus, the positivist rejection of the atomic theory in the late 19th century, on the grounds that no one had ever "seen" an atom, did not stop chemists and physicists from then laying the groundwork for our present understanding of microscopic matter. However, in the human sciences, particularly in psychology and sociology, the situation was quite different. Here positivism was to have a most profound effect. One reason for this is that practitioners of the human sciences are much more dependent on philosophical support of their work than are physical scientists. For in contrast to the clearly definable research aims of physical science, it is often impossible to state explicitly just what it really *is* about human behavior that one wants to explain. This in turn makes it quite difficult to set forth clearly the conditions under which any postulated causal nexus linking the observed facts could be verified. On the one hand, positivism helped to bring the human sciences into being in the first place, by insisting that any eventual understanding of man must be based on the observation of facts, rather than on armchair speculations. On the other hand, by limiting inquiry to such factual observations and allowing only propositions that are based on direct inductive inferences from the raw sensory data, positivism constrained the human sciences to remain taxonomic disciplines whose content is largely descriptive with little genuine explanatory power. Positivism clearly informed the 19th century founders of psychology, ethnology and linguistics. Though we are indebted to these founders for the first corpus of reliable data concerning human behavior, their refusal to consider these data in terms of any propositions not derived inductively from direct observation prevented them from erecting a theoretical framework for understanding man.

Structuralism transcends the limitation on the methodology, indeed on the agenda of permissible inquiry, of the human sciences imposed by positivism. Structuralism admits, as positivism does not, the possibility of innate knowledge not derived from sensory experience. Furthermore, structuralism not only permits propositions about behavior that are not directly inducible from observed data but it even maintains that the relations between observed data, or *surface structures,* are not by themselves explainable. According to this view the causal connections which determine behavior do not relate to surface structures at all. Instead, the overt behavioral phenomena are generated by covert *deep structures,* inaccessible to direct observation. Hence any theoretical framework for understanding man must be based on the deep structures, whose discovery ought to be the real goal of the human sciences.

Probably the best known pioneer of structuralism is Sigmund Freud, to whom we owe the fundamental insight that human behavior is governed not so much by the events of which we are consciously aware in our own minds or which we can observe in the behavior of others, but rather by the deep structures of the subconscious which are generally hidden from both subjective and objective view. The nature of these covert deep structures can only be inferred indirectly by analysis of the overt surface structures. This analysis has to proceed according to an elaborate scheme of psycho-dynamic concepts that purports to have fathomed the rules which govern the reciprocal transformations of surface into deep and of deep into surface structures. The great strength of Freudian analytical psychology is that it does offer a theoretical approach to understanding human behavior. Its great weakness, however, is that it is not possible to verify its propositions. And this can be said also of most other structuralist schools active in the human sciences. They do try to explain human behavior within a general theoretical framework, in contrast to their positivist counterparts that cannot, or rather refuse to try to do so. But there is no way of verifying the structuralist theories in the manner in which the theories of physics can be verified through critical experiments or observations. The structuralist theories are, and may forever remain, merely plausible, being, maybe, the best we can do to account for the complex phenomenon of man.

For instance, positivist ethnology, as conceived by one of its founders, Franz Boas, sought to establish as objectively and as free from cultural bias as possible the facts of personal behavior and social relations to be found in diverse ethnic groups. Insofar as any explanations are advanced at all to account for these observations, they are formulated in *functionalist* terms. That is to say, every overt feature of behavior or social relation is thought

to serve some useful function in the society in which it is found.
The explanatory work of the ethnologist would be done once he
had identified that function and verified its involvement by
means of additional observations. Accordingly, the general aim of
this approach to ethnology is to show how manifold and diverse
the ways are in which man has adapted his behavior and social
existence to the range of conditions which he encountered in set-
tling the Earth. By contrast, structuralist ethnology, according
to one of its main exponents Claude Levi-Strauss, views the concept of functionality as a tautology, devoid of any real explanatory power for human behavior. All extant behavior is obviously
"functional" since all "disfunctional" behavior would lead to the
extinction of the ethnic group which exhibits it. Instead of functionality, so Levi-Strauss holds, only universal and permanent
deep structural aspects of the mind can provide any genuine understanding of social relations. The actual circumstances in which
different peoples find themselves no more than modulate the
overt behavior to which the covert deep structures give rise. In
other words, the point of departure of structuralist ethnology is
the view that the apparent diversity of ethnic groups pertains only to the surface structures and that at their deep structural level
all societies are very much alike. Hence, the general aim of that
other ethnology is to discover those universal, deep mental structures which underlie all human customs and institutions.

Positivist linguistics, as conceived by its founders such as Fer-
dinand de Saussure and Leonard Bloomfield, addresses itself to
the discovery of structural relations among the elements of spoken language. That is to say, the work of that school is concerned
with the surface structures of linguistic performance, the patterns which can be observed as being in use by speakers of various languages. Since the patterns which such classificatory analysis reveals differ widely, it seemed reasonable to conclude that
these patterns are arbitrary, or purely conventional, one linguistic group having chosen to adopt one, and another group having
chosen to adopt another convention. There would be nothing that
linguistics could be called on to explain, except for the taxonomic
principles that account for the degree of historical relatedness of
different peoples. And if the variety of basic patterns of various

human languages is indeed the result of arbitrary conventions, study of extant linguistic patterns is not likely to provide any deep insights into any universal properties of the mind. By contrast, structuralist linguistics, according to one of its main proponents, Noam Chomsky, starts from the premise that linguistic patterns are *not* arbitrary. Instead, all men are believed to possess an innate, *a priori* knowledge of a *universal grammar,* and despite their superficial differences, all natural languages are based on that same grammar. According to that view, the overt surface structure of speech, or the organization of sentences, is generated by the speaker from a covert deep structure. In his speech act, the speaker is thought to generate first his proposition as an abstract deep structure which he transforms only secondarily according to a set of rules into the surface structure of his utterance. The listener in turn fathoms the meaning of the speech act by just the inverse transformation of surface to deep structure. Chomsky holds that the grammar of a language is a system of transformational rules that determines a certain pairing of sound and meaning. It consists of a *syntactic component, a semantic component* and a *phonological component.* The surface structure contains the information relevant to the phonological component, whereas the deep structure contains the information relevant to the semantic component, and the syntactic component pairs surface and deep structures. Hence, it is merely the phonological component of grammar that has become greatly differentiated during the course of human history, or at least since the construction of the Tower of Babel. The semantic component has remained invariant and is, therefore, the "universal" aspect of the universal grammar which all natural languages embody. And this presumed constancy through time of the universal grammar cannot be attributable to any cause other than an innate, hereditary aspect of the mind. Hence, the general aim of structuralist linguistics is to discover that universal grammar.

Now, in retrospect, at a time when positivism and its philosophic and scientific ramifications appear to be moribund, it seems surprising that these views ever did manage to gain such a hold over the human sciences. Hume, one of the founders of positivism, already saw that the positivist theory of knowledge has a near-fatal logical flaw. As he noted, the validity of inductive reasoning—which, according to positivism the basis of our knowledge of the regularity of the world, and hence for our inference of causal connections between events—can neither be demonstrated logically nor can it be based on experience. Instead, inductive reasoning is evidently something that man brings to rather than derives from experience. Not long after Hume, Immanuel Kant showed that the positivist doctrine that sensory impressions are the sole source of human knowledge derives from an inadequate understanding of the working of the mind. Kant pointed out that sensory impressions become experience, i.e., gain meaning, only after they are interpreted in terms of a set of innate, or *a priori* concepts. Induction (or causality) is merely one of these concepts, time and space being others. But why was it that although Kant wielded an enormous influence among philosophers, his views had little currency among scientists? Why did the positivism of Hume, rather than the "critical idealism" of Kant, come to inform the explicit or implicit epistemological outlook of much of 19th and 20th century science? At least two reasons can be advanced for this historical fact. The first reason is simply that many positivist philosophers, especially Hume, were lucid and effective writers whose message could be readily grasped after a single reading of their works. The texts of Kant, and of his mainly Continental followers, are, by contrast, turgid and hard to understand.

The second reason for the long scientific neglect of Kant is more profound. After all, it does seem very strange that if, as Kant alleges, we bring such concepts as causality, time and space to experience *a priori*, these concepts happen to fit the world of our experience so well. Considering all the ill-conceived ideas one *might* have had about the world prior to experience, it seems nothing short of miraculous that our innate notions just happen to be those that fit the bill. Here the positivist view that all knowledge is derived from experience *a posteriori* seems much more reasonable. It turns out, however, that the way to resolve the dilemma posed by the Kantian *a priori* has been open since Darwin put forward the theory of natural selection in mid-19th century. Nevertheless, few scientists seem to have noticed this until

Konrad Lorenz drew attention to it thirty years ago. Lorenz pointed out that the positivist argument that knowledge about the world can enter our mind only through sensory experience is valid if we consider only the *ontogenetic* development of man, from fertilized egg to adult. But once we take into account also the *phylogenetic* development of the human brain through evolutionary history, it becomes clear that individuals can also know something of the world innately, prior to and independent of their own sensory experience. After all, there is no biological reason why such knowledge cannot be passed on from generation to generation via the ensemble of genes that determines the structure and function of our nervous system. For that genetic ensemble came into being through the process of natural selection operating on our remote ancestors. According to Lorenz, "experience has as little to do with the matching of *a priori* ideas with reality as does the matching of the fin structure of a fish with the properties of water". In other words, the Kantian notion of *a priori* knowledge is not implausible at all, but fully consonant with present mainstream evolutionary thought. The *a priori* concepts of causality, time and space, happen to suit the world because the hereditary determinants of our highest mental functions were selected for their evolutionary fitness, just as were the genes that give rise to other innate behavioral acts, e.g., sucking the nipple of mother's breast, which require no learning by experience.

The importance of these Darwinian considerations transcends a mere biological underpinning of the Kantian epistemology. For the evolutionary origin of the brain explains not only why our innate concepts match the world but also why these concepts no longer work so well when we attempt to fathom the world in its deepest scientific aspects. This barrier to unlimited scientific progress posed by the *a priori* concepts which we necessarily bring to experience was a major philosophical concern of Niels Bohr. Bohr recognized the essentially semantic nature of science, pointing out "as the goal of science is to augment and order our experience, every analysis of the conditions of human knowledge must rest on considerations of the character and scope of our means of communication. Our basis [of communication] is, of course, the language developed for orientation in our surroundings and for the organization of human communities. However, the increase of experience has repeatedly raised questions as to the sufficiency of concepts and ideas incorporated in daily language". The most basic of these concepts and ideas are precisely the Kantian *a priori* notions of causality, time and space. The meaning of these terms is intuitively obvious and grasped automatically by every child in the course of its normal intellectual development, without the need to attend physics classes. Accordingly, the models which modern science offers as explanations of reality are pictorial representations built of these intuitive concepts. This procedure was eminently satisfactory as long as explanations were sought for phenomena that are commensurate with the events that are the subject of our everyday experience (give or take a few orders of magnitude). For it was precisely for its fitness to deal with everyday experience that our brain was selected in the evolutionary sequence that culminated in the appearance of *homo sapiens*. But the situation began to change when, at the turn of this century, physics had progressed to a stage at which problems could be studied which involve either tiny subatomic or immense cosmic events on scales of time, space and mass billions of times smaller or larger than our direct experience. Now, according to Bohr, "there arose difficulties of orienting ourselves in a domain of experience far from that to the description of which our means of expression are adapted". For it turned out that the description of phenomena in this domain in ordinary, everyday language leads to contradictions or mutually incompatible pictures of reality. In order to resolve these contradictions, time and space had to be denatured into generalized concepts whose meaning no longer matched that provided by intuition. Eventually it appeared also that the intuitive notion of cause and effect is not a useful one for giving account of events at the atomic and subatomic level. All of these developments were the consequence of the discovery that; the rational use of intuitive linguistic concepts to communicate experience actually embodies hitherto unnoticed presuppositions. And it is these presuppositions which lead to contradictions when the attempt is made to communicate events outside the experiential domain. Now, whereas the scope of science was enormously enlarged by recognizing the pitfalls of everyday language, this was achieved only at the price of denaturing the intuitive meaning of some of its basic concepts with which man starts out in his quest for understanding nature.

In addition to explaining in evolutionary terms how the human brain and its epiphenomenon, the mind, can gain possession of *a priori* concepts that match reality, modern biology has also shown that the brain does appear to operate according to principles which correspond to the tenets of structuralism. By this statement I do not mean that the neurological correlates of any of the structuralist theories, particularly not of Freud's subconscious, or of Levi-Strauss' ethnological universals, or of Chomsky's universal grammar have actually been found. Such a claim would be nonsensical, inasmuch as it is not even known in which parts of the brain the corresponding processes occur. What I do mean, however, is that neurological studies have indicated that, in accord with the structuralist tenets, information about the world reaches the depths of the mind, not as raw data but as highly processed structures that are generated by a set of stepwise, preconscious informational transformations of the sensory input. These neurological transformations proceed according to a program that preexists in the brain. The neurological findings thus lend biological support to the structuralist dogma that explanations of behavior must be formulated in terms of such deep programs and reveal the wrong-headedness of the positivist approach which rejects the postulation of covert internal programs as "mentalism".

One set of such neurological findings concerns the manner in which the nervous system of higher vertebrates, including man, converts the light rays entering the eyes into a visual percept. For the purpose of this discussion it is useful to recall that the nervous system is divisible into three parts: (1) an input or *sensory* part that informs the animal about its external and internal environment; (2) an output, or *effector,* part that produces motion by commanding muscle contraction, and (3) an *internuncial* part that connects the sensory and effector parts. The most elaborate portion of the internuncial part is the brain. The brain does much more than merely connect sensory and effector parts, however: it processes information. This processing consists in the main in making an *abstraction* of the vast amount of data continuously gathered by the sensory part. In order to abstract, the brain destroys selectively portions of the input data and thus transforms these data into manageable categories, or *structures* that are meaningful to the animal. It is on the basis of the perceived meaning that the international part issues the relevant commands to the effector part which then result in an appropriate motor response.

For vision, the input part of the nervous system is located in the retina at the back of the eye. There a two-dimensional array of about a hundred million primary light receptor cells — the rods and the cones — converts the radiant energy of the image projected via the lens on the retina into a pattern of electrical signals, much as a television camera does. Since the electrical response of each light receptor cell depends on the intensity of light that happens to fall on it, the overall activity pattern of the light receptor cell array represents the light intensity existing at a hundred million different points in the visual space. The retina contains not only the input part of the visual system, however, but also the first stages of the internuncial part. These first internuncial stages include another two-dimensional array of nerve cells, namely the million or so *ganglion cells*. The ganglion cells receive the electrical signals generated by the hundred million light receptor cells and subject them to information processing. The result of this processing is that the activity pattern of the ganglion cells constitutes a more abstract representation of the visual space than the activity pattern of the light receptor cells. For instead of reporting the light intensity existing at a single point in the visual space, each ganglion cell signals the light-dark *contrast* which exists between the center and the edge of a circular *receptive field* in the visual space. Each receptive field consists of about a hundred contiguous points monitored by individual light receptor cells. The physiological mechanisms by means of which the input point-by-point light intensity information are more or less understood. They can be epitomized simply by stating that the light receptor cells reporting from points at the center or the edge of the receptive field make respectively excitatory or inhibitory connections with their correspondent-ganglion cell. Thus the ganglion cell is maximally excited if the field center receptors are struck by bright light while the field edge receptors are in the dark. In this way, the point-by-point fine-grained light intensity information is boiled down to a somewhat coarser field-by-field light contrast representation, thanks to an algebraic summation of the outputs of an interconnected ensemble of a hundred contiguous light receptor cells. As can be readily appreciated, such light contrast information is essential for the recognition of shapes and forms in space, which is what visual perception mainly amounts to.

For the next stage of processing the visual information leaves the retina via the nerve fibers of the ganglion cells. These fibers connect the eye with the brain, and after passing a way station in the midbrain the output signals of the ganglion cells reach the cerebral cortex at the lower back of the head. Here the signals converge on a set of cortical nerve cells. Study of the cortical nerve cells receiving partially abstracted visual input has shown that each of them responds only to light rays reaching the eye from a limited set of contiguous points in the visual space. But the structure of the receptive fields of these cortical nerve cells is more complicated and their size is larger than that of the receptive fields of the retinal ganglion cells. Instead of representing the light-dark contrast existing between the center and the edge of circular receptive fields, the cortical nerve cells signal the contrast which exists along straight line edges whose length amounts to many diameters of the circular ganglion cell receptive fields. A given cortical cell becomes active if a straight line edge of a particular orientation—horizontal, vertical or oblique—formed by the border of contiguous areas of high and low light intensity is present in its receptive field. For instance, a vertical bar of light on a dark background in some part of the visual field may produce a vigorous response in a particular cortical nerve cell, and that response will cease if the bar is tilted away from the vertical or moved outside the receptive field. Actually, there exist two different kinds of such nerve cells in the cerebral cortex: *simple* cells and *complex* cells. The response of simple cells demands that the straight edge stimulus must not only have a given orientation but also a precise position in the receptive field. The stimulus requirements of complex cells are less demanding, however, in that their response is sustained upon parallel displacements (but not upon tilts) of the straight edge stimuli within the receptive field. Thus the process of abstraction of the visual input begun in the retina is carried to higher levels in the cerebral cortex. The simple cells, which evidently correspond to the first cortical abstraction stage, transform the data supplied by the retinal ganglion cells concerning the light-dark contrast within small circular receptive fields into information concerning the contrast present along sets of circular fields arranged in straight lines. And the complex cells carry out the next cortical abstraction stage. They transform the contrast data concerning particular straight line sets of circular receptive fields into information concerning the contrast present at parallel sets of straight line sets of circular receptive fields.

It is not clear at present how far this process of cerebral abstraction by convergence of visual channels can be imagined to go. Nerve cells have already been found in the cerebral cortex which respond optimally to *straight-line ends* or *corners* in the receptive fields. Evidently, the output of these cells represents an even higher level of abstraction than the parallel straight lines of a given orientation to which the complex cells respond. But should one suppose that the cellular abstraction process goes so far that there exists for every meaningful structure of whose specific recognition an animal is capable (e.g. "my grandmother") at least one particular nerve cell in the cerebral cortex that responds if and only if the light and dark pattern from which that structure is abstracted appears in its visual space? This could very well be the case for lower vertebrates, with their limited behavioral repertoire. For instance, there is neurological evidence that the visual system of the frog abstracts its input data in such a way as to produce only two meaningful structures, "my prey" and "my predator", which, in turn, evoke either of two alternative motor outputs, attack or flight. But in the case of man, with his vast semantic capacities, this picture does not appear very plausible, despite the fact that the human brain has many more nerve cells than the frog's brain. Somehow, for man the notion of the single cerebral nerve cell as the ultimate element of meaning seems worse than a gross oversimplification; it seems qualitatively wrong. Yet, so far at least, it is the only neurologically coherent scheme that can be put forward.

Here we encounter what could turn out to be a barrier to the scientific effort to understand man. I think it is highly significant that in working out his structuralist linguistic theory, Chomsky has encountered the greatest difficulty with the semantic component. Thus far, he has been unable to spell out how that presumably universal component manages to extract meaning from the informational content of the deep structure. It is over just the problem of meaning that disputes have arisen between Chomsky and some of his students, and it does not seem that any solution is presently in sight. The obstacle in the way of giving a satisfactory account of the semantic component appears to reside in defining clearly the problem that is to be solved. That is to say, for man the concept of "meaning" can be fathomed only in relation to an even more elusive notion, namely that of the *self*, which is both ultimate source and ultimate destination of semantic signals. But the concept of the self, the cornerstone of Freud's analytical psychology, cannot be given an explicit definition. Instead, the meaning of "self", or of its old-time, pre-scientific equivalent "soul", is intuitively obvious. It is another Kantian *a priori* concept, one which we bring to man, just as we bring the concepts of space and time to nature. The concept of self can serve the student of man as long as he does not probe too deeply. However, when it comes to explaining the innermost workings of the mind—the deep structure of structuralism—then, just as microscopic physics or cosmology, this attempt to increase the range of understanding raises, in Bohr's terms, "questions as to the sufficiency of concepts and ideas incorporated in daily language". From this ultimate insufficiency of the everyday concepts which our brain obliges us to use for science it does not, of course, follow that further study of the mind should cease, no more than it follows from it that one should stop further study of microscopic physics. But I think that it is important to give due recognition to this fundamental epistemological limitation to the human sciences, if only as a safeguard against the psychological or sociological prescriptions put forward by people who allege that they have already managed to gain a scientifically validated understanding of man.

Marius Jeuken

Commentary

It was a pleasure for me to comment on Dr. Stent's paper, for in it I found some ideas which I myself had been thinking over in my reflections on the relation between philosophy and natural science, especially biology. My commentary is divided into three items, each of which is a praiseworthy element of Dr. Stent's paper.

These items are:

1. The decline of positivism
2. The emphasis on the so-called deep-structure
3. The reference to the problem of the mind-matter relation.

1. As regards the decline of positivism (in its dual form: the positivism of Hume and the neo-positivism of Wiener Kreis) Stent sees structuralism as an answer to modern problems, and illustrates it, referring to the role of the subconscious (Freud), to ethnology (Levi-Strauss) and to linguistics (Chomsky). I would like to point out that structuralism is not the only answer to positivism. Stent too says that there are philosophical alternatives, and it is my opinion that they must not be underestimated.

That positivism was one-sided was already acknowledged in philosophies more or less in the positivist tradition, especially in so-called analytical philosophy. Some examples:

a. *Moore* emphasized the common sense idea. Common sense is expressed in ordinary everyday language. In his ethics, common sense and intuition are basic concepts. Some innateness must be assumed.

b. *Russell* on the contrary had not much confidence in common sense, and ordinary language, but sought after an ideal logical language. Maybe there is some relationship with Chomsky's deep structure of language. The co-author of *Principia Mathematica*, Whitehead, became the great metaphysicist of Harvard University, and certainly cannot be called a positivist.

c. *Wittgenstein* wrote his *Philosophical Investigations* during his Cambridge period (1953) in which he proposed his theory of language games. The statements which in the positivist's theory were senseless, such as statements on aesthetics and metaphysics, got sense by means of the language games principle.

Other reactions on positivism are known as well, more from outside the positivist tradition:

a. Reactions of philosophers of dialectical materialism, as Marcuse. His criticism of the one-dimensional man who in his alienation is incapable of realizing his real self-development, his responsibility and his freedom, is an indication that Marcuse cannot be called a positivist. He expects little or nothing from science, it is true. According to him science is too much tied to the study of existing reality, whereas the not-yet-existing must also be explored.

b. The position of the renewed Aristotelian philosophy is far removed from positivism.

c. The idea of structure is not a new one. In biology we have the holist theory, already brought forward by Smuts. Afterwards followed organicism, being Von Bertalanffy's solution for the mechanicism-vitalism controversy. "The whole is more than the sum of its parts." In cybernetics the functioning organized structure is the central idea. In psychology we have Kohler's Gestalt theory. We can say: what organicism in in biology, is structuralism in ethnology and linguistics.

However, I think that the main reason why Dr. Stent emphasizes structuralism is that in structuralism we find the idea of the so-called deep structure, innate in man, *a priori* given. And this brings me to the second item.

2. *The emphasis on the so-called deep structure.*

In biology the need for philosophical reflection and for a sound philosophical basis has always been felt. There is a famous saying:

"When you scratch a biologist, you find a philosopher under the skin." Contrary to theoretical physics, theoretical biology was from the beginning philosophy of biology. Only later did biomathematics come into existence.

Likewise contrary to modern physics, where mathematical explanation is almost the only explanation admitted, we have in biology various kinds of explanation, such as causal explanation, teleological explanation, historical explanation, morphological explanation etc. So in the study of animal and human behavior we know the idea of the innate, and it is precisely the innate where the deep structures lie. Innate can be explained as: "given with our being". Maybe this notion of the innate in biology has been transferred to other fields of thinking like ethnology and linguistics. One can call the innate also the *a priori*, but in my opinion it is not necessary to refer to Kant. Other modern philosophical systems know the contents of this notion too. In connection with this I would like to indicate some points in which I disagree with Stent —a disagreement however that may enliven the discussion.

• When Stent uses the term "verification" he seems only to have in mind the positivist's conception of verification. However, I think that nowadays the term verification tends to the generic meaning on "making true in general"; so that in the various fields of knowledge—biology, philosophy, theology—the concomitant specific kind of verification must be sought out.

• When Stent discusses Bohr's and Levi-Strauss' ideas on ethnology, he seems to agree that functionality has no explanatory power. This is not in accordance with data of modern biology. Here we acknowledge the value of functional or teleological explanation, not as a substitute for causal explanation, but as another way of seeing the phenomena. So functional explanation cannot be opposed to causal explanation; both explain the whole phenomenon in one of its aspects. The total explanation of the phenomenon is the result of all the aspects together: causal, teleological, mathematical, historical, morphological and maybe more still.

• The structure of our chromosomal pattern and the structure of cytoplasmic elements are the basis of our being Homo

Sapiens. That natural selection is conditional for the coming
into existence of this pattern, is a valid theory. However, the
question is whether natural selection, if it is a necessary condition, is also a sufficient condition in evolutionary theory.
Natural selection certainly leads us to a historical explanation, but I doubt whether it is also a causal explanation, I
think, however, that evolutionary theory is not necessary to
explain our *a priori* concepts.

• In his interesting desciption of the way our visual pattern works, Stent finally points out the structures in our
brain cortex. He calls them "the depths of mind", but the
question is whether this notion of the "deep" is the same as
in "deep structures". And are these structures necessarily
correlated with the deep structures of the mind? Of course
in the unity of mind and matter, there must be a material
correlate for our mental activities, but it seems premature
to me to indicate already certain structures as the material
basis for the mental deep structure. Moreover the term
"structure" has a different meaning in the various language
games of biology, ethnology and linguistics. And this leads
me to the third item.

3.   *The problem of the mind-matter relation.*

Stent indicates this problem at the end of his paper. The real
problem for our knowledge is how concrete, individual representations and perceptions of the object in the brain cortex can yield
abstract universal ideas in our mind. This is the problem of
extracting general meaning from concrete information.

In my opinion Chomsky is on the wrong track looking for an
explanation in brain structures. Not only is the language of natural science insufficient, it is incapable. For an explanation we
have to change over to another language game, the language of
metaphysics. The concept of meaning belongs to the metaphysical language, whereas the description of brain structures is on the
level of scientific language. Maybe a renewed positive metaphysical understanding of matter can give a clue for solution.

Daniel N. Robinson

c2 Some Thoughts on the Matter Of the Mind/Body Problem

Abstract

Every major philosopher since Descartes has devoted a portion of his work of a "solution" of the Mind/Body problem. The major psychologists of the nineteenth century also offered a variety of solutions. A temporary and largely unproductive halt in speculation was achieved by the half century of Behaviorism, but the issue is once more attracting the attention of serious scientists and neuropsychologists.

Unfortunately, the modern revival has tended to ignore the rich history of discourse on this issue and has, as a result, been given to committing a number of the old blunders. Some spokesmen, perhaps owing to a lower threshold for frustration, have abandoned the problem, and have dismissed the entire affair as a "pseudo-issue", destined to evaporate in a purer linguistic climate.

It can be shown, however, that the Mind/Body problem is a bona fide issue for science — though not necessarily for experimental science — and one which is likely to determine, in principle, the degree to which the "unity of sciences" is likely to become a reality. At a more specific level, the MIND/BODY problem serves as the acid-test of those theoretical attempts in the biological and psychological disciplines which seek to assimilate *homo cogitans*.

* * *

In his oft-cited and regularly misunderstood *De Anima*, Aristotle sought to establish the boundary-conditions within which a purely naturalistic science might address itself to the facts of life. As every undergraduate learns, Aristotle found little difficulty in relating the nutritive, sensitive, reproductive, and locomotor functions of the soul to the physiological processes of the organism. However, on the question of *intellect*, he is found to be rather more diffident. It was Aristotle's thesis that there must be some common elements shared in any causal sequence. Or, as his Scholastic commentators put it, nothing can be the cause of anything unless the two events have a likeness. On this construction of causation, the empirical knowledge of man and brute pose no difficulty for the materialist. A knowledge of *things* can, somehow, be acquired by anything capable of being impressed or otherwise stimulated. But the rational knowledge of man — a knowledge which includes *universal* truths — cannot be imparted by things, or by particulars of any kind. Thus, such knowledge is not the gift of our sensitive faculty.

Aristotle's relaxation of this epistemological tension was to accord transcendental status to the rational faculty, and to render intellect "impassable". This summit of mental achievements was, on his account, attained only by human beings, and represented a condition of mind which was indestructible. After all, to be destroyed or to undergo degeneration, an entity must be material; to be material, it must be particular; but to be particular, it cannot partake of the universal. Accordingly, and with the legislative authority of the syllogism, Aristotle was able to conclude that the feature of mind which communes with "universals" is, itself, eternal. Lest this analysis make a modern audience too hopeful, it is sadly necessary to note that the eternal life granted here is not a *personal* survival after the death of the body. Persons, after all, are *individuals!*

Even in this very sketchy summary of *De Anima*, we begin to see the scientific implications of the Mind/Body problem, and also the complexity of the web of suppositions surrounding the problem. It is clear, for example, that Aristotle was forced to his position on the "impassability" of reason by the prior position he had taken on the question of causation. As I shall discuss further on, there is still a close connection between the two issues in modern scholarship, although it is a different sort of connection from the one established by Aristotle. It should also be clear that at least since the Hellenistic period, philosophers have recognized that the pecular properies of *mind* would constitute the acid-test of any naturalistic metaphysics.

Since Aristotle's day, countless figures in the history of ideas have faced the Mind/Body problem, and a fair share of them were persuaded that they solved it—once and for all! A review of their efforts is beyond the scope of this treatment. Instead, it will be sufficient to summarize the several categories into which all these attempts can be placed.

At the coarsest level of classification, the entire history of speculation can be reduced to the two headings, "Monism" and "Dualism". Monists and dualists, however, present themselves in a variety of forms. There are, for example, *mentalistic* monists such as George Berkeley, and *materialistic* monists such as La Mettrie. There is also the rarer species — the so-called "neutral monist"—who will not commit himself either to a universe that is exclusively spiritual or to one that is exclusively material, but who rejects duality. In his formative years, Bertrand Russell was pleased to espouse this position, but even his charisma could not attract many disciples to this position.

Perhaps the most popular form of monism is that which serves as the foundation of "double-aspect" theories. This is the monism of many of the great names in nineteenth century science: Thomas Huxley, C. Lloyd Morgan, Ernst Haeckel, Alexander Bain (on certain accounts). The "double-aspect" theorist has the laudable penchant for conciliation. He insists that the organism is unitary, but that it displays two aspects; a mental and a physical. Neither is completely reducible to the other; neither is more valid than the other. Indeed, there are not two *realities,* but two *aspects* of a single reality. Here, of course, we have a monism almost shamelessly courting dualism.

As for dualism, it, too, has been served up in various fashions and has enjoyed the support of famous and accomplished figures in science and philosophy. The most common form of dualism, and the form which seems to dominate our contemporary metaphysics, labors under the title, "epiphenomenalism". Aherents of this thesis accept the validity of Mind, but insist that all mental events, states, and processes are uniquely caused by physical events, states, and processes. The physical work required by this thesis is generally regarded as taking place in the brain, or in the nervous system at large—thus, the Mind/Brain problem instead of the more ambiguous Mind/Body problem.

The two remaining major categories of dualism are "two-way interactionism" and "psychophysical parallelism". In polling my own students from time to time, I have ascertained that the former is most popular among upperclassmen majoring in psychology. The latter enjoys some support from our Theology majors. But the latter also was adopted by Leibniz and by Wilhelm Wundt and, opinion-polls aside, has something to recommend it.

Each of these traditional solutions to the Mind/Body problem has its own body of facts, convictions, and hunches to back it up. Berkeley's *Immaterialism* — as odd as it is irrefutable — begins with the indubitable claim that we can know only the contents of our own minds, and that these are *ideas*. Every knowledge-claim we make which contains non-ideational elements can only be an inference, and cannot be tested except ideationally. Accordingly, the knowable universe is furnished exclusively with ideas. (I put aside the more Delphic entity of "spirit" in the interest of brevity). A thoroughgoing refutation of Berkeley must begin, then, with a demonstration of material existence independently of any *idea* of the putative matter. This, of course, is impossible. The shortest refutation on record is that registered by the foot of Dr. Johnson. Perhaps in kicking the stone, this impatient genius of the *Enlightenment* acted for legions of practical men and women who would find it easier to ignore or ridicule Berkeley than to rebut him. We do, however, find echoes of Berkelean metaphysics in the *phenomealism* of J.S. Mill, where matter is defined as the "permanent possibility of sensation".

Leaving Berkeley—for we must—we arrive at his polar- opposite, *materialistic* monism. In its modern dress, it is called the "Identity Thesis", and is closely associated with the works of J.J.C. Smart. If I were to permit myself a bold speculation, I would insist that the question of the "unity of sciences" will be settled completely by the fate of this thesis. If, as Professor Smart maintains, sensations are not caused by processes in the brain but are, in fact, these very processes, then there would seem to be no reason for psychology not to prepare itself for imminent absorption by physics. The dream of Epicurus will be a reality, and the song of Lucretius a veritable Book of Knowledge. But if, as I suspect, the thesis is either wrong or unintelligible, then the disunity of sciences is likely to be a very long season.

What can be said for the "Identity Thesis" and its older cousins is that they are parsimonious. The history of physics, from the seventeenth century until a few decades ago, lent credence to the antique belief that Nature is not profligate in her laws and operations. For many centuries, scientists have groomed their sensibilities with Ockham's razor and, for the past century, psychology has followed suit on the strength of Lloyd Morgan's famous *canon.* It is less clear, however, what else might be said in favor of *materialistic* monism. The facts of neurophysiology and clinical neurology—to the extent that they are relevant to the issue—will support *epiphenomenalism* and *two-way interactionism* as well as they are said to support the "Identity Thesis". And there are other facts which the "Identity Thesis" cannot confront without embarrassment. There is, for example, the uncontestable authority of percipients in the matter of their first-person reports of sensations. When Mr. Jones insists that he has a toothache, we discover that, in principle, there is nothing we can do to refute the claim. If we assume that Jones is not a liar, we accept without hesitation not only that, indeed, he has a toothache, but that his sensation will serve as our only means of ever developing impersonal methods of detecting such events. Thus, even if we choose to test Jones's credibility—for example, by recording the discharge-patterns from his dental nerves—we can only do so with instruments which have been "calibrated" against the claims of other Joneses.

This status which attaches to cooperative (i.e., non-deceptive) first-person reports of sensation is unique. There is no statement which Jones might make about nerves, brains, or glial cells which, in principle, cannot be proven to be wrong. But what Jones says about his aches, hopes, and passions is, in principle, irrefutable. The implication of this to the "Identity Thesis" should be obvious. If everything one might say about processes in the brain is, in principle, refutable, and if nothing said by Jones about his sensations is, in principle, refutable, then Jones's brain processes and sensations are not identical.

This is not the only problem which infects the "Identity Thesis". In an almost perverse way, the thesis pushes its adherent firmly in the direction of Berkeley's curious metaphysics. It converts all mental events to events in the brain, and all reports of mental events into reports of processes in the brain. It is not at all clear that an external world can survive this analysis. And, as in the case of Berkeley's argument, it revives the vexing problem of "other minds". It does this by converting the problem of "other minds" to that of "other brains", but it offers us no means by which our brains can be conversant with these other brains. Nor does it tell us how, given a nervous system which is probably never in the same state on any two successive occasions, there can be continuity of "self", or of "self-identity".

With respect to this latter problem the "Identity Thesis" is hardly alone in its awkwardness. All materialistic accounts of "self", when examined closely are found to be incredible. This is due principally to the historical tendency of materialistic metaphysics to ally itself with empiricistic epistemologies. The usual argumentative chain is as follows: (a) all we know is furnished exclusively by experience; (b) experiences are the consequence of sensory events which are impressed upon the nervous centers; (c) a history of experience is possible as a result of residual *traces* or chemical codes formed in these nervous centers pursuant to stimulation; (d) one's sense of "self"—as a continuing personal identity—is but these memories.

It was Descartes who introduced the fashion of doubting one's own existence, but it has had a longer life than most fashions in philosophy. Locke was the first of many to settle the issue by taking recourse to memories, but Thomas Reid's utter devastation of this theory has not prevented others from following in Locke's footsteps. Examining the proposition that "self" is identical to "memories", Reid offered this illustration:

1. There is a brave officer who remembers being the small boy punished years earlier for stealing from the orchard.
2. There is a decorated General who recalls being the brave officer, but who has no recollection of the small boy punished in the orchard.

On Locke's account, the small boy is identical to the brave officer; and the brave officer is identical to the decorated General; but the small boy and the decorated General are not identical. In other words, A ^{5} B and B ^{5} C, but A $^{5/}$ C. Thus, the thesis bears the double-burden of implausibility and self-contradiction. I might note that the modern Lockeans who would use the findings resulting from surgical separation of the hemispheric connections to challenge the concept of a "unified self", fall into the same trap. The patient never doubts his "personal identity", but does provide conflicting responses on tests of memory. For such facts to sustain the claim that multiple identities are involved, it would be necessary to reduce "self" to "memory"—and we see that this cannot be done with logical impunity.

Berkeley's *Immaterialism* is something we have agreed to praise and to bury, and the "Identity Thesis" is bloated with difficulties even when it is expressed coherently. Thus, among the *monisms,* we are left with the Double-Aspect theory. It promises to give us the same parsimoniousness and it also allows us to continue speaking intelligibly and scientifically about minds. Moreover, it seems to be at least metaphorically related to that lingering dualism in physics whose demon has been named the *wavicle.* But the metaphor cannot be said to be entirely apt. There are electromagnetic phenomena which are best explained in terms of quantum-effects; others in terms of wave-mechanical effects. But both classes of effects are amenable to identical procedures of quantification, and both classes fit into that matrix of explanatory devices known as the laws of radiation and matter. The *wavicle* in physics should, on the "double-aspect" account, have a corresponding entity—let us call it the *mentasome*—in the realm of Mind/Body. But the plain fact is that virtually *none* of the predicates ordinarily assigned to mental events can be plausibly assigned to somatic events. Merely on the face of it, there would seem to be no two entities drawn from the universe of realities which are less similar than the mental and the somatic. All the events in one are explicable in the scientific language of *causation,* but most of the truly interesting events in the other seem not to be. This is not to say that the actions of psychological beings are inexplicable; only that the explanations are not of the scientific, causal sort.

What I mean by "truly interesting" are those events which, for want of a clearer term, might be called *historical.* These are the events which have significant effects on the personal or social history of a species—and here I am considering only our own species. When we attempt to provide an explanation for such events, we generally take recourse to the language of *reasons,* not the language of *causes.* This gets us back to the remarks I made regarding Aristotle, and the connection between the Mind/Body problem and theories of causation. If we ask, "Why did Pericles urge Athenians to destroy their possessions on the eve of battle with the Spartans?", we surely do not want to be told, "Because of neuromuscular discharges in his tongue and larynx". The question seeks to penetrate the *reasons* Pericles had for making such a speech, and not the physical causes by which speech of any kind is produced.

Here we have another difference between the *wavicle* in physics and the *mentasome* in psychology. Whether the physicist is concerned with waves or particles, the fundamental logic of explanation is the same. But those who would seek to understand why Pericles spoke as he did, or why Smith sold his properties in Wales, or why Jack chose the train over the airplane, will only be satisfied with a *rational* account of such actions. If treated to a *causal* account, they will assume their correspondent is being droll. It is like being told, when asking why so many men have died in war, that their blood pressure dropped.

This is not to say, however, that no form of Double-Aspect theory is likely to be satisfying. Over the past decade, Professor Pribram has attempted to develop a *holographic* theory of perception and memory; a theory which, like its *Gestalt* ancestors, proposes an isomorphic resemblance between the structure of psychological events and the structure of neural correlates. Professor Pribram is not to be faulted for the historic habit of modelling the human nervous system after the most current productions of technology. Descartes had his hydraulic pumps, J.S. Mill his "mental chemistry", Sherrington his cables, and Hebb his "assemblages". Why should we deny Dr. Pribram his holograms! But the point, of course, is not whether holograms are apt. The point is that a Double-Aspect theory which goes no further than the one bequeathed by the nineteenth century is little more than religious science. Pribram has set forth a *substantive* rather than a polemical theory and has, in my view, given Double-Aspect theories a new lease. More importantly, he is to my knowledge the only Double-Aspect theorist who has stated the case in a manner which, at least in principle, is amenable to experimental refutation. This will be no easy trick, but it is not arrantly impossible, whereas experimental refutation of the "Identity Thesis" is.

It is probably all too evident from what I have said that I judge the historic attempts to reduce Mind to Body as failures, and that—from my own reading of this literature—I do not see much by way of encouragement on the horizon. It is by no means clear, however, that even if my own estimations are correct, the "unity of sciences" is a casualty. Behaviorism and its twin—associationism—diverted the intellectual energies of psychology for far too many years. All sorts of facile and occasionally agile evasions were promoted by this perspective such that, even today, many otherwise serious scientists accept reductionism as the official method of the sciences. The leaders of the behavioristic schools— and these schools are ancient—have always tied their claims to the achivements in physics and biology; often corrupting the facts and theories established in these other disciplines. Ironically, behaviorism has always leaned on evolutionary biology for support. Yet, there is nothing in the theory of evolution which requires all species to develop the same adaptive mechanisms. Quite the contrary. Evolutionary biology leaves as much room for the appearance of *mind* in the natural world as it does for prehensile forelimbs or for feathers. Thus, psychology need not fear that, in accepting the *facts* of human mental life, it somehow is cutting itself loose from Darwin's science.

Associationism infected modern psychology with a quieter but equally lethal notion. It convinced a woeful number of psychologists that the final product of associative learning contained all the elements involved in all the stages leading to the final product. On the traditional associationistic account, then, we should expect the accomplished pianist to repeat all the errors made in the course of his training! This was the line of reasoning that led to the otherwise incredible notion that the richest expressions of human cognition were, in principle, reducible to elemental forms of associational learning. Let us agree that there are good and bad forms of reductionism, and that the bad form invariably asks us to eliminate facts for the sake of the theory.

I noted that a failure on the part of reductionism does not, *ipso facto* spell doom for the "unity of sciences". Doom can be averted by the expansion of the established sciences to embrace the logical and geometric coherence of *homo cogitans*. Physics, after all, can trace as many of its triumphs to an expansion of the conceptual bandwidth as to a narrowing. Not everything in physics must be *reduced* to principles of sub-atomic interactions. And if astrophysics can proclaim its scientific status even while ignoring xi-zeta particles, one would think that psychology can proceed scientifically even if it cannot cram a thought into a neuron. Moreover, we already have refined models of human cognition, although we have yet to come to think of them as models. Let me mention a few: Euclidean Geometry, Model logic, Constitutional Law, Algebra, Music. In reciting this short list I do not intend to display my "humanistic" credentials, nor am I offering a veiled defense of romanticism. In as hard-nosed a fashion as is possible, I am suggesting that these subjects and achievements are veritable working-diagrams of human mental organization. They are star-charts for astronomers of the mind and blueprints for architects of the mind. They tell us far more about the intrinsic "design" features of the human nervous system than can be gleaned in a millenium of bar-presses and key-pecks. Like the geological records which waited for a Darwin, these records of mental evolution are already there. It requires no experiment to unearth them, no technology to assess them. What is required is that nemesis of so-called "objective psychology", a *theory*. And, in light of the manner in which psychologists have approached this mission over the past fifty years, there would seem to be no reason for physicists to be sheepish.

Juan Antonio Gomez

C3 Neurological Correlations of Some Universal Principles

It has been said many times that the knowledgeable are beings and that the being who knows is man. Even though, this last statement may constitute only a partial truth, in our case, it is valid and pertinent, because this particular form of knowledge that we refer to as science and its possibly unity, is the subject of this conference. Although, it has not been clarified, if the different sciences can be "reduced",[1] following the example of chemistry and atomic physics, or "unified"[2] by the creation or encountering of a common language, or "articulated"[3] in a hierarchical structure, we can begin with the assertion that the universal instrument of sciences is the human brain. With that in mind, we can restate the question of unity among the sciences on a physiological ground.

It is natural, therefore, that we initially inquire into the way that sensations are registered and compared in a cortical or subcortical level, although, it is not necessary to know completely the functioning of the central nervous system to analyze the final product of its activity. On the contrary, the observations of regularities in the handling of sensible representations or concepts can provide many clues of the organization of neuronal networks. It is, therefore, preferable to compare what is known of neurophysiology and what is observable in the form of thought, in order to establish correlations.

There must be a conformity of structures[4] if translation is possible from outside events to inner ideation and from reasoning to outside facts as when an hypothesis is tested.

Piaget[5] justifies the psychologist's interest, in logic in the way that it permits building a pure model of thought structures.

Similar reasoning could be used by the neurophysiologist in searching after psychological events, because they have all been correlated with the whole or the parts of the encephalon and the mounting neurological and neuropathological evidence indubitably points in favor of those assertions. Clinical records and experimental data support this indisputably. Minor mental disorders and abstract thinking, space and time concepts and all forms of language have been related casually with the functioning of the nervous system. Lesions in restricted cortical regions can produce motor or receptive asphasias, different types of agnosias, apraxia, amnesias, dyscalculia, disorientation and inability in the use of symbols. It is not necessary to take part in the issue of holistic vs. limited cortical localizations, because in either case the parallelism between brain and psyche is implicit.

Besides these functions there are elements in our intellectual activity of a general nature not ascribable to any particular area, that we may consider as keystones for the analysis that we are trying to pursue. The first one and the one that has concerned philosophers more, is the presence of truth and falsity in thought. Since ancient Greece, it has been accepted that such values do not belong to things but to propositions and that error and knowledge imply combinations and separations.

The second element is that apparently we can only comprehend in terms of relations. The third element, similar to the previous one is that all psychological phenomena are surrounded by an associative halo, or, according to the simile used by James[6] any definite image is embedded in and colored by the free waters that flow around it, being blood and bone of its bone and flesh of its flesh. The fourth element that must be accepted is that learning is conditioned by developmental stages[7] and the fifth is that thinking tends to generalizations. Finally, it should be pointed out that oppositions seem indispensable for reasoning.

The principle of contradiction, a case of the more general idea of opposition, has been used in logic to test the truth. Combinations and separations are closely linked to language and imply relations, associations and generalizations, which are part of the process of learning.

Ubiquity of Contraditions in Intellectual Activity

The problem of opposition not only has caused difficulties to philosophers, logicians and mathematicians, but it reappears anywhere, in simple phrases and every day wisdom, as well as in elaborated scientific theories and reflects itself persistently in the pages that narrate the great scenes of mankind's historical drama.

In the beginning with the most elementary cases, let us take, as an example the ancient beliefs that cold and hot were like two antagonistic forces, that heaven and earth were opposed regions, that brutes and men are essentially opposites, that man and woman or male and female are opposed, that love and hate are contradictory, that the white race is intrinsically different to the negro race, that our culture is in contradiction to primitive cultures, that philosophy and sciences are opposed disciplines, that humanistic studies are opposed to natural sciences and that there is a dilemma between environment and inheritance.

The oriental civilization has been presented as a counterplot to western tradition. Bloody battles have been fought for a white rose or a red rose, for catholic belief or protestant ritual, or for belonging to the Right or to the Left. If these tragic consequences of the principle of contradiction did not occur, it would not have been worthwhile to question ourselves about the possible anatomical substratum, or to consider the philosophical meaning.

Wise men have seen in the struggle of contraries a general principle for the organization and evolution of the universe. The Epicurians stated the issue as creation vs. destruction, the Chinese as yin and yang and some theologians in the polarity between good and evil. Many evolutionists were dominated for a while by the generalization of fighting among opposed species as the principal explanation for biological change, and Marxists have taken contradiction and its resolution by violent struggle as one of their fundamental beliefs. If we go back for a while in history to look for guides we can find that in the dawn of western knowledge, Plato systematically utilized opposition to clarify notions, to define statements by dichotomy and to seek the truth by reducing ultimately the arguments to contradictory pairs. According to him every thing has one opposite and no more than one.[8] The Platonic dialogues are beautiful examples of these methods used rigorously in scientific investigation, and even today, it is the most trusted scheme for learning and for problem solving.

But bipartite divisions, objected Aristotle, cannot be applied in many cases because they, necessarily, produce breaking up and dislocation of natural groups.[9] Since then, the concept was refined and framed in the classical square of opposition: correlative opposites in which each term implies the other; contrary opposites as cold and hot; privative opposites as blindness and vision, and the contradictory opposites, or, opposites of affirmation and negation.

The first three cases can be considered as parts of the continuous scale. Only the last case, which is contradiction and, perhaps some of the contrary opposites as even and odd, can be accepted as criteria for truth, because they seem to exhaust all possibilities by an alternative in which there is no room for the more subdivisions.

But even in the case of even and odd there is an unresolved position in the fractional numbers.

Kant restricted more the principle of contradiction since, according to him, only in analytic propositions (affirmative or negative) the truth can always be proved by such a principle that in this case is sufficient and general for all types of knowledge. However, its usefulness and authority cannot be permitted to extend to synthetic propositions because in analytic judgment we can only predicate the concept that is already there, and in synthetical judgment one has to go beyond a given concept and bring another together that is different from what is contained in the first. In this case "we have nothing in the judgment in itself by which we can discover its truth or its falsity."[10] Many contradictions, and precisely the more important ones, belong to the last category and because of that cannot be solved in such a manner and do not belong to the domain of certain knowledge.

By taking one step forward, Hegel[11] denied in fact the principle of contradiction, when he built his doctrine on the synthesis between contradictions. The German thinker found that the terms of a contradiction coexist in reality and that for each judgment there is a contradiction because one implies the other. Even in the case of being and not being, this is true since one contains the notion of the other and can be resolved with the introduction of time element: they are unified in becoming.

Unfortunately, some of his followers have acted thereafter as if instead of resolution of the principle of contradiction the important part of his theories were the contradictions in themselves and the practical consequences that so often result in conflicts. In that case, it could be pointed out not every struggle leads to a synthesis but there can be an absolute conqueror and a complete defeat. The brief enumeration that precedes opposition seems to be present in every form of thinking. The humble phrase and the proud argument, the simple deduction of the forward hypothesis carries its shadow of contradiction.

Physiological Correlations

Let us go back once again to the neuronal level with this enlightenment in order to investigate possible correlations that may help in clarifying our point of concern.

The forms of energy that produce our sensations or reflexes stimulate first the nerve endings of the primary sensory neurons. At that very moment there is already certain modifications of the signals. For example, the type of sensation sometimes depends more in the pathway affected than in the stimulus itself. A light pressure with the point of a pen can be perceived as such or as a cold spot according to the cutaneous region in which it is applied. Even the quality of superficial touch (coarse or fine) is related more to the nature of the neuronal relays than to the type of receptors.

Through the peripheral nerves the signals transformed and coded in the dry language of action potentials, reach the secondary sensory neurons that are located in the gray matter of the cord or in the nuclei of the brain stem. The action potentials are produced by depolarization under the all-or-nothing law. From the secondary sensory neurons the signals relay to the tertiary sensory neurons which project to the cortex where the final analysis is made in the corresponding areas arranged in a somatotopic sequence. But this, of course, is an over simplification because often small neurons are placed between the primary neurons and the tract cells of second order, or between secondary and tertiary neurons. At all levels there is facilitation and inhibition, and the influence of impulses coming from various regions in the central nervous system (including the cortex) is evident. Therefore, any transmission of a message is, in a way, continuously "edited" at the different levels. The coding of a message is achieved by the frequency of action potentials in a given fiber (limited by the refractory period) and by the somatotopic arrangement in the peripheral nerve or in the central pathway. By a general rule, the increase in stimulus strength produces higher rates of discharge, but approximately in a linear function of the logarithm of the stimulus. Correspondingly, the intensity of a sensation is perceived also in logarithmic relation to the magnitude of the stimulus.

Therefore, it seems clear that a process of reorganization and, perhaps true alteration, occurs all along the conduction of a message through successive relays and different pathways until it reaches the cortex. This involves coding and uncoding of signals, inhibition and facilitation, unequal delays that change the time sequence, and convergence, which is one of the more general characteristics of pathway structures in the nervous system. Convergence produces summation of stimuli, which reduces the discriminative quality, but assures a low threshold of sensibility.

The Auditory System

The auditory system may be taken as a significant sample for concrete analysis of the events leading to perception and recognition of given message, because it is the most important pathway for language, a fundamental part of all sciences. The sound waves produce vibrations in the tympanic membrane that are transmitted by the three ossicles to the oval window of the middle ear. They are transformed in pressure waves that finally stimulate the nerve endings in the organ of Corti.

In the simple mechanical transmission through the ossicles there is already a change because they function as a lever, which produces a vibratory force in the oval window 10 times greater than in the tympanic membrane. Inside the organ of Corti the basilar membrance responds to pressure waves by vibrations which occur maximally in different parts of it, according to the pitch of the sound. The vibrations, by a process of transduction in the hair cells produce stimulation of dendritic terminals of cells in the cochlear ganglion. There is overlapping of dendritic fields and also convergence of several hair cells into one ganglion cell.

with the suppressor nerve efferents this arrangement helps in discrimination and localization of stimuli. The region of maximal vibration is interpreted as tone of the sound and this is reinforced by feed back circuits in the central nervous system.

An increase in intensity produces activation of more neurons and also augmentation of the frequency of discharge. The auditory pathway has one or several synaptic relays to the medial geniculate nuclei and from these projects, via the auditory radiation, to the cortex where the signals are analyzed.

Language

Let us take language under the bilateral point of view of neurology and communication theory, in order to show the relations of the different structures involved.

Sound waves that carry the signals, and therefore, subjected to the entropy law, or progressive degradation, have to be transduced and analyzed first in the ear, and then coded, as we have seen, in the binary system of the nerve fiber conduction. Any interference at this level can produce great difficulties of interpretation. The chain of events continues with the transmission, through the auditory pathways, of the signal information complex to the brain where, we believe, must be compared with pre-existing models. In other words, the complex is analyzed by successive stages where the information is restructured to some degree.

At all levels the risk of degradation is critical. Perhaps, this is the fundamental reason why any human language is a communication system highly redundant. In this way, the wealth of information is maintained in spite of a massive aleatory interference acting at the sound end as well as in the consecutive coding and uncoding in the nervous system.

Each word is composed of primary elements called phonemes, that, when heard in a conventional sequence, form a mental image of the word which must be compared, if it is to be comprehended, with a previous experience.

We shall not divide further the phoneme in this occasion but the question of how the brain recognizes each one as a particular entity may be risen since every person pronounces the phonemes in a different way. It is needed, therefore, an analyzer of phonemes as well as one for words, according to Lord Brain.[12] We may add to his general conception of speech that, in our opinion, each mental model (or scheme in his terminology) discharges in a fixed and total manner when it is activated by a variable combination of some characteristic signals of the incoming stimulation. Let us suppose, for example, that three out of five typical elements of an afferent image are necessary to open, in a figurative sense, the lock. In the case of a word, it may be that a phoneme heard from the beginning and one heard at the end, are sufficient to discharge the whole mental model of this particular verbal representation. This variable combination of characteristic signs may be referred to as the essence of a particular set of stimuli coming from outside or from inner representations.

When the minimal necessary conditions are present an impulse or new signal is released and goes on to activate (or to "inform") the next level or model. Then the basic mechanism is repeated: the word (not the word that was heard that could have been incorrectly pronounced or dimmed by noise but the inner symbol, complete, total and simultaneous of the word discharged in response to a special set of impulses) forms a new unity that together with others is recognized by the intellect as a phrase according to its temporal organization. Neither is it necessary that all words in the sentence be present: it can be understood by being aware of only a few important parts of the proposition. Here, we have an explanation that we could advance for the Gestalt psychology.

It is important to add that mental models are dynamic and changeable according to the frequency of the use and with other variables. They include not only the structure with which the combination of the stimuli that we are referring act upon, but also several relations of continuity, similarity (essential or not essential), simultaneity, and perhaps other forms of association with different schemes or mental events even of emotional type.

Now, we can go back to the phrase. When it is recognized or comprehended (that is, compared with models of grammatical or syntactical type) it is important to grasp its meaning which is done in the same manner; by comparing with the structure of the inner or central language where the afferent cycle is completed.

There, in the central language, we find a common ground for both the expressive and receptive speech.

This consecutive decoding by comparison with models more and more general or complex is done in the central nervous system in a simultaneous way at each stage, according to indirect data. Therefore, we have to call for a short memory system to transform the time organization into one of a spatial nature.

It is not necessary to comment on the implications of the theory that we have just finished sketching with respect to the philosophical issue of essences and universal ideas.

All we have left is to emphasize, that, as in any given information analysis, the probability of the message is basic for its comprehension. The probability is conditioned by the relative frequency of the words in speech and by their syntactical arrangement. When one does not understand a sentence for some reason, there is the tendency to assimilate it with the mental scheme more similar and more frequently used. We agree with Broadbent[13] in that the "dictionary units" of the central nervous system are controlled by the last active stimulus and by the present stimulus in a statistical way.

In the expressive side a symmetrical process is postulated. The idea that a person is trying to express at first is conceived as a whole and is present in the mind simultaneously, but perhaps organized in a special structure. Then, the syntactic schemes that we have encountered in the afferent side are used. The words are searched for (sometimes we cannot find them) arranged in a temporal order and finally the process ends in a motor discharge through the complicated mechanisms carried up by the phonetic organs. A small voluntary part puts into action a large unconscious co-ordination without which the performance is not possible.

But the cycle is not yet completed. The last part of it is a feed back through the ear that acts as a controlling link on the spoken word.

The overall significance of the mechanism described is to establish, with the greatest precision the correspondence between the two systems, one primary and the other subordinated, through a series of symbols and with several feed back cycles of positive or negative action.

Thought, in itself, is different from language or at least it is what is suggested by observations of aphasic patients. A similar conclusion can be reached by studying the pauses in every day speech that, according to several authors, are in direct correspondence with selection and stratification of language.

We may add, by the way, that there seems to be intellectual deficit when a patient is aphasic (even though his I.Q. remains above average). It must be accepted as well, that language helps thought, not only because it is the vehicle of information not easily obtained by other means, but because it carries with it the structured experiences of a given human culture and because the use of symbols facilitates mental operations.

From what has been already said it can be inferred that all intellectual activities are structured in one way or another. This is true for the simple reflexes or for abstract cogitations, for feelings and for emotions.

All mental structures are related in successive links although not necessarily by unidirectional connections. In the inferior levels predominate stereotyped reactions to stimuli, but there is already certain analysis and influence of previous experiences. When we ascend in the Jacksonian sense, in the upper levels, the responses to stimuli are more flexible and can be delayed more. At the cortical level the structures are somehow more fluid and the schemes and models become the key elements of intellectual activities.

The first step in the formation of schemes could be the simple association by proximity in space or time of group of stimuli. A given scheme can be composed by visual, tactile, auditive impressions plus coincidental emotions and memories. But the associative body in such a manner formed may not correspond at all to logical relations or formal thinking. The repetition of the same aggregates or stimuli slowly fixes the scheme until it becomes something that we may call a model. The majority of them have an associated word that in a given case can act as its symbol.

If we take a person that sees one or several implements for writing consisting of a slender cylinder containing a solid marking substance, we may assume that he forms in his mind the scheme of a pencil, in which there may be associated qualities irrelevant to the strict concept of pencil, as the yellow color or the circumstance that he only has observed such implements in connection with lined paper. By observations of increasing numbers of similar objects the most common properties are reinforced and the less generalized are weakened (although they do not disengage completely from the scheme) until a concept of a pencil is constituted or, following the terminology used before, a model is formed. According to what we have suggested, a variable combination of a few of the common and perhaps some of the less frequent attributes of the object, would be able to arouse the complete and general idea with all the characteristics considered essential and surrounded by the associated representations that, even though vague and imprecise, remained attached to it like an aureola.

These latter types of loose associations are used poetically with highly gratifying and aesthetic consequences (sometimes) and involuntary in organic brain syndromes, common lapses, subconscious representations, dementia, intoxications, extreme fatique and other occasions where there is a defit in reasoning. Only vigilant attention prevents a model from discharging by irrelevant associations that always exists in the free waters, as James would call it, of the stream of thought. It is possible that attention may act by peripheral inhibition and perhaps secondary facilitation of the signals more frequently related to a given model which are what we call commonly the essential attributes.

In practice any pair of stimuli can be linked seemingly in a rather mechanical way, if they are close in time. The Pavlovian school may show many examples which have been analyzed carefully with remarkable productivity results for psychology.

Once the model is established it is used actively in new situations and applied to new objects for the sake of comparison. Consequences are inferred from it, but in many occasions we may recognize an implement bearing some similarity to it as a pencil which in fact may not be. The new concept leads to generalizations and generates new lines of thinking becoming a totalizer model. The mental models slowly become more regular and tend to great symmetry, as has been shown with memories. A totalizer model may be used indefinitely until by experience more often or by thought, infrequently, a similar but not equal assembly of signals is found which would be inconvenient to assimilate with the pre-existing model. The previous model is in a situation of direct inapplicability, but retains its utility by serving as a comparative base against which the new scheme can be brought together for the purpose of noting points of lightness and difference. Here we have to augment our attention in order to distinguish signals that before were linked to another scheme or model. This can be achieved by dividing them into two categories: one being the old model and the other, the new representation which usually is the same old model plus some negative condition about a few of the attributes that before were considered essential, plus elements from the new model.

In the world of reality there are no negative facts, but the brain, when it distinguishes, may introduce a negation which often creates a position in its more extreme case.

Not only because of the all or nothing law that governs conduction along nerve fibers, but also for what we have postulated for the functioning of mental models and for the last consideration about the tendency to oppose when a distinction is made, we can explain the omnipresence of opposition in the intellectual realm. The fight that against the opposition has been a permanent struggle of the spirit. We should remember finally that an inadequate representation can be true, as Hessen has declared[14] because even if it is incomplete it can be exact if the notes that it contains are really in the object. But if we take as a starting point an incomplete representation as is true of all objects represented in our mind, it is possible and easy to err. With the purpose of constant correction of the correspondence between the thought system and the real relations in events or things that the intellect aspires to reproduce, the different ways of establishing truth or falsity in judgments were introduced.

The process of modeling, synthesis and differentiation generates wider and wider circles of mental associations that may bring about many errors but also lead to universal concepts and finer distinctions. In experimental sciences the latter tendency predominates but we should not lose sight of the inherited structure of our brain which imposes limitations upon us like the tendency to understand by opposition. The dialectic controversies that have obstructed progress in the unity of sciences may not be real but a projection of our gusto for contradiction.

BIBLIOGRAPHY

1. Neurath, *Unified Science as Encyclopedic Integration.* In International Encyclopedia of United Sciences, Chicago, 1938.
2. Carnap, *Logical foundations of the Unity of Sciences.* In International Encyclopedia of United Sciences, Chicago, 1938.
3. Federici C., *Elements de Logica y Metodologia.* Universidad Nacional de Colombia, 1974.
4. Russell B., *El Conocimiento Humano.* Editorial Taurus, Madrid, 1968.
5. Piaget J., *Traite de Logique.* Paris, Colin, 1949.
6. James W., *Compendio de Psicologia.* Editorial Emece, Buenos Aires, 1951.
7. Piaget J., *Le developpment de la notion de temps chez l' enfant.* Paris, P.U.F., 1946.
8. Plato, *Protagoras.* Obras Completas. Editorial Omeba, Buenos Aires, 1967.
9. Aristotle, *Prior Analytics.* Obras Completas. Editorial Aguilar, Madrid, 1967.
10. Kant E., *Critica de la Razon Pura.* Obras Selectas. Editorial Ateneo, Buenos Aires, 1950.
11. Hegel, *Philosophy of History.* Oxford University Press, 1952.
12. Lord Brain, *Speech Disorders.* In Disorders of Language. Spencer and Churchill, London.
13. Broadbent, D.E., *Perceptual and response factor in the organization of Speech.* In Disorders of Language. Spencer and Churchill, London.
14. Hessen J., *Teoria del Conocimiento.* Editorial Losada, Buenos Aires, 1967.
15. Locke, *An Essay concerning human understanding,* Ch. XXII, sect. 5, Oxford University Press, 1952.

J.W.N. Watkins

c4 A Basic Difficulty in the Mind-Brain Identity-Hypothesis

§1   The hypothesis that every mind-event or process is, as a matter of fact, identical with some brain-events or processes, is popular today. I think that one reason for its popularity is this. It is still widely held that dualist interactionism is quite implausible. Those who hold this can avoid the depressing doctrine of epiphenomenalism (roughly: mind-events are but the shadows or echoes of brain-processes) and retain their belief in 'the causal efficacy of the mental', that is, the belief that what we think makes a difference to what we do, by adopting the Identity-hypothesis; for this allows one to hold that our bodily behavior is strongly influenced by our beliefs, values, and decisions just because these mental entities *are* at the same time causally efficacious brain-processes.[1]

For my part, I hold that there are no insuperable objections to dualist interactionism, but I will not argue for that here.[2] I shall argue only for the negative thesis that there is a seemingly insuperable objection to the Identity-hypothesis.

An early statement of that hypothesis was given by Moritz Schlick.[3] I am going to take this as my starting-point for several reasons. First, it remains to this day one of the clearest and boldest statements of the hypothesis. Second, it has been largely ignored in the rapidly expanding literature on mind-brain identity.[4] My third and main reason is this. Schlick treated *both* sides of the mind-brain divide with the utmost seriousness. Some contemporary identity-theorists are like Schlick in this respect. I am thinking especially of David Armstrong[5] and Grover Maxwell.[6] But others take the mind-side of the divide less seriously. It has been claimed that Ryle in *The Concept of Mind* succeeded in reducing nearly all allegedly private and ghostly inner happenings to publicly observable behavior, leaving only tickles and other 'raw feels' to be mopped up. In earlier times there were identity-theorists who did not take matter altogether seriously, but only paid it a kind of lip-service. I am thinking of Russell's neutral monism and his idea that matter is a logical construction from sense-

data, and of Mach's sensationalism and his idea that some configurations of sensations constitute minds while others constitute
material objects.

By contrast, Schlick was both an unrepentant mentalist and
an unrepentant physical realist (to begin with, at least; he re-
neged on his physical realism later). He held that the last thought
of a dying man is something *real*, though private and without
causal effects. He also held that, for instance, an unobservable
physical atom is real (as real as a loaf of bread). Moreover he was
an eager explorer of both sides of the divide. He came to philosophy from theoretical physics (he had studied under Max Planck and written a book on space and time in contemporary physics). At the same time he was fascinated by various features of
human consciousness, especially the peculiar *unity* of consciousness. Although highly critical of many of Kant's ideas, Kant's
doctrine of the 'synthetic unity of apperception' was one which,
considered as a psychological thesis, he wholeheartedly endorsed,
reinforcing it with striking arguments of his own.

In short, my main reason for going back to Schlick is that,
instead of softening up the problem for the Identity-hypothesis
by first so redescribing one side of the mind-matter divide that it
becomes not unlike the other, he hardened the problem by going
out of his way to highlight features on one side which seem to
have no analogue on the other. He presented a contrast between
mind and brain which was strong and stark, and then boldly
claimed that, notwithstanding this, each item on the mind-side is
actually identical with some item on the brain-side. I shall argue
that the peculiar features of consciousness which he rightly highlighted do in fact constitute a basic difficulty for the Identity-
hypothesis.

One formulation he gave to that hypothesis was the following:

> . . . in place of the dualistic assumption we introduce the much simpler
> hypothesis that the concepts of the natural sciences are suited for designa-
> ting every reality including that which is immediately experienced. The re-
> sulting relation between immediately experienced reality and the physical
> brain processes is then no longer one of causal dependency but of simple
> *identity*.[7]

He also called his view 'psychophysical parallelism', making it
clear that the parallelism was only *linguistic:* there is the lan-

guage of psychology and the language of physics and physiology (not necessarily as it is today but as it would be if these sciences were in a final form); and any mental event which can be designated by an expression in the former language can also be designated by an expression in the latter language; the two expressions designate the same thing:

> . . . the expression 'psychophysical parallelism' is entirely suitable for characterizing our view that one and the same reality — namely, that which is immediately experienced — can be designated both by psychological concepts and by physical ones.[8]

[8]2   In this section I will try to arrive at a rather more precise formulation of the Identity-hypothesis as adumbrated by Schlick. I will begin by distinguishing three different types of non-analytic identity-statements, which I will call respectively: (i) singular; (ii) universal and one-one; (iii) universal and one-some. (i) A contingent singular identity-statement has the form 'a^5b', where 'a' and 'b' are both uniquely designating phrases, as in 'The Morning Star is the Evening Star'. An example of (ii) is: 'Each President of the USA is the Commander-in-Chief of the US forces'. Let 'P_1', 'P_2', 'P_3' . . . denote respectively the first, second, third . . . President of the USA, and 'C_1', 'C_2', 'C_3' . . . the first, second, third . . . C in C US forces; and let 'i' be a variable which ranges over the indices of 'P' and 'C'. Then this universal one-one identity-statement could be formulated thus:

$$(Ai)\,(P_i{}^5C_i) \qquad \text{for } i^5 1, 2, 3 \ . \ . \ .$$

In words: the i-th US President is always the i-th US C in C. As an example of (iii) I take this feature of the British peerage: at any given time there is *one* Earl Marshal and *several* Dukes, and the Earl Marshal is always one of the Dukes. Let 'M_1', 'M_2', 'M_3' . . . denote respectively the first, second, third . . . Earl Marshal; and assume that all past and present Dukes are numbered off (say, according to their date of accession) and denoted by 'D_1', 'D_2', 'D_3' . . .; and let 'i' and 'j' be variables which range over the indices of, respectively, 'M' and 'D'. Then this universal one-some identity-statement could be formulated thus:

$$(Ai)\,(Ej) \qquad (M_i{}^5D_j) \text{ where } i^5 1, 2, 3 \ . \ . \ . \text{ and } j \quad i.$$

In words: each i-th Earl Marshal is always some j-th Duke.

I have dwelt on this last type because Schlick's version of the Identity-hypothesis concerns type (iii) rather than type (ii) or type (i) identity-statements. For him, as for other identity-theorists, a mental state is not identical with a total brain state: 'Certainly the correlate is not the total brain process, but only *some part* of it' (my italics).[9]

To formulate Schlick's Identity-hypothesis I will invoke the idea of a psychological language M which is complete in the sense that, for any mental event or process, M can provide an expression which denotes it, and likewise a physiological language B which is complete in the sense that, for any brain event or process, B can provide an expression which denotes it. To make things more manageable I will relativise M and B to a particular person, who may as well be myself; and I will restrict the denoting expressions in M and B to those which actually succeed in denoting, respectively, a mental event or process in my consciousness, or a physical event or process in my brain.

However, the Identity-hypothesis cannot be formulated *within* M and B. To formulate it we need to postulate a metalanguage above M and B which is complete in the sense that it can provide a name for each denoting expression in M and in B. Assume that the names in the metalanguage for these denoting expressions in M and B are lexicographically ordered, and let them be 'm_1', 'm_2', 'm_3' . . . and 'b_1', 'b_2', 'b_3' . . . Let 'i' and 'j' be variables which range over the indices of, respectively, 'm' and 'b'. We can now formulate the Identity-hypothesis in this metalanguage as follows:

$$(Ai)(Ej)(m_i{}^s b_j)$$

In words: for any mental event or process of mind depicted by a psychological expression m_i there is an event or process in my brain depicted by a physiological expression b_j such that what b_j denotes *is* what m_i denotes.

[8]3   I now turn to two conditions which any contingent identity-statement must satisfy for it to be possible that the statement is true. I begin with type (i) statements.

For it to be possible that a singular statement of the form '$a^s b$' is true, one condition is that 'a' and 'b' are both denoting phrases each of which, at least in principle, picks out or individuates one definite person, thing, object, event, process, etc. (I say 'in principle' because we do not want to exclude phrases like 'the tallest man in Tibet' which may fail in practice to pick out one definite individual.) A second condition comes into operation where 'a' and 'b' are neither of them purely denoting phrases but also have some descriptive content; or, to put in in Frege's terminology, where each of them has a sense as well as a reference. In that case it must be conceptually possible that the thing as (denoted and) partially characterised by 'a' is the thing as (denoted and) partially characterised by 'b'. Let us consider these two conditions in their application to the following putative identity-statements:

(1) Sir Isaac Newton is the author of *The Compleat Angler;*
(2) The Noble Savage is the author of *The Compleat Angler;*
(3) The mountain called Mount Everest is the tallest man in Tibet.

Sentence (1), though false, satisfies both conditions: 'Sir Isaac Newton' picks out one person and so does 'the author of *The Compleat Angler*', and it is not conceptually impossible that the former is the latter. Sentence (2) violates the first condition: 'The Noble Savage' is not a genuine denoting phrase; it does not, even in principle, pick out one individual. Sentence (3) violates the second condition: it is conceptually impossible that a mountain is a man.

We can extend the above considerations to type (ii) statements, like our 'Ai $(P_i{}^5C_i)$', by requiring them to be such that our two conditions are met by the singular statements which can be obtained from them by dropping the quantifier and putting a particular value on i; for instance, '$P_{10}{}^5C_{10}$' must satisfy our two conditions. And we can likewise extend them to type (iii) statements, like our 'AiEj $(M_i{}^5D_j)$' by requiring these to be such that our two conditions are met by the singular statements which can be obtained from them by dropping the quantifiers and putting particular values on i and j; for instance, '$M_{10}{}^5D_{100}$' must satisfy our two conditions.

§4   I now turn to Schlick's striking ideas about human consciousness. One way to introduce them is by contrast with Hume's psychological atomism. As well as declaring that a self is 'nothing but a bundle or collection of different perceptions' Hume declared that

> All perceptions are distinct. They are, therefore, distinguishable, and separable, and may be conceiv'd as separately existent, and may exist separately.[10]

On this view, a perception occurring in a bundle of perceptions is similar to an atom located in an aggregate of atoms in that it could exist separated from the others. (Notice that this psychological ontology promises well for the Identity-hypothesis: for the left-hand side of the equation it provides neat units waiting to be picked out by m-expressions, which would then await pairing with b-expressions.)

As Schlick pointed out, Hume's view implies that a sequence of such unit-like perceptions occurring in one individual could be conceived 'as being distributed among different individuals'.[11] So let us in imagination despatch the first perception in the sequence to one oyster, the second to another oyster, and so on; and let us suppose that each oyster has just this one momentary perception in its life. We could hardly say that the oysters attained *consciousness* in virtue of a momentary sensation (of light, sound, pain or whatever) which then vanished totally. Let us now, instead of despatching each perception to a different oyster, despatch them one at a time to the same oyster but with intervals of total blackout between each perceptual unit. Clearly, the oyster's condition would differ only numerically from its previous condition: if it did not attain consciousness from one momentary sensation with a blackout on either side of it, the oyster will not attain consciousness from a sequence of momentary sensations with a blackout on either side of each of them. Now let the blackout intervals become shorter and shorter. This again will not change the oyster's condition in any significant way, *even if the intervals become vanishingly short.* For the oyster will not be having a continuous flow of experience, but only a chopped up series of unit-sensations. (Schlick acknowledged that Wundt had already stated that momentary "consciousness" is not really consciousness.)

Schlick's view could be summed up thus: no *consciousness* without *unity* of consciousness. He wrote:

> And where there is unity of consciousness, the individual moments of consciousness then exist not for themselves but, as it were, for each other. That is, they cannot be considered independently of their neighbors. Torn from their interconnection with them, they would no longer be the same; the interconnection is of their *essence.*[12]

This 'indescribable interconnection', as he at one point called it,[13] is both intersensual and temporal. Although he did not actually use the term 'specious present' he endorsed the idea: we 'experience temporally adjacent elements of consciousness not merely as succeeding one another but also as being simultaneous'.[14] The conscious *present* always has '*some* duration'.

[8]5 Let us now consider the bearing of Schlick's unity of consciousness thesis on his Identity-hypothesis. It will help to have a simple example before us. Yesterday evening I was, let us suppose, at an official dinner. The port having been circulated the presiding officer rose, rapped on the table, raised his glass and said: 'Ladies and gentlemen, let us drink a toast to Her Majesty the Queen'. A tape-recording was made of this performance: it took ten seconds. What does the Identity-hypothesis say concerning what went on in my mind/brain during those ten seconds? Presumably something like this: — It would in principle be possible to give, in that ideally complete physiological language *B*, a full description of all the changes that took place in my brain during the first, second, third . . . tenth second. And in the psychological language *M* there are expressions to denote what I was experiencing during the first, second, third . . . tenth second. For convenience, suppose these expressions to be numbered m_1, m_2, m_3 . . . m_{10}. Then within the physiological description of my brain during the first second there will be something which denotes what m_1 denotes, and so on for each subsequent second. We could express this by:

$$(Ai)(Ej)(m_i {}^5 b_j) \text{ for } i {}^5 1, 2, \ldots, 10$$

Let us now ask whether this putative one-some identity-statement meets the first of the two conditions presented in [8]3 above: if we form a singular identity-statement from it by dropping the quantifiers and putting a value between 1 and 10 inclusive on i and some value on j, will both the m-expression on the left and the b-expression on the right of the identity-sign be genuine denoting phrases?

So far as I know there is no reason why the b-expression should not be. Admittedly, it might need to be enormously long and complicated. According to Eccles, one fifth of a second of neuronal activity is already

> . . . . very long indeed. The time for transmission from one nerve cell to another is no longer than 1/1000th of a second; hence there could be a serial relay of as many as 200 synaptic linkages between nerve cells before a conscious experience is aroused. Many thousands of nerve cells would be initially activated, and each nerve cell by synaptic relay would in turn activate many nerve cells. The immensity of this patterned spread throughout the neuronal pathways of the brain is beyond all imagining.[15]

But length and complexity do not debar an expression from being a denoting phrase. Imagine a faithful stone-by-stone description of Westminster Abbey, prefaced by 'The building which satisfies the following description:' that would constitute a genuine denoting phrase, even if it ran to millions of words.

But what about the left-hand side? Let us consider my experience in the light of Schlick's unity of consciousness thesis. This suggests that it would be most misleading to say that I had a sequence of visual perceptions (of a man rising, raising his arm and moving his lips) running alongside a sequence of aural perceptions (of a rap on the table followed by vocal sounds). I perceived someone proposing a toast. And it would be quite wrong to say that I heard 'Ladies and' during one second, then stopped hearing that and heard 'gentlemen' during the next second, and so on. What I first heard lingered on and merged into what came after. I was still in a way "hearing" 'Ladies and gentlemen' when he got to 'the Queen': I did not have to *recall* how his sentence began.

To make things definite let us select m_9, which is supposed to denote what I experienced during the ninth second. Erasing the first eight seconds and the tenth from tape we find that the ninth consists of ' . . . to her Maj . . .' Schlick's unity of consciousness thesis clearly implies that my flow of experience did not provide any distinguishable unit for m_{90} denote some (no doubt very complicated) process which went on in my brain during that ninth second. Then

$$m_9{}^5b_{90}$$

is a putative identity-statement; but I say that it does not meet our first condition: the left-hand term is not a genuine denoting phrase.

I do not say that there are no denotable and, as it were, unitary items in human experience. There surely are: hearing a click, a stab of toothache, feeling a pinprick, the first taste of an iced drink, and so on. Rather surprisingly, Schlick seems to have regarded such essentially *simple* experiences as the main threat to his Identity-hypothesis. Suppose that a sleeper is half-awakened by, say, a steady drone which he drowsily hears for a while and then sinks back into sleep. Then he briefly has an essentially simple experience. But its physiological correlate

> . . . . is apparently extremely complex. The physical processes . . . are enormously complicated. From among the innumerable cells of which the brain is composed, a goodly number go into action when a sensation takes place . . . And now the concept of a brain process . . . is supposed to designate a single quality, namely, this simple sound! Is this not a truly unsolvable contradiction? This objection is so basic that there seems to be no escape from it.[16]

Actually, there is a fairly easy escape from this objection, and Schlick had no difficulty in finding it. Given an m-expression which, as in this case, succeeds in picking out a definite item ('this simple sound'), the Identity-hypothesis makes the merely existential claim that there exists a b-expression which denotes what the m-expresson denotes. This claim is irrefutable, a fact of which Schlick took advantage in answering his own objection:

> But we do not know *which* [brain] process is to be associated with a simple sensation as its physical correlate . . . Thus it may be a very small partial process, one that is extremely simple.[17]

But Schlick would have been the first to agree that simple sensations, raw feels, episodic perceptions of bangs, flashes, and the like do not constitute a major part of ordinary experience. If I look back over my experience during the last hour to find how many isolable, denotable episodes it contained, how many instantiations it provided for the 'm_i' in (Ai) (Ej) ($m_i{}^5b_j$), I find hardly any: the telephone rang and I heard the front-door open and shut; otherwise there was practically nothing of that kind.

In order to secure something definite for his m-expressions to denote, the identity-theorist might take as his unit a person's entire experience from each first awakening until he next falls into unconsciousness. (This would exclude dreams, but let us ignore that complication here.) Let us allow that m-expressions thus conceived constitute genuine denoting phrases. And let us take m_n to denote all that I experienced yesterday between 0715 and 2340. Applied to this particular chunk of experience the Identity-hypothesis will now say

$$Ej\,(m_n{}^5b_j)$$

This is not itself an identity-statement. It is analogous to 'Ex ($x^5$the author of *The Compleat Angler*)' which promises that a true identity-statement could be got by dropping the existential quantifier and correctly specifying x. Similarly, '$Ej\,(m_n{}^5b_j)$' promises that a true identity-statement could be got by dropping the existential quantifier, and correctly specifying j. Suppose that '$m_n{}^5b_m$' is proposed as a candidate for being this true identity-statement, where 'b_m' is a denoting phrase somewhat analogous to the one for Westminster Abbey we imagined earlier: that is, it is prefaced by 'The brain which satisfies the following description:' after which follows what is in fact a faithful record of certain processes that took place in my brain during the period between 0715 and 2340 yesterday.

We are assuming, now, that 'm_n' and 'b_m' are both genuine denoting phrases, so that '$m_n{}^5b_m$' meets the first of our two conditions. Does it meet the second? Is it conceptually possible that what is (denoted and) partially characterized by 'm_n' *is* what is (denoted and) partially characterized by 'b_m'? If '$m_n{}^5b_m$' were *true*, every property of what is denoted by 'm_n' would be a property of what is denoted by 'b_m'; or

$$(A\ \ )(\ \ m_n \quad b_m).$$

But let us now recall some of those peculiar properties of consciousness highlighted by Schlick. Assume that the 'day in the life of JW' to which 'm_n' refers was relatively free of bangs, flashes, etc. Then this stretch of experience will contain few elements that are, in Hume's words, 'distinguishable and separable'. It is not easy to give a verbal characterisation of its general properties. One wants to say that neighboring elements in this experiential flow interfuse and color each other; but one also wants to say that the interfusing leaves no elements to interfuse with one another. This difficulty shows itself in Schlick's statement, quoted earlier, that we 'experience temporarily adjacent elements of consciousness not merely as succeeding one another but also as being simultaneous'. One sees what he meant: I heard 'Ladies-and-gentlemen' *both* as one contemporaneous unit and as a short temporal sequence. One understands why Schlick called the interconnectedness *indescribable.*

Schlick himself recognized that this interconnectedness posed a problem for his Identity-hypothesis (though he seems to have regarded it as less threatening than that posed by simple sensations). He wrote:

> Mental qualities have that special relationship which, as the interconnection of consciousness, has so often occupied us. And in this way they are distinguished from all other qualities . . . Does this not represent a dualism . . . ?[18]

He met this objection with the cheerful prophecy that science will eventually come up with physiological correlates for the unity of consciousness. To this I will only say that *if* physiology were ever to show that the abovementioned properties of consciousness are *also* properties of the brain, then the brain would be utterly different from the brain as described by contemporary physiology and, indeed, from *any* physical system so far known to us.

Identity-theorists drew encouragement from Frege's 'The Morning Star is the Evening Star', which showed that a contingent and even surprising statement of identity may nevertheless be true. Yes, but a star that is the last to become invisible in the morning is the sort of thing that could be a star that is the first to become visible in the evening. To claim that certain control processes *are* conscious experience seems to me like claiming that the Morning Star is the evening stillness.

NOTES

1. I came to see the Identity-hypothesis in this light after discussion with Ted Honderich. I am grateful to David Armstrong for his patient criticism of an earlier version of this paper.
2. I have argued for it elsewhere, in §5 of my 'Three Views Concerning Human Freedom' (in R.S. Peters, ed: *Nature and Conduct,* Macmillan, London, 1975).
3. Moritz Schlick, *Allgemeine Erkenntislehre,* 1918; revised edition 1925. Now translated by A.E. Blumberg as *General Theory of Knowledge,* with an Introduction by A.E. Blumberg and H. Feigl; Springer-Verlag, Wien-New York, 1974.
   I have reviewed this work in *Brit. Jour. Phil. Sc.,* 28, December 1977.
4. There are some passing references to Schlick in H. Feigl, *The "Mental" and the "Physical";* I have found no other references to him in the contemporary literature, which often gives the impression that the Identity-theory was first invented in Australia in the late 1950s.
5. See D.M. Armstrong, *A Materialist Theory of Mind,* Routledge, London, 1968, especially pp. 92 f.
6. See Grover Maxwell, 'Rigid Designators and Mind-Brain Identity' in C. Wade Savage (ed): Perception and Cognition: Issues in the Foundations of Psychology; *Minnesota Studies in the Phiosophy of Science,* Vol. IX, University of Minnesota Press, Minneapolis, forthcoming 1978.
7. *General Theory of Knowledge,* p. 299.
8. Ibid., p. 310.
9. Ibid., pp. 320-1.
10. *Treatise* (ed. Selby-Bigge), p. 634.
11. Ibid., p. 123.
12. Ibid., p. 125.
13. Ibid., p. 126.
14. Ibid., p. 127.
15. J.C. Eccles, *Facing Reality,* Springer-Verlag, 1973, p. 71.
16. *General Theory of Knowledge,* p. 320.
17. Ibid., pp. 300-1.
18. Ibid., p. 332.

Grover Maxwell

c5 Unity of Consciousness and Mind-Brain Identity

I had planned not to read the written reply that I had made to Professor Watkins' paper, but to make a few informal off-the-cuff remarks instead. Unfortunately, most of these remarks were made in the earlier session by people like Professor Wigner, Professor Melvin and others. Because of this, I intend to do something very much like reading the original reply that I wrote, so you won't think that I'm plagiarizing from the morning session. Before I do that, however, since I didn't make clear in the written reply (as my wife Mary Lou pointed out) exactly what I was up to, I think I'll put all of my cards on the table at the onset so that it doesn't come as a complete shock at the end.

I am here to *defend* the mind-brain identity thesis as a thesis of strict identity; by 'identical' I mean *one and the same thing* or *one and the same event*, such that the Leibniz law is at least a necessary condition for identity to hold. One other preliminary remark: Professor Watkins and I have a remarkable amount of agreement; in fact we start from virtually the same premises but, unfortunately, reach contradictory conclusions. Now this is not to impugn John's abilities as a logician; rather, I think that there is a suppressed premise operating in his argument, and I'll just say briefly what I think it is. It's something to the effect that the brain really *is* pretty much like the picture we get from common sense plus the picture we get from people like Karl (Pribram), Sir John Eccles, and other brain physiologists, and eventually what we get from physics. I think this suppressed premise entails that, if the identity theory implies that the brain is different from this, then the identity theory is in serious trouble. I shall challenge this premise, and now I shall try to clarify somewhat the way in which I do it. I like to tell of the time when I heard Benson Mates remark that it makes about as much sense to try to identify a billy goat with a quadratic equation as it does to try to identify a mental state with a brain state. In a perhaps less colorful but suitably more elegant and reasoned approach, Watkins reaches a similar conclusion. Now I have a great deal of sympathy *and* empathy with these sentiments of Watkins, Mates, Sir John and many others, including myself at times.

The difficulty that Watkins poses for the mind-brain identity is an ingenious, highly developed instance of the more general argument, the argument that is by far the most cogent against the identity hypothesis. Let me put it briefly and crudely: Premise -1: we know from direct observation, from common sense, and from physics, chemistry, neuro-physiology, etc., *what* the brain *is*, what it is *like*, what its *properties*, *states*, and *processes are*, etc. Premise -2: we also know from common sense, from direct acquaintance, and perhaps from the science of psychology *what* the mind or mental states or mental events *are*, and what *they* are *like*. Intermediate conclusion: this knowledge entails that mental events have properties that brain events lack, and conversely. Conclusion: it follows from the Leibniz law, to say nothing of good old everyday horse sense, that mental events cannot be brain events.

Traditionally materialists have countered this argument by denying premise -2. They hold that our knowledge of the mental is so defective that it can be pretty much disregarded, indeed that, in the sense advocated by mentalists, there is no such thing as the mind or the mental, no such thing as mental events, etc. Rightly, Watkins rejects this. I applaud his appreciation of the fact that Schlick does the same. Such a rejection, however, entails that the identity theorist must deny premise-1; that is the identity theorist must deny that we know enough about brain events to be sure that they can't be mental events. Now this already strongly suggests Professor Watkins' contention that, if the identity hypothesis were true, then the brain would be utterly different from the brain as described by contemporary physiology, and indeed different from any physical system so far known to us. And this is already the case before we consider the difficulty Watkins raises about the unity of consciousness. For the identity theorist must contend that among the constitutents of the brain are pains, tickles, joys and sorrows, beliefs that $2^2 2^5 4$, etc., in all of their qualitative, mentalistic richness. Surely a brain that numbers such entities among its constitutents *is* utterly different from the brain and from all other physical systems as they are ordinarily conceived, even, for *most* of us, when the results of contemporary physiology are taken into account.

Now as Professor Watkins knows, Schlick not only recognized this, he emphasized and insisted upon it. More specifically, he insisted that contemporary scientific knowledge virtually forces us to change drastically our beliefs about the nature of the brain, and about all physical systems, and that this is independent of the mind-brain identity thesis. Scientific knowledge forces us to change our customary *interpretation* of *scientific knowledge itself,* and this is, moreover, independently urged upon us prior to consideration of mind-brain identity. Moreover, this holds with full force for the picture of the brain that *seems* to result from contemporary physiology.

The general thesis that Schlick emphasizes (along with the late Bertrand Russell) may be put as follows: physical science provides us with knowledge about the structural properties of physical systems, but it leaves us entirely ignorant as to what the intrinsic or the qualitative properties of these systems are. In particular, physiology leaves us entirely ignorant as to what the intrinsic properties of the brain are, and thus ignorant as to the intrinsic nature of the brain events. Regarding any specific brain event, physiology tells us no more than where it is located in that portion of the spatio-temporal, causal network that we ordinarily call the brain. This is utterly different from our ordinary conception of the brain, which misguidedly involves intrinsic properties, even when it seems to take physiology and physics into account. When we correct this and realize that our best knowledge to date, the knowledge from physiology, physics, etc., leaves the intrinsic nature of brain events entirely unspecified, the way is entirely open for speculating that some brain events just are our joys, sorrows, pains, thoughts, etc., in all of their qualitative and mentalistic richness. So Watkins is mistaken, I believe, in intimating that such a speculation is wrong just because it entails that the brain is utterly different from what we and physiologists ordinarily believe it to be, since reflection on the nature of scientific results *from* physiology, physics, etc., suggests very strongly that the brain *is indeed* very different from what our ordinary beliefs entail.

However, the difficulty he poses concerning the unity of consciousness remains a genuine and acute one for the identity theorist, for it becomes apparent upon reflection that some of the differences between mental events involving the unity of consciousness on the one hand, and brain events on the other, are differences in structure rather than differences in intrinsic properties. Specifically his arguments are that, for example, the causal structure of our auditory experience involved in hearing and understanding a phrase such as "Her Majesty the Queen," is very different from the spatio-temporal, causal structure of events treated by physics, physiology, etc. I want to suggest two possible ways to deal with this. The first, if only it would work, would be far simpler. I'm going to abbreviate this very much. It would be to resort to something like short-term memory traces, say something like a reverberating circuit or synoptic microstructure activity. For example, at a given instance the auditory trace on the cortex might have a structure isomorphic to the following:

...HER MAJES... etc.

Now the size of the letters is supposed to correspond structurally to the intensity of the trace on the cortex, and their order corresponds to an order that is exemplified in the auditory space of the sensorium, or whatever you want to call it. Although such an order is sensed at an instant, it is interpreted at that instant by a scanning mechanism, say in another part of the brain, as temporal succession analogously to our instantaneous visual perception of the symbol, "ICUS", in which you see "ICUS" in an instant and *at that instant* you perceive that "I" precedes "S" in your visual space.

Now even if my account of this less drastic approach is intelligible, I'm not very optimistic about its success. For reasons that include Watkins' unity of consciousness objection, as well as other ones besides, I think it is likely that the existence of the genuinely mental events that both Watkins and I champion neccessitates the existence of spatio-temporal, causal structures quite different from those with which contemporary physical science operates. Far from reacting to this with despair, I find it encouraging and exciting, both as an identity theorist and as a student of the physical sciences. For one thing, I am far from satisfied with the current state of physics. In spite of many impressive accomplishments, quantum theory seems to me to be largely a conceptual and scientific mess. Our other current fundamental theory, general relativity, also leaves much to be desired. And finally, I believe that it is generally agreed that all attempts to integrate fully quantum theory and general relativity with each other have been rather abject failures. Perhaps a radically new space-time theory is just what physics needs at this time. I do not find it too fanciful, even, to contemplate that neurophysiologists and bridge scientists, such as neuro-psychologists and psychophysiologists, in their attempts to implement an identity theory, may be led to propose bold new theories of spatio-temporal, causal relationships, theories that may alter fundamentally and irrevocably the course of *all* physical theory. In any event, I have no doubt that neuroscientists must make such attempts and not be too intimidated by current physical theory. It would be a happy circumstance if physicists, philosophers and others were to join them in such attempts. I'm encouraged by the remarks of Professor Wigner, Professor Melvin and others at this conference to feel this may not be a forlorn hope.

Sir John Eccles

c6 A Critical Appraisal of Brain-Mind Theories

From Greek times to the present an enormous intellectual effort has been made in the attempt to understand how the inner illumination which we may refer to as a conscious state is related to the material world. At first this internal world was restricted to the body of the experiencing subject, so defining the body-mind problem. But now on the basis of our brain science we can refer to it as the brain-mind problem. The prevailing philosophy of materialism or physicalism offers four more or less independent theories on the brain-mind problem. Three of the theories admit the existence of states of consciousness, but relegate it to an impotent role, hence they are classified as materialistic. A brief outline of each will be followed by their critical examination.

Materialist Theories of the Brain-Mind Problem

1. Radical Materialism. There is a denial of the existence of conscious processes and mental states. Radical behaviorism provides a complete explanation of behavior including verbal behavior and the dispositional states that lead to this. I do not think that many neuroscientists hold such an extreme view. It is however attractive to many philosophers because of its simplicity and because it eliminates not only the brain-mind problem, but also the problem of the origin of mind. The cosmos is reduced to the pristine simplicity that it had before the origin of life. While this may appeal to reductionist philosophers, neuroscientists must find this extreme reductionism absurd, so it will not be further discussed.

2. Panpsychism. This is a very ancient theory developed by the earliest Greek philosophers, who proposed that "soul is mingled with everything in the whole universe." Such philosophers as Spinoza and Leibniz espoused various forms of panpsychism. Essentially their belief was that all things had an inner psychical aspect and were material in their outer aspect. Panpsychism has even attracted modern biologists such as Waddington and Rensch because it offers such an attractive solution to the problem of the evolutionary origin of consciousness, namely that consciousness was associated with all matter in some protopsychic state and was merely developed with the increasing complexity of the brain to appear as the self-consciousness associated with the human brain. However, modern physics does not admit memory or identity to elementary particles — electrons, protons, neutrons — hence the panpsychist doctrine of the "protoconsciousness" of such particles must be rejected.

3. *Epiphenomenalism.* Epiphenomenalism differs from panpsychism in that mental states are attributed only to animals that exhibit mindlike behavior, such as learning and reacting intelligently and purposively. All varieties of epiphenomenalism have as a central tenet the thesis that the mental processes are completely ineffective in controlling behavior. The neural machinery works without any influence from consciousness, just as, according to T.H. Huxley, the work of a steam locomotive is uninfluenced by the sound of the steam whistle! Yet is it proposed that at a certain stage of evolution these ineffective mental states emerged and were then greatly developed in the evolutionary process to the full human self-consciousness.

4. *The psycho-physical identity theory or the central state theory.* Like panpsychism this theory was first developed by Greek philosophers and the two theories have often been linked, as for example by Spinoza and Rensch. The most subtle and acceptable form of the theory has been given by Feigl. Several analogies have been used in illustrating the postulated identity, but all are unsatisfactory because both components are in the materialist mode. For example there is the much overworked analogy: evening star, morning star achieving identity in the planet Venus. Other analogies are: cloud and fog, achieving identity in water droplets of the atmosphere; or a flash of lightning [5] electric discharge; or genes [5] DNA. Nevertheless there are attractive and important features in the identity theory. Mental proces-

ses are regarded as real or things in themselves. They are conjectured to be a property of a very small and select group of material objects, namely neural events in the brain, and probably in special regions of the brain. The conscious experiences are known within, *knowledge by acquaintance,* whereas the "identical" physical events are known from without by description, *knowledge by description,* of the neural events in the brain. These events described by the neuroscientist turn out to be the experiences consciously perceived. Thus the key postulate is essentially a parallelism or an inner and outer aspect.

Neuroscientists find the identity theory attractive because it gives the future to them. It is admitted that our present understanding of the brain is quite inadequate to provide more than a crude explanation of how the brain provides all the richness and wonderful variety of perceptual experiences, or how the mental events or thought can have the immense range and fruitfulness that our imaginative insights achieve in their action on the world. However, all this is taken care of by the theory that Popper has named *promissory materialism.* This theory derives from the great successes of the neurosciences, which undoubtedly are disclosing more and more of what is happening in the brain in perception, in the control of movement and in states of consciousness and unconsciousness. The aim of these research programs is to give a more and more complete and coherent account of the manner in which the total performance and experience of an animal and of a human being are explicable by the action of the neural machinery of the brain. According to promissory materialism the scientific advance will progressively restrict the phenomena that appear to require mental terms for their explanation so that in the fullness of time everything will be describable in the materialist terms of the neurosciences. The victory of materialism over mentalism will be complete. I regard this theory as being without foundation. The more we discover scientifically about the brain, the more clearly do we distinguish between the brain events and the mental phenomena and the more wonderful do the mental phenomena become. Promissory materialism is simply a religious belief held by dogmatic materialists who often confuse their religion with their science. It has all the features of a Messianic prophecy, with the promise of a future freed of all problems — a kind of Nirvana for our unfortunate successors. In contrast the true scientific attitude is that scientific problems are unending in providing challenges to attain an even wider and deeper understanding of nature and man.

General Discussion of the Four Materialist Theories in Relation to Dualist-Interactionism

A simple formulation of the similarities and differences may be given on the basis of Popper's terminology:

World 1 is the whole physical world, the world of matter-energy;

World 2 is the world of mental phenomena, the subjective states.

For *Radical Materialism* all is World 1, World 2 does not exist.

For *Panpsychism* all is World 1-2, neither World 1 nor World 2 has any independent existence.

For *Epiphenomenalism* World 1 has two components: World 1_P, all the world of physics without mental states; and World 1_M, the world of physics with mental states as an epiphenomenon. So it may be written that: World 1^5World $1_P{}^5$World 1_M, where World 1_M — World 2.

For *Identity theory* World 1^5World $1_P{}^5$World 1_M and World 1_M ^{5}World 2 by virtue of the identity relationship.

For *Dualist interactionism* World 1 and World 2 are independent entities and it is proposed that in special sites in the brain, the liaison brain (LB) there is reciprocal interaction. World 1_{LB} — World 2 where World 1_{LB} is the part of World 1 that forms the liaison brain.

I propose now to consider the biological implications of the three materialist theories that admit the existence of consciousness or mental states (World 2). Despite the differences in detail with respect to the relationship of World 2 to World 1, all are in agreement that the physical events in the brain (World 1) are alone causally effective in bringing about actions. In panpsychism the mental accompaniments of brain events are given no more causal effectiveness than in epiphenomenalism. They are merely the necessary concomitants of the on-going brain activities. At first it seems otherwise with the identity theory where

World 1 can interact with World 1_P because both are components of the neural machinery in the brain. Thus we have:

World 1_P — World 1_M and World 1_M [5] World 2.

Nevertheless the performance of the brain in controlling behaviour is entirely within the physical structures of the brain. No causal effectiveness of World 2 is admitted other than that of pertaining to World 1_M. Thus the closedness of World 1 is as absolute as with panpsychism or epiphenomenalism.

These three theories assert the causal ineffectiveness of World 2 and hence fail completely to account for the biological evolution of World 2, which is an undeniable fact. There is firstly its emergence and then its progressive development with the growing complexity of the brain. In accord with evolutionary theory only those structures and processes that significantly aid in survival are developed in natural selection. If World 2 is impotent, its development cannot be accounted for by evolutionary theory. It has not been recognized by the proponents of panpsychism, epiphenomenalism and the identity theory that they are advocating a theory that is in contradiction with the theory of biological evolution. According to that theory mental states and consciousness (World 2) could have evolved and developed only if they were *causally effective* in bringing about changes in neural happenings in the brain with the consequent changes in behavior. That can occur only if World 1 of the brain is open to influences from the mental events of World 2, which is the basic postulate of the dualist-interactionist theory.

The Dualist-Interactionist Theory

This theory is the most ancient formulation of the mind-body problem being in some form generally accepted by Greek thinkers from Homer onwards. It was developed by Descartes who attempted to define a detailed mode of operation that led to it being rejected in favor of some form of parallelism. In its modern form it is distinguished from all parallelistic theories precisely by the requirement of the openness of World 1 to World 2 events. As formulated above:

World 1_{LB} — World 2, World 1_{LB} being the liaison brain.

Since World 1LB is some part of the brain, it is of course in an intimate and intense reciprocal interaction with the rest of the brain,
but, over and above that, it is open to the mental influences of
World 2, which are of a non-physical kind. The causal effectiveness of these mental influences is apparent in countless actions of
everyday life where thoughts become expressed as actions or in
the recalls of memory on demand. It is reassuring to find that the
causal effectiveness of mental states can be deduced from evolutionary theory.

The self-conscious mind is conceived to be an independent
entity, a World 2 existence, which has a status in reality equivalent to that of the brain with its World 1 existence. This is a
strong dualism.

A brief outline of the hypothesis may be given as follows. The
self-consciousness mind is actively engaged in reading out from
the multitude of active centers at the highest level of brain activity, namely the liaison modules that are largely in the dominant
cerebral hemisphere. The self-conscious mind selects from these
modules according to attention and interest, and from moment to
moment integrates its selection to give unity even to the most
transient experiences. Furthermore the self-conscious mind acts
upon these neural centers modifying the dynamic spatiotemporal
patterns of the neural events. Thus it is proposed that the self-
conscious mind exercises a superior interpretative and controlling role upon the neural events.

A key component of the hypothesis is that the unity of conscious experience is provided by the self-conscious mind and not
by the neural machinery of the liaison areas of the cerebral hemisphere. Hitherto it has been impossible to develop any neurophysiological theory that explains how a diversity of brain events
comes to be synthesized so that there is a unified conscious
experience of a global or gestalt character. The brain events remain disparate, being essentially the individual actions of countless neurones that are built into complex circuits and so participate in the spatiotemporal patterns of activity. This is the case
even for the most specialized neurones so far detected, the feature
detection neurones of the inferotemporal lobe of primates. The
present hypothesis regards the neuronal machinery as a multi-

plex of radiating and receiving structures: the experience unity comes, not from a neurophysiological synthesis, but from the proposed integrating character of the self-conscious mind. It is conjectured that in the first place the self-conscious mind was developed in order to give this unity of the self in all of its conscious experiences and actions.

REFERENCES

Armstrong, D.M. (1968) *A Materialist Theory of the Mind*, Routledge, London.
Barlow, H.B. (1972) *Perception*, 1, 371-394.
Eccles, J.C. (1978) in *Cerebral Correlates of Conscious Experience*. Buser, P. and Rougeul-Buser, A. eds., Elsevier, Amsterdam.
Feigl, H. (1967) *The "Mental" and the "Physical"*, University of Minnesota Press, Minneapolis.
Laszlo, E. (1972) *Introduction to Systems Philosophy*, Gordon and Breach, New York and London.
Pepper, S.C. (1960) in *Dimensions of Mind*, Sidney Hook, ed., Collier-MacMillan Ltd., London.
Place, U.T. (1956) *Brit. J. Psych.*, 47, 44.
Polten, E.P. (1973) *A Critique of the Psycho-physical Identity Theory*, Mouton Publishers, the Hague.
Popper, K.R. and Eccles, J.C. (1977) *The Self and its Brain*, Springer Verlag, Heidelberg, New York, London.
Quine, W.V.O. (1960) *World and Object*, M.I.T. Press, Cambridge, Mass.
Rensch, B. (1971) *Biophilosophy*, Columbia University Press, New York.
Schlick, M. (1974) *General Theory of Knowledge*, Springer Verlag, Heidelberg, New York.
Smart, J.J.C. (1962) in *The Philosophy of Mind*, V.C. Chappell, ed., Prentice-Hall, Englewood Cliffs.
Szentagothai, J. (1975) *Brain Res.*, 95, 475-496.
Waddington, C.H. (1961) *The Nature of Life*, Allen & Unwin, London.

Hardin B. Jones

Commentary

Sir John Eccles has given examples of the differences between the cerebral hemispheres with regard to the location of self. It provides a basis for understanding mind-brain relationships. I wish to extend the examples.

Some forms of mental impairment are not perceived by the person affected. He needs the very part of the brain now suppressed in order to realize the deletion. Some effects of drugs are of this sort. The active ingredient of cannabis accumulates in the body and in the brain. This explains the progressive changes in the personality and behavior of the marijuana smoker, and the point is that the user has little or no insight to the altered mental function even if it is so severe that he becomes indolent. During months of abstinence, however, the former user becomes aware of many steps in recovery. This process may last several years in heavily affected persons.

Persons using opiates gradually develop faulty memory and a curious defect in mental process that denies them comprehension of the significance of many of the facts available. This is particularly true of the deductions that would allow the opiate user to realize the threat of harm or to know the consequence of an act. These changes from taking opiates occur prior to addiction and are reversed only slowly during months of abstinence.

When enough cocaine has been taken to induce euphoria, the sensation is often reported by the observer as a sensation of clear-headedness. This is illusion, for the person is usually hallucinating at the same time. Also from animal studies it has been shown that although a state of hyperactivity is induced by administration of cocaine the metabolism of the brain is not increased, rather it is decreased approximately by one-third.

These examples suggest that the self of the mind is complex; perhaps self is divisible into many subparts. For a more complete discussion of the effects of drugs on the mind see *Sensual Drugs* by Hardin and Helen Jones, Cambridge University Press, 1977.

Karl H. Pribram

c7 The Mind/Brain Issue As A Scientific Problem

John Eccles, in his opening address, noted that the Mind/Brain problem is at the center of a revolution *necessitated* by the relatively recent discoveries of modern physics. However, as Daniel Robinson has reviewed for us, philosophers have been concerned with this problem for some time and have provided us with a variety of answers which are encapsulated by the labels dualism and monism. Dualistic theories are ordinarily distinguished as parallelist or interactionist and monism has engendered multiple aspects and identity proposals. Philosophers have also stated, and this view was affirmed here by Robinson and Watkins, that scientific experiment and observation will yield little, if any, resolution of the question as to which of the philosophical positions is the correct one. These thoughtful scholars suggest that what is needed is more philosophical analysis, or perhaps the acceptance of one viewpoint because of its overwhelming logical persuasion.

As a scientist I cannot accept either the premise that scientific experiment and observation are irrelevant to an issue of such fundamental import nor the view that therefore we should continue the analysis much as philosophers have done for almost three millenia.

When in science a question arises that appears to be unresearchable the scientist asks whether that question has been properly phrased. As Medawar has stated so succinctly "science [in common with politics] is the art of the possible." Ordinarily, problems that appear to be resistant to research are so either because the appropriate technical (and that includes analytical techniques such as forms of mathematics) resources have as yet not been invented or because the question has not been broken down into meaningful (i.e. precisely interrelated) subquestions.

Scientists using the techniques of behavioral psychology, information engineering and brain physiology are addressing problems on the interface between brain and mind. Thus, the difficulty with the Mind/Brain issue appears to be conceptual rather than technical (as our philosophical contributors suggest). But rather than continue the century old debate as to which philosophical position is correct, I will approach the problem from a different vantage.

The logical possibility exists that the Mind/Brain issue consists not of one global problem but a set of specific and interrelated questions. If that should prove the case, then experimental observations might well become relevant to one or another of these questions. Further, it could turn out that each of the more global philosophical "positions" is correct with respect to one or another of these specific questions.

Using this approach it is possible to discern at least three very different questions that compose the Mind/Brain issue. These questions are: 1) how to characterize existential reality 2) how to characterize the transactions between an organism and its environment and 3) how to characterize the organization of the universe (including the biological universe).

Philosophical inquiry has approached the first question, the nature of existential reality through introspection. Scientists have approached the same question by making experiments and observations on the physical universe. Both introspection and physical science have yielded the same result: one must take into account both the observer and the observed. As an example, in philosophy Brentano characterized the essence of self-report to be the ability to distinguish between perceiver and the perceived and between intent and act. This principle is usally referred to as "intentionality." In physics Heisenberg and Wigner (e.g. 1969), among others, have clearly stated that the science of physics deals primarily with probability correlations among *observations,* and that the referents of those observations must be inferred.

Thus both philosophy and science arrive at an existential dualism. The scientist investigating the material universe is thrown back upon his own observation as critical; the introspective philosopher finds "self" only when he can distinguish a difference between intention and that which is intended.

Questions as to the "existence" of each of these "realities" and whether the one can be "reduced" to the other are subsidiary questions to which I shall return shortly. For the moment it is sufficient to understand that dualism is composed of a duality in which neither the material nor the mental can ultimately be examined (at least at present) without recourse to the other.

Are there any observations or experiments that are relevant to this issue? I believe there are. One such question concerns the evolution of intentionality. Are apes self aware? If so, are monkeys? Other mammals? What will the results of answers to these questions have on our existential experience of intentionality? Will the centrality of intentionality to the Mind side of the Mind/Brain issue be jeopardized if animals other than man can be shown to possess intent?

Another relevant experimental observation concerns the specialization of function of the hemispheres of the brain, as Eccles (e.g. 1970) has repeatedly pointed out. If both hemispheres display intentionality and their behavioral output can be separated, are there then two selves? And if there are, does that not mean that a two hemispheres-two minds correlation becomes established? And if not, then the quest for what brain process does correlate continues and doesn't it make a difference to the Mind/Brain issue whether total brain hemisphere processes or e.g. linguistic processes correlate with mental processes? Aren't precise definitions of Mind dependent on such observations?

It is, of course, with just such precise definitions that questions about the Mind/Brain issue must be asked. So far we have asked about the existence of Mind and Brain—their reality in experience. Mind so defined becomes identified with intentional being, with "self"—self-awareness, self consciousness. Being, awareness and consciousness can however be conceived either as states (relatively enduring configurations) or as functions (relationships among relatively enduring configurations). Two very different theoretical frames are derived depending on which conception is pursued.

Gilbert Ryle first defined mind in terms of minding, a function. Minding is behavior. Minding is paying attention. And there is a considerable body of scientific knowledge concerning behavior and attention. The consequences of behavior (technically these are called acts when they rearrange environmental configurations and reinforcements when they rearrange organismic states, e.g. Pribram 1971;) and of paying attention (or not paying attention) are well documented scientifically. When these consequences are framed within the Mind/Body issue they lead to an interactionist view.

Popper and Eccles in their recently published book "The Self and its Brain" (1977) develop the case for such an interactionist viewpoint. Unfortunately, they do not clearly distinguish between Mind as state and Mind as function so that the thrust of their argument often loses force and the experiments described by Eccles do not address the specific problem to which they are appropriate.

It should not be surprising that Popper as one of the most influential heirs of Mach's emphasis on sensory experience and the consequent positivism of the Vienna Circle espouses a position in which Mind as function — as minding — acts upon the physical universe which in turn influences Mind as state through the senses. But note also that other equally perspicacious philosophers of the Vienna Circle such as Feigl (e.g. 1960) could bring to flower an identity position from the same roots.

Perhaps this difference between philosophical views stems from the confounding of Mind as state and Mind as function already noted. If emphasis is placed on minding as function, its interactive properties become paramount. If, on the other hand, emphasis is placed on Mind as state, correspondences, identities between states (configurations) will be sought. In biology and physics, Helmholtz (e.g. 1863) and Hertz, (e.g. 1956) for example, looked for such correspondences e.g. between the physical stimulus as described by instruments, and the resulting experience as described by verbal response. Hertz used the terms *Bild*, image, and *Darstellung*, representation, as a construction or model of reality which is best described in mathematical terms. Whereas Machian functionalism leads to interactions by way of the senses and behavior, Helmholtz and Hertz's structuralism leads to modelling, a cognitive constructional activity which searches for identities.

Popper combines these historical traditions by making his third world (Mind as function) the medium for interaction between

Brain (World 1) and Mind as state (World 2). But he fails to point out, as does Hertz, that interaction occurs only to the extent that World 3 identifies World 1 with World 2 — i.e., the limits of interaction are described by the limits of the *identity* between model and what is being modelled ("reality").

Further, by creating World 3 as apart from World 2, World 2 the mental world, becomes restricted to the sensory world of Mach, from which cognitive activity is derivative (Mach) rather than integral (as proposed by Kant, 1963), Neuropsychological research (Pribram, 1971, Chap. 17) has indicated that the Kantian view must at least be seriously considered.

Max Jammer, in this conference, has given a superb account of these differences between Mach's functionalism and the scientific approach developed by Helmholtz and Hertz. Toulmin (in Janik and Toulmin's "Wittgenstein's Vienna," 1973) also gives a detailed account of these developments. Feigl's views and those derived from them such as Grover Maxwell's thoughtful and thought provoking paper presented at this conference appear to me to be kin to the structural approach. "Multiple aspects" of some partially perceived identity are not altogether different from the "models" of reality espoused by Hertz.

I am inclined to accept this structuralist approach to the Mind/Brain problem because it can subsume the others and bring to bear additional scientific evidence. The concept "structure" in this sense is not to be confused with morphology or anatomical structure. Structure here means the structure of process, the meaning used by Hertz, Levi-Strauss (1963) and by Merleau-Ponty (1963). Process involves one state becoming another. Functional interactions are thus encompassed.

A structural approach to the Mind/Brain issue discerns systems of states some of which are hierarchically related, others are processed in parallel, while still others interact to produce new states. Examples of such systems are information processing devices. There is a hierarchy of configurations — at the lowest level are electrical circuits which are organized into flip-flops, then into "and" "or" gates and "nand" and "nor" configurations. From these more complex computational elements are constructed. These are then combined into the hardware "brains" that we call computers. To operate, i.e. to function, these "brains" must interact with an appropriate environment through input-output devices (hardware sense organs and effectors). Without such devices the computer does not function, nor does it function without programs which constitute its appropriate interactive environment. One might say that without programs computers won't mind. They won't attend, they won't change their configurations, their states. Programs and hardware are certainly different in function and realization—perhaps as different as Mind and Brain.

Still there are identities, as well. There is a truism in the information sciences that anything that can be realized in a program can be constructed in hardware—and vice-versa.

What is it that shares this identity? It is called the "structure" of the process. It is this structure which we recognize functional program and functioning computer to have in common. It is the same commonality as that which characterizes the structure of a symphony which we recognize whether it is realized as an experience in the concert hall or as the score in sheet music. A variety of realizations—score, tape, disc, performance, shares an identity in structure which we can experience in appropriate circumstances.

The structural approach therefore does not deny an apparent dualism in Mind/Brain. It does, however, suggest that a better description might be that of a duality (a set of symmetry relationships) which has certain properties in common. It can explain the apparent dualism in terms of a hierarchy of knowledge systems (Sociology, Psychology, Physiology, Chemistry, Physics) which, when explored in a reductive direction, yields ever more material descriptions until the limit is reached in microphysics where such descriptions become almost totally mathematical—i.e. descriptions of relationships among observations rather than of relationships among observables. (There is therefore an ultimate paradoxical circularity to the hierarchy). When, by contrast, the explorations are performed in an upward direction in the hierarchy, conventions must be established in order that the exploration may proceed. The theories of relativity established the role of such conventions in physics, the periodic table based on atomic number is such a convention in chemistry, and *mental* language (consensually i.e. socially validated) provides this convention for psychology (Pribram, 1965).

Note that with this view, intentionality is derived by looking upward in a hierarchy which is comprised of the biological organism is his eco-system. The convention becomes established that the organism can distinguish between himself and his environment and that this distinction characterizes mental life, or mind. Other conventions adopt other distinctions. For example, the functional approach is characterized by the convention that mind is to behaving biological *bodies* as force is to *masses* in motion (i.e. behaving).

It is this conventional aspect—the fact that one must choose a frame within which exploration proceeds—that makes plausible the varieties of philosophical approaches to the Mind/Body issue. I have tried here to make explicit which frame, which convention, proscribes which philosophical position. I have also therefore attempted to show that each position has merit and to discern that merit. In short, the Mind/Body issue appears to me to yield to a set of *complementary* theories, each of which has explanatory power and limits.

Unity is therefore to be achieved when the relationships between the complements that characterize the theories are clarified. Ultimately understanding the complementarities may devolve on understanding what goes on at the limits of the theories. Thus, does the fact that microphysical theory is a description of observations rather than of observables mean that "ultimately" the universe is made up of observations, i.e. Mind, or does it mean that we simply cannot in this instance, use the ordinary neurophysiological mechanisms of "projection" (e.g. Bekesy 1967) to construct an apparent physical reality as we normally do for the mechanistic universe? As a scientist I believe it is this type of question that can now supplant the earlier philosophical analyses. As a scientist, also, I believe that experiment and observation will have a high yield of contributions to make in answer to such specific questions.

REFERENCES

Bekesy, G. von. *Sensory Inhibition.* Princeton: Princeton University Press, 1967.

Eccles, J.C. *Facing Reality,* New York, Heidelberg, Berlin: Springer-Verlag, 1970.

Feigl, H. Mind-Body, not a pseudo problem. In S. Hook (Ed.) *Dimension of Mind.* New York: Collier Books, 1960.

Helmholtz, H. von. Die, *Lehre von den Tonempfindungen.* Braunschweig: Vieweg, 1863.

Hertz, H. *The Principles of Mechanics Presented in a New Form.* trans. by D.E. Jones and J.T. Walley, with Preface by H. von Helmholtz and Introduction by Robert. Cohen, New York: Dover, 1956.

Janik, A. and Toulmin, S. *Wittgenstein's Vienna.* New York: Simon and Schuster, 1973.

Kant, I. *Critique and Pure Reason.* (N. Kemp Smith, trans.) New York: Macmillan, 1963.

Levi-Strauss, C. *Structural Anthropology.* New York: Basic Books, 1963.

Merleau-Ponty, M. *The Structure of Behavior.* Boston: Beacon Press, 1963.

Popper, K.R. and Eccles, J.C. *The Self and Its Brain.* New York, Heidelberg, Berlin: Springer-Verlag, 1977.

Pribram, K.H. Proposal for a structural pragmatism: some neuropsychological considerations of problems in philosophy. In B. Wolman and E. Nagle, (Eds.) *Scientific Psychology: Principles and Approaches.* New York, Basic Books, 1965, pp. 426-459.

Primbram, K.H. *Languages of the Brain: Experimental Paradoxes and Principles in Neuropsychology.* Englewood Cliffs, New Jersey: Prentice-Hall, Inc., 1971.

Wigner, E.P. Epistemology of Quantum Mechanics: Its Appraisal and Demands. In M. Grene (Ed.) *The Anatomy of Knowledge.* London: Routledge and Kegan Paul, 1969.

Roger Sperry

c8 Bridging Science and Values: A Unifying View Of Mind and Brain

Introduction

General acceptance of the inadequacy of science in the realm of ethics and moral judgment is reflected in the old adage that "Science deals with facts, not with values," and its corollary that "Value judgments lie outside the realm of science." In other versions it is stated that science may tell us *how* but not *why* or that science may show us how to achieve defined goals, but not which are the right goals to aim for. A further pronouncement holds that science can tell us what *is* but not what *ought* to be: science *de*scribes but cannot *pre*scribe.

Although this time-honored dichotomy between science and value judgment has not gone unchallenged[1, 2, 3], the great majority in science, philosophy and related fields continue today to accept the tradition that science as a discipline must by its very nature operate in the realm of objective fact and that science, either as a method or as a body of knowledge, can neither formulate value standards nor resolve issues in the domain of subjective value. When it comes to value conflicts and ethical validation, we are told that we must seek our answers elsewhere — in the humanities, in ethics and philosphy, and particularly in religion, long held to be the prime custodian of human value systems. In what follows, my aim, in large part, is to try to show that this traditional separation of science and values and the related limitations it has implied for science as a discipline are no longer valid in the context of current mind-brain theory.

The issues at stake, even by the most hard-nosed, pragmatic standards, are neither trivial nor ivory tower. Human values, in the framework to be spelled out below, become a practical concern of concrete consequence. In addition to their commonly recognized significance from a personal, religious, or philosophic standpoint, human values can also be viewed objectively in scientific terms as universal determinants in all human decision making. All decisions boil down to a choice among alternatives of what is most valued — for whatever reason; and are determined by the particular value system that prevails at the time. Viewed objectively, human value priorities stand out as the most strategically powerful causal influence now shaping events on the surface of the globe. More than any other causal system with which science now concerns itself, it is variables in the human value factor that will determine the future.

I have rated human values as a social problem above the more concrete crisis conditions like poverty, population, energy or pollution, on the following grounds.[3]: First, all these crisis conditions are man-made and very largely products of human values. Further, they are not correctable on any long-term basis without first changing the underlying human values involved. And finally, the more strategic way to remedy these conditions is to go after the social value priorities directly in advance, rather than waiting for these value changes to be forced by changing environmental conditions. Otherwise we are doomed from here on to live always on the margins of intolerability, because it is not until things get rather intolerable that the voting majority gets around to changing its established values.

The importance of value issues is apparent also in other perspectives. From the standpoint of brain function, it is clear that a person's or a society's values directly and constantly shape its actions and decisions. Any given brain will respond differently to the same input, and will tend to process the same information in quite diverse ways depending on its particular system of value priorities. In short, what an individual or a society values determines very largely what it does. As human numbers increase, and science and technology advance, the regulative control role of the human value factor (that directly determines how all this growing human impact will be applied and directed) will become correspondingly more powerful.

In a different vein we are informed that the prevailing social neurosis of our times is a growing sense of valuelessness, apathy, a sense of hopelessness and loss of purpose and ultimate meaning. One is reminded of the generalized disintegration of long established values and belief systems and the grasping in all directions for new answers, new life styles, and the reviving in radical form of some of the old answers. From still other directions come warnings that we need a whole new system of social value guidelines if civilized man is to survive, "new ethics for survival" as Hardin[4] puts it, that would act to preserve man's world instead of destroying it.

Accepting the enormous control power of human values and the critical key role their shaping will play in determining the future, it follows that if science is inherently inadequate to deal with value problems, we are indeed confronted with a profound shortcoming in science and all it stands for. On these terms perhaps it is for the best that government should be tightening the screws on the funding of science, especially pure science; and that public confidence in science generally should be in question, while the forces of antiscience gain new ground fostered by the eloquent and often cogent writings of critics like Roszak[5] and Mishan[6]. Certainly the future of science will be very different depending on whether science is, or is not, recognized in the public mind to have competence in the realm of values. Of greater importance, the future of civilized society and of the ecosystem generally will also be very different, depending on the extent to which future social values are shaped from the world view of science or from various alternatives.

Grounds for Reappraisal

While the epistemological separation of science and values has seemed logically justified in the past, especially with respect to physical science, and still applies in practice to many aspects of scientific methodology, new grounds can be seen today to directly question the main philosophic validity of the science-vs.-values dichotomy. Recent developments, especially in the behavioral sciences, reopen central questions and greatly strengthen arguments for a revised, almost diametrically opposed philosophy in which modern science is advanced as man's prime hope in the quest for new values and a sense of meaning. Problems of values, ethics and morality (questions, i.e., of what is *good, right* and *true* and of what *ought* to be) become, on these revised terms, something to which science can, in the most profound sense, contribute fundamentally and in which science should be actively and responsibly involved.

Although proposals along similar lines since Francis Bacon have failed to gain any wide acceptance and have been largely written off under the label "scientism" by detractors, conceptual developments during the last decade in the area of mind-brain relations introduce an interpretation of conscious mind and a related philosophical framework that substantially alter the picture. The scope of science in respect to mental activity and its qualifications for dealing with subjective experience are directly affected. A modified concept of the relation of subjective experience to brain mechanisms and to external reality has emerged, that involves a direct contradiction of the central founding thesis of Behaviorism in this country and of the materialistic philosophy in Russia and elsewhere[7-10]. Important departures from long-established determinist and materialist doctrine follow with extensive implications for the philosophy of science and derivation of values.

Current mind-brain theory no longer dispenses with conscious mind as just an "inner aspect" of brain activity, or as some passive "epiphenomenal", metaphysical, or other impotent by-product, as has long been the custom; nor does it reject consciousness as merely an artifact of semantics or as being identical to the neural events. Consciousness, in these revised terms, becomes an integral, dynamic property of the brain process itself and a central constituent of brain action. Subjective experience is viewed in operational terms[11] as a causal determinant in brain function and acquires emergent control influence in regulating the course of physico-chemical events in brain activity. No metaphysical interaction in the classical sense is implied; the causal relation primarily involves the power of the whole over its parts. In a sense, mind moves matter in the brain just as an organism moves its component organs and cells, or a molecule governs the molecular course of its own electrons. In the case of conscious phenomena, it is the dynamic enveloping power of conscious high order cerebral processes over their constituent neural and chemical elements[12]. As an emergent interpretation of mind, it differs from the concepts of Gestalt psychology[13] in that the conscious effects are not ascribed to isomorphic field forces, nor are they considered to be mere correlates of neural activity. The conscious mind is put to work and given a reason for being and for having been evolved in a material world.

Although inseparably tied to the physical brain process, conscious awareness is conceived to be something distint and special in itself, "different from and more than" the collected sum of its physico-chemical components. Values and other mental phenomena, though built of neural events, are no longer conceived to be reducible to, nor identifiable with, those events, nor to be mere parallel correlates.

This modified approach to the status of mind emerged largely out of efforts to account for the unity and/or duality and related aspects of conscious experience in split brain studies. I described the scheme initially[7] as a swing toward mentalism that puts conscious mind in the driver's seat in command over matter, gives ideas and ideals control over physico-chemical interactions, and recognizes conscious mental forces as the crowning achievement of evolution. It provides a conceptual explanatory formula for the interaction of mind with matter that does not violate the principles of scientific explanation and is expressed in terms acceptable to modern neuroscience. Conscious mind is reinstated in the brain of objective science and scientific theory is squared with common sense on the mind-controlling-behavior issue.

A New Outlook

The involved change in the status of conscious mind in objective science carries with it a renunciation of much of the mechanistic, behavioristic, deterministic, and reductionistic thinking that formerly has characterized behavioral science and scientism. Long-standing epistemological paradoxes involving the separation of mind and matter, subjective and objective, fact and value, free will and determinism, and *is* and *ought* that have long puzzled and polarized ethical and scientific thinking, seem now to begin to resolve in principle. The current interpretation brings together selected aspects of prior materialist, mentalist, gestalt, monist and dualist doctrine. Some of its implications are explored here, not with any presumption that the present view offers definitive solutions, but only that it seems to represent an advancement containing certain features that differ from those on which value-belief systems have previously been built.

On the present terms it becomes increasingly impossible, among other things, to accept the idea of two separate realms of knowledge, existence, or truth: one for objective science and another for subjective experience and values. Old metaphysical dualisms and the seemingly irreconcilable paradoxes that have prevailed in psychology between the realities of inner experience on the one hand and those of experimental brain research on the other[14], disappear in a single continuous hierarchy. Within the brain, we pass conceptually in a hierarchical continuum from the brain's subnuclear particles on up through atoms, molecules, and brain cells to nerve circuit systems without consciousness, and finally to cerebral processes with consciousness. Objective facts and subjective values become parts of the same realm of discourse. The hiatus between science and values is erased in part by expanding the scope of science to encompass inner experience, and also by altering the status of subjective values so that they are no longer set off in an epiphenomenal or other parallelistic subjective domain beyond the reach of science[8]. "Science" is used broadly here to include the knowledge, insight, perspectives, beliefs, and understanding that come from science as well as the relative validity, credibility, and reliability of the scientific method itself as an approach to truth so far as the human brain can know it. Also, one needs to remember in this connection that modern science includes the behavioral, political, social and related sciences and does not on the above terms imply the traditional hardcore materialism and strict objectivity of a decade ago[15].

So long as science was lacking a plausible account of mind in relation to matter, and excluded on principle the whole realm of inner subjective experience, the worldview of science remained incomplete and inadequate to provide answers in the realm of subjective moral value or higher meaning. Alternative world views built around more wishful metaphysical dimensions were not only more appealing to the public majority, but also remained competitive in credibility. With the value-rich world of inner experience no longer excluded on principle from the realm of science, scientism (i.e. the search for values and higher meaning through science) takes on added humanistic dimensions and a whole new look. On these revised terms the emotional, interpersonal, and aesthetic dimensions in ethical systems no longer exclude a scientific approach nor are they either excluded from an ethic based on science. Many of the antiscience and counterculture objections leveled against materialistic science no longer apply.

From the outset it has been recognized that this compromise operational interactionist approach to consciousness would provide in theory a long sought unifying view of mind, brain and man in nature and would go far to restore to the scientific image of man some of the freedom, dignity, and other humanistic attributes of which it has long been deprived.[7] An antireductionist worldview and interpretation of reality are also implied in which the qualitative pattern properties of all entities are conceived to be just as real and causally potent as are the properties of their elements or their quantitative measurements and abstractions. This preservation of the qualitative value and pluralistic richness of reality helps to counter antiscience views[5] that correlate science with reductionism.

The reductionist approach that would always explain the whole in terms of "nothing but" the parts leads to an infinite nihilistic regress in which eventually everything is held to be explainable in terms of essentially nothing. By our present interpretation, it is better science to conceive wholes and their properties as real phenomena with their own meaning and causal efficacy. This means essentially that the pattern relationships of the component parts to each other in time and space are recognized to be of critical importance in causation and in determining the nature and meaning of all things and that these configurational relationships are not reducible to properties of the parts alone. The message will not be found in the chemistry of the ink. Thus, the search in science for a unifying explanatory formula for the universe is discouraged in favor of the recognition and sanction of pluralism.

Further Implications

A substantially altered picture of scientific determinism is also implied[7, 16]. Subjective values of all kinds, even aesthetic, spiritual and irrational come to be recognized as having causal control potency in the brain's decision-making process—along with all other components of the world of inner experience. Even such factors as one's subjective feelings about predicted outcomes anticipated to result from a given choice as long as 25 or 100 years in the future, may be entered proactively as causal determinants in the cerebral operations that lead to a given choice. In terms of the degrees and kinds of freedom of choice introduced thereby into the causal sequence of decision making, the human brain is clearly set apart above all other known systems, at an apex post in the deterministic universe of science.

Issues raised in the foregoing are central and fundamental to ethics and value questions at all levels. Value priorities especially in the ideological, religious, and cultural areas, are heavily dependent, directly or by implication, on concepts and beliefs regarding the properties of the conscious mind, and on the kinds of life goals and worldviews which these permit. Directly and indirectly, the latter depend on whether consciousness is believed to be mortal or immortal, or reincarnate or cosmic; and whether consciousness is conceived to be localized and brain-bound or essentially universal as in pan-psychism or Whiteheadian theory—or perhaps capable of "supracoalescence" in a megamind. Where formerly there were seemingly unlimited degrees of freedom for speculation in these areas, advances in neuroscience during the last few decades substantially narrow now the latitudes for possible realistic answers. In modern neurology it is no longer a question of whether conscious experience is tied to the living brain, but rather to what particular parts of the brain, or to which neural systems and under what physiological conditions.[17].

As the brain process comes to be understood objectively, all mental phenomena, including the generation of values, can be treated as causal agents in human decision making. The origins, directive potency, and the consequences of values all become subject, in principle, to objective scientific investigation and analysis. This applies at all levels, from that of the brain's pleasure-pain centers and other reinforcement systems on up through the forces that mold priorities at the societal, national, and international plane. Modern behavioral science already treats value variables and their formation as important causal variants in behavior, and it also deals analytically with goals, needs, motivation, and related factors at individual, group, and societal levels. Value variables are in principle reproducible through replication of similar brain states. What amounts to a separate science of values in the context of decision theory becomes conceivable, extending into all branches of behavioral science and forming a skeletal core for social science. Any advances in our understanding of the origins and logical structure of value systems can be expected to result in wiser selection and ordering of social values, and better value judgments and decisions generally.

Remaining Obstacles

Once it is possible, in principle, to resolve epistemological differences between mind and brain, subjective value and objective fact, determinism and free will, and to treat values objectively in the context of decision making, it then follows that other remaining obstacles and objections to an approach to values and meaning through science tend to disappear. The old argument of professional philosophy that it is logically impossible to determine what *ought to be* from what *is,* or to derive ethical values from scientific facts may hold on paper in the abstract. It carries little practical significance, however, when values are viewed pragmatically as above in a brain-behavior framework. Human values are inherently properties of brain activity and it invites logical confusion to try to treat them as if they had independent existence artificially separated from the functioning brain. In the operations of the brain, incoming facts regularly interact with and shape values. In terms of cerebral processing, it is difficult to see a better way to determine "what ought to be" than on the basis of factual information, especially facts and deductions therefrom that have been scientifically verified. History and common observation confirm that nothing tells better than science what ought to prevail in order to achieve any defined aim, whether the aim be a landing site on Mars, improved health or whatever.

The human brain comes already equipped in advance with established value determinants and with inbuilt logical constraints that have their origins partly in biological heritage, partly in prior experience, and may even come through formal acceptance of ethical axioms. In practice, therefore, it is not a question of deriving values from the facts per se. Incoming factual information interacts as a cofunction with intrinsic cerebral value determinants in hen-egg fashion in the building of one's sense of value. The value system of any adult or society is determined in large part by objective facts. The mutual interactions through time between the inbuilt systems of values inherent in human nature and the developing worldview determinants form a complex manifold. Value judgments will never be made simple by a scientific approach and in some respects promise to become more complicated. One can hope only for improved value judgments through error correction and advanced insight. The worldview of science includes, of course, a growing understanding of the origins and structure of the inherent value functions and of their chronological shaping during development.

The question at issue may thus be framed more usefully in terms of the impact of a set of facts upon ongoing brain processes wherein values and related logical determinants already are operative. If one asks accordingly whether a set of facts can shape value priorities, the answer, of course, is "yes." We are constantly adjusting our values to conform logically with new factual information. The advance of science historically has always had a deep inevitable influence on social value systems. For present purposes, the innate primal system of values inbuilt in human nature (the personal and social aspects of which tend to form a large common denominator for any human value system) is treated largely as constant in order to focus on the more extrinsic variables that involve science and its alternatives. Our concern here is specifically with those value system variables introduced by acceptance of the method and worldview of science. Many advances of past teachings in the area of personal and interpersonal relations would not be changed. The related problem of starting axioms or premises and prime determinants in ethical systems is considered separately below.

Science, as man's number one source of factual information, may be enlisted in the realm of value judgment on the simple and straightforward rationale that an informed judgment is generally preferable to one that is uninformed or misinformed. Merely to close the value gap that currently exists around the world between the informed and the uninformed might in itself go a long way to help counter current disaster trends. Similarly, if judgments about right and wrong are best arrived at on the basis of what is true, avoiding what is false, science would seem on this count as well to deserve a lead role in determining ethical values instead of being disqualified.

Some of the arbitrariness and endless complexity of human values that have always seemed forbidding to any approach through science disappear in part if one agrees to exclude the metaphysical and mythological, and to hold to a frame of reference supported by science. Societal values of the category that get written into law can be shown to be largely goal-dependent directly or by implication and arrangeable into logical hierarchical systems with major and subsidiary goals superseded by ultimate goals and conditioned throughout by inherent traits and needs of the species[3].

A quite different view would renounce any rational approach to ethics through science, not because social values should be left to the humanities, the church, the courts, or to Karl Marx, but rather on grounds that it is wiser that values be left to themselves to change spontaneously, by collective intuition as it were, in response to changing environmental conditions. Some economic realists assert that this is the only way that values change and eschew any moral philosophizing and idealizing as ineffectual. This latter overlooks the strong reciprocal interaction between mental concepts and environmental conditions and the tremendous impact that ideology and value systems have always had on the course of human history. It overlooks also the fact that social

values formed merely on this situational feedback basis as a
reflection of prevailing conditions tend in the democratic process
to be locked to levels of tolerability.

Science and the Prime Determinants of Value

It is not only the value systems of formal religion that have
been found wanting today, but also those based in humanist,
communist, existentialist, and even in common humanitarian
persuasions. Contemporary recourse to alternatives like the
"lifeboat ethic" or that of "triage" hardly offer inspired solutions. The global ecospheric nature of current world problems
calls for value perspectives built on something higher than just
the human species or its societal dynamics, something that will
include the welfare of the entire biosphere and ecosphere on a
long term basis[4]. It becomes a logical necessity also in efforts to
perceive any higher meaning or purpose, that humanity see itself
in terms of a meaningful relation to something more important
than itself.

The more critical value issues that must be faced in the near
future will involve decisions that ultimately require appraisals of
the relative worth of human life in various contexts. As terrestrial crowding conditions get tighter, for example, the value of
human life must be balanced increasingly against that of other
species. Having already destroyed the natural meaning and dignity of life for a number of subordinate species and permanently
extinguished others, man will be forced to judge how much farther the violation of species' rights should be carried and by what
ethic. Many more examples can be listed where scientific advance-
ments, coupled with mounting population and related pressures,
raise a growing host of moral dilemmas that resolve finally
around the question of the ultimate worth and meaning of life
itself. Possible answers become relative with alternatives that
call for assessment within some larger ethic yet to be found.
What is needed ideally, of course, to make decisions in these areas
is a consensus on some supreme comprehension and interpretation of the universe and the place and role within it of man and
the life experience.

The same position is reached by way of abstract value theory, in which values are shown to depend largely on goals, and that any concept or belief regarding the goal and value of life as a whole, once accepted, then logically supersedes and conditions values at all subsidiary levels. Value priorities become ordered and ethical issues judged in accordance with the conceived ultimate goal. This latter will imply in turn an associated "worldview" or universal scheme that is consistent.

By one route or another, then, we come down to these prime determinants of value priorities — these "life-goal", "worldview" concepts and beliefs, explicit or implied, that lie at the heart of the problem of values and pose the central challenge for a scientific or any other approach. This is where the great unknowns lie and also where the great differences of opinion are found. This is where answers are most needed and where any answers once accepted, right or wrong, have the greatest impact. And it is here also that the competence of science in the arena of values and any new ethic must eventually prove itself. The scientist, trained to rigorous reasoning and skepticism, to checking against empirical evidence, and above all, to avoiding false conclusions, may easily be persuaded at this point that value problems are not for science. It must, however, be remembered that final, absolute, or perfect answers are not demanded, only improved ones; and that society has in the past and probably will continue in the future to find and abide by some kind of answers from somewhere.

Actually, modern science, with its concepts of cosmology, evolution and the nature of conscious mind, reaching into all levels and aspects of the natural order from subnuclear particles on up through galaxies millions of light years away, has considerable to say about most of those fundamental cornerstone concepts upon which man's great mainline value systems have built through history. The worldview of modern science renders all previous schemes simplistic by comparison and provides man's most reliable understanding of, and rapport with those forces that move the universe and control creation. What has been accepted most commonly in the past as the highest reference for ethical standards and moral authority, man's creator, becomes in the eyes of science the vast interwoven fabric of all evolving nature. Each new scientific discovery and insight increases by that much more man's comprehension of the total design of evolving nature which, as indicated, implicates value and meaning in our current concept of mind and makes a final referent and framework for any ethical or moral system.

Some of the kinds of social value changes that might inhere in an ethic founded in science can be foreseen in broad outline[2, 3], but these remain for the most part still to be developed. Social decisions on ethical issues, however, do not require and frequently do not involve, nor wait on precise logical answers. Decision making proceeds commonly on the basis of vague impressions, inclinations, doctrinal perspectives, emotional leanings and convictions, personal biases, and the like. Even a slight shift in the ethical norms of society, as along the science-antiscience axis, could set in motion, through a vast complex of decisional differences, changes affecting population policy, global conservation, and ecosystem planning generally, the overall future impact of which would make that of other top goals in science, like a cure for cancer, appear insignificant by comparison. Progress along the above lines could be greatly speeded on many fronts if we can merely clear the way by making it intellectually respectable and scientifically sound to think that "Science deals with values as well as with facts."

REFERENCES

1. Clyde Kluckhohn, *Proc. Am. Philos. Soc.* 102, 469 (1959).
2. Ralph W. Burhoe, *Zygon* 4, 65 (1-69); *Zygon* 8, 412 (1973).
3. R.W. Sperry, *Persp. Biol. Med.* 16, 115 (1972); reprinted in *Zygon* 9, 7 (1974).
4. Garrett Hardin, *Exploring New Ethics for Survival* (Viking, New York, 1972).
5. Theodore Roszak, *Where the Wasteland Ends: Politics and Transcendence in Postindustrial Society* (Doubleday, Garden City, New York, 1973).
6. Ezra J. Mishan, *The Costs of Economic Growth* (Preager, Inc., New York 1969). See especially Chap. 12, sections *d* and *e.*
7. R.W. Sperry, *Bull. Atom Sci.* 22, 2 (1966); Joh Platt, *New Views of the Nature of Man,* Chap. 4 (University of Chicago Press, Chicago, 1965).
8. R.W. Sperry, *Psychol. Rev.* 76, 532 (1969).
9. R.W. Sperry, *Psychol. Rev.* 77, 585 (1970).

10. R.W. Sperry, in *Consciousness and Brain*, Gordon Globus, G. Maxwell, I. Savodnik, Eds. (Plenum, New York, in press).
11. R.W. Sperry, *Amer. Scientist* 40, 291 (1952).
12. For an expanded discussion of holistic causality see Edward Pols, *Internat. Philos. Quart.* 11, 293 (1971).
13. Wolfgang Kohler and Richard Held, *Science* 110, 414 (1949).
14. T.W. Wann (Ed.) *Behaviorism and Phenomenology: Contrasting Bases for Modern Psychology* (Univ. of Chicago Press, Chicago, 1965).
15. (See also Michael Polanyi, *The Tacit Dimension* (Doubleday and Co., New York, 1966).
16. R.W. Sperry, *Problems Outstanding in the Evolution of Brain Function*, James Arthur Lecture, American Museum of Natural History, New York, 1964.
17. John C. Eccles, *The Understanding of the Brain* (McGraw-Hill, New York, 1973), *Brain and Conscious Experience* (Springer-Verlag, New York, 1966).

J. W. S. Pringle

C9 The Mechanism of Knowledge: Limits to Prediction

The title of this group discussion is "The New Physics and Absolute Values." I cannot claim full familiarity with the new physics and I am not sure if I can define absolute values, but the topics in Group IV suggest that this conference has wide terms of reference. I will therefore start on the central theme of my paper by means of a diagram (Figure 1, solid lines) summarizing some of the intellectual problems that have troubled mankind. There are no doubt many others, but I don't think there will be much doubt that these problems are very much discussed and that they have not been resolved. Thinking men and women everywhere consider and discuss these problems and have done so for a very long time without, in my opinion, making much progress in their understanding.

This word 'understanding' seems to me to lie at the root of all the problems. Fourteen years ago, when I was preparing my Inaugural Lecture at Oxford University, it occurred to me that maybe we have been trying to do the wrong thing. That great physical scientist, Sir Arthur Eddington, once wrote[1] that we have no need to define knowledge. I cannot agree. What we are trying to do in all these problems is to establish a state of inter-relatedness between our brains which are the medium for our thinking and our observation and interpretations of phenomena outside ourselves. So we ought not to be surveying the problems from a pedestal external to them, but ought to take as our material for study the system of ourselves studying and considering things. So Figure 1 is completed with the portion drawn with dotted lines, by the insertion of the human brain interacting with the problems. This at once looks more promising, since it becomes obvious that the block to progress may lie in our failure to understand how the human brain works. If we knew how the human brain worked and what was the physiological process that is cor-

Figure 1

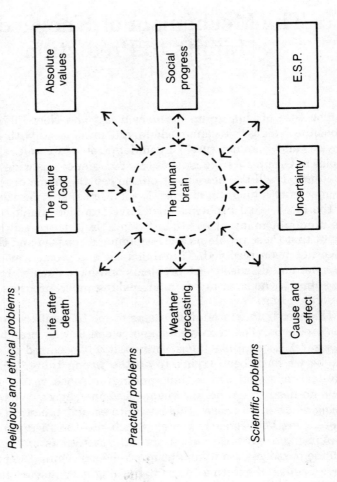

related with our conscious thoughts, then we might be able to judge whether the problems are soluble or not. If they are not then we could stop worrying about them and get on with things that are practicable.

Now I am no more an expert in the functioning of the brain than I am an expert in modern physics or philosophy. I am a zoologist and I suppose that the one field of which I can claim to have some understanding is the process of evolution. My thinking on this subject has developed from considering the process of evolution by natural selection and as this is a rather unusual starting point from which to consider either brain physiology, psychology, modern physics or philosophy, it is just possible that I may have something worthwhile to say.

In 1951, I published a paper with the title "On the parallel between learning and evolution."[2] The argument went as follows. It is common ground among biologists that as organic evolution proceeded, the structure of animals became more complex. What, however, does this mean? If one examines critically the concept of complexity, it is clear that it is a term that can validly be ascribed only to statements about things, not about the things themselves without some further qualification. It certainly appears to be necessary to make more complex statements in order to describe the structure of higher animals than of lower animals, but is there any way in which it can be valid to state that the animals themselves are more complex. I suggested that, in relation to structural complexity, the necessary further condition was that repeated observations should require statements with the same degree of complexity; that is, that the structural features should have some order or permanence in time.

Things that one can describe as structures must have some permanence in time, but this permanence can be a dynamic steady state, as in a lenticular cloud which stays in one place although the wind blows through it. The process of evolution by natural selection preserves thermodynamically improbable states of organization in the molecular complexes of which organisms are composed. The stability derives from the ability of certain molecular assemblies to replicate: that is, to produce more states of organization like themselves. The whole process of evolution occurs because certain molecular assemblies have this property of replication and because the replication is slightly imperfect. Assemblies which survive longer or which replicate more rapidly under the given conditions are preserved in competition with other assemblies for the available raw materials. This is the process of evolution by natural selection of intrinsically variable replicating molecular assemblies. The most recent semi-popular discussion of the subject is a book by Richard Dawkins entitled, "The Selfish Gene."[3]

Now it appears to students of animal behavior that complexity also increases when the phenomenon of learning takes place in animals. Learning is the modification of behavior which occurs due to events during the lifetime of the animal. All animals possess a behavioral machinery which is part of their genetic inheritance and has been naturally selected with due regard to events happening during the life-times of their ancestors. This is the innate component of behavior which provides the background upon which the learned changes take place. I explored the different manifestations of the process of learning as classified by Thorpe and it became clear that more complex statements were indeed required to describe the final state of affairs than the state before the learning had occurred.

Is it then possible to transfer the concept of complexity from the description of the time pattern of animal behavior to the time pattern itself? Not, obviously, by using the same criterion of permanence in time, because a time pattern is what is being described. I suggested that the criterion to adopt is permanence in space; that is, that simultaneous observations in different places should yield descriptions with the same measure of temporal complexity.

I then tried to see if one could find a type of process which would show an "evolution" of time patterns with the same characteristics as organic evolution except that the parameters of space and time were interchanged. It was necessary that the process should show the essential features of natural selection of intrinsically variable replicating phenomena; otherwise it would not evolve. The simplest time pattern is a sinusoidal oscillation, which has only one frequency component. Loosely coupled sinusoidal oscillators have a tendency to lock to the same frequency if

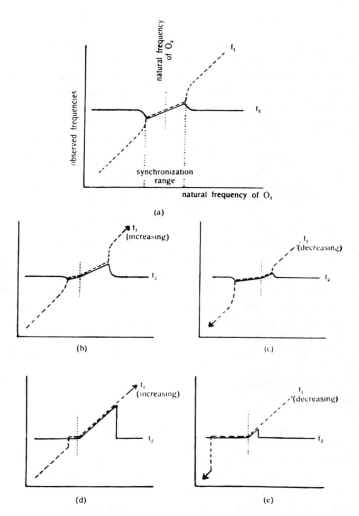

Fig. 2. Diagrams, based on experiments with electronic oscillators, to illustrate the phenomenon of synchronization. The graphs show the observed frequencies f_1 and f_2 of two coupled oscillators. O_1 and O_2 as the natural frequency of O_1 is varied.

a) Linear oscillation
b) Non-linear oscillation: frequency of O_1 increasing.
c) Non-linear oscillation: frequency of O_1 decreasing.
d) Relaxation oscillation: frequency of O_1 increasing.
e) Relaxation oscillation: frequency of O_1 decreasing.

their natural frequencies of oscillation are sufficiently close together. The interaction is, however, symmetrical and this is not a satisfactory model since there is nothing in the nature of selection, which requires some asymmetry. The genes which survive in a population are those that have better means of propagating themselves than do other genes. If, however, the oscillations are non-linear, then when they lock in frequency the interactions are asymmetrical (Figure 2). An oscillator O_1 whose natural frequency is swept through the natural frequency of oscillator O_2 has more effect on the frequency of O_2 if its own natural frequency is increasing than if it is decreasing; its own oscillation frequency is displaced less when its natural frequency is increasing than when it is decreasing. The effect is particularly obvious in the case of relaxation oscillators, which are extremely non-linear. If now one adds the further postulate that, when an oscillator has been forced through the synchronization process to oscillate at a frequency different from its natural frequency, its natural frequency is changed in the same direction, then there is a "replication" of a time pattern. In a population of such oscillators, those that sweep through another frequency in the upward direction will gradually "capture" those through whose natural frequencies they sweep and there will subsequently be more oscillators in the population with that natural frequency. The total population with a particular time pattern has replicated in the space occupied by the population.

This looked promising and I therefore went on to two further discussions. First, to what extent could the detailed features of the learning process in animals be explainable on the basis of a model in which the information was contained entirely as time patterns? I showed that all the five forms of the learning process described by Thorpe could, indeed, be modelled in this way and that, for example, the particular relationships between stimuli found experimentally in conditioned reflexes would be expected in the models. Secondly, I considered whether there was any evidence for self-sustaining oscillators in those parts of the brain where it is thought that the learning process takes place, and what was the most plausible neural mechanism of such oscillators. Since much more evidence is available now than was available in 1951, I will expand this part of the argument.

Much of the literature on this subject does not use the language of the animal behaviorist who talks about learning, but refers to memory. This is the same thing, since when behavior depends on the previous experience of the animal, it can be considered to have acquired a memory of the previous events. The most important type of evidence that memory must involve time patterns is that it is not localized in space, although this is not usually explicitly recognized. Professor Eccles summarised one of his contributions to a symposium[4] as follows, "We may summarize this discussion of the structural basis of memory by stating that memory of any particular event is dependent on a specific reorganization of neuronal associations (the engram) in a vast system of neurons widely spread over the cerebral cortex. Lashley has convincingly argued that the activity of literally millions of neurons is involved in the recall of any memory. His experimental study of the effects of cortical lesions on memory indicates that any particular memory trace or engram has multiple representation in the cortex. Furthermore, Lashley concludes that any cortical neuron does not exclusively belong to one engram, but on the contrary, each neuron and even each synaptic junction would be built into many engrams. We have already seen that the systematic study of the responses of individual neurons in the cortex and in the subcortical nuclei is providing many examples of this multiple operation."

In the input channel for information from sense organs, there clearly is spatial localization. Each sensory nerve carries information about one sensory quality. Similarly in the output channels, each motor nerve fibre carries the commands to a particular muscle. But as physiologists study the ascending nervous pathways through which information passes on its way from the sense organs to the cerebral cortex, the localization gets less and less precise at each synaptic layer, so that finally a very large number of cortical neurons are influenced by a message in any given sensory channel. Again on the output side, the further back one goes in the motor pathways, the more does any local excitation produce output in several muscles. There are large areas in the human cerebral cortex called by Penfield the uncommitted cortex which have no function that can be defined in terms of localized effects. Yet the information is not lost in this whole process. The logical conclusion is surely that the information is being transformed into some other form, such as a pattern in time rather than in space, and back into spatial patterns on the way out again. Eccles talks about "spatio-temporal patterns" being important; I suggest that one should leave out the "spatio-" altogether.

Experimental evidence about the nature of spontaneous oscillatory activity in cortical neurons is intrinsically difficult to obtain, because of the fact that any recording system must be spatially localized. The electroencephalogram is the record of electrical activity as recorded with electrodes placed externally on different parts of the head; this does indeed show spontaneous oscillations which have been much studied in an attempt to correlate particular frequency components with states of cerebral activity as described subjectively or observed behaviorally. The fact that anything at all can be recorded with superficial electrodes from a brain containing about 10^9 neurons implies that a great deal of synchronization must be taking place. Records using microscopic electrodes inside individual cortical neurons are dominated by the discrete impulses which are the way in which information is transmitted without loss down the long axon connections between cells some distance apart and are not the components contributed by each cell to the overall electroencephalogram. The individual component potentials are very small continuous fluctuations in membrane potential which are so small that they are almost undetectable against the noise background of the recording apparatus. So with our present techniques it is probably impossible to determine the exact nature of the oscillators whose frequency of activity may be carrying the information at the time when it is subject to the analytical processes involved in learning phenomena, particularly as, if there is indeed no significant spatial localization, the particular structures which are manifesting the significant frequencies of oscillation may be changing from instant to instant. Waves of electrical activity at a particular frequency do pass over the surface of the cortex.

I suggested in 1951 that the unit of rhythmic activity consists of a closed loop of neurons which oscillates because of a small amplification and phase shift introduced by each neuron. Since each cell in the cortex has synaptic connexions to a large number of other cells, the spatial localization of such a loop oscillator will be extremely plastic, depending on the amplification and phase shifts of every cell in the network. One cell can be a component part of more than one oscillating loop at the same time, providing the means for coupling between them. The change demanded by my model when a neuronal loop has been forced to oscillate at a frequency other than its natural frequency, by synchronization to a driving oscillator, is a small change in the amplification or phase shift contributed by the cells. There is no need to postulate any change in the pattern of connectivity between cells and the model is therefore different in essentials from all models of memory which involve synaptic growth or regression. I have been surprised at the way in which neurophysiologists seem to take it almost as an axiom that memory must necessarily involve a change in synaptic connexions in the central nervous system. A model in which the information is represented as a complex of time pattern with no spatial localization makes this assumption unnecessary.

I just do not know how to proceed to test further the value of a model of this sort and it is in the hope of obtaining some suggestions and help that I have described the model rather fully. Dr. Brian Goodwin,[5] who has considered oscillating systems in the biochemical machinery of cells, has suggested that it may be possible to develop a sort of statistical mechanics of interacting oscillators and he has even defined macroscopic parameters of such a system which bear some similarity to the parameters of temperature and free energy of classical statistical mechanics, coining for them the adjective *"talandic"* from the Greek world for oscillation. This sort of thing is well beyond my capacity.

Consciousness

The earlier part of this paper restates in outline a hypothesis about the physiological mechanism by which the associative processes of the central nervous system take place and locates the memory trace within a large number of neurons instead of in the synaptic connexions between them. In the rest of the paper I shall make some highly speculative suggestions which depend on the general correctness of the hypothesis. If the hypothesis is false, these suggestions have no value; if it is correct, they constitute a possible way of making progress with several problems which have hitherto defied scientific analysis. The first of these problems is the nature of consciousness.

Professor Penfield, as a result of his experience as a surgeon operating on the brains of conscious patients, has written[4] "Consciousness is not something to be localized in space. Nevertheless, if we assume that it is a function of the integrated action of the brain, there is placed before us a challenging problem of physiological localization." Penfield is unable to escape from the assumption that some form of localization must be necessary and is driven to involve a sub-cortical region of the brain. I would like to make a concrete suggestion, which cannot be more than a speculation but which might be testable. It is that consciousness occurs when complex time patterns spread over a sufficiently large region of space. The physiological correlate of consciousness does not need to be localized at all, since the information which a conscious thought contains is represented in the brain as a time pattern. The clarity and preciseness of the conscious thought could correlate with the extent of spatial spread of the time pattern, and "vague" or imprecise thoughts—half-thoughts—could correlate with time patterns which do not have a large enough spatial spread.

Now it is sometimes suggested that only half of the human cerebral cortex containing the speech center, normally the left side, is capable of conscious thought. Normally the two sides of cortex are extensively connected together by nervous tracts so that the whole functions as a single unit, but in patients in whom these tracts have been severed, Sperry in particular has described[4] how the patient is only able to describe objects presented in the half of the visual field which projects on to the left cortex. Correct motor movements can be made in response to stimuli presented to the other half of the visual field and these may depend on previous experience, but the patient is not conscious of what he is doing, in the sense that he cannot later describe in words what he has done. Conscious thought need not, however, be accompanied by actual speaking and conscious patients whose speech center is stimulated electrically are still capable of thought although they cannot speak while the electrical stimulation lasts. A thought is clarified and made more precise by describing it in words, but it exists in some form before it is spoken. I know of no better statement of this than a little known poem by an anonymous author that I will quote in full. It was published in 1949 in the Oxford Magazine over the signature "X" and was entitled "Words."

I lag behind, my words go on before
  And tell me what I did not know I knew,
And yet I knew it, but I know it more
  When I have said it too.

Dark mystery of words that can reveal
  Even to the speaker what were else obscure,
Can on the soul's dim searching set a seal
  And mark them clear and sure.

Deceiving mystery of seal and word:
  The inarticulate escapes them still:
The caged is not the glancing, half-seen bird:
  You have not yet your will,

You must go on to seek the bird you sought,
  Yet count as gain, as gain unpriceable,
This which the mystery of words has caught,
  Which sings, is beautiful.

I leave the subject of consciousness with this suggestion. It is conceivable that the hypothesis might be testable by stimulating the surface of the cortex with a sufficiently complex time pattern, with particular phase relationships between different regions. If there is no spatial localization, it should not matter just where the stimulus is applied, since the information is in the time pattern.

The Evolution of Consciousness

In large parts of the nervous systems of many animals, there is

probably complete functional localization, even to the extent
found in insects where a single cell always serves one particular
function. There is also no reason why the particular mechanism
for learning proposed above should be the only mechanism found
in the nervous systems of animals. It is only in the vertebrates
and especially in the mammals that we have *evidence* of the
gradual loss of localization that occurs in ascending pathways. It
is by no means unthinkable that this particular method of analyzing sensory information is peculiar to the vertebrates, which
show more plasticity of behavior than most invertebrates and
rely more on learning during the animal's own lifetime and less on
innate patterns of behavior inherited from previous generations.
Alternatively, it could be that we do not yet know enough about
other types of animals to have found evidence for loss of localization. A corollary of the hypothesis put forward in the previous
section would be that only those animals are conscious in which
the transformation of spatial information into time patterns proceeds to a sufficient extent. Furthermore, there could be degrees
of consciousness depending on the extent to which the time patterns achieve spatial spread. A zoologist does not readily accept
the emergence of a new character suddenly in evolution. I myself
prefer to think that consciousness evolved gradually and that it
developed particularly in man when his vocal apparatus developed to the point where it could be used for symbolic expression.
The speech center may be unique in that it is located in the cerebral cortex and provides a direct organizing output for the cortical processes; centers for the group control of other, innate movements are located in evolutionarily lower parts of the brain.

Human evolution is peculiar in that the original process of genetic selection has been largely superseded by cultural selection involving the formulation of ideas in the brain and their replication
through the population by means of the spoken and written word.
This is a much more rapid process than genetic evolution and it
demands that there be a form of natural selection different in essentials from the original one. The natural selection of time patterns in the brain could be such a mechanism and something
ought to be discoverable about the operation of the process by
adapting the knowledge that we have of the dynamics of natural

selection.

Emotions

We do not start our thinking lives with an unbiased reasoning machine in our brains. In our adult mental processes as in our adult structural organization, our starting point is the organization that we have inherited our genetic constitution and our individual developmental history. In the model that I have suggested, the initial time patterns for any thought, the input channels which determine the conditions in which the temporal selection process takes place and the output channels through which the selected time patterns are re-expressed in spatially localized movements are all part of the given situation for any individual brain. There is, I understand, some evidence that the neural circuits involved in long-term memory are different from those involved in short-term memory and that the establishment of new long-term memories can be prevented by localized lesions without affecting consciousness and short-term memory. Emotional states probably involve the coupling in to the cortical circuitry of still more primitive regions of the brain so that the time patterns and the resulting conscious states of mind incorporate other than purely logical determinants.

When we are presented through our sense organs with a situation, we are consciously aware of a mental process that we describe as coming to a conclusion about the action that we will take. We are aware of trying to take into account in arriving at the conclusion, our previous long and short-term memories and our emotions which may introduce bias as between alternatives. What sort of physical processes are involved in this mental process? I suggest that a way of looking at the problem is to treat the sensory input, the memories and the emotional bias as the "environment" within which a process of selection takes place. Coming to a conclusion represents the establishment of a new dynamically stable equilibrium which then determines the output results.[6] In my model the new equilibrium is the new set of time patterns which result from the synchonization process. The more far-reaching is the conclusion, the more have the complex time pat-

terns representing the initial state been resolved into a simpler
set of time patterns. Since no new information is generated by
this process, the new state of organization is consistent with the
original state. I suggest that our mental satisfaction depends on
the extent of the process of resolution and that we call this pleasure when the initial state of the "environment" contained a
large component from the innately determined input. Certain inputs will be mutually incompatible and no simpler dynamic equilibrium will then result; if the sensory input is incompatible with
the innately determined inputs, then the situation is unpleasant,
cannot be resolved and is avoided if possible in the future.

I hope that the previous paragraph makes clear the way in
which I think some of these problems can be tackled. It is almost
impossible to avoid the use of terms whose meaning is incompletely defined and this means that there may be flaws in the logic. If so, I should be glad to have them pointed out. If not, then I
hope I have established that concepts derived from the study of
natural selection could have value in considering human mental
problems.

Uncertainty and Purpose

Our thought processes do not stop when there is not sensory
input. Volunteers undergoing prolonged sensory deprivation
usually develop, after two or three days, states of extreme mental
awareness and their thought processes are liable to become uncontrolled to the point where they become intolerable.

My model leaves room for the possibility that quantum uncertainty can be the "cause" of changes in the time patterns through
the ability of the brain mechanism to amplify the effects of thermal fluctuations in inidividual cells. The possible role of "random" phenomena has been explored by Gomes in the context of
the problem of free-will but, as Mackay has shown, it is probably
irrelevant to this. What is relevant here is the fact that uncertainty on a micro scale need not lead to macroscopic uncertainty in a
mechanism that is dominated by selection. In organic evolution,
mutations are random in their occurrence in time but they provide the background against which evolution takes place and,

apart from exceptional circumstances, it is the forces of natural selection which determine the direction of evolutionary change. Normally in the brain, the sensory input establishes "environmental" conditions sufficiently precise to ensure that the effect of thermal noise is negligible. Sensory deprivation, however, produces a condition when the state of brain organization can drift, using the term in the same sense as it is used in organic evolution. The fact that the uncontrolled mental states that occur under these conditions are unplesant suggests that the effect of random drift may then be sufficient to override the innate determinants.

In organic evolution, the negative feedback involved in natural selection can give the impression of purposefulness. Animal communities evolve so as to appear to be "trying" to make the best use of their environment. Purpose in human mental processes could have the same origin and be due to the selection of time patterns that accompanies the reaching of a conclusion or decision. Ethologists call this type of process "insight learning" and speak of it as involving an internal process of trial and error, operating on some formal representation of the external world in the brain of the animal and making it unneccessary to go through an actual process of trial and error by overt behavioral acts, so avoiding the dangers inherent in failure. It is because of the much greater rapidity of the selection of time patterns that this mechanism is superior to other alternatives, making man the dominant form of life on the planet.

Predictability and Understanding

We can now return to the basic thesis of this paper, that many intellectual problems can only be understood on the basis of an interaction between the human brain and the external world (Figure 1). Let me deal with practical problems first.

Because the speed of the internal selection mechanism of the brain is so much faster than any process in nature that involves selection, the human brain can hope to make predictions about the future course of events, provided that it can set up within itself a formal representation of all the factors which condition that selection process in the external world. The difficulty arises from the fact that in many such natural situations, there is a near infinity of factors which are capable of influencing the natural selection that occurs, and that some of these factors are themselves the result of a selection process. Drift in an evolutionary development occurs when conditions are such that the intrinsic variability of micro phenomena is magnified to a macroscopic scale without the restraining influence of limiting factors. Ultimately, there is always a limit on the magnification process but if the restraints are reduced, as in organic evolution in the fresh colonization of a new habitat, then drift occurs and the situation is fundamentally unpredictable. It is a moot question whether or not true drift occurs in synoptic meteorology, due to the inherently unstable conditions of atmospheric circulation along the polar front. The exact time and place of formation of an individual cyclonic circulation may be theoretically unpredictable, since even if an exactly similar formal set of conditions was set up in the human brain, the evolutionary development in the two cases might be different. The same may be true of social progress, since here many of the conditions which determine the natural selection are human brains themselves performing "evolutionary" decisions. In such situations, the best that can be hoped for is a statistically probable prediction, but even this may be doubtful, since statistics hold good only for ensembles of similar units. Since in both the examples chosen for Figure 1 some of the most important predictions are those relating to a particular time and place, complete predictive certainty may be unattainable.

Rather different considerations apply to the religious and ethical problems of Figure 1. Here we are trying to decide the validity and degree of understanding which can be expected of abstract concepts which are themselves the product of our thinking processes. It is worth considering why we establish these concepts in the first place. This can, I think, only be answered in relation to our past evolutionary history as social animals, which has determined the starting organization of the brains which we use for the processes of thought. One can ask the question: what survival value was conferred on man by the selection of a human brain machinery which leads to the formulation of such concepts? This is a problem for social anthropology, but it may be that any mechanism that has evolved with the function of performing insight learning must formulate such concepts when it reaches a certain degree of perfection just because its inherent tendency to try to forecast the future and to make the assumption that all external events have a cause, as a basis for its predictive activities. Our search for absolute values could stem from this feature of the brain mechanism which makes a single concept a more stabled state than a mixture of two concepts; if my model of the brain mechanism is correct, this is ultimately a problem in talandic thermodynamics.

The problem of why we try to perform certain feats of mental analysis is, of course, different from the problems themselves. I suggest that the former is scientifically more interesting; at any rate, to a biologist, it appears to offer more chance of solution, and it is always possible that if and when we know why we try to do certain things it may be easier to do them. I am not myself very hopeful of this, but it is the only suggestion I can offer to the search for absolute values which is the title of this conference.

Coming finally to the scientific problems, the question to be answered is whether our knowledge of the mechanism of the human brain does or does not suggest that we may ultimately be able to understand the phenomena. I think that progress will be made with this only if my model of the functioning of the brain proves to be useful and if someone else thinks it worth while to explore more fully some of its implications, particularly from a mathematical standpoint.

REFERENCES

1. Eddington, A. (1949). *The Philosophy of Physical Science.* Cambridge Univ. Press.
2. Pringle, J.W.S. (1951). On the parallel between learning and evolution. *Behaviour,* 3, 173-213.
3. Dawkins, R. (1976). *The Selfish Gene.* Oxford Univ. Press.
4. Eccles, J.C. (1966) (editor). *Brain and Conscious Experience.* Springer-Verlag. Berlin.
5. Goodwin, B.W. (1963). *Temporal Organization of Cells.*
6. Pringle, J.W.S. (1963). *The Two Biologies,* p. 26. Clarendon Press, Oxford.

B.D. Josephson

Commentary

Professor Pringle has presented us with a fascinating discussion of the possible mechanisms involved in understanding, and of the deeper question of what influences these mechanisms may have on the possibility of our being able to resolve certain long standing and very difficult problems in the future. In my commentary I should like to give first some of my own thoughts on the question of understanding, and then return to discuss Professor Pringle's ideas in detail.

It may be useful for us to divide the process of understanding into two parts, namely the understanding itself and a process which we may call *learning to understand*. Let me illustrate the difference with a particular example, involving students attending a lecture course on quantum mechanics. Someone who knows quantum mechanics can fairly readily follow a derivation such as that of the spectrum of hydrogen. This is an example of what I call the understanding itself. Now before a person can perform this act of understanding he must first of all have grasped certain essential ideas — those special ideas which distinguish quantum mechanics from its predecessor classical mechanics. Such a process of grasping essential ideas may fairly be called learning to understand, since firstly it involves learning and secondly its result is an ability to understand.

The process responsible for the really major advances in science, and the process to which Professor Pringle chiefly addressed himself in his talk, is the one of learning to understand. To give an example, it was the learning and acceptance by scientists of Einstein's concept that space and time are not absolute but depend on the observer that allowed them to develop all the consequences of special relativity: one key idea permitted an enormous number of phenomena to be discovered and understood. The problems to be considered now are, what similar advances may lie ahead in the future, and how (following Professor Pringle's theme) is our ability to make such advances dependent on the way our brains function?

Here is one more point I should like to make before I comment on detailed mechanisms. This is to the effect that both a person's ability to discover a new idea and his ability to understand one are very much affected, often adversely, by his previous prejudices and beliefs. A classic example from the past relates to the law of conservation of parity in physics (the assertion that the laws of nature make no distinction between left and right).

Until about twenty years ago the idea that the laws of nature did not distinguish between left and right was such a firm belief among physicists that it was not considered necessary to test the belief by experiment, while the slight experimental evidence that the symmetry assumptions was not true was disregarded. Eventually certain phenomena caused Yang and Lee to re-examine the situation. They concluded that for certain kinds of process evidence for conservation was lacking. Following this, measurements showed that for these processes the assumption of parity conservation was indeed false. From such examples we can conclude that however much the design of the human nervous system may make possible in principle grand synthesis such as those of quantum theory and relativity, the ability of an individual to make use of such a capability in practice may be reduced considerably by his tendency to adhere quite rigidly to his previously acquired beliefs. I shall return to this problem later.

I should now like to comment on some details of Professor Pringle's discussion of mechanisms of understanding. He described a model involving a system of coupled non-linear oscillators, which had the capacity of undergoing evolution. Such a kind of model is one I find quite attractive, though I do not believe that it is the whole story.

It is important to realize that the process of grasping a new idea, the one I have called learning to understand, consists in fact of two parts, one of discovery and one of memory. Understanding can be regarded as discovering a point of view from which the solution to a problem becomes transparently clear, and the remembering how one came to that viewpoint. Without subsequent acts of memory and reconstructions, many moments of illumination may be experienced to no avail. I would suggest that Pringle's mechanism of coupled oscillating systems or something similar could account for the processes of discovering a new viewpoint and exploring its potentialities, but that long-term storage to make the understanding permanently available is probably due to the conventional mechanisms involving synaptic modification. The latter mechanisms seem to me to be much more suitable for providing the necessary stability of memory.

The detailed working out of Pringle's proposed mechanisms for understanding must doubtless be very complicated. It is possible that the ideas of Prigogine,[1] relating stability in dissipative systems to states of minimum entropy production, may well prove to be the key to understanding what is going on.

I should like to give now some personal opinions on our prospects of understanding the particular problems listed by Pringle (in his Fig. 1). I shall leave aside those problems designated as practical problems, since it seems to me that in these cases the difficulties are not primarily those of coming to an understanding. In the other cases, however, — the religious, ethical and special scientific problems — I suspect that the prime difficulty is not in the inherent capacity of our brains to solve the problems but in the effects of our previous conditioning. We are in a similar situation to that of those physicists who could not bring themselves to question the assumption that parity in physical processes was conserved.

What are the beliefs that may be holding up understanding in our present situation? I will make two suggestions as to what some of them may be. One, which has relevance concerning the possibility of ESP and other psychic phenomena, is what could be called the myth of the perfect reproductability of natural phenomena. Present scientific method rests on the assumption that one can design experiments such that similar conditions will always produce similar effects. We already know that such an assumption runs into difficulties in the quantum domain; perhaps trying to force such an assumption upon the world at large may be causing us to miss some crucial aspect of reality.

A second possibility limiting belief is the almost universal working rule of scientific workers that no natural phenomena, even those of human behavior or of evolution, should include religious concepts such as the existence of God as a component of their explanation. As far as I am aware, present-day physics does not in any way exclude the possibility of some configuration of matter or energy having the qualities normally ascribed to God, any more than it would exclude the discovery tomorrow of a new kind of charmed particle. It is true that science has not yet found it necessary to postulate the existence of God, but this can reasonably by ascribed to the fact that science has not yet been able to study the situations in which God might be expected to assert an influence with adequate precision.

Finally, I should like to discuss the question of whether there are any specific actions which might be able to allow us to make better use of the problem-solving capability of the brain of man.

Descriptions by creative thinkers have indicated that getting an original idea involves a special state of consciousness, in which the person is aware of the problem to be solved and of that part of his knowledge which pertains to the general nature of the problem, but he has suspended his beliefs or prejudices as to what the solution to the problem might be. It has been suggested that certain techniques such as biofeedback and meditation can enhance the ability to produce such a state. At the moment the situation is not completely clear, but should systematic enhancement of creativity prove to be possible to any significant extent, we have in prospect a situation in which original scientific theories may be frequently produced which are not the direct descendants of any previous theories, and enter the minds of their creators simply because they are the correct answers to those problems most in need of solution at that particular time.

REFERENCE
1. P. Glansdorff and I. Prigogine, *Thermodynamic Theory of Structure, Stability and Fluctuations*, Wiley, 1971.

— D5 —
Death and the Meaning of Life
Kai Nielsen

— D6 —
Death and the Meaning of Life in the Christian Tradition
W. Norris Clarke

— D7 —
Death and the Meaning of Life—A Hindu Response
Ravi Ravindra

— D8 —
Natural Theological Speculations on Death and the Meaning of Life
Sir John Eccles

W.H. Thorpe

D1 Science and Man's Need for Meaning

In recent years a group of psychoanalysts in this country, and others elsewhere, have described how one of the major threats to health and sanity today is what they call the 'existential vacuum' experienced by vast numbers of their patients: a feeling of inner emptiness, of aimless lives set down in a desert of meaninglessness. This is claimed as characteristic of modern scientifically oriented society — the result, in a word, of the widespread assumption that science is the only 'philosophy' in which one can believe. The existential vacuum is regarded as due to the frustration of the most basic motivational force in man — the will to meaning. (In contrast to the Adlerian 'will to power' and the Freudian 'will to pleasure.') The argument is that people do not care for pleasure or for the avoidance of pain; but that they do crave profoundly for meaning. This need or demand for meaning is regarded as one of the most basic features of man.

Science, of course, as we all know, answers the need for 'understanding' in the more limited sense, and is opening ever enlarging vistas of the stupendous complexity and beauty of the created universe. But in general, this does not, by itself, help to assuage the need for meaning. Belief in 'meaning' in this sense, rests on religious faith or on an accepted philosophy or system of myths as to the nature of the world and the relation of man to it.

From the biological point of view the modern crisis was mainly generated by the theory of evolution by natural selection. I think that there is no doubt that, in Western countries, the retreat from organized religion is, in the long term, mainly based on the slow dissemination of the changed world picture, especially that originating from Darwin's work with the overwhelming evidence it *seemed* to supply of the importance of chance in the origin and development of man. For obviously mankind, before the nineteenth century, was by no means denied a measure of satisfaction of his

needs: he had it of course in Western countries as a result of the
Judaeo-Christian vision which gave man a clear place in the
world system and a faith and hope in the future. But not only
this: in Western Europe there was a very wide basic belief in (and
acceptance of) a world system and man's place in it which could
be held with or without the Judaeo-Christian picture and which
in general reinforced some of the most important of its beliefs and
attitudes. This was 'The Great Chain of Being' — which served to
express the unimaginable plenitude of God's creation, its unfalt-
ering order, and its ultimate unity. This 'chain' or 'ladder,' if one
likes to regard it so, was thought of as stretching from the foot of
God's throne to the meanest of inanimate objects. Every speck of
creation represented a link in the chain. But its importance for
my story now is that the top of every inferior class touched the
bottom of a superior one — so that where the steps were in contact, as at the boundary between rocks and plants or between
plants and animals or between animals and man there were
transitional forms in which both higher and lower grades co-oper-
ated. And so at the top the noblest entity in the category of
bodies, was the human body which touches the fringe of the next
class above it — namely the human soul which occupies the lowest
rank in the spiritual order.

As late as Elizabethan times awareness of this sophisticated
system was widespread and basic. But by the eighteenth century
the scheme was beginning to reveal flaws and was breaking down
under philosophical and scientific criticism. And so the coming of
evolution theory in the nineteenth century can in a way be regarded as ushering in the final destruction of that which had sustained man's thought for many centuries and had given him comfort in a mysterious world: indeed since Plato; from whose teaching the mighty plan originally grew.

I need not try to trace the process further; for threats to meaning are obvious everywhere — not least of these being the widespread monistic views of so many scientists and humanists of the
present day; views which make man's spiritual side appear to be
merely the superficial by-product of a material process. Again at
the present day many scientists, and particularly scientific popu-
larizers, have a lot to answer for in the way they have exhibited

what has been called 'the compulsive urge to disenchant,' by being irresponsibly and irrepressibly smart and clever; often seeming to deliberately 'bamboozle' the 'common man' and his beliefs by shock and ridicule. The result has, I think, contributed to a sense of helplessness, a loss of nerve; indeed a sense of boredom and a failure to see (because life seems so complicated) that all the vast developments in science — dangerous as they are as threatening the very existence of life on this planet — have their beneficent side; and, if properly used and understood, can be, indeed must be, the means of progress to a new world order and re-awakening.

But how does today's scientific world picture affect man's view of himself and of his place in the universe? It seems to me that a very subtle and important series of changes has been taking place in recent years — changes which bear closely on our ideas of the emergence of new properties and values in the world. This is after all the key question — how and how far does quantity and complexification become quality? What is the real relation between wholes and parts? Emergent properties are the properties of a whole system not possessed by its parts. This is what one may call the *orthodox* scientific view. The program with which scientists commence, is that in principle, though not yet by any means in practice, the whole should be entirely explicable in terms of their parts; and for many branches of physical science it is indeed a sound research tactic. So it seems to me that this basic program of the physicist, though being very far from complete, is undoubtedly the one which he must pursue. But we all know that physical theorizing often leads to what seem to be absurdities — for instance the modern view is that, against all intuition (based on the special theory of relativity), there is no role for the 'flow of time' or 'now' in the physical world.

But before coming to biology I wish, at the risk of trespassing in the fields of the two other speakers today, to point out the extraordinary way modern cosmology seems to come nearer to asserting that the universe is, in some surprising ways, far more appropriate for life than was at one time thought. That although, as far as we *know*, life is only present in this solar system and on this planet, living beings, including ourselves, are perhaps more 'at home' in the cosmos than we hitherto had reason to believe.

The first point that can be made with certainty is that if the universe were not much as it is, neither ourselves nor other forms of life could have come into existence. If the universe were not expanding, if there were no stars, if the proton-proton force were slightly different—without a certain ratio between the basic forces of interaction and a certain relationship between the fundamental constants—without all the space and time in the world, the 'universe' would be dead. In particular the present theory of the periodic system explains the production of the heavier nuclei through the fusion of several hydrogen nuclei. These heavier elements, such as iron, are essential to life. All evidence at present points to the conclusion that it is only under the circumstances of intense gravitational contraction, which leads to supernova outbursts, that the heavier elements can have been formed; and it is only as another result of supernova explosions that these elements can have been spewed out into space and so made available to stars with solar systems such as ours. So it is this chain of events which during an estimated $10 \cdot 2$ billion years, that has provided us with the heavy elements which we all of necessity carry around in our bodies. It is indeed the astounding coherence of the universe as a whole which had led to the present state of the cosmos being (according to current theory) due to events which took place a minute fraction of a second after the 'big bang'—the very onset of time!

I have just said that the idea of the flow of time, of the present, and of 'now,' appear to be an emergent property of ourselves, and to have no counterpart in theoretical physics. Yet in the mental world such concepts have the unshakeable validity of direct experience. So here science seems to have brought us to the boundary between the material and mental worlds where there does seem to be an unbridgeable gap. Now the property above all properties which demarcates this gap is that of consciousness or self-awareness. So, in company with some neurophysiologists and philosophers, I see some form of dualism between 'Matter' and 'Mind' to be unavoidable in the future program for biology. Karl Popper for instance sees that no explanation of the physical world can be valid which regards the self-consciousness of man as being merely an epiphenomenon—an accidental outcome of the mechanical workings of a machine which we call the brain. This amounts to saying that there must in fact be two worlds—the world of self knowing and the physical world which is known by the operations of the scientific method as used by the physicists and biologists. The miracle is that the 'big bang' created a situation such that thousands of millions of years later a part of the universe could study the rest of itself!

Now let us return to consideration of the evidence for what, if we are dualists in the sense above used, we are forced to describe as 'Mind' or 'The Mental' or 'The Quality of Awareness' in the biological realm, apart from man himself.

In recent years the problem as to whether or not we are justified in the assumption that some animals have some kind of mental experiences—certainly not comparable in quality and scope to our own—but evolutionarily continuous with it—has come to the forefront of biology as the result of new and highly important experiments.

There are a number of lines of research which have provided new evidence, indeed key evidence, for this question of the 'mentality' of animals; all of them concerned with the modern study of communication and an increased understanding of what the word can signify, when we are considering the co-ordination of behavior between individuals of the same species. It similarly arises from much modern work on the nature of animal orientation—in particular, studies of the hearing of bats, the orientation of the flights of migratory and homing birds, the underwater hearing of fish, whales, and, above all (in bats and fish), their ability to orient themselves by responding to echoes of their own 'voices' (i.e., by echolocation). But because of lack of time I must restrict myself to a very brief summary of recent work in two fields— namely the ability of primates such as the chimpanzee to acquire languages taught them by human beings; and secondly, the ability of the social insects, particularly the worker honey bee (*Apis mellifica*) to transmit information to other members of the colony with a subtlety and precision which hitherto had been regarded as quite unthinkable.

The first, and by now widely famous, study of the language learning of chimpanzees is that of R.A. and B.T. Gardner, who achieved remarkable success in teaching a young female animal in captivity the gesture language known as the American Sign Language (A.S.L.). This language is composed of manually produced avisual signals called 'signs' which are strictly analogous to words used in speech. These are arbitrary but stable meaningless signal elements which are arranged in a series of patterns constituting minimum meaningful combinations of those elements. Not only did the Gardners' first chimp 'Washoe' but also other chimps since studied, achieve surprisingly good learning of the varieties of signs; they also developed signs which can best be described as 'straight inventions,' in that they were quite different from signs which had, until then, been the models provided for them by their teachers. Moreover it is possible for such experimental animals to use pronouns appropriately. The animals can also combine previously learned signs into small groups in meaningful ways and apply them appropriately to new situations. For example the sign for 'open,' which was originally learnt in regard to doors, was later used correctly in requesting the opening of boxes, drawers, brief-cases and picture books. All this provides clear evidence for elementary purposiveness.

The significance of these new results is strengthened enormously by the fact that there are at least three series of experiments (with different animals and using different techniques) in which the same results have been reached. One of the reasons why it has been necessary to consider so carefully the question of animal language is because it relates to the arguments put forward by Chomsky and others that the possession of language is indubitable evidence of mentality and of some basic and innate mental structure without which the acquisiton of true language and its purposive use, whether by animals or men, in inconceivable.

There has of course been a great deal of pungent criticism of the results of these studies and their interpretation. But I think the experimenters have now gone a long way, if not the whole way, towards giving satisfactory answers. As a result of the totality of chimpanzee experiments nearly all the critical objections raised by scientists and philosophers against crediting animals with true linguistic developments have been answered by at least one animal and most of them by several. These objections amounted to the demand for the fulfilment of five criteria, namely that an animal must:

1) Demonstrate an extensive system of names for objects in the environment.
2) Sign about objects which are not physically present.
3) Use signs for concepts; not just objects, actions and agents.
4) Invent semantically appropriate combinations, and
5) Use correct order when it is semantically necessary.

Over and above the fact that all these questions have now been answered in the affirmative; still yet more relevant activities are coming to light. It has been shown that captive chimpanzees can communicate fairly complex information by some combinations of gestures or expressive movements that human investigators have not yet deciphered. In the light of these results it is very interesting to look at some of the more recent statements of philosophers and linguists; (who have argued that human language is closely linked with thinking, if not basically identical and inseparable from it). In 1968 (M. Black) we were assured that it would be astounding to discover that insects or fish, birds or monkeys are able to talk to one another—because man is the only animal which can talk and can use symbols, the only animal that can truly understand and misunderstand. Again: —'Language is an expression of man's very nature and his basic capacity . . . animals cannot have language because they lack this capacity. If they had it they would no longer by animals—they would be human beings.'

Now let us look for a moment at the communication of bees. The general story of the communication of the distance, the situation and the direction of a food source by the dances of the returning worker bee on the vertical comb of the hive, has been known in general outline from the work of Karl von Frisch in the middle 1950s. Philosophers and linguists have made the same kind of objection to the attempt to regard this as language as I have just referred to in relation to the use of ASL by apes.

The basic correctness of the original conclusions has now been amply confirmed and established. But, far more than this, recent observations have shown overwhelmingly how adaptable, flexible and 'purposive' is the use of these signs. For instance it has been argued that the use of the dances is rigidly controlled by the circumstances (such as the absence or presence of food). This is not so. For the dances though most frequently used to signal the location of a food source, are, under special conditions, also applied to other requirements of the mutually inter-dependent members of the colony of bees. After all they are not *rigidly* used for foraging flights. When food is plentiful returning foragers often do not dance at all. The odors conveyed from one bee to another always help to direct recruits to new sources and often they alone are sufficient. Independent searching by individual foragers seems to be adequate under many conditions. Thus the dance-communications system is called into play primarily when the colony of bees is in great need of food; but it is not tightly linked to any one requirement; on the contrary it may be used for such different things as food, water and resinous materials from plants (propolis). Moreover when a colony of bees is engaged in swarming, the scouts search for cavities suitable to serve as the future home for the entire colony and report their location by the same dances —which are now performed when crawling over the mass of bees which makes up the swarm cluster (von Frisch 1967 and Lindauer 1971). When Lindauer observed the scouts of a swarm of bees which had moved only a short distance away from the original colony he found that the same marked bee would sometimes change her dance pattern from that indicating the location of a moderately suitable cavity to one signalling a better potential site for a new hive. This occurred after the dancer had received information from another bee and had flown out to inspect the superior cavity. Thus the same worker bee can be both a transmitter and receiver of information within a short period of time; and in spite of her motivation to dance about one location, she can also be influenced by the similar but more intense communication of another dancer. As Griffin (1976) says, 'There is no escape from the conclusion that, in the special situation when swarming bees are in serious need of a new location in which the colony can continue its existence, the bees exchange information about the location and suitability of a potential hive site. Individual worker bees are swayed by this information to the extent that after inspection of alternative locations they change their preference and dance for the superior place rather than for the one they first discovered. Only after many hours of such exchanges of information, involving dozens of bees, and only when the dances of virtually all the scouts indicate the same hive site, does the swarm as a whole fly off to it.' (Lindauer 1971a). This consensus results from the communicative interactions between individual bees which alternately 'speak' and 'listen.'

Here again the sweeping negativisms of Chomsky have been thrown into the arena. His main thesis as to the pre-eminence of human reason is sound and important and needs constant reiteration in these days when it is the fashion to denigrate man and all that is transcendental in his nature. But Chomsky does poor service to his cause, and merely weakens his case by scorning the proven abilities of animals. He says (Chomsky, N. 1972), 'Human reason in fact is a universal instrument which can serve for all contingencies, whereas the organs of an animal or a machine have need of some special adaptation for any particular action . . . no brute (is) so perfect that it has made use of a sign to inform other animals of something which had no relation to their passions . . . for the word is the sole sign and the only certain mark of the presence of thought hidden and wrapped up in the body; now all men . . . make use of signs, whereas the brutes never do anything of the kind; which may be taken for the true distinction between man and brute.'

One of the philosophers (Terwilliger, R.F. 1968) who argues specifically against the evidence from honey-bees in his efforts to support his view of the animals as Cartesian machines, says, 'No bee was ever seen dancing about yesterday's honey (he means of course *nectar*) not to mention tomorrow's . . . Moreover bees never make mistakes in their dance.'

One of the many facts that Terwilliger, and other authors of a similar persuasion ignore is that bees can be stimulated, by extreme food deficit, to dance during the middle of the night (a thing which they normally very rarely do) about a food source they have visited the day before, and will almost certainly visit again the next morning. In these circumstances a bee which has been dancing right up to sundown will, as soon as the morning comes, fly out to the same source, now, of course, *taking a very different direction relative to the sun, in its morning position.*

It is not so very surprising to find true linguistic ability in a primate with a brain-construction so similar to that of ourselves. But it is indeed in a sense 'shocking' to find it in an insect, with its vastly simpler central nervous system.

A prominent student of 'machine intelligence' has said 'an organism which can have intentions is, I think, one which could be said to possess a mind, provided that it has the ability to form a plan and make a decision to adopt the plan.' (H.C. Longuet-Higgins). And to 'decide on and adopt a plan' implies purpose. From all this it appears that the presence of mental images and an ability to provide introspective reports on self-awareness and intentions or purposes emerge as criteria of mind. So again we must ask ourselves, do these studies of animal language show evidence of purpose or 'intention'? It seems to me extremely difficult to support a negative answer. M.J. Adler (1967) argues that if it were discovered that animals differ from men only in degree and not radically in kind, this would destroy our moral basis for holding that all men have basic rights and individual dignity. It would seem that Adler, now confronted with the present situation, would conclude that the study of communicative behavior in animals has more dangerous political consequences than nuclear physics had in the 1930s (Griffin 1976).

Such views raise the whole question of 'emergence' which is, at rock bottom, what all this discussion is about. We have been considering the emergence of new properties in complex systems through physics up to the mind of man. In the physical sciences such emergence can often be fully accounted for in terms of the individual properties of the component particles in isolation. In a very large number of other cases this cannot be done — though it is the widely accepted research strategy to assume that, as the science develops further, it will prove possible to do so. As we proceed to biology and up towards the higher reaches of the subject, this goal appears increasingly remote and unattainable. So many are forced to the conclusion, that at least when we come to the development of the behavioral abilities of the 'higher' animals and man himself, this reductive view can never suffice and we must perforce envisage truly unpredictable and unforeseeable events (emergents) for which no refinements of physical technique or theory can ever be able fully to account. If this conclusion is accepted and absorbed into the culture and consciousness of mankind — that there are real and what can only be defined as sacred values in the world which must *never* be denigrated or relinguished — then the dangerous moral and political consequences referred to just now can and must be avoided.

A.N. Whitehead said in 1938 (*Modes of Thought*) 'The distinction between man and animals is in one sense only a difference of degree. But the extent of the degree makes all the difference. The Rubicon has been crossed.' I believe this must be taken with the greatest seriousness.

To summarize, very briefly, the two aspects of the present world picture as it affects our estimate of our own situation:

1. I have little doubt that the cosmological revolution, provisional though it may be, has shown us a deep relationship between ourselves, the stars and space; and so has provided us with a universe more concordant with the life and aspiration of man than any which preceded it up to the 1930s. And although I have used the presently favoured 'big-bang' model, I believe the same could be argued for a 'steady-state' model; or indeed a combination of the two. This is not to say that there is now a sound basis for a new argument from design. But (to quote Dr. Carling) 'It is a rather strong kind of coherence that can relate the present appearance of the universe back to events a minute fraction of a second after the 'big-bang' — approximately ten thousand million years ago.'

2. When we come to realise the strength of the present evidence for the continuity of mental experience, we are led to postulate a real predisposition in the world for the evolution of mental awareness. And this brings us to contemplate a supreme miracle — 'That the universe created a part of itself to study the rest of itself.' (J. Lilly).

All this presents us with the great task of formulating the new prospect in a manner which the majority will welcome and understand. In this connection I cannot do better than paraphrase some remarks of Polanyi (1959). So far as we know we are the supreme bearers of thought in the universe. After five million centuries of evolution, we have been engaged for only fifty centuries in a literate process of thought. It has all been an affair of the last hundred generations or so. If this perspective is true, a supreme trust is placed in us by the whole creation; and it is sacrilege even to contemplate actions which may lead to the extinction of humanity or even its relegation to earlier or more primitive stages of culture. To avoid this is the particular calling of literate and scientific man in this universe.

In this task of re-formulation perhaps the key lies in the modern development of Process Philosophy and Process Theology— based upon the thought of Alfred North Whitehead.

During these three days we have been considering the human brain and have come to realize that, in spite of its overwhelming complexity, it has ultimate limitations as a machine. But I believe with Whitehead that in spite of these limitations the human mind and soul which operates in liaison with it, has latent possibilities and capacities for further emergence and transcendence—capacities to which we can set no limit.

And in conclusion I would like to paraphrase some words of Louis Pasteur: 'Infinity stares us in the face, whether we look at the stars or search for our own identities. A true science of life must let infinity in and never lose sight of it.' Hold fast to this and we shall find that the infinity of mind seems to encompass us everywhere.

ACKNOWLEDGEMENTS

I have been indebted to many colleagues and friends in the preparation of this paper. Among them it is an especial pleasure to acknowledge the following:

The late Dr. E.M.W. Tillyard was the first to introduce me to the subject of the Great Chain of Being. His book *The Elizabethan World Picture* (1945. London: Chatto and Windus) and the admirable earlier work of the American scholar Professor A.O. Lovejoy, *The Great Chain of Being* (1936, Cambridge, Mass: Harvard), proved of much value.

For the section on Cosmology I became acquainted with facts and theories from a number of astronomer colleagues at Cambridge University— particularly Dr. W. Saslaw, Professor M.J. Rees and Professor Antony Hewish. But for the first part of the section I am especially indebted to Mr. C.D. Curling, Sub-Dean of the Faculty of Natural Science of King's College, University of London. However none of these may be blamed for any errors; which are mine alone.

While I was engaged in writing, a new book, *The Question of Animal Awareness* (1976. Rockefeller University Press, New York) by a friend of many years. Professor Donald R. Griffin, landed on my desk. This was remarkably fortunate in that it enabled me to substantially improve the section on mind and mentality and provided me with some new references.

REFERENCES

A. **General:** In addition to the work by Donald Griffin mentioned above the following may be found useful as providing general summaries:

Thorpe, W.H. *Animal Nature and Human Nature.* (1974) Methuen, London and Doubleday-Anchor, New York.

Cobb, J.B. and Griffin, David Ray (Eds.) *Mind in Nature: Essays on the Interface of Science and Philosophy.* (1977) University Press of America, Washington, D.C. (This constitutes a general summary of the present position of Process Philosophy. Readers may find the contributions of J.B. Cobb, Theodosius Dobzhansky, Charles Hartshorne, R.H. Overman, C.H. Waddington and Sewell Wright of particular relevance.)

Thorpe, W.H. *Purpose in a World of Chance,* (1977) Oxford University Press, London. (Written from a biological viewpoint.)

B. **Specific:**

Adler, M.J. *The Difference of Man and the Difference it Makes.* (1967) Holt, Rinehart and Winston, New York.

Black, M. *The Labyrinth of Language.* (1968) Praeger, New York.

Chomsky, N. *Language and Mind.* (1972) Harcourt/Brace, Jovanovich: New York.

Frisch, K. von *The Dance Language and Orientation of Bees.* (1967) Cambridge, Mass: Harvard Press.

Lilly, J.C. *The Centre of the Cyclone.* (1973) Paladin: London. (see p. 215)

Lindauer, M. *Communication among Social Bees.* (1971, revised edition) Harvard University Press: Cambridge, Mass.

Longuet-Higgins, H.C. in Kenny, A.H.P., Longuet-Higgins, H.C. Lucas, J.R. and Waddington, C.H. *The Nature of Mind.* (1970) Edinburgh University Press: Edinburgh.

Polanyi, M. *The Study of Man.* (1959) University of Chicago Press, Chicago and London.

Terwilliger, R.F. *Meaning and Mind, A Study of the Psychology of Language.* (1968) Oxford University Press: London and New York.

Whitehead, A.N. *Modes of Thought.* (1938) Cambridge University Press: Cambridge and London.

Duke L.V.P.R. de Broglie

D2 The Scientist at His Last Quarter of an Hour

When we have reached the end of our lives (and which of us, whatever his age may be, is sure of not being about to reach it?), it is only natural that we should try to understand the meaning of life and to pass judgment on the activities we may have carried out during our existence. In particular, anyone who has devoted the greater part of his time in scientific research must of course be led during his "last quarter of an hour" to consider the material and spiritual value of Science, the place it occupies in the progress of civilization and in the general evolution of the human race, the prospects which we may see as to the significance and the destiny of the Universe and of Thought. On the assumption that we have come to our last quarter of an hour, let us therefore ponder over these grave problems.

A few billion years ago, Life appeared on the surface of the Earth, no doubt in a very humble form in which living matter was hardly distinguished from inert matter. Then over the centuries and millenaries, driven by a mysterious force whose true nature we are still far from understanding, it spread through the waters, into the air and on firm land, producing more and more complicated organisms, which were better and better adapted to very diverse conditions of life. According to the data of Paleontology, it is most probable that all the species have arisen from one another, although we do not know by what continuous or discontinuous processes (progressive evolution of sudden mutations) have successively come about the living forms which have existed or still exist on the earth. During this long and astounding history of the development of Life on our planet, of this grandiose epic which Mr. Jean Rostand has given the striking name of "the adventure of protoplasm", living organisms have adapted themselves with incredible flexibility to the conditions of existence offered to them and have reached that degree of prodigious complexity and admirable precision to be found in the evolved species and, in particular, in the higher vertebrates. Apart from the astonishing physico-chemical mechanisms that ensure the continuation of life in individuals and its perpetuation through successive generations, how can one fail to admire the perfection of those "sense organs" which allow a living being to know its environment and, thanks to its mobility, to find there what can be useful to it and to avoid as far as possible the dangers which may lie in wait for it. The marvelously precise structure, the extraordinary sensibility of organs such as the eye and the ear of the higher animals stagger the imagination and it seems incredible that such organs could have been produced by mere chance, even over enormous periods of time. The realizations of Life seem to result from a kind of organizing force which does not manifest itself inert matter and whose true nature is totally unknown to us.

Linked to the mobility of living beings and to their faculty of perception, there appeared one of the most astonishing phenomena in the world such as we know it; I am referring to the phenomenon of "consciousness", that is, to the fact that living beings, at least those whose organization is sufficiently high, are aware that they constitute a unit endowed with autonomy in the physical world and consciously "perceive" the messages sent to them from the outer world through their sensory organs and which, so to speak, are reflected on their autonomy. A deeply mysterious faculty! We clearly understand how, for instance, light may be collected by our eye, act on our retina, induce in our optic nerve an electrical influx which excites certain nerve cells in our brain, but the transformation of these purely physical phenomena into the conscious perception of a luminous sensation remains astounding and almost inconceivable.

The appearance of thought marked a new and prodigious step forward in Life, linked to the existence of consciousness which is its necessary condition. Thought is superior to it. Its higher forms which tend, by abstraction and generalization, to break away from the always limited and particular data of perception, go far beyond simple consciousness. Whilst consciousness no doubt already exists in an elementary state in relatively inferior species, thought is certainly still only very rudimentary even in the most intelligent higher vertebrates. It really appears in all its fullness in man only and, as has often been said, it is that which constitutes Man's eminent dignity and gives him the exceptional place he holds in nature.

The appearance of Man on earth, the development in him, thanks to a prodigious complexity of the cerebral mechanisms, of thought and reason, have marked a decisive turning-point in the history of Life on our planet and a new phase of that history began as human intelligence improved. Having acquired the capacity for reasoning, man endeavored to understand what we observed, to classify the phenomena, to discover their regularity. He has unceasingly acquired knowledge through this rational observation of things and his knowledge has been preserved in the individual by memory, soon to be assisted by books, and handed down from generations to generations by oral or written teaching — such knowledge increases continually. In its endeavor to discover laws and causes, the human mind wants to understand the "how" and the "why" of things, and this noble aspiration, though an audacious one, has led man to tackle scientific and metaphysical problems which are both a credit to him and a torment.

If one thinks of it, it is most surprising and incomprehensible as well, that this progressive appearance of consciousness and thought should have occurred in the midst of a physical world which, it would seem, might well have remained totally and eternally unconscious and inert. Is it not a strange fate for the small pieces of animated matter that we are to have succeeded, at the cost of long efforts often pursued for generations, to reconstitute laboriously a few elements of that Nature from which however we derive? Our body is made up of atoms teeming with electrons, protons and other elementary particles, and in which quantic transitions follow one another unceasingly; our nervous system, the essential tool of our activities, is the seat of innumerable electrical phenomena required for its functioning, the whole balance of our body and of the processes that ensure the continuation of our existence depends upon the action of hormones, vitamins and a large number of complicated organic substances. And yet, it needed the whole slow development of modern science to make known to us all these things *which are in us!* Scientific work therefore consists in a kind of strange "reconquest" whereby, by reflecting itself in men's consciousness and reason, the World learns to know itself. An astonishing outcome of the adventure of protoplasm!

Thus is revealed the outstanding value of human thought in general, of scientific thought in particular. Through it, the Universe becomes slightly conscious of itself, and to a certain extent, we are the consciousness of the Universe and each advancement in our Science marks an advancement in that consciousness.

That is what reveals the grandeur of Science in its disinterested aspect. But there is another way of considering things when seen from the standpoint of action. We have said that as there appeared on the earth more complicated organisms in which consciousness showed itself more and more clearly, Life entered upon a new course. Sprung from inert matter and undergoing incessantly its obsessing pressure, living matter breaking up into units conscious of their autonomy began in turn to exert a voluntary action on the exterior environment and thus to modify somewhat the evolution thereof. Furthermore, man endowed with consciousness, intelligence and liberty may influence the material world surrounding him. To acquire a deeper knowledge of the physical world and to act upon it, man uses means totally different from those used by the other living beings. Until the appearance of man, Life, which had already launched forth on the conquest of the World by the organizing impulse that characterizes it, had increased its means of perception and its possibilities of action through anatomical and physiological channels thanks to a complexity and gradual refinement of the living structures and their organs.

With the intervention of human intelligence, Life will extend its power by other means—in man, the sense organs no longer evolve perceptibly, but instruments which science enables him to design and bring into being will considerably extend the field of his perceptions. The telephone and radio enable him to hear at great distances, optical instruments enable his eyes to scan the depths of the heavens and the innermost part of matter. A still more extraordinary process because more subtle principles are involved, the electron microcscope further extends indirectly his field of vision in the realm of the infinitesimally small. Whilst his power of perception is constantly increasing and gaining in refinement, man also acquires through science means of action which formerly could never have been imagined. The railway, the steamer, the submarine, the car, the airplane enable him to travel at increasing speeds on land, on the sea, under water and in the air. The steam-engine, the production and transport of electric power make considerable energies available to him whenever and wherever he wishes. Chemistry by supplying him with an ever increasing number of bodies with diverse properties offers wider and wider possibilities to his industry. Sustained by the rapid progress of physiology and the natural sciences, Medicine and Surgery hold back sickness and death, whilst Biology is beginning to cast a somewhat disturbing beam of light on the mysteries of Life itself and particularly on the mechanism of heredity. And in the recent and remarkable developments of biology, we again see, in accord with previous remarks, how Life by applying itself to its own study, is beginning to understand itself.

Thus, thanks to Science and its technical applications, man is going to domineer over the Earth and transform its history. He knows its whole surface, goes across it rapidly and can act more and more on it as well as on the flora and fauna that cover it. Through atomic energy and other discoveries to be made, man will be more than ever the Master of the Earth—no one knows how far his work will stop in this field. And who knows whether one day, perhaps in the not too distant future, some mutation either accidental, or brought about by man himself, may give rise to a superman with a far greater intelligence than ours who, with means of which we have no idea, will pursue the work we have begun and carry still further the triumphs of Life.

Fired with the enthusiasms for the prospects disclosed to him by such thoughts, the scientist may grow excited at the idea that he participates more than anyone to this progressive evolution of the World. He will be tempted to cry out with Jean Perrin: "Thanks to the more and more differentiated living beings in which its structure is building up, the Universe is gradually rising to an ever extending Thought, so much so that it may become a Will governing its own history".

And yet, there is a formidable argument which may make us fear that our hopes are vain and our enthusiasm is ingenuous. Life, Thought, Will, we know these only on the surface of the Earth, this small planet, and then on limited regions of its surface. No doubt we can imagine that in other solar systems there exist other planets where Life may appear, where perhaps being somewhat similar to us and likewise endowed with thought pursue a task akin to ours. It may also be presumed (not in the near future no doubt) that man may succeed in leaving the Earth, in extending his presence or at least his influence to more or less vast parts of the solar system. But how insignificant all this is in comparison with the immensity of the heavens, with the illimitable dimensions of that Universe where the galaxies float like isolated islands at distances of hundreds of millions of light-years! The progressive evolution of Life on Earth, the achievements of our intelligence and of our will, all these things which formerly made us feel proud and confident now appear to us as having been reduced to nothing by the immensity of space. Moreover, there is the immensity of time, the final death which threatens the Earth, the solar system, the whole present or future theatre of our activities. We are oppressed by such thoughts and are tempted to sink into despair.

We are perhaps the victims of an illusion and give too much importance to space and time, which are just the *frames* of our perceptions. Maybe we are wrong to admit implicitly that the value of a thing is to be measured according to the volume it occupies in space or to its duration in time. Perhaps the whole Universe which we know by our perceptions from the atom to the spiral nebula is only a very small fraction of a much greater Reality which some superman may succeed one day in knowing partially. Within the framework of this vaster Reality, our effort, which from the standpoint of Sirius seems to us so localized and so temporary, might resume all its value. The worker who, facing the reverse side of his work, weaves a high-warp tapestry, may not realize the real work he is performing, but he would perceive this day when he could turn the tapestry back and contemplate it. Thus, when human thought has reached a higher stage of its development, it may perceive some day, beyond the reaches of

Space and Time, the true meaning of the work which, extending and crowning Life's effort, it will have endeavored untiringly to accomplish. Such is the supreme hope, which, at the close of his existence, may comfort the scientist who has reached the end of his task.

H.D. Lewis

D3 Persons in Recent Thought

This is a very wide topic. It is, however, in my view, altogether central to our main concerns today, especially as they are focused for us at this conference and its like. It will therefore not be inappropriate to direct attention to the main issues involved in our thought and about persons and outline what I take myself to be most important in the way we should think about persons.

First of all there is the long debate about dualist and monist views of persons. Are we two things, or perhaps two streams of events, in some peculiar relation, or is there just the one type of reality which may be viewed in some respect mental and in another material or physical—or perhaps even more simply just one mode of being, as far as we are concerned and perhaps the entire universe?

All these views have been held. Indeed, they have a long and fairly continuous history from as early as we have records of reflective and speculative thought—and they figure in diverse cultures. The most popular form of monistic view—that is the doctrine that there is only one type of being—in our times is materialism. All reality must be thought to be material or physical, including our thoughts and purposes. But while this is a highly fashionable doctrine in our times we do well to remember that this has come about by a very massive swing of opinion early in this century. The philosophical thinking, and with it related attitudes, which dominated almost every aspect of thought, not only in the English-speaking world but elsewhere including the Orient, at the turn of the century and for some decades before that, was idealism, which, in an astonishing variety of ways, proclaimed the view that in one way or another all reality was thought or mental, usually along the lines of the many variations on the Hegelian theme of the one absolute being appearing in many forms. 'The real is the rational' was the famous text, and for many this was understood to mean that all existence is mental or some kind of experience. The confidence with which this view was held at one time, the strong belief that all future philosophy must be some variation on it, may seem astounding today, but it is salutary to recall it when we note the surprising assurance with which some other fashionable views have since been held.

There are other forms of idealism, some to my mind more attractive, than post-Hegelian idealism, much though we have to learn from the latter and much though we appreciate the revival of Hegelian studies pioneered by John Findlay, H.B. Acton, W.B. Walsh, T.M. Knox and a host of others in many countries. There is the idealism of Berkeley and the monadology of Leibniz, to name some of the obvious examples, and some forms at least of recent phenomenalism.

The fashionable monism today is some form of materialism, although it was not from that quarter, but from the very different realism of Cook Wilson and G.E. Moore, that the initial drastic inroads were made on nineteenth century idealism. There are many forms of materialism, and not all exponents of it favor the term, but they are all agreed in maintaining that there can be no mental existence which is altogether distinct from physical reality or wholly real in its own right.

The more outright form of this is what is usually known as 'old-fashioned' materialism. This took the extraordinary line of maintaining that all that we are apt to take as distinct mental reality, thoughts, sensations, etc., are states or processes in our bodies conditioned solely by material events in the world around us. Thought itself is just movements in our vocal chords and hopes and fears are tensions in our breasts or stomach. It is a constant source of wonder to me that highly intelligent people should have adhered seriously to this view. Yet at one time it was strongly held, not only by ingenious behaviorists like J.B. Watson but also as a cardinal feature of communist philosophy.

My own reaction here is a very simple one. If nothing exists other than these dispositions of our bodies, almost everything to which we attach importance loses its significance. The attitudes of many highly intelligent adherents to strictly materialist communist philosophy, which is not the same thing as saying that material needs are basic or decisive in human responses — a more modest though still very questionable form of materialism — are often ambivalent. They stress the advantages which, in their views at least, follow from communist systems, better living conditions, better education, art and music. But even if all this could be established, what would it matter if this new happiness or more creative existence could be reduced to purely physical states.

The materialist in more recent times is more subtle. He insists that he holds nothing to bring into question or discredit the obvious facts of everyday existence, that we do think and purpose and feel pain and other sensations. What he claims is somehow to dissolve the difference, in Gilbert Ryle's famous terms, between the dualist and the materialist account of thought and existence, Ryle, with his exacting standards in thought and expression, would not want to say that we never think and that it does not matter how sound and clear is our thought and its expression. He could not have been one of the most famous editors of our time if he held such a view. At the same time, when we look carefully at what Ryle, and his many followers, actually hold it is very hard to see what difference, in essentials, there is between their ingeniously held positions and the simpler less ambiguous materialism of J.B. Watson. So strongly entrenched in some quarters is the 'corporealist' view of persons that many do not seem to think it necessary even to argue for it, and such people include some of the ablest and most scholarly writers. Thus Mr. Jonathan Barnes, of Oriel College, Oxford, after one of the most learned and incisive surveys of the many ingenious forms of the famous 'ontological argument'[1], disposes, in direct consideration, of the idea of God on the ground that 'Gods are persons' and it is 'becoming increasingly clear that persons are essentially corporeal'[2]. All the same, however ingenious the defesces, or however firm and widespread the conviction, nothing seems more certain to me, as a matter of obvious immediate experience, than that thoughts, purposes, sensations, etc., have a character as experience which is quite radically different in essential nature, a quite different mode of being altogether, from all corporeal or physical or observable reality. I also hold that recognition of what seems here a simple fact of common sense and immediate apprehension is vital for all good sense in the treatment of all other major issues and our basic attitudes. In practice, it all may seem to make little difference. Corporealists live and argue like the rest of us, but in the long run I cannot but believe that failure to recognize the distinctness of mental states and processes will lead to an impoverishment and enervation of all our distinctive activities and the very will to live as civilized communities.

There is one point that needs to be very much stressed here. The essential appeal in these matters must be to the immediate awareness we have of what it is like to have thoughts or sensations. Defenders of materialism are apt to confront us with the need for argument, and they vigorously reject the view that we can appeal to 'private access' or 'private detection'[3]. We must not be dogmatic and just lay down the law, we must provide a proper argument. This is the ploy, disconcerting enough in its way, to which Mr. Roger Squires has recourse in his very gifted and spirited defense of materialism in the paper from which I have just quoted. But this is the issue which I have also discussed at length in my own paper 'Ultimates and a Way of Looking' originally prepared for the Oxford International Symposium arranged by the late Professor Ryle and first published under his editorship as *Contemporary Aspects of Philosophy* (Oriel Press) and now reproduced in my own book *Persons and Survival of Death* (Macmillan 1978). In this paper, as in other essays in this volume, I insist that philosophers must be prepared to recognize the limits of argument. It is hard for us to do so, for at once we seem to be opening the door to dogmatism and blind assertion—what is philosophy without argument? Nonetheless I think Wittgenstein, with whom I do not often agree, was altogether right in insisting that 'philosophers must know when to stop'. There is a point beyond which further argument is not possible, and there are certain 'given' features of experience, however baffling, which we must simply recognize as being the case. This is a delicate and tricky issue which I cannot discuss as carefully here as I have done in my book. It seems to me all the same of quite crucial importance for good sense in philosophy, and, however easily abused, indispensable for a sound understanding of ourselves and the world around us. We have to cultivate the sense of when we have reached this kind of ultimate, and the flair for this appears to be one of the major requirements of sound philosophy.

In my own writings on these subjects, in *The Elusive Mind* and *The Self and Immortality* for example, I have tried to come closely to terms with an array of formidable arguments from Ryle, Passmore, Hampshire and others, but in the last analysis, when all the ground has been cleared in this way, we come down to our claim to recognize, or fail to recognize, the inherent distinctness of mental existence, for man and brute, and the radical difference between it and the reality about which we learn in sensible observation. If this appeal to what we seem to find to be the case is denied us, there is nowhere else to which we may turn. I can only invite those who disagree to think again or look again. When Ryle, for example, declares that the surgeon's skill lies in his hands making the correct movement, I cannot but remain convinced that something vital is left out here from the total picture. Nor will dispositions supply the defect. There is something going on *all the time* besides the work of the 'skilled hands' as such. And there I must leave this matter as far as this short paper is concerned.

There are not in fact many who would persist today in denying that mental processes are inherently different from physical ones, and that we have in this way an 'inner life' to which we have some sort of immediate access. So far the battle has swung round fairly firmly in favor of the dualist. But this is only half the battle. Two main things in particular may be maintained. Firstly, it will be argued that while mental states and processes are not strictly reducible to states of the body, they are conditioned throughout or at least essentially dependent on physical states, ultimately the brain. That there is peculiarly close dependence on the body will not, I think, be in serious dispute. Any change in my bodily state, most of all some serious malfunctioning, immediately brings about a corresponding change in my state of mind, a fever or brain damage seriously disrupts my thinking and experience in general. These obvious facts of experience need not be amplified. But it does not at all follow, as some suppose, that the state of the body is the sole determinant of my mental states. Sensitivity and understanding prescribe their own course and reactions, subject, normally at least, to physical conditions. I answer the telephone because I *hear* and *understand* what is said. To deny the influence of our own apprehension of meaning in the course of our activities is again to run against the plain evidence of normal experience.

A more plausible position is to hold that, in view of the close correlation of mental and physical events, it cannot be allowed that mind can function at all without its bodily correlate. This does not seem to me, however, in any way inevitable. Under present conditions of existence the dependence on the body is close, but that does not preclude the possibility of mental existence without the present physical correlates. How this may be conceived, and how communication etc. would be possible is one of the main topics of my *The Self and Immortality* (Macmillan).

There is however a second major submission which the critics of dualism are apt to make, and this is the one to which most importance would be ascribed today. It is the real crux in these matters in the present state of the discussion. This is the question of ownership of experience and continued identity. Critics of my own view, see my forthcoming *Persons and Life After Death — Essays by Hywel Lewis and his Critics* (Macmillian), are apt to stress especially the difficulty of accounting for personal identity without bodily continuity. In my own replies the following points are made.

Firstly, I accept the substance of the Kantian argument that our awareness of an objective world around us presupposes a subject which transcends our passing experience and gives us a unified world which we can understand, and within limits change. But I take the argument further than this and maintain that the Kantian argument itself would be very hard to understand without some more direct awareness of oneself as subject and agent. My second main contention then is that, at any time, everyone is aware of himself as the being that he is, unique and irreducible. This is very different from the more specific knowledge that I have of myself as the particular kind of person that I am, my likes and dislikes, my aptitudes, skills and dispositions etc. I am better placed in many ways to know these than my friends, but in some ways they may know me better at this level (and so might a psychiatrist if I consulted him). But all these properties characterize me, and no other, and it is this *me* (*being me* is Professor Roderick Chisholm's recent phrase) that I know, so I claim, immediately as the being that I am essentially and which at this level cannot be characterized further. Self-awareness in this sense is one of the *ultimates* to which I give prominence in my forthcoming book.

But there remains the question of continued identity. How do I know that the distinct being I am now is the same as the being who came into this room and started to write an hour ago? Very briefly, and this is the third point I am noting now, the Kantian argument will take us a long way here. But I supplement and strengthen it by recourse to what I have elsewhere called 'strict memory'. Most that we may be said to remember about ourselves and the world around us, depends on elaborate evidence and extends well beyond the sphere of our own immediate experience — sometimes to remote times — I remember that Plato lived from 427 to 347 B.C. But I do not strictly remember this — I was not alive at the time; I do not remember the battle of Arginusiae because I was not there. But I remember coming into this room in a sense which would not be intelligible if I had not actually done this myself. My claim is that there are cases where we do directly, and independently of supporting evidence, remember such things as coming into the room visiting places in Israel a few weeks ago and some things very early in my life. If this is so, then the being that I know myself to be, having these experiences now, just has to be the being who experienced other things and did certain things in the past, however much I may have changed in other ways, physical appearances, skills and interests etc. This does not apply to all that has happened to me or which I have done. I am very far from strictly remembering all my life. But if there are cases and I think they are extensive, when we strictly remember our past, then we have very firm assurance of continued identity around which we may build the other things we know less directly about ourselves. The question of the fallibility of memory presents difficulties with which I have tried to cope elsewhere.

We have thus, in outline here, the notion of persons as essentially non-corporeal and continuing as the distinct beings that they are, ultimate and irreducible, through changes of circumstances and fortune, including physical appearance. Such persons do not of necessity outlive the destruction of the body, they are no more inevitably immortal or indestructible than other finite existences. God alone exists by necessity of his nature. But there is no inherent reason why we should not exist and be the same persons essentially without the present body—or indeed any body at all. I have indicated elsewhere[4] what reasons I think there are for believing that we shall so exist.

Personal identity, on this view is absolute and not relative. This contrasts sharply with positions, like those of post-Helgelian idealists like T.H. Green and Bosanquet, who find the identity of persons in partial continuity of characteristics and circumstances. If a tree is cut down into logs and burnt, the ashes (or what grows out of them) would not be regarded as the same entity as the tree. Just where we draw the line is arbitrary in the last resort, though not independent of continuities in the course of events. Location and spatial contiguities play an important part here. A suit that is so patched over that none of the original material remains might still be said to be the same suit. But this is relative and arbitrary. In the case of persons the identity is strict and not partial, however completely we may change. A man who is converted and abandons erring or evil ways is the same being as the one he was before, although we may say at another level, or for rough and ready purposes, that he is 'not the same person' anymore. This is where I differ radically from an idealist, like Bosanquet at one extreme, and many fashionable thinkers of today at the other, for they would say that after a lapse of time I cease to be responsible for what I did long ago—or at least my responsibility is much diminished—because it is not the present 'I' who did what I am to be praised or blamed for in the past—I am no longer the same person. My submission is that I am essentially the same person through all changes of circumstance and fortune and in all my actions.

This distinct being that I am is normally dependent on physical conditions, and the experiences that I have are entensively, though by no means wholly, conditioned by physical factors, especially the state of my brain, but it also acts upon the world around us, normally and perhaps always through the brain and the body—causation at a distance, if it happens, as some maintain, would make an exception. What we have therefore is an essentially mental entity, which has a unique and final identity, which is nonetheless in continuous interaction with the physical world, mainly at least through one's own body. The relation with the body is peculiarly close, as I have also stressed (see the chapter in 'The Importance of the Body' in *The Self and Immortality*), but we are not essentially corporeal beings, however much we may for rough and ready purposes, identify ourselves as or through our bodies.

This is an essentially Cartesian position, with antecedents from Socrates through Plato and Augustine and Kant and many others, in Eastern as in Western thought. To establish it seems to me of first importance for all our major concerns and issues today.

I had meant to take up most of my space on the implications of holding this notion of the distinct and ultimate identity of persons. In the little that remains to me I can only make the briefest reference to what I take to be the significance for us of this doctrine today. Some of the matters of the greatest importance here have been reflected in some things I have already said. For example the question of moral responsibility. In terms of the view I have advanced it is possible to conceive of *some* of our actions as being cases of genuinely open choice where our action is in no sense at all determined. To reinstate the sense of our own ultimate and unquestioned responsibility is, in my view, a matter of the utmost importance — and on this I have also ventured to say much in other writings.

Then there is the question of life after death and the genuineness of our identity in any postmortem existence which we may have reason to expect. Many aspects of personal relationships, and the values which center upon them, are affected in the same way — to recognize the 'other' as genuinely other and have due regard to what Bertrand Russell, in somewhat surprising terms for him, described as 'our somber solitude, the genuine inner existence and essential privacy of everyone, is one of the major conditions of healthy personal and social relations'.

Likewise, in religion, much that is travestied and distorted in traditional doctrine, like the notion which some have seriously held, of an angry God who sentences sinners to eternal torment, comes to be seen in its right meaning and context when we reflect on the consequences for our inner existence and solitude of much that we actually do. There is no need for trivializing or attenuation of traditional doctrine but the terms of it have to be thought out afresh and its meaning, in times past as today, properly appreciated on the basis of a sound understanding of what makes us the creatures we actually are. So also, for the vexed question of mysticism, and the claims often made for it. There is no doubt of the profound spiritual experience reflected in mystical writings and the lives of the mystics. But the sense in which this involves the extinction of the self is a further moot point. There are few things more central in contemporary religious and metaphysical thinking than this matter of the possible fusion of person as against the view that, even in the finest and holiest relationships, each remains the person he is and no other. The real divide, in the great religions, begins here, and if we are to find what I have elsewhere called 'the points of convergence' in modern thought and civilized existence, we just have to face up to this basic question of how we are to think of individual existence. This is where it is hardest to find agreement, and it is for this reason above all that I direct attention to it in this paper. My view is that nothing important is lost, for any of the great religions, if the finality of the distinctness of persons is allowed. On the contrary, it is in the light of this, I would contend, that we can properly grasp what is vital in the main traditions, appreciate differences where they remain, and rethink our way to the appreciation of the most creative ways in which religious traditions may correct and enrich one another. This seems to me the most urgent concern for our times, and I regret that exposition of my own stance, for those not familiar with it, has been allowed to take up most of my space. In the discussion we can perhaps advert more to these implications and significance of the issues I have raised and the view of them I have outlined.

FOOTNOTES

1. *The Onotological Argument*, Macmillan 1972
2. op. cit. 84
3. Cff. Roger Squires in 'Zombies vs. Materialists' in *Proceedings of the Aristotelian Society* supp. vol. XLVIII p. 162-163
4. *Persons and Survival of Death*

Mary Carman Rose

Commentary

Psycho-physical dualism which Professor Lewis wisely associates with the thought of Socrates, Plato, Augustine, Descartes, and Kant has had few explicit defenders in twentieth century Western philosophical thought. Hence, our thanks are due to Lewis for his unequivocal attempts to draw our attention to this position. Those of us who are dualists will certainly be grateful to Lewis. But those who are not dualists ought to be grateful to Lewis also. For we hear so little in defense of dualism these days that those who oppose it are in danger of forgetting what it is they are opposing. Also valuable is Lewis' brief noting of metaphysical materialism and idealism as positions opposed to dualism. Lewis argues fairly and congently with his materialist opponents. And perhaps on their part materialists have argued honestly according to their rights; though I agree with Lewis that they have not argued wisely from their own and others' experience as persons.

There are, however, others whose opposition to psycho-physical dualism is to some extent covert. That is, their arguments pertaining to personhood and embodiment are enthymemes, and their conclusions depend on premises that are not explicitly examined nor even articulated. Two such thinkers Lewis mentions — i.e., Ryle and Wittgenstein. An academic generation which sometimes pays too little attention to courtesy will do well to think highly of Lewis' generosity to these thinkers. Clarity and courtesy are compatible, however; and philosophical advance requires the assessment of covert premises. I suggest that Ryle's insufficiently examined premise is that what cannot be said behavioristic or operational language has no role in the study of mind. And Wittgenstein seems to be arguing always from the premise that what words pertaining to mind, personhood, and embodiment mean to him they will mean to all of us and that where he finds 'muddles' in these words all of us will.

There are, however, opponents of dualism whose arguments against that position are more formidable because they are more nearly totally covert. These are Husseralian phenomenology; Heideggarian ontology; and secular existentialism as practiced by Sartre, Camus and Merleau-Ponty. Husseralian phenomenology does not encompass all data pertaining to personhood and embodiment because of its assumption that all concepts, intentionalities, and data which pertain to these topics are fully open to inspection and can be fully explicated and articulated by the thinker who has been trained exclusively along Husseralian lines. Clearly, however, on the one hand, many aspects of mind-body inter-relations are not open to direct inspection and, on the other hand, the spiritual development of the investigator determines what he will find in his own experience as a person and embodied consciousness and how he will interpret the reports of others concerning their experiences. *Mutatis mutandis* similar criticisms are to be made of Heidegger's 'fundamental ontology' with its insufficiently examined assumption that 'being is unconcealed'— e.g., the being of mind and of its *de facto* dependencies on and various apparent independencies of body. *A fortiori* this is true of the secular existentialists' deliberately idiosyncratic decisions, discoveries, and interpretations of their own experiences as persons and embodied consciousness. Further, Lewis himself is implicitly contributing to a phenomenology of personhood and embodiment. This is clear, for example, in his concern with the content and import of certain given features of experience. Five conclusions may be drawn from the data pertaining to personhood and embodiment which are provided by Lewis and all the others.

First, the data pertaining to personhood and embodiment in the life of any one individual and his mode of interpreting these data depend to some extent on his world view and convictions concerning human ethico-religious potentialities and the human predicament. Thus, Lewis wisely draws our attention to Eastern views on personhood. And some experiences of personhood and embodiment as known to Buddhism, Hinduism, and Zen Buddhism will support Lewis' observations and conclusions. On the other hand, perhaps the Indian thinker for whom reincarnation is a fact will not agree with Lewis' understanding of 'strict memory' as essential to the continuity of the person. Second, persons with different world views will differ in their conclusions concerning the phenomenology of personhood and embodiment. Third, persons with different world views will come to some of the same phenomenological conclusions if they share some experiences, commitments, and hopes. Thus, Lewis finds common ground with Bertrand Russell on the importance of the individual's 'essential privacy' and 'genuine inner existence'.

Fourth, it is not only the investigator's intellectual integrity and training which have necessary investigative roles in his inquiry concerning personhood and embodiment. His spiritual or ethico-religious development, experiences, convictions, and commitments have also investigative roles in this enquiry. Fifth, there is necessarily a coherence among the individual's experiences and interpretation of embodiment and his world view. This means, as I indicated above, that his experiences and interpretations of the many facets of his own being are in part at least determined by his world view. It also means that his experiences reinforce, illumine, and lead to the further development of his views concerning man, reality, and the relations between them. Further, I wish to emphasize the fact that I am not here drawing attention to coherence among various aspects of philosophical thought as a possible ideal of philosophical work. That is another topic altogether. Rather, I am drawing attention to the *de facto* limitation or support given to an individual interpretation of personhood and embodiment by his metaphysical, ontological, axiological, and epistemological convictions.

Because of the coherence among beliefs, commitments, and aspirations which inform any situation where an individual reflects on personhood and embodiment I am uneasy about Lewis' appeal to Wittgenstein. To be sure, in some philosophical contexts it is wise to stress resemblances among thinkers who are in some ways very different in their interpretations of philosophical work, philosophical commitments, modes of inquiry, and conclusions. Yet it is important to be cautious in this philosophical generosity and cooperativeness. For two thinkers who are diametrically

opposed may use the same words although, because of the fundamental differences in their philosophical views, their respective
uses of these words may have very different meanings. In fact,
the introduction on the basis of a superficial similarity of meaning of a philosophical dictum which is fundamentally alien to the
view into which it is introduced may be dangerous or even
destructive to the latter.

Such, I suggest, is the case with the manner in which Lewis
has introduced Wittgenstein's thought into his own defense of
dualism. I take it that Lewis is referring to Wittgenstein's famous dictum, 'Whereof we cannot speak let us be silent'. Of course,
virtually all aspects of Wittgenstein's thoughts are controversial.
Yet I think there is ample ground for concluding that when, as
Lewis expresses it, Wittgenstein says, 'philosophers must know
when to stop', Wittgenstein is working in the tradition of Gorgias
rather than in that of Socrates.

Further, the Sophist and the Socratic traditions are diametrically opposed. Gorgias is speaking from the point of view for which
it is useless to seek knowledge of an objective order—e.g., to seek
facts concerning mind-body relations, personal survival of physical death, or the fundamental universal nature of personhood. This
is not the tradition of Socrates, Plato, Augustine, or Descartes.
And while Kant introduces a fundamental agnosticism in respect
to the ontological and metaphysical aspects of these topics, his
ethico-religious thought which draws attention to the universally
human spiritual needs, potentialities, and legitimate hopes is
very definitely in their tradition.

Yet these two traditions share dicta to which they give opposed
interpretations—e.g., Protagoras' reinterpretation of 'Man is the
measure of all things'. Another example is Wittgenstein's 'Whereof we cannot speak let us be silent' which Lewis introduced into
his own inquiry. When used in any defense of dualism, however, it
must be given a meaning consistent with the spirit of Socratic
inquiry. Perhaps in this role it is a new form of the Socratic admo-
nition to be aware of the limits of our knowledge. Thus the dualist
who believes that he is not identical with his body and that he will
survive physical death not only may, but must, remind the materialist, metaphysical naturalist, and secular existentialist and

phenomenologist that their experiences of personhood and embodiment are not the measure of all human experiences which pertain to these. The presence in our midst of representatives of all the great world religions who know at first hand the existential import of the hope for survival provides ample evidence for this last statement. And at the very least this evidence also establishes the import for philosophical study of personhood and embodiment of the thinker's spiritual commitment and aspiration which provide him with data and insights that he can achieve in no other way.

Bradley T. Scheer

D4 Individual Existence

Lewis begins by listing metaphysical bases for consideration of persons, under the classical headings of idealism and materialism. I consider that the prevailing metaphysics of natural scientists, and of all those multitudes whose thought is formed on theirs, may be designated monistic naturalism. This is the position that nature, defined as the sensible universe accessible to human senses, aided or supplemented by suitable instruments of known mechanism of operation, is the only reality. This is a form of materialism in that, according to the prevailing reductionist ontology, all nature can be understood in terms of a single entity, matter-energy, and therefore nature, and all reality, are comprehended in this single entity.

Henry Margenau, in a treatment[1] which has had less notice than it deserves, presents a different metaphysics, and Weisskopf, in a recent article,[2] has joined the small heretical party of those who recognize some limitations of natural science in understanding nature. According to Margenau, physical reality consists in those sets of verifacts (deductively verified mental constructs) categorized as systems, observables, and states. I consider this to be a form of idealism, though Margenau attempts to refute any such intention. In his system, reality does not reside in the "P-plane" of perceived objects and phenomena, but rather in the "C-plane" of, as I should put it, mappings of perceptions into constructs, using accepted epistemic rules. We may, however, apply Margenau's system to our consideration of Lewis' question as to the meaning of individual existence. From a naturalistic point-of-view—which is by no means my only personal viewpoint—the question is whether the system designated "person", and the states of that system, can be fully defined by a limited set of observables.

A person may be thought of as a member of the larger category of living systems. I shall consider three properties of living systems under the headings of individuality, continuity, and ectropy.

Individuality is apparent in the common observables of size or mass, color, and form. For legal purposes, a single feature of form, the fingerprint, is considered sufficient to identify a person, and for many purposes a signature, which is a product, is sufficient. Evidently, however, to say that we know a person, in the sense of the French verb *connaitre*, we require much more information and long acquaintance or observation. All these modes of knowing clearly reveal individuality or observation. All these modes of knowing clearly reveal individuality as a characteristic of persons. The basis of individuality of all living systems is a genome or set of genes, a unique body of information constituted, in all species with a sexual process in the life history, at the moment of conception when one gene set, from one parental strain, is united with another from the other parental strain to constitute the genome of the individual.[3] I should not wish to be interpreted, however, as proposing a genetic determinism of persons, for individuality is also a matter of the history of the individual.

Weisskopf[2] notes that living systems are different from most physical systems in that the properties of a living system reveal the history of the system. The genome of every member of a species contains something of the entire history of the species and its predecessors from The Beginning. This is expressed in the biochemical and physical properties of individuals which constitute the taxonomic characteristics used by systematists in classification. On these common specific properties, incorporating a large element of variance introduced by random processes in the transmission of a genome from one generation to the next, is imposed the record of the history of the individual from the moment of conception. The expression of genes in the biochemical and physical characteristics of the individual is subject to a variety of environmental influences, and heredity is much less determinate than some writers would have us believe.

Beyond these developmental influences, the brain, once it begins to function, preserves the record of a large part of the history of the individual, including not only external stimuli and their perception, but also a record of the responses to those stimuli and their interpretation. The identity of a person, and the sense of continuity as Lewis notes, is rooted in memory. Psychological experimentation has shown that the erasure of the past by post-hypnotic suggestion results in the immediate appearance of schizophrenic symptoms, loss of identity and modification of personal expression in behavior. Our identity is in the past, and not only in our personal past but in that of our ethnic, regional, and national forebears. I am an American, not only because I was born in this state and nation, but because my ancestors for at least nine generations were born in some part of this nation.

We come then to the matter of the states of the system we have denoted by person. In the interests of brevity, I shall only consider the states of consciousness and its opposite, unconsciousness. These states are evident in terms of the observables of activity and responsiveness. Sir Charles Sherrington[4] has given us an unforgettable picture of the spread of nervous activity through the "great ravelled knot" of nerve fibers we call the brain, during the process of awakening. Since he wrote, we have learned more than he knew about the localization of the events he described, and with the elaborate instrument known as an encephalograph electrical correlates of nervous activity in the brain can be detected in the wavy lines and spikes of an encephalogram. Although the nerve impulse itself, the source of these electrical events is now fully understood in terms of events at the level of atoms and molecules, we still do not understand the connection between the functions of the brain and the electrical events detectable with the encephalograph. This is a scientific mystery which, in Weisskopf's terms, evades our understanding because it is too complex, rather than because we have no principles of explanation. In effect, we have more principles than we can usefully employ. The "higher functions" of the brain in a state of consciousness are not understood in naturalistic terms, even though we have a working model of the memory and logical functions in electronic computers. There thus remain important aspects of the system person which are not defined by common physical observables, and are not explained by known physical principles. In my opinion, the mystery of the person is of the sort for which the requisite explanatory principles have not yet been discovered. My intuition, for I can claim no more than that, is that the key to our understanding of persons will be found in the concept of informa-mation, at the interface between thermodynamics and information theory, and I shall outline the sketch of my thinking here. Information is a matter of pattern or order. The information which I may convery in my speech is conveyed by means of elaborate patterns of sounds in time. The same or other information may be conveyed in an elaborate pattern of conventional marks on paper, or in any suitable code, even the system of dots and dashes in the traditional telegraphic code.

The information which I attempt to convey has its source and seat in my brain, where it has been assembled by the organization and integration of elements from perception and from memory. When I say "my brain" I am manifesting that property of proprietary self-awareness mentioned by Lewis as an important characteristic of persons. I hope that I am also manifesting two other characteristics, namely spontaneity and self-transcendence. Spontaneity is the creative property of persons, whereby we create new patterns of order by the manipulation of objects, symbols, or constructs. The property of self-transcendence, a term I owe to the late Reinhold Niebuhr,[5] is the ability to "stand outside oneself and look at oneself."

The history of a person is a history of the expression, reception, creation, and transmission of information. The information that is transmitted from one generation to the next in the genome is expressed materially during the process of development, which continues througout life from conception to death. Development is epigenetic, in that each stage or step is dependent on those that precede it, and provides the necessary conditions for those that follow.

The genome of an individual may be described as a program for the life processes and development of the individual, written in the genetic code, which has a well-defined material basis. The expression of that program depends to a considerable degree on external influences. During the lifetime of the individual there is a continuing process of reception, selection, integration, and accumulation of information beyond that contained in the genome,[3] and the creation of information by rational construction and imagination beyond that contained in the input from the environment. Some of this accumulated information is transmitted during the lifetime of the individual, and the ultimate question concerning persons is that of the survival of the distinctive pattern of information that characterizes the individual after the death and disintegration of the material vehicle of that information. I have defined the person in terms of individuality, historicity, and information, and concluded that the body of information carried in and by the body of a human person defines that person as a continuing entity, and the question is primarily one of continuity. The psychological experiments I mentioned earlier showed that, when the future was erased by post-hypnotic suggestion, the result was lethargy and a complete lack of interest in the life of the present. And when both past and future were erased in a single suggestion, the subject fell into a coma. Our identity as persons is in the past, and our hope is in the future. Many of the symptoms of society at the moment can be traced to the absence from the information content of many persons of any definite constructs of the past or of the future, and the fear of death so markedly evident in western society today results from the absence of future, and is, in effect, the fear of ceasing to exist as a person.

Information is immaterial, though it is ordinarily carried by or embodied in a material medium or vehicle. The challenge to non-idealistic philosophies is the undoubted reality of information, independent of its medium or vehicle. The production of information — order, pattern, negentropy, or ectropy— has been recognized as the distinctive property of living systems, and pre-eminently of persons, by Auerbach,[6] Schrodinger,[7] Schoffeniels,[8] and the present writer.[3, 9] Weisskopf[2] has suggested that the principle according to which a flow of energy from high to lower potential, with increase in entropy, engenders a smaller decrease in internal entropy (increase in ectropy) could be called the fourth law or principle of thermodynamics. This is a form of the principle stated by Prigogine[10] as the principle of minimum entropy production.

Even the monistic naturalist, who regards only the material expression of information and not its content, sees in the fundamental and universal laws or principles of natural science, invariant in time, something of absolute value. In the contemplation of these principles and their operation we come in touch with eternity. The theist may, as I do, regard these principles as the expression of the Will of the Creator. From either viewpoint, it is possible to envision a philosophy of values, comprising ethics and esthetics, founded on the ectropy principle. I can see no difficulty, on that foundation, with the conclusion that the information content or ectropy which defines a person has the property of eternity, and is of the highest absolute value.

FOOTNOTES

1. Margenau, H., The Nature of Physical Reality, McGraw-Hill, New York, 1950.
2. Weisskopf, V.F., The Frontiers and Limits of Science, American Scientist, 65 -4, 405-411.
3. Scheer, B.T., Patterns of Life. Harper's College Press, New York, 1977.
4. Sherrington, C., Man on his Nature. Cambridge U. Press, 1940.
5. Niebuhr, R., The Nature and Destiny of Man, vol. I, Human Nature, Scribner's, New York, 1941.
6. Auerbach, F., Ektropismus oder die Physikalisches Theorie des Lebens, Englemann, Leipzig, 1910.
7. Schrodinger, E., What is Life? MacMillan. New York, 1945.
8. Schoffeniels, E., L'Anti-Hasard, Gauthier-Villars, Paris, 1973.
9. Scheer, B.T., A Universal Definition of Work, BioScience *26* -8, 505-506, 1976.
10. Prigogine, I., Introduction to the Thermodynamics of Irreversible Processes, Thomas, Springfield, 1955.

Kai Nielsen

D5 Death and the Meaning of Life

I

For intellectuals, at least, the effects of the posture of modernity is very pervasive. It characteristically leaves us with a fear of being caught out in trivialities and with a fear of saying the obvious.[1] This leads us to indirect discourse, to a penchant for being clever and, because of that very fear of saying the obvious, into trivialitiy. Certainly on a topic such as our present one such anxieties readily surface and no doubt have a reasonable object. However, without any posturing at all, I shall simply brush them aside and plunge into my subject.

Most of what I say here I have said before and it has, as well, been said before by many others.[2] Moreover, it is my belief that most of the claims made here should be a series of commonplaces, but, given the direction of our popular culture, they are not. I repeat them because they seem to me to be true, to be truths which are repeatedly avoided and which need to be taken to heart.

J.M. Cameron, a distinguished Roman Catholic philosopher whose work I admire, has remarked that more and more people today think "that to die is to be annihilated".[3] Particularly for very many of us who are intellectuals and are touched by modernity and the swarth of our secular culture, belief in the survival of bodily death is an impossibility. It seems to many of us at best a groundless bit of fantasy and at worst a conception which is through and through incoherent.[4] It is an interesting point, a point which I shall not pursue here, whether the philosophical arguments purporting to establish these thoroughly secular beliefs are sound or whether they simply reflect the *Weltbild*—itself without grounds—of the dominant secular culture with its deeply scientistic orientation.[5] Whatever we should say about this, it remains the case that among the intelligentsia, and to a not inconsiderable degree elsewhere as well, belief in the survival of death is either a very considerable stumbling block or something dismissed out of hand as something which is simply "beyond belief" for anyone who can look at the world non-evasively and think tolerably clearly.

Even Cameron, who presumably does believe in some form of the survival of the death of at least our present bodies, recognizes that for most men "the hypothesis of survival" is "impossibly difficult".[6] Annihilation seems plainly and evidently to be our end. Yet he thinks that the "full terror of death" and the need to give some significance to our lives will drive us, if we are honest with ourselves and probing, to such an at least seemingly implausible belief.[7]

I want to resist this. I shall argue that, even if death is, as I believe it to be, utter annihilation, we can still find significance in our lives and that, if we will think carefully and indeed humanly— from the emotions or existentially if you will—we need not, and indeed should not, feel death to be such a stark terror. Cameron, like Kierkegaard, seems to take it as almost true by definition that to be fully human is to react to death. But why should we accept this conventional wisdom?

I shall, for a moment, as seems to me appropriate in this context, speak personally. Even though Tolstoy, Dostoevsky and Pascal have deeply touched my life, I do not feel terror when I dwell on death. Yet I know full well it must come and I firmly believe—believe without a shadow of doubt—that it will mean my utter annihilation. Yet I am without such a dread of death, though, of course, when I think of it, I feel regret that I must die, but, unlike Ivan Ilyitch, I do not feel that "before its face" all life is meaningless: nothing is worth experiencing or doing. As I am now in possession of the normal powers of life, with things I want to do and experience, with pleasure in life and with people I very much care for and who care for me, I certainly do not want to die. I should very much like, in such a state, to go on living forever. Yet plainly I cannot. In the face of this, it seems to me both a sane response and a human response to that inevitability to rather wistfully regret that fact about our common human lot and to want to make the most of the life one has. But I see no reason to make a mystery of death. And I see no reason why reflecting on my death should fill me with terror or dread or despair. One takes rational precautions against premature death and faces the rest stoically, as Freud did and as Samuel Johnson came to, and as I am confident countless others have as well. Death should only be dreadful if one's life has been a waste.

By a conventionalist's sulk such an attitude, as I have just evinced, is thought to be a shallow one devoid of the depth and the *angst* that Cameron evinces or that he finds in Ernest Becker's *The Denial of Death* or that we find in the existentialists. (I do not speak here of Nietzsche.) John Austin, when he was dying of cancer and knew that he was dying of cancer, but when others did not, was reported to have responded to a talk by Gabriel Marcel on death by remarking "Professor Marcel, we all know we have to die, but why do we have to sing songs about it?" The conventional wisdom would make this a shallow response, but, coupled with an understanding of the integrity and importance of Austin's work and with a knowledge of Austin's fierce determination to work right up to the end, it seems to me to be just the opposite. We know we must die; we would rather not, but why must we suffer *angst*, engage in theatrics and create myths for ourselves. Why not simply face it and get on with the living of our lives?

II

There is a tradition, finding its most persistent expression in Christianity, which contends that without life everlasting, without some survival of the death of one's present body and without the reality of God to ensure that such a life will have a certain character, life will be pointless and morality without significance. I shall now argue that these beliefs, common as they are, are not true.

It is indeed true that moral perplexity runs deep and moral ambivalence and anguish should be extensive. A recognition of this should be common ground between morally sensitive believers and skeptics. But there is no need to have the religious commitments of Christianity or its sister religions or any religious commitment at all to make sense of morality. Torturing human beings is vile; exploiting and degrading human beings is through-and-through evil; cruelty to human beings and animals is, morally speaking, unacceptable; and treating one's promises lightly or being careless about the truth is wrong. If we know anything to be wrong we know these things to be wrong and they would be wrong and just as wrong in a Godless world and in a world in which personal annihilation is inevitable as in a world with God and in which there is eternal life.

There is indeed a philosophical problem about how we know these things to be wrong, but this is as much a problem for the believer as for the skeptic. I would say that for anyone—for believer and skeptic alike—if he or she has an understanding of the concept of morality, has an understanding of what it is to take the moral point of view, he or she will, *eo ipso*, understand that it is wrong to harm others, that promises are to be kept and the truth to be told. This does not mean that he or she will be committed to the belief that a lie *never* can rightly be told, that a promise *never* can be broken or that a human being in *no circumstance* can rightly be harmed. But, if there is no understanding that such acts always require very special justification and that the presumption of morality is always against them, then there is no understanding of the concept of morality. But this understanding is not intrinsically or logically bound up with knowing God or knowing about God or the taking of a religious point of view or knowing or even believing that one will survive the death of one's "earthly body".

It might be responded that such an understanding does imply a knowledge of the reality of God because we *only* know these things to be wrong because we know they are against God's will and something is only good because God wills it and is only wrong because God prohibits it. Leaving aside skeptical questions about how we can know, or whether we can know, what God does and does not will, the old question arises whether something is good simply because God wills it or does God will it because it is good? What is plain—leaving aside God for a moment—is that something is not good simply because it is willed or commanded; indeed it is not even morally speaking, a good thing to do simply because it is willed or commanded by an omnipotently powerful being, unless we want to reduce morality to power worship, as has one rather well known but (on this issue) confused philosopher.[8] But might—naked power—doesn't make right. And there is no implication that it will become right even when conjoined with faultless intelligence. There can be—and indeed are—thoroughly ruthless, exploitative, manipulative people who are very intelligent indeed. Neither omnipotence nor omniscience imply goodness.

However, it is still not implausible to say that it is *God's* willing it which makes all the difference, for God, after all, is the supreme, perfect good. But I in turn ask, how do we know that or do we know that? If we say we know it through studying the Scriptures and through the example of Jesus, then it should in turn be responded that it is only in virtue or our own quite independent moral understanding of the goodness of his behavior and the behavior of the characters in the Bible that we come to recognize this. Moral understanding is not grounded in a belief in God; just the reverse is the case: an understanding of the religious *significance* of Jesus and the Scriptures presupposes a moral understanding.

If, alternatively, we claim that we do not come to understand that God is the supreme and perfect good in that way but claim that it is a necessary truth—a proposition, like "Puppies are young dogs", which is true by definition—then we still should ask: how do we understand that putatively necessary proposition? But again we should recognize that it is only by having an understanding of what goodness is that we come to have some glimmering of the more complex and extremely perplexing notions of supreme goodness or perfect goodness. The crucial thing to see is that there are things which we can recognize on reflection to be wrong, God or no God, and that we can be far more confident that we are right in claiming that they are wrong, than we can be in claiming any knowledge of God or God's order.

Finally, someone might say that since God is the cause of everything, there could be no goodness or anything else if there were no God. But this confuses *causes* and *reasons*, confuses questions about causally bringing something into existence or sustaining its existence and justifying its existence. If there is the God of the Jews and the Christians everything causally depends on Him, but still, even if there were no God who made the world, it would still be wrong to torture little children, and even if there were no people to be kind, it would be timelessly true

that human kindness would be a good thing and that the goodness of human kindness does not become good or cease to become
good by God's fiat or anyone else's. And it is in no way dependent
on whether we live out our fourscore years and ten or whether life
is everlasting.

In terms of its fundamental rationale, morality is utterly independent of belief in God or a belief in immortality. To make sense
of our lives as moral beings there is no need to make what may be
an intellectually stultifying blind leap of religious faith or to in
any way believe in an afterlife. Such a moral understanding, as
well as a capacity for moral response and action, is available to us
even if we are human beings who are utterly without religious faith.

Furthermore, it does not follow that our lives are pointless,
empty or meaningless if there is no God and if death is unequivo-
cally our lot. There is no good reason to believe that because of
these things we are condemned to an Oblomov-like, senseless
existence. There is no reason why we must despair if God is dead
and if life must come to an end. If there is no God, it is indeed true
that we are not blessed with the questionable blessing of being
made for a purpose; furthermore, if there is neither God nor
Logos, there is no purpose to life, no plan for the universe or prov-
idential ordering of things in accordance with which we must live
our lives. Yet, from the fact, if it is a fact, that there is no purpose
to life or no purposes for which we are made, it does not at all follow that there are no purposes *in* life that are worth achieving,
doing or having, so that life in reality must be just one damn
thing after another that finally senselessly terminates in death.
"Purpose of life" is ambiguous: in talking of it we can, on the one
hand, be talking of "purpose to life", or, on the other, of "purposes
in life" in the sense of plans we form, ends we seek, etc. that result
from our deliberate and intentional acts and our desires, including
our reflective desires. The former require something like a god or
a *Logos*, but the latter most certainly do not. Yet it is only the latter that are plainly necessary to make life meaningful in the sense
that there are in our lives and our environment things worthwhile
doing, having or experiencing, things that bring joy, understanding, exhilaration or contentment to ourselves or to others. That
we will not have these things forever does not make them worth-

less any more than the inevitability of death and the probability of decay robs them, or our lives generally, of their sense. In a Godless world, in which death is inevitable, our lives are not robbed of meaning.

III

Some might concede all this and still respond that I am leaving out something crucial from the religious traditions. They could agree I have shown that life for an atheist can very well have meaning. But what I have not shown is that with the loss of the kind of hope and the kind of perspective that have gone with Judaism, Christianity and Islam something has not been irreparably taken from us, the loss of which is increasingly felt as the managed society of the Twentieth Century closes in on us.

What I am alluding to can perhaps best be brought forward if I turn to a famous trio of questions of Kant's: "What can I know?", "What ought I to do?" and "What may I hope?",[9] Max Horkheimer, in commenting on them, remarks that an examination of the "third question leads to the idea of the highest good and absolute justice".[10] He then adds that the "moral conscience . . . rebels against the thought that the present state of reality is final . . ."[11] In the struggles of our everyday life, in the world as we know it, our hopes for a realization, or even approximation, of a truly human society, a society of human brotherhood and sisterhood, a just society or even a rational society are constantly dashed, constantly defeated. This led Kant, Lessing and even Voltaire to postulate immortality in order to make some match between our aspirations and what is realizable. Such postulations are indeed easy to satirize and indeed it is folly to try to argue from such hopes to any likelihood at all that such a reality will obtain.[12] But one can understand it as a hope—a hope which a person who truly cares about his fellows and has lost all faith in anything like a Marxist humanist future, might well keep close to his heart. If we believe, as Horkheimer and Adorno do, that we live in a world where we grow lonelier, more isolated, more caught up in meaningless work routines, more passive, more and more incapable of seeing things as a whole and of having any believable sense of where we come from, who we are or where we are going, we may perhaps rightly become "knights of faith" and make such an otherwise absurd postulation.

Yet, if we can rightly live in hope here, can we not, even more rightly, live in accordance with the less intellectually stultifying hope that we humans can attain a certain rationality and come to see things whole and in time make real, through our struggles, a truly human society without exploitation and degradation in which all human beings will flourish? Even *if* this hope is utopian — another dream of the "dreamers of the absolute" — it is still far less utopian, and far less fantastical, than the hope for "another world" where we will go "by and by". Moreover, such secular hopes are in the various Marxisms (reified and otherwise) as alive in traditions as are the otherworldly conceptions of Christianity.

NOTES

1. The sense of this is very acute in Stanley Cavell's *Must We Mean What We Say*, (New York: Charles Scribner's Sons, 1969) and this sense is further astutely conveyed in Francis Sparshott's discussion of it in *The Times Literary Supplement*, July 22, 1977, p. 899.

2. My *Ethics Without God*, (London: Pemberton Books, 1973), *Scepticism*, (London: Macmillan, 1973), "Linguistic Philosophy and 'The Meaning of Life'", *Cross-Currents*, Vol. XIV (Summer 1964), "Linguistic Philosophy and Beliefs", *Philosophy Today*, No. 2, Jerry H. Gill (ed.), (London: Collier Macmillan Ltd., 1969), "An Examination of the Thomistic Theory of Natural Moral Law", *Natural Law Forum*, Vol. 4 (1959) and "God and the Good: Does Morality Need Religion", *Theology Today*, Vol. XXI (April 1964).

3. J.M. Cameron, "Surviving Death", *The New York Review of Books*, Vol. XXI, No. 17 (October 1974), pp. 6-11.

4. Antony Flew, "Is There a Case for Disembodied Survival?" *The Journal of the American Society For Psychical Research*, Vol. 66, (April 1972), pp. 129-144, part III of Antony Flew, *The Presumption of Atheism*, (New York: Barnes & Noble, 1976), Terrence Penelhum, *Suvival and Disembodied Existence*, (London: Routledge & Kegan Paul, 1970) and my "Logic, Incoherence and Religion", *International Logic Review*, forthcoming.

5. Ludwig Wittgenstein, *On Certainty*, translated by Denis Paul and G.E.M. Anscombe, (Oxford: Basil Blackwell, 1969) and G.H. von Wright, "Wittgenstein on Certainty", *Problems in the Theory of Knowledge*, ed. by G.H. von Wright, (The Hague: Martinus Nijhoff, 1972) pp. 47-60.

6. J.M. Cameron, *op. cit.*, p. 11.

7. *Ibid.*

8. Peter Geach, *God and the Soul*, (London: Routledge & Kegan Paul, 1969), pp. 117-129.

9. Immanuel Kant, *Critique of Pure Reason*, tr. by J.M.D. Meiklejohn, (New York: Dutton, 1934), p. 457.

10. Max Horkheimer, *Critique of Instrumental Reason*, (New York: The Seabury Press, 1974), p. 2.

11. *Ibid.*

12. J.L. Mackie, "Sidgwick's Pessimism", *Philosophical Quarterly*, (1976), pp. 326-7.

W. Norris Clarke, S.J.

D6 Death and the Meaning of Life In the Christian Tradition

The purpose of this morning's symposium is to discuss what light death, or more precisely the meaning of death, sheds on the meaning of life. And my particular task is to present this as interpreted by the Christian tradition in contrast with Professor Nielsen, who will discuss it, I presume, from a naturalist viewpoint. I must say it caused me some surprise at first that such a topic should be on the program at a non-theological conference, since up to the very recent years in most American intellectual and social circles death was a subject that was ordinarily veiled in a conspiracy of silence and brushed under the rug as much as possible; it was considered bad taste to bring it up, at least in any personal existential way, i.e. in any way other than as a practical technical problem concerning practical adjustments among those on this side of death. A striking example of this technical viewpoint was given me by one of my students recently, who is doing a PhD thesis on the philosophical dimensions of death. He was interviewing a distinguished doctor at the famous Sloan-Kettering Institute for the treatment of cancer in New York, and was trying to get at the doctor's own personal attitude toward death as a human experience, since he was dealing with it in his patients every day. When he was asked, "Doctor, what does death mean to you personally?" the answer was: "To me, death is the ultimate challenge to my expertise." Hardly a personalist response. But in recent years there has been a sudden and dramatic rise in interest in the subject, as we all know. Courses in colleges and universities proliferate on it, books pour out, symposia are held, etc. This is quite a healthy sign, it seems to me, since it would appear all too obvious that the end of human life should throw a great deal of light on the significance of what has gone before. Hence I welcome our frank discussion of the subject in the context of this conference on ultimate values and their relation to the work of science.

I shall treat the question primarily from the point of view of the Roman Catholic side of the Christian tradition, since it is this that I know best,[1] though I suspect that most of it will apply, *mutatis mutandis,* to the other branches of Christianity. I shall examine first the meaning of death itself in the Christian view of human destiny, then the light that this sheds on the meaning of life itself this side of the grave.

I. The Meaning of Death

Let us go at once to the heart of the matter. The essence of the Christian teaching on death is that it proclaims the victory over death through the life-giving power of the risen Christ. As St. Paul cries out in those exultant phrases that have echoed and reechoed all down through Chrisitan history, "Death is swallowed up in victory. O death, where is thy victory? O death, where is thy sting? Thanks be to God who has given us the victory through our Lord Jesus Christ" (I Cor. 15:54-57). In this conception death in its present painful form is viewed as having exercised domination over man even since the sin or fall of early man, personified in Adam and Eve. It is thus looked on as a punishment for sin. This reign of death over mankind is overthrown by the voluntary death of Jesus on the Cross and his resurrection by the power of the Father, who now appoints him as the Giver of Life—eternal life— to all who believe in him (and indeed to all who seek God with a sincere conscience and thus implicitly believe all that God wishes them to believe).

The exact meaning of the doctrine that death is the punishment of sin is veiled in considerable obscurity. Contemporary theological speculation is more or less agreed that it does not mean necessarily that man would not have died at all without the sin of Adam. Karl Rahner speculates that even without sin man would have had to pass through death as an end to his biological life, but a death chosen by his free decision as the completion of his life and not a painful death forced upon him from without and veiled in fear and obscurity as at present.[2] We do not wish to delay any further here on this more technical question but will concentrate on the more positive Christian vision of victory over death at least in its present human modality, whatever the latter's origin.

Death has always haunted the consciousness of man, as a source of fear, of sadness at the threat of ultimate defeat and extinction, or at least the uncertainty of what lies beyond this impenetrable veil. The Greek elegiac poetry, with its muted but deeply moving chords of resigned sadness over the death of a loved one or the anticipation of one's own death, bear eloquent witness to man's sense of profound disappointment and frustration at the apparent ultimate victory of death over all his projects, his loves, his life itself. Death, as Rahner puts it, is "the point where man in the most radical way becomes a question for himself, a question which God himself must answer."[3]

Most, if not all, religions promise man some victory over death, some form of immortality, even though not always by the preservation of his own distinct individuality (as in some Hindu and Buddhist traditions). But the distinctive character of the Christian vision of the victory over death is that not only does it preserve the individuality of each person in the future life, but this overcoming of the domination of death is brought about by the special intervention of God himself become incarnate in the man Jesus, through his voluntary acceptance of death as taking on the burden of the sins of all mankind, and then breaking the power of death as the last word in man's destiny by rising from the dead in a transformed state beyond the reach of death to enjoy the fullness of eternal life with God his Father. And it is by voluntary participation in the death and resurrection of Christ that each man can pass over to eternal life with Christ. As St. Paul often says, just as we have died with Christ in baptism, so too we have risen with him, and our life is now hidden with Christ in God,[4] and, as St. John adds, we now have within us the seeds of eternal life, though they will not blossom fully till the resurrection.[5]

One could put this same central message more precisely by saying that the victory of Christ over death is not so much a destruction of death itself, since all men must still pass through death, as a transvaluation of its meaning. Death now becomes no longer the ultimate darkness, the end without issue, but rather the gateway to a new and indestructible fullness of life. Death is no longer the end of the journey but a passage to a new and definitive chapter of life.

Before we pass on to consider the light shed upon the meaning of life by this vision of death as the passage to eternal life by participation in the death and resurrection of Christ, we would be failing in our duty if we did not point out one implication of the traditional Christian view of death. This is the rejection of any literal doctrine of *reincarnation* of the human soul in other bodies after the present life. The grounds of this tradition are as follows: (1) the clear text of St. Paul: "It is appointed for man to die once, and then the judgement" (Hebrews 9:27), though the import of this canonical text may be somewhat weakened by the fact that the *Epistle to the Hebrews* is now widely acknowledged not to have been written by Paul himself; (2) a clear implication of the doctrine of redemption through Christ: those who die "in Christ," as St. Paul says, are definitively saved and sure of their ressurrection to eternal life in and through him (one might also mention the indelible mark of baptism: once baptized, always baptized): (3) a long tradition of the Church reaffirming this, although not explicitly mentioning reincarnation. This long but still sparse documentary tradition is summed up admirably by the unofficial summary of the main doctrines of the Christian faith in a Schema presented by the theologians of the Second Vatican Council but which for lack of time never came to an official vote:

> Those who die in this grace (of Christ) will, with certainty, obtain eternal life, the crown of justice, and just as certainly, those who die deprived of this grace will never arrive at eternal life. For death is the end of our pilgrimage, and shortly after death we stand before the judgement seat of God "so that each one may receive what he has won through the body according to his works, whether good or evil" (II Cor. 5:10). And after this mortal life there is no place left for repentance or justification.[6]

As Karl Rahner puts it, commenting on this text and the foregoing tradition in his recent *Encyclopedia of Theology:* "In this way any doctrine of transmigration of souls is rejected as incompatible with the conception of the uniqueness and decisiveness of human history and the nature of freedom as definitive decision."[7]

Despite the solidarity of this tradition, which some, however, think may not be quite as airtight as it seems, I must note that in very recent years a small but growing number of Christians, especially those interested in Eastern religions, are raising the question again as to the absolute incompatibility of Christian doctrine with that of reincarnation—including some in this room, if I am not mistaken. Although I do not share this view, it might well be a subject for discussion.

II. Implications for the Meaning of Life

1. Optimistic View of Human Life. One implication of seeing death as a passage of eternal life and ultimate human fulfillment is that one also sees our present human life as a prelude and preparation for this same eternal life. This sets the short and precarious span of our earthly human existence in a much vaster framework that should take away the sting of most of our fears, anxiety, a frustration in the face of a precarious existence whose course and outcome we can only partially control and which is doomed to be cut short eventually, unpredictably, and ineluctably by death as the end of all our projects. Seeing this present life as a prelude and preparation for eternal life where total and truly authentic human fulfillment can be ours if we sincerely will it (coming at once as a gift of God and yet as matched to our own good will and moral effort) illumines our present life with the light of a magnificent destiny extending far beyond it, of which the uncontrollable accidents and even mistakes of this life cannot rob us unless we stubbornly cling to them. All this gives both a profound meaning and purpose and an indestructible hope to the project of the earthly part of our existence. This lifts from us the burden of either desperate urgency to achieve as much happiness and fulfillment as possible in this life or the sad, bitter resignation at seeing it slip from our hands or recede beyond our reach—attitudes all too natural to fall into—if we believe that this short life is all that there is for this self-conscious "I" with its inexhaustible reach of longings and desires.

The positive vision of man thus becomes that of an image of God, in process of development toward transformation and final union with Infinite Intelligence, Goodness, and Love. This vision and the hope that it nourishes makes of man's earthly life a project of immense dignity and eternal importance for which death is

no longer the cruel and inscrutable end to all hopes, the passage
to final extinction, but the passage to a new and definitive chapter of fulfillment. As a result, the ultimate importance in themselves of our possessions and achievements, whether successes or
failures, in this earthly chapter of our history becomes profoundly
relativized, so that we do not have to seek for or cling to them
desperately, as though it is all or nothing in this life alone, as
though failure here is ultimate and unredeemable. An authentic
Christian should thus be characterized by a certain liberating
freedom and detachment from the fruits of his earthly efforts,
which should also give him a special readiness and willingness to
sacrifice without anxiety not only his possessions but even his
physical life for the sake of some proportionate value, even if it be
for the welfare of another. It is not clear to me how the readiness
to sacrifice one's own life for another, no matter how much one
may admire the courage and generosity of the person acting thus,
can make truly good sense, satisfying sense, if one believes that
death is the absolute and total end of oneself. But this too is a
point open for the most fruitful discussion. It seems to me that it
is a crucial test for the viability of any ethics and overall vision of
the dignity of man that one should be able to make good sense of
the act of giving up one's life for another.

Before we leave this point, it should be noted that man's earthly
life, viewed in this Christian perspective of the meaning of death,
appears as at once a project of man's own self-development and
fulfillment and at the same time the carrying out in loving obedience of a project first conceived and given to us with our being by
our Creator, the Father of life, hence a project not subject merely
to our own arbitary will. This existential synthesis of authentic
self-interest and loving obedience to a Higher Will, where loving
obedience and service become in fact identical with our own
authentic self-fulfillment, is one of the hallmarks of the Christian
vision of the meaning of human life. Life for a Christian is both
his own and God's project.

2. *The Urgency of Living Well This Present Life.* We have
said above that the perspective of an eternal life after death implies
a notable relativization of our achievements in this life, whether successes or failures, since our definitive fulfillment far transcends

them, and all their immediate fruits must be let go of as we pass through the purifying emptiness of death. Yet on the other hand there is a peculiar urgency to our moral life on this earth resulting from the fact that we have only this one life to live, this one preparation for eternal life, since there is no reincarnation or second chance. Although our outer historical achievements and possessions are indeed relativized, the inner quality of our moral life, of our pursuit of and response to primary values, which depends on our own free decision, takes on an enhanced import and urgency because of the eternal significance of what we do with our freedom in time. Even though one's external successes and failures in this life can and should be taken lightly, the moral portrait which we slowly forge out of our truly authentic acts of free moral decision during our lives, and which receives final and definitive ratification at the moment of death, is to be taken with the utmost seriousness. Yet even here, because of the Christian doctrine of forgiveness available to every man for even the most evil act, through the salvific death and resurrection of Christ, the moral portrait of every man remains unfinished, capable of even the most drastic remodeling, up to the moment of death. As you perhaps may know, though it is not a question of official Catholic doctrine one way or the other, and opinions are about equally divided over it, many Catholic theologians today hold for a theory of *final option* at the moment of death. This means that at the time of death, either at the moment before or at the moment of actually leaving the body, each person has the opportunity to pull together the meaning of his whole life, which may never have been clear to him before, and decide definitively in full clarity and self-possession just what he wishes the radical meaning and commitment of his life to be, which at this point would be a commitment either to God as the center of value and meaning, or to oneself as the center, or perhaps to meaninglessness and despair. There is much to be said both for and against this appealing doctrine, and I am not too sure just where I stand on it, though I do lean toward it. In any case, it would be highly imprudent even for someone who believes in it to bet on the chance that his final option would, with no prior preparation, be somehow radically different from the freely and deliberately forged moral portrait characteristic of his whole prior life.

It seems to me that here, if one compares this view of human
life and death with the traditional Hindu and Buddhist belief in
reincarnation, insofar as this doctrine is to be taken literally—as
most ordinary Hindus and Buddhists seem to do—we come face
to face with at least one clear-cut point of difference between
these two great traditional views of human life and death. And
there is no doubt that the practical ethical and religious consequences of this difference are considerable. The belief that we
have only one life to live, and that our eternal destiny depends on
how we live it, insofar as this comes under the control of our freedom, invests each human life-span and one's personal moral decisions within it with a unique dignity, decisiveness, and urgency.
For the Christian, this life is an all or nothing deal, not an indefinitely repeated series of new starts and new chances, both for
good and evil. But this again is a fine subject for discussion. How
different in practice is the moral pressure exerted by the desire to
escape the wheel of *karma* from the urgency for the Christian to
live his one life well? Surely there must be a difference in the psychic and spiritual tonality of one's inner life, as one lives within
one or the other of these two spiritual universes.[8]

3. *Mindfulness of Death in the Midst of Life.* Since the meaning of death, as we have seen, plays such an important role in
determining the meaning of life for a Christian, one of the characteristic spiritual attitudes that should mark the entire life of an
authentic Christian—though this is more honored in the breach
than in the observance by most, I fear—is the *mindfulness of
death* as a guide for life, rather than a deliberate forgetfulness of
it, as has become the custom in our contemporary secular culture.
For the Christian, death is one of what have been traditionally
called "the four last things"—namely death, judgement, heaven,
and hell—which should be kept permanently on his mind as part
of the abiding background or horizon of his spiritual consciousness, as a positive beacon to guide his way on this earth. Thinking of these "last things," rather than being an escape from the
present, has a way of illuminating and setting in proper perspective all that is prior to them. In the tradition of Christian spiritu-
ality it has always been a potent device for preventing us from

being hypnotized by the often apparent urgency and absorbing fascination of the immediate moving present, for cutting through the insidious spell of self-deception, and for arranging our practical priorities in harmony with our deepest beliefs—in a word, for testing the Christian authenticity of our moral decision-making. Thus St. Ignatius uses it as one of his key rules in his famous *Spirtual Exercises* for making an important decision in one's life. He recommends that one put himself in his imagination on his death-bed and ask himself: "How at that moment would I feel disposed towards the present decision now facing me? Which alternative would I feel better then, as I am about to face God in judgement, about having made now?"

4. *The Spirit of Detachment.* Another key spiritual attitude that flows immediately from the above is a certain permanent spirit of inner freedom from attachment, that is, possessive clinging attachment, to any of the created goods (possessions, projects, pleasures, modes of enjoyment even of persons) that will pass away with death. This does not mean that we have nothing to do with them, which would be impossible anyway, or that we do not respect and love them according to their value, enjoy them as temporary gifts of God, and use them to help us along the way to Him. But it does mean that we do not *cling* to them tenaciously, anxiously, as though we could not do without them, as though God alone were not enough for us. In a word, we are spiritually *free* with respect to them, can take them or leave them according to the will of God as manifested in our lives at the time. Another traditional name for this is "poverty of spirit": "Blessed are the poor in spirit, for theirs is the Kingdom of Heaven" as the First Beatitude in Jesus' Sermon on the Mount puts it. The purpose of such "detachment" is not purely negative, emptying for the sake of emptying. It is a form of self-emptying in order to open ourselves more fully to the fullness of God Himself, who wishes to give Himself to us as fully as we are able and ready to receive.

Seen in the light of the Christian meaning of death, this spirit of detachment from all creatures during life appears as a progressive, freely willed preparation throughout one's life for negotiating well what should be the supreme *act* of a human life for a Christian, that is, death itself. For death by nature is that radical moment which forces upon us a total self-denudation of all the possessions, projects, and modes of activity and relationship we have enjoyed upon earth, a total emptying and withdrawal of all that seemed to support us here, to be left naked and alone in the presence of the living God. This cannot help but awaken a certain natural fear in us. But this unavoidable moment can be met either as something undergone purely passively, as something we are dragged reluctantly into, desperately and vainly trying to hold on to as much of our possessions as possible; or it can be accepted freely, willingly, even joyously, as a deliberately willed act of total detachment, self-emptying, in order that we may open ourselves as fully as possible for the final gift of Himself that God alone can give, in whom alone we believe and hope our total fulfillment will lie. There is no other way, really, it seems, for man as a creature of the earth to prepare himself adequately for the final gift of God than by passing through this freely accepted moment of total self-denudation as condition to his transformation to a new mode of life unrestricted by the bonds of space and time-bound matter. The same held true for Christ himself as man, whose freely accepted death in loving obedience to his Father was the very instrument for making available to all men the final victory over death by transforming it into a passage to eternal life.

Here the marvelous yet fearful paradox of death comes fully to light as mystery-filled coincidence of opposites. As Karl Rahner puts it so strikingly: "Consequently in death the act of human life . . . finally comes to its sharpest contradiction, the simultaneity of highest will and extreme weakness, a lot which is actively achieved and passively suffered, plenitude and emptiness."[9] That we prepare well and with eyes open to meet this supreme challenge and opportunity at our best, rather than stumble into it terrified and unprepared, is surely a significant part of the meaning of human life for a Christian — as also, I might add, for a sincere Hindu or Buddhist.

5. *The Intrinsic Value of Man's Earthly Activities: Two Christian Views.* What has gone before I think would find fairly wide acceptance in all Christian traditions. Let me conclude now with a more controverted question among Christians regarding the Christian meaning of man's secular activities during his earthly

life. What is the intrinsic value of man's work in the world such as culture, civilization, science, technology, art, etc., in a word, the work of building the human city on this earth? Secular humanists of various kinds, including Marxists, have often criticized Christianity for being as preoccupied with the next life as to have little real interest in or wholehearted commitment to the betterment of this world, compared to the secularist for whom this life is the only one and hence deserving of his total attention and commitment. It is true that Christian thought has shown a certain ambivalence on this point down the ages, tending to oscillate between two different if not opposed attitudes.[10] One has been called the *eschatological* view (i.e. focused primarily on the *eschata*, the last things) for whom this world and all its activities are merely the theater or testing ground for man's inner moral and spiritual growth, which alone has intrinsic permanent value. In themselves apart from their purely instrumental character they have no value in the eyes of God and no intrinsic relation to man's true goal, eternal life.

The other attitude, called the *incarnational* view, so called from its focus on the incarnation as God's act of assuming, consecrating, and conferring intrinsic value forever to the world of matter, regards man's work of culture in the world as having not merely instrumental but intrinsic value of its own in the eyes of God, and hence some direct proportion and significance even for man's eternal life. Secular history is not merely an external foil or framework for sacred history but bears an intrinsic relation to it as built in to the latter's own growth and destined to be not merely swept away as useless straw at the end of history but to be somehow assumed in a transformed way into the eternal life itself of man. St. Augustine may be taken as a type of the first attitude, Teilhard de Chardin of the second.

The second naturally appeals more to contemporary Christian man, with his strong commitment to social action, and gives him a more secure stance in meeting the challenge of the secular humanists. I must admit it appeals more to me too. And it is, I think, one genuine Christian view of the world and the meaning of human life, though the dyed-in-the-wool eschatologist looks on it as a compromise with worldliness. But it is not the only authentic Christian view, one reason being that the basic Christian sources

360   W. Norris Clarke, S.J.

give no sufficient grounds for a clear-cut choice between them. It
may be that for the full dimensions of the Christian mystery to
remain intact and not be arbitrarily truncated by our limited
human wisdom, both attitudes must remain in vital and creative
tension within Christian thought, so that each will help to keep
the other honest and humble in not believing too easily that it has
mastered the mystery of the total meaning of human life, as seen
in the partly revealing, partly concealing light of death.

NOTES

1. Here are few key references from which one can follow up with bibliography: Karl Rahner, *The Theology of Death* (New York: Seabury, 1961),
   together with his excellent condensation of its main points in the *Encyclopedia of Theology* edited by him in 1 volume (New York: Seabury,
   1975), article on "Death." See also Ladislaus Boros, *The Mystery of
   Death* (New York: Seabury, 1965); M.M. Gatch, *Death: Meaning and
   Mortality in Christian Thought and Contemporary Culture* (New York:
   Seabury, 1969); E. Kubler Ross, *Death and Dying* (New York: Macmillan,
   1969); M. Simpson, *Theology of Death and Eternal Life* (University of
   Notre Dame, 1971). See also the magisterial work of the Protestant
   theologian, John Hick, *Death and Eternal Life* (New York: Harper and
   Row, 1976).
2. Article "Death" in *Encyclopedia of Theology*, p. 329.
3. Article cit., p. 329.
4. Colossians 2:22-3; 4.
5. I John 2-3.
6. In *The Church Teaches:* Documents of the Church in English translation, ed. by J.F. Clarkson *et al.* (St. Louis: Herder, 1955), no. 891, pp.
   352-53; it should be noted that this text comes from the *Schema* prepared by the theologians of the Council as a summary of the principle
   mysteries of faith, but the Council ended hastily before the *Schema*
   could be brought to the floor of the Council for formal approval; hence
   it is not an official document but clearly reflects Catholic teaching. The
   more official documents through history can be found in the same book
   under the heading "The Last Things," esp. nos. 878, 881, 883-84, 886,
   887, 889; these maintain that we rise in this flesh in which we now are
   and not some other, that soon after death, or the purification needed in
   Purgatory—during which there is no more place for merit, increase of
   charity, or loss of salvation—the souls of those who die in Christ receive
   the beatific vision forever, while the souls of those who die in mortal sin
   go to eternal punishment.
7. Art. on "Death," p. 330.

8. Cf. F.H. Holck, ed., *Death and Eastern Thought* (New York: Abingdon, 1974).

9. *Art. cit.*, p. 333.

10. A spirited controversy on this aspect of the theology of history broke out in the 50s and 60s; a few samples are: H. Urs von Balthasar, *A Theology of History* (New York: Sheed & Ward, 1965); J.V.L. Casserley, *Toward a Theology of History* (New York: Holt, Rinehart, 1965); H. Butterfield, *Christianity and History* (New York: Scribner, 1950); O. Lewry, *Theology of History* (Notre Dame: Fides, 1969).

Ravi Ravindra

D7 Death and the Meaning of Life — A Hindu Response

Since the "Hindu Response" covers a wide spectrum, I shall base my remarks mainly on the *Bhagavad Gita;* this, however, being the most popular scripture in India may fairly be taken to be representative of Hindu views. There is, first of all, a relativity of life and death, and a definite continuity across the barrier represented by physical death, a barrier which appears permanent and massively opaque. What really is, cannot cease to be; just as death is certain for those who are alive, rebirth is certain for those who are dead. Man's existence thus includes both sides of the apparently uni-directional divide called death. Therefore, the problem of death is not essentially different from the problem of life.

What changes is the form of manifestation: from gross to subtle and back to gross, and so on endlessly. This process will go on forever according to the laws of nature, which revels in the subtle no less than in the apparent, and all beings, human as well as others, are compulsively born again and again, and die repeatedly. This process of repeated births and deaths, that is, a continual change of form, is an outcome of cosmic causal necessity and operates for all existences, at all scales, for all time. This is what is called *sam sara.*

To be free of the entire inherent compulsion of sam sara is the only real freedom. This freedom is no more in "death" than in "life," these being the two sides of the same ceaselessly changing coin. From this point of view, death lends no more immediacy to the question about the meaning of life than life does itself. What then is the meaning of life? The general Hindu response is that the meaning of life consists in the opportunity it affords for this radical liberation — deliverance from the endlessly repititious, unconscious nature, outside as well as inside man, driven by mechanical necessity.

This unconscious nature includes not only our bodies but also our minds. But man is more than that. He is spirit as well. According to most Hindus, man is essentially nothing but spirit, which by some illusion identifies itself with a part or the whole of his psycho-somatic complex (*sarira*). The real man (*puru sa*, spirit) is incarnated, that is he takes on a *sarira*, for the explicit purpose of seeing through the illusion that keeps him in bondage; and he gives up the *sarira* when it is no longer able to be useful to him in his essential purpose. It is *sarira* which is born and which dies, and we mistakenly think that it is the real man who is born and who dies. At "death" what is said is that the person has given up the *sarira* (in contrast to saying that he has given up the ghost).

This process of birth and death will go on, for millions of lives if necessary, until the spiritual principle in man realizes its true nature and is freed. Then there will be no more need of being born or dying. Until then "death" is as necessary for the purposes of the spirit as "life."

Sir John Eccles

D8 Natural Theological Speculations on Death and The Meaning of Life

On all materialist theories of the mind there can be no consciousness of any kind after brain death. Immortality is a non-problem.
But with dualist-interactionism it can be recognized from the
standard diagram (Fig. 2 of Section B1) that death of the brain
need not result in the destruction of the central component of
World 2. All that can be inferred is that World 2 ceases to have
any relationship with the brain and hence will lack all sensory
information and all motor expression. There is no question of a
continued shadowy or ghost-like existence in some relationship
with the material world, as is claimed in some spiritualist beliefs.
What then can we say?

Belief in some life after death came very early to mankind, as
is indicated by the ceremonial burial customs of Neanderthal
man. However in our earliest records of beliefs about life after
death it was most unpleasant. This can be seen in the Epic of Gil-
gamesh or in the Homeric poems, or in the Hebrew belief about
Sheol. Hick (1976) points out that the misery and unhappiness
believed to attend the life hereafter very effectively disposes of
the explanation that such beliefs arose from wish-fulfilment!

The idea of a more attractive after-life is a special feature of
the Socratic dialogues, being derived from the Orphic mysteries.
After the poignant simplicity of Socrates' messages before death,
it is quite an experience to contemplate the many kinds of immortality that have been the subject of speculation. The idea of
immortality has been sullied over and even made repugnant by
the many attempts from earliest religions to give an account that
was based on the ideologies of the time. Thus today intellectuals
are put off by these archaic attempts to describe and depict life
after bodily death. I am put off by them too.

A more interesting and meaningful disputation concerns the recognition of self after death. We normally have the body and brain to assure us of our identity, but, with departure of the psyche from the body and brain in death, none of these landmarks is available to it. All of the detailed memory must be lost. If we refer again to Fig. 2 of Section B1, memory is also shown located in World 2. I would suggest that this is a more general memory related to our self-identity, our emotional life, our personal life and to our ideals as enshrined in the values. All of this should be sufficient for self-identity. Reference should be made to the discussion on the creation of the psyche by infusion into the developing embryo (Eccles, 1980, lecture 10). *This divinely created psyche should be central to all considerations of immortality and of self-recognition* (cf. Lewis, 1978).

Our life here on this earth and cosmos is beyond our understanding in respect of the Great Questions. We have to be open to some deep dramatic significance in this earthly life of ours that may be revealed after the transformation of death. We can ask: What does this life mean? We find ourselves here in this wonderfully rich and vivid conscious experience and it goes on through life; but is that the end? This self-conscious mind of ours has this mysterious relationship with the brain and as a consequence achieves experiences of human love and friendship, of the wonderful natural beauties, and of the intellectual excitement and joy given by appreciation and understanding of our cultural heritages. Is this present life all to finish in death or can we have hope that there will be further meaning to be discovered? In the context of Natural Theology I can only say that there is complete oblivion about the future; but we came from oblivion. Is it that this life of ours is simply an episode of consciousness between two oblivions, or is there some further transcendent experience of which we can know nothing until it comes?

Man has lost his way ideologically in this age. It is what has been called the predicament of mankind. I think that science has gone too far in breaking down man's belief in his spiritual greatness, as examplified in the magnificent achievements in World 3, and has given him the belief that he is merely an insignificant animal that has arisen by chance and necessity in an insignificant planet lost in the great cosmic immensity. I think the principal trouble with mankind today is that the intellectual leaders are too arrogant in their self-sufficiency. We must realize the great unknowns in the material makeup and operation in our brains, in the relationship of brain to mind and in our creative imagination. When we think of these great unknowns as well as the unknown of how we come to be in the first place, we should be much more humble. The unimaginable future that could be ours would be the fulfillment of this our present life, and we should be prepared to accept its possibility as the greatest gift. In the acceptance of this wonderful gift of life and of death, we have to be prepared not for the inevitability of some other existence, but we can hope for the possibility of it.

This is the message we would get from what Penfield (1975) and Thorpe (1962) have written; and I myself have also the strong belief that we have to be open to the future. This whole cosmos is not just running on and running down for no meaning. In the context of Natural Theology I come to the belief that we are creatures with some supernatural meaning that is as yet ill defined. We cannot think more than that we are all part of some great design, which was the theme of my first Gifford series (Eccles, 1979). Each of us can have the belief of acting in some unimaginable supernatural drama. We should give all we can in order to play our part. Then we wait with serenity and joy for the future revelations of whatever is in store after death.

REFERENCES

Eccles, J.C.: *The Human Mystery.* Berlin, Heidelberg, New York: Springer International (1979)

Eccles, J.C.: *The Human Psyche.* Berlin, Heidelberg, New York: Springer International (1980)

Hick, J.: *Death and Eternal Life.* London: Collins (1976)

Lewis, H.D.: *Persons and Life after Death.* London: Macmillan (1978)

Penfield, W.: *The Mystery of the Mind.* Princeton, New Jersey: Princeton University Press (1975)

Thorpe, W.H.: *Biology and the Nature of Man.* London: Oxford University Press (1962)

Index

A

adaptation, 13, 18-21, 23, 25, 45f, 48-49, 54, 59, 61
Adler, A., 295
Adler, M.J., 304
Adorno, T., 345
ape and man, 29, 32-33, 71, 74
Aristotle, 63, 113, 197, 198, 204, 210
Armstrong, D., 221, 232
atheism, 5, 339-346
auditory system, 212f
Augustine, 325, 327, 330
Austin, J., 341
autokinesis, 119-120

B

Bacon, F., 113, 258
Barnes, J., 319
Becker, E., 341
behaviorism, 113-114, 197, 205, 258
Berkeley, G., 199, 200, 201, 203, 318
Bernard, C., 116
biology of consciousness, 4, 9f, 13f, 26-27
Bloomfield, L., 182
Boas, F., 181
Bohr, N., 185, 186, 194
Bosanquet, B., 324
brain, abilities of, 94, 95, 96, 97
Brain, Lord, 214
brain transplants, 107-112
Buddhism, 328, 351, 356, 358
Burch, G., 116

C

Cameron, J., 339, 340
Camus, A., 328
Cannon, 116
Carnap, R., 173, 174, 219
causality, 56, 62, 127, 184, 186, 194, 262, 311

chain of being, 296
chance, 47, 53, 55, 56, 310
Chisholm, R., 322
Chomsky, N., 183, 191, 192, 195, 300, 303
chunking procedure, 14f
conditional reflex, 116, 117, 118, 119, 120, 121, 151
consciousness, cerebral correlates, 2, 79f
cybernetics, 60, 105, 106

D

Darwin, C., 29, 30, 31, 41, 45, 184, 185, 204, 206, 295
Dawkins, R., 274, 287
death, 4-6, 73, 173f, 339f, 349f, 365
Descartes, R., 113, 115, 169, 197, 202, 243, 327
Dewey, J., 122
Dostoievski, F., 340
double aspect monism, 199, 204
drugs, effects of, 246f
dualism, 199, 208f, 298f
dualist interactionism, 199

E

Eddington, A., 271, 287
Einstein, A., 122, 288
empathy, 35-36
encephalization, 23, 30-32, 54, 68
epiphenomenalism, 199, 240, 258
eschatological view, 359
ESP, 4, 290
evolution, 1, 9f, 13f, 24f, 26-27, 41-44, 46, 73, 168, 185, 195, 267, 273, 309
existential vacuum, 295

F

Fiegl, 250, 254
final option, 355

O

organ system responsibility, 120f

P

panpsychism, 171, 239, 240, 242
Pascal, B., 340
Pavlov, 2, 104, 114, 115, 117, 119, 217
Pasteur, L., 306
Penfield, W., 149, 150, 277, 280, 367
Perrin, J., 313
person, religious view, 5, 74, 75, 317-331, 333-338
personhood and brain, 82
Piaget, J., 207, 219
Pierce, 122
Planck, M., 122, 127, 152, 222
Plato, 209, 296, 323, 325
Polanyi, M., 305, 307
Polten, E., 67, 152, 154, 245
Popper, K., 65, 67, 68, 72, 85, 97, 103, 104, 105, 150, 167, 172, 241f, 250, 298
positivist linguistics, 182f
positivism, 3, 179f, 184, 192
pragmatism, 122
prediction, 271f, 285f
Prigogene, 290, 291, 337
psychological parallelism, 199-200, 222
psi, 172
purposiveness, 45f, 57, 58, 60, 68, 284f, 344, 353

R

Rahrner, K., 350, 351, 352, 358, 360
reality, construction of brain, 17, 187f
rebirth, 352, 363f
Rostand, J., 309
Roszak, T., 257, 268
Russell, B., 192, 199, 325
Ryle, G., 221, 249, 319, 321, 327

S

Sartre, J.P., 328
Saussure, F. de, 182
schizokinesis, 118
Schlick, M., 221-223, 226-230, 231, 234, 235
Schroedinger, 127, 132, 338
science and values, 255f, 260f
self-awareness, 10-11, 33, 36f, 43, 66, 72, 81f, 191, 279, 281f, 310
Shashua, V., 142, 146
Sherrington, C., 67, 115, 123, 127, 132, 149, 168, 171, 335
Skinner, B.F., 114, 151, 152
skin stimulus, 100-101
Smart, J.J.C., 200
Sperry, R.W., 160
Spinoza, B., 240
Squires, R., 320, 326
states of consciousness, 9, 10
structuralism, 3, 4, 180f, 183, 187, 191

T

Teilhard de Chardin, 171, 359
telepathy, 172
Terwilliger, 303
Thorndike, 114
Tolstoi, 340
transcendental consciousness, 11

V

Voltaire, 345

W

Walter, G., 114
Washburn, 173
Watson, J., 114, 318
Weisskopf, 333, 334, 338
Whitehead, 192, 305, 306, 307
Wigner, E., 174, 248, 254
Wittgenstein, 320, 327, 330
women and evolution, 29-39, 41-44
world of culture, 66f, 68f
Wundt, W., 200, 226

Y

yin-yang, 209

Paragon House Publishers and the International Conference on the Unity of Sciences (ICUS) are divisions of the International Cultural Foundation, Inc. The International Cultural Foundation is an independent, non-profit organization dedicated to promoting academic, scientific, religious and cultural exchange among the countries of the world. Founded in 1972 by the Reverend Sun Myung Moon, the Foundation is now headquartered in New York with branch offices located throughout the world.

Avian Genetics
A Population and Ecological Approach

Avian Genetics
A Population and Ecological Approach

Edited by

F. Cooke and P. A. Buckley

With a Foreword by

John Maynard Smith

1987

ACADEMIC PRESS
Harcourt Brace Jovanovich, Publishers
London   Orlando   San Diego   New York   Austin
Boston   Sydney   Tokyo   Toronto

ACADEMIC PRESS INC. (LONDON) LTD.
24/28 Oval Road, London NW1 7DX

United States Edition Published by
ACADEMIC PRESS INC.
Orlando, Florida 32887

British Library Cataloguing in Publication Data

Avian genetics: a population and ecological
approach.
1. Birds—Genetics
I. Cooke, F. II. Buckley, P. A.
598.2'15   QL673

ISBN 0-12-187570-9

Typeset and printed by Galliard (Printers) Ltd, Great Yarmouth, Norfolk

Contributors

GEORGE F. BARROWCLOUGH, *Department of Ornithology, American Museum of Natural History, Central Park West at 79th Street, New York, New York 10024, USA.*

PETER T. BOAG, *Biology Department, Queen's University, Kingston, Ontario, Canada K7L 3N6.*

PAUL A. BUCKLEY, *Graduate Ecology Faculty, Center for Coastal and Environmental Studies, Rutgers University, New Brunswick, New Jersey 08903, USA.*

FRED COOKE, *Biology Department, Queen's University, Kingston, Ontario, Canada K7L 3N6.*

KENDALL W. CORBIN, *Department of Ecology and Behavioral Biology, 318 Church Street, South East, University of Minnesota, Minneapolis, Minnesota 55455, USA.*

PETER G. H. EVANS, *Edward Grey Institute, Zoology Department, Oxford University, South Parks Road, Oxford OX1 3PS, UK.*

C. SCOTT FINDLAY, *Department of Zoology, University of Toronto, Toronto, Ontario, Canada M5S 1A1.*

PAUL J. GREENWOOD, *Department of Adult and Continuing Education, University of Durham, Durham DH1 3JB, UK.*

PETER O'DONALD, *Emmanuel College, University of Cambridge, Cambridge CB2 3AP, UK.*

DAVID T. PARKIN, *Department of Genetics, University of Nottingham, University Park, Nottingham NG7 2RD, UK.*

TREVOR D. PRICE, *Department of Biology, C-016, University of California, San Diego, La Jolla, California 92093, USA.*

TOM W. QUINN, *Biology Department, Queen's University, Kingston, Ontario, Canada K7L 3N6.*

ROBERT F. ROCKWELL, *Department of Biology, The City College and The Graduate School, City University of New York, New York 10031, USA.*

GERALD F. SHIELDS, *Institute of Arctic Biology and College of Natural Sciences, University of Alaska, Fairbanks, Alaska 99701, USA.*

ARIE J. VAN NOORDWIJK, *Zoologisches Institut der Universität Basel, Rheinsprung 9, CH-4051 Basel, Switzerland.*

BRADLEY N. WHITE, *Biology Department, Queen's University, Kingston, Ontario, Canada K7L 3N6.*

v

To our Parents and our Teachers

Foreword

There was a time, not all that long ago, when the "modern synthesis" of evolutionary biology consisted, not of a synthesis of ideas from palaeontology, taxonomy, genetics and ecology, but of a synthesis based on the palaeontology of marine molluscs, the genetics of *Drosophila*, and the taxonomy and ecology of birds. Indeed, there is still more truth in such a picture than we would wish. The species of *Drosophila* that are genetically best known are virtually unknown as wild animals. Most of our quantitative knowledge of the fossil record is of marine invertebrates, or rather of shell details whose adaptive significance is usually obscure. This has had the unfortunate effect of persuading some recent theorists that Darwin's emphasis on adaptation was excessive: it is not an accident that the attack on the "adaptationist syndrome" was launched jointly by an invertebrate palaeontologist and a molecular geneticist.

As the present volume demonstrates, the birds may offer the best chance for a genuinely synthetic theory of evolution. Their ecology, demography, geographical distribution and behaviour is better known that that of any comparable animal group (although students of the flowering plants might claim that they, and not the ornithologists, have the ideal material for evolutionary studies). In recent years, studies of the genetics of wild birds have begun to correct a major gap in our knowledge of bird evolution. The House Sparrow and the Great Tit will never rival *Drosophila* or *E. coli* as tools for genetic analysis. But we are beginning to acquire the information we need as evolutionary biologists. Three main lines of approach have contributed. The first is the study of plumage polymorphism: work on the Snow Goose and the Arctic Skua illustrates how what might seem rather pedestrian information about single gene effects can be used to study more general questions, such as sexual selection, gene flow, and imprinting. Second, by combining biometrical methods with the marking of individuals and the collection of pedigree data, it is possible to study the inheritance of, and selection on, quantitative traits in natural populations. The data collected in this way on birds will never be as extensive or detailed as are the comparable data on our own species, but the bird data have the advantage, for an evolutionary biologist, of referring to species that are living in an environment not too different from that in which they evolved.

The third, and most extensive, type of information is molecular. Bird taxonomy is already being revolutionized by DNA hybridization data. In the long run, however, I think the most valuable contribution of molecular techniques will be to tell us about the genetic structure of populations, past and present. There has been considerable controversy among population geneticists about the most effective ways of investigating genetic structure. Are direct methods (e.g. measuring how far individuals move) or indirect ones (e.g. measuring the "genetic distance" between populations) the most effective? The great virtue of birds, in this context, is that both methods are possible. As ringing and molecular data become available on the same species, we shall be better able to test the theories of population genetics.

Today, I think that the greatest threat to continued progress in biological understanding lies in the increasing tendency to separate our subject into "ecology and evolution" on the one hand, and "cell and molecular" on the other. For an evolutionist, such a separation is even sillier than the old division between botany and zoology, which, happily, is beginning to disappear. A major merit of this book is that it helps to unify biology.

John Maynard Smith

Preface

In the mid-1960s, P.A.B. was approached by the publishing house Lea & Febiger about preparing a brief summary of what was then known about the genetics of wild and captive birds (excepting domesticated fowl and game birds) for a book Margaret Petrak was preparing on *Diseases of Cage and Aviary Birds*. The short chapter that resulted reflected the scanty literature at that time, much of which was anecdotal. Almost twenty years later, when the chapter was revised, it had become ninety large-format pages long, and yet still was only a review. In the course of writing that chapter, P.A.B. had extensive correspondence with F.C., and it soon become apparent that a broader-based book-length treatment of the expanding field of avian genetics was in order.

We agreed we wanted the ecological/population approach we used in our own research, and that if such a book were ever to see the light of day, a compendium of carefully refereed chapters written by invited experts was essential. A suggested outline of topics and possible authors was circulated on several continents, input was received and incorporated, and finally manuscripts solicited. Each went through at least one revision after receipt of referees' and editors' comments.

Topics in this book follow what can be considered the historical evolution of work in avian genetics, as in genetics generally, proceeding from a discussion of Mendelian (i.e. classical) genes through quantitative genetics, chromosomal genetics, biochemical genetics, to extensive treatment of population genetics, and concluding with some examples of long-term studies.

Our intended audience is ecologists, population biologists and ornithologists wanting to learn genetics techniques that are applicable to wild birds. We hope to stress what is known, but perhaps more importantly, to identify large gaps in knowledge that capable scientists, especially those with opportunity for field work, can help fill. We assume our readers have a knowledge of basic genetics, of statistical testing, and of population biology algebra and notation. Our authors have hewn well to keeping their text discursive and low on extensive mathematical modelling. Concentration has been more on intra- than on inter-specific variation; in that sense, the approach has been more genetic than evolutionary or taxonomic. However, the two areas are becoming increasingly interconnected, as several chapters make clear.

While this book was not designed as a take-into-the-field manual, or laboratory workbook, we do hope readers will get ideas for new approaches to old problems, will appreciate areas needing research attention, will understand that some very basic genetic principles remain only weakly demonstrated in birds, and will in general consider the largely heretofore unappreciated significance of the genetics of natural populations of birds in modifying what have sometimes been facile, even dogmatic, explanations of population and evolutionary phenomena. We also hope it will help lay to rest well intentioned but impermissible attempts to infer genetic control or inheritance patterns without breeding data, another trap into which too many, who otherwise know better, have fallen.

To avoid misunderstandings, prevent disappointment and remove a few arrows from reviewers' quivers, we should point out that this book is not intended to be an encyclopaedia of avian genetics knowledge, but rather an intentionally eclectic sampler emphasizing areas we feel are most important to ecological and population biologists working with wild birds. Nor is it in any way representative of the vast literature on domesticated birds: fowl, Mallards, Rock Doves, turkeys, *Coturnix*, various doves, Budgerigars, canaries, estrildids, etc. It also almost entirely omits discussion of the growing body of work on the inheritance of postural and vocal behaviour in birds, on non-Mendelian inheritance, on disease and teratological inheritance patterns and on reproductive physiology, to name but a few areas that might be covered in a hypothetical handbook. Such a volume remains to be written—but not by us.

Any success we may have achieved in putting this book together has been made possible by the high quality of the manuscripts our authors provided, as well as by their willingness to incorporate suggestions for change or clarification. Reviewers of manuscripts, and referees on our early outlines kept all concerned on a true course. Andrew Richford at Academic Press helped clear many logjams, and his professional training in genetics stood us all in good stead on many occasions. Extensive technical, editorial, illustrative and other assistance was provided by Anna Sadura and Lauraine Newell at Queen's University; heroic MS support from Patricia Eager at Rutgers University is also acknowledged. Lastly, we thank John Maynard Smith for his insightful Foreword and we are honoured he chose to recognize the efforts of all concerned by his contribution.

Kingston, Ontario, Canada   F.C.
New Brunswick, New Jersey, USA   P.A.B.

Contents

Part III   Genetic Case Histories

Part IV   Coda

Introduction

As a cohesive scientific field, avian genetics is a relatively new one, although incidental contributions were beginning to appear outside the poultry and cage/domesticated bird literature in the 1940s, and occasionally before. Generally, though, major genetic studies involving wild birds were very rare, as birds were assumed to be unfit subjects for field work because of long generation times, the difficulty of ascertaining lineages, and so forth. Indeed, it was not until the mid-1960s that it was known for certainty that sex determination was by a pair of sex chromosomes, initially called X and Y, but now usually Z and W. Most genetics texts reported correctly, from poultry work, that males were homogametic and females heterogametic, although usually as XX and XO, respectively. Cytogeneticists avoided avian chromosomes as impossibly difficult, and karyotypy in birds was all but non-existent.

That began to change in the 1960s when Rothfels *et al.* (1963) first demonstrated avian Z and W chromosomes using new staining techniques. Lowther's (1961) astonishing discovery of morphological and behavioural polymorphism in a common North American bird, White-throated Sparrow (*Zonotrichia albicollis*), was soon followed by the first important cytogenetic study of a wild bird, that of Thorneycroft (1966), also of White-throated Sparrow, where he was able to associate the morphological polymorphism with a chromosomal polymorphism. That pioneering demonstration remains unique in birds.

Not surprisingly, much early and present work on avian genetics involved plumage polymorphisms, a convenient genetic handle and a topic on which there is a substantial literature, although little of it involved birds. A conspicuous exception was Julian Huxley's 1955 summary paper describing [poly-] morphism in birds for the first time. His paper was amplified by E. B. Ford's two landmark texts on the same topic (1965 and 1975) and was tied into a conceptual framework, however much subsequently modified, by Mayr's (1963) classic, *Animal Species and Evolution.* That book was especially felicitous for the field of avian genetics: it came at the same time that avian cytogenetics was born, and Mayr was an ornithologist who used innumerable avian examples in his massive volume.

It was probably not accidental that the field of avian genetics generated momentum shortly thereafter, and that, moreover, two of the four longest-term natural population genetics studies of birds—those of Cooke and Rockwell on Snow Geese and of O'Donald (1983) on Arctic Skua—began at that time. And as graduate training increasingly recognized the importance of genetics, and the first detection of extensive biochemical variation was reported in the mid-1960s (Lewontin and Hubby 1966, Hubby and Lewontin 1966), students of avian biology began to pay attention to the genetics of wild bird populations.

In the mid-1970s the techniques of quantitative genetics, long used by fowl geneticists, began to be applied to wild birds, initially to determine simple heritabilities of various morphological traits (Garnett 1976, Boag and Grant 1978), and other components of fitness such as clutch size (Perrins and Jones 1974), and then more complex aspects of life history and fitness such as dispersal, continuously varying traits and ontogenetic–environmental interactions (Greenwood *et al.* 1978, Grant and Price 1981, van Noordwijk *et al.*, unpublished).

Also in the 1970s were made the first applications of allozyme techniques in the search for cryptic genetic variation in birds (Klitz 1973, Corbin *et al.* 1974). Research in this area mushroomed by the end of the decade, persisting unabated at present (e.g. Johnson and Zink 1985). The logical outgrowth of allozyme analyses were the DNA–DNA hybridization studies of birds pioneered by Sibley and Ahlquist (1980) and continuing to the present (Sibley and Ahlquist 1985). Actual DNA base-pair sequencing has not yet been done with wild birds, but the studies of Quinn and White (Chapter 5) using DNA restriction fragment length polymorphisms are almost to that point.

Needless to say, all the while, work was still being done on the more traditional aspects of avian genetic analysis, albeit with increasingly refined techniques, such as on chromosomal analyses (Shields 1983), and avian plumage polymorphisms (O'Donald 1983). Theoretical population geneticists such as Lande, Arnold, Templeton and others were making great strides, especially on the vexing problems of quantitative genetics, and in the last few years, their results have begun to be applied to natural bird populations, and particularly to life history variation, with exciting results (Grant 1985, Price and Grant 1985). Thus, as perusal of the Literature Cited sections of virtually all chapters in this book affirm, it was not really until the later 1970s and beyond that enough progress had been made to allow an overview of the field.

This first book-length treatment of avian genetics is divided into three long sections and one short section. To a large degree paralleling historical work, Part I considers the finding, measuring and assaying of genetic variation, proceeding from Mendelian genes through quantitative genetics, chromosomal variation, allozyme variation and DNA sequence variation, and concluding with a brief synthesis. Part II analyses the factors modifying and shaping the genetic structure of natural avian populations, including inbreeding and philopatry, selection, gene flow, non-random mating and speciation processes, also concluding with a short synthesis. Part III provides four different but complementary approaches to the unravelling of the genetics of natural populations of birds via detailed long-term studies involving marked individuals. Four organisms with different life history characteristics provide a counterpoint to the various techniques used. Species examined include: (*a*) a loosely colonially nesting, migratory, polymorphic, carnivorous seabird (Arctic Skua, *Stercorarius parasiticus*); (*b*) a densely colonially nesting, highly social, migratory, polymorphic, herbivorous waterfowl (Snow Goose, *Anser caerulescens*); (*c*) a solitary, dispersive, woodland, sexually monomorphic, temperate-zone, insectivorous passerine (Great Tit, *Parus major*); and (*d*) a social, sedentary, loosely colonially nesting, sexually dimorphic, human commensal, granivorous passerine, widely introduced around the world (House Sparrow, *Passer domesticus*). Each species presents its own opportunities and problems for genetic research; each provides instruction to the avian geneticist considering field work. The fourth and briefest part of this work treats some topics not covered elsewhere, and offers suggestions for future research directions.

Our approach has been from the start to stress that data can be obtained in the field from natural populations, with perhaps later additional laboratory analyses, in an attempt to explain the ecological or evolutionary phenomena characterizing the species under study. If we are to understand the evolution of birds, we must know their genetic architecture, and the constraints thereby placed on, or the opportunities thereby provided to, the species. We hope this volume will aid in developing that knowledge.

REFERENCES

Boag, P. T. and Grant, P. R. (1978). Heritability of external morphology in Darwin's Finches. *Nature* **274**, 793–794.

Cooke, F. and Rockwell, F., "Natural Selection in the Lesser Snow Goose". Princeton University (to be published).

Corbin, K. W., Sibley, C. G., Ferguson, A., Wilson, A. I., Brush, A. H. and Alquist, J. E. (1974). Genetic polymorphism in New Guinea starlings of the genus *Aplonis*. *Condor* **76**, 307–318.

Ford, E. B. (1965). "Genetic Polymorphism". Faber & Faber, London.

Ford, E. B. (1975). "Ecological Genetics". Chapman & Hall, London.

Garnett, M. (1976). Some aspects of body size in tits. Unpublished D.Phil. Thesis, Oxford University.

Grant, B. R. (1985). Selection on bill characters in a population of Darwin's Finches: *Geospiza conirostris* on Isla Genovesa, Galapagos. *Evolution* **39**, 523–532.

Grant, P. R. and Price, T. D. (1981). Population variation in continuously varying traits as an ecological genetics problem. *Am. Zool.* **21**, 795–811.

Greenwood, P. J., Harvey, P. H. and Perrins, C. M. (1978). Inbreeding and dispersal in the Great Tit. *Nature* **271**, 52–54.

Hubby, J. L. and Lewontin, R. C. (1966). A molecular approach to the study of genic heterozygosity in natural populations. I. The number of alleles at different loci in *Drosophila pseudoobscura*. *Genetics* **54**, 577–594.

Huxley, J. (1955). Morphism in birds. *Acta XI Int. Ornithol. Congress.*, Basel, 1954, pp. 309–322.

Johnson, N. K. and Zink, R. M. (1985). Genetic evidence for relationships among the Red-eyed, Yellow-green and Chivi Vireos. *Wilson Bull.* **97**, 421–435.

Klitz, W. J. (1973). Empirical population genetics of the North American House Sparrow. *In:* "A Symposium on the House Sparrow (*Passer domesticus*) and European Tree Sparrow (*Passer montanus*) in North America" (ed. S. C. Kendeigh). *Ornithol. Monogr.* No. 14, pp. 39–49.

Lewontin, R. C. and Hubby, J. L. (1966). A molecular approach to the study of genic heterozygosity in natural populations. II. Amount of variation and degree of heterozygosity in natural populations of *Drosophila pseudoobscura*. *Genetics* **54**, 595–609.

Lowther, J. (1961). Polymorphism in the White-throated Sparrow *Zonotrichia albicollis* (Gmelin). *Can. J. Zool.* **39**, 281–292.

Mayr, E. (1963). "Animal Species and Evolution". Belknap Press of Harvard University, Cambridge, Mass.

O'Donald, P. (1983). "The Arctic Skua: A Study of the Ecology and Evolution of a Seabird". Cambridge University Press.

Perrins, C. M. and Jones, P. J. (1974). The inheritance of clutch size in the Great Tit (*Parus major* L.). *Condor* **76**, 225–228.

Price, T. and Grant, P. (1985). The evolution of ontogeny in Darwin's Finches: a quantitative genetic approach. *Am. Natur.* **125**, 169–188.

Rothfels, K., Aspden, M. and Mollison, M. (1963). The W-chromosome of the budgerigar, *Melopsittacus undulatus*. *Chromosoma* **14**, 459–467.

Shields, G. (1983). Bird chromosomes. *In* "Current Ornithology" (ed. R. F. Johnston). Vol. I, Chap. 7, pp. 189–209. Plenum, New York.

Sibley, C. G. and Ahlquist, J. E. (1983). Phylogeny and classification of birds based on the data of DNA-DNA hybridization. *In* "Current Ornithology" (ed. R. F. Johnston). Vol. I, Chap. 9, pp. 245–292. Plenum, New York.

Sibley, C. G. and Ahlquist, J. E. (1985). Phylogeny and classification of New World suboscine passerine birds (Passeriformes: Oligomyodi: Tyrannides). *In* "Neotropical Ornithology" (eds P. A. Buckley, M. .S. Foster, E. S. Morton, R. S. Ridgely and F. G. Buckley), pp. 396–428. A.O.U. *Ornithological Monographs* No 36.

Thorneycroft, H. B. (1966). Chromosomal polymorphism in the White-throated Sparrow, *Zonotrichia albicollis* (Gmelin). *Science* **154**, 1571–1572.

van Noordwijk, A. J., van Balen, J. H. and Scharloo, W. Heritability of body size in a natural population of the Great Tit, and its relation to age and environmental conditions during growth (unpublished).

Part I

Assaying Genetic Variation

1

Mendelian Genes

P. A. Buckley

Ecology Graduate Faculty and Center for Coastal and Environmental Studies,
Doolittle Hall, Rutgers University, New Brunswick, New Jersey 08903, USA

1 INTRODUCTION

It is useful to begin any discussion of the large field of avian genetics by considering the simple single-gene effects first discerned by Gregor Mendel, and which bear his name. Even though a great deal is known about the inheritance, action and interaction of Mendelian genes, thanks to studies with Drosophila and other classical genetics subjects, surprisingly little information is available about the Mendelian genetics of wild birds.

We here distinguish between Mendelian or major genes and polygenes because even though both obey Mendelian laws of assortment and segregation, different analytical techniques are used to discern each. Major

1

genes might equally well be called "qualitative genes", for they are largely responsible for differences in *kind* between phenotypes, while polygenes (chapter 2) are responsible—acting in concert—for differences in *degree* between phenotypes.

Because discrimination of individual genes' action becomes difficult when more than two loci are involved, it is customary to use the methods of quantitative genetics at that point, dealing with genetic effects on a population level, statistically, rather than with individuals and their specific progeny. And while the notion of differences in kind versus degree is a useful one, it does not always hold. Mammals differing in, say, coat colour hue may control that hue by one or by many genes, while differences in, for example, lizard tail length (a quantitative, mensural character) and the numbers of medial dorsal scales (a semi-qualitative, meristic character) are both the kinds of characters controlled polygenically.

Most work on the inheritance of external (as opposed to biochemical) characteristics in wild birds comes from reports of natural hybridization between closely related species, augmented by captivity hydridization records, and suggests that polygenic is more common than single-gene inheritance. From an evolutionary point of view this is not surprising, since the additive genetic components of heritability (see chapter 2) are the raw material on which natural selection acts. Thus, many common Mendelian gene phenomena have rarely or never been reported in wild birds. Those that have been analysed usually involved normal and aberrant plumage, the occurrence and maintenance of plumage polymorphisms, the effects of domestication, and vocalizations. The inheritance of chromosomal and biochemical genetic variation is discussed in chapters 3 and 4, respectively. While I use examples from wild-bird populations whenever possible in order to illustrate certain genetic phenomena in birds, I occasionally must refer to the poultry and cage-bird literature. This should serve as a goad for future researchers to replace these examples with evidence of similar effects in wild birds.

Certain important topics have been excluded from discussion for considerations of space, or because they are covered far more adequately elsewhere. In these categories are gene frequency analysis (cf. Wilson and Bossert 1971; Hartl 1981; Ayala 1982), statistical testing of various genetic hypotheses (cf. Kempthorne 1957, Sokal and Rohlf 1981; Fleiss 1981) and linkage mapping (cf. Hutt 1964, or any other good recent genetics text). Likewise, relatively little mention will be made, in this chapter, of the Mendelian genetics of Lesser Snow Geese (*Anser c. caerulescens*) studied so effectively by Cooke and colleagues, or of Arctic Skua (*Stercorarius parasiticus*), analysed in detail by O'Donald and associates; they are treated in their own chapters (13 and 14).

I assume the reader has a knowledge of basic genetic principles and terminology, even though the first major part of this chapter is a refresher mini-course, with those principles and terminology applied to wild birds. The second part summarizes what is known about Mendelian inheritance patterns in wild birds, and the last part looks at actual procedures and approaches to be used, and which have been used, in analysing Mendelian inheritance in (mostly) wild birds. The chapter concludes with some recommendations for future research on the inheritance, expression and detection of Mendelian genes in wild birds.

2 PRINCIPLES AND PROCESSES

Any analysis of inheritance patterns involves breeding or pedigree data. Obvious as this may sound, these have not always been available. While one can make testable predictions about probable inheritance patterns, they can only be demonstrated by breeding tests or observations. In this section, I give a synopsis of phenomena to look for, tests to be made, and finally known effects that are capable of obscuring or confounding expected results.

2.1 Phenomena and concepts

As the characters whose inheritance is controlled by Mendelian genes are essentially qualitative (and in wild birds mostly concern plumage), the basic genetic concepts of dominance and sex-linkage are usually easily demonstrable. Thus, initial genetic analysis should rely heavily on detection of (*a*) ratios of phenotypes, (*b*) their frequency within sexes of progeny and (*c*) significant reductions in clutch or brood size—usually an indication of lethality.

2.1.1 Autosomal genes

The first step after compilation of breeding data is analysis of phenotype ratios. If F_1 progeny are all like one of the two different parental types, and F_2 progeny show both parental types in the ratio 3:1, one can assume the character is controlled by one autosomal gene pair (two alleles) showing complete dominance. If the F_1s show a phenotype intermediate between the two parental types, and the F_2s segregate into three phenotypes in the ratio 1 (first parental type):2 (similar to F_1s):1 (other parental type), then inheritance is by one autosomal gene pair (two alleles) showing no dominance. In such cases one often needs to determine whether an individual showing the dominant character is homozygous or heterozygous. This is done by crossing the unknown genotype with a known homozygous recessive (a testcross). If all progeny (with a suitably large sample size) are phenotypically dominant, the test animal was homozygous dominant; if both parental types segregate in the progeny in a 1:1 ratio, then the test animal must have been heterozygous ($AA \times aa = 100\%$ Aa; $Aa \times aa = 50\%$ Aa; 50% aa).

Even sketchy data can be used to infer likely patterns of inheritance that can later be tested with fuller, and carefully chosen data sets. For example, Johnson and Brush (1972) reported a case of plumage polymorphism in Sooty-capped Bush-Tanagers (*Chlorospingus pileatus*). Although they had casual observations on only two breeding occurrences, these few data allow a conclusion to be drawn about the inheritance of this polymorphism. The first incident involved two begging juveniles (one yellow, one grey) following two yellow adults; the second involved a mixed pair (one yellow, one grey) attending a juvenile yellow. The first case suggests that both parents were likely heterozygous (Yy) because one of each young was produced (Y- and yy), grey being recessive. The second case is consistent with this interpretation, one parent (grey) being yy, the other (yellow) being Y-, and the single yellow offspring being heterozygous (Yy). These meagre data sets do provide a testable hypothesis for future workers, namely that ventral colour in this species is controlled by a single gene, with the allele for yellow completely dominant to that for grey. We can say nothing about whether the gene might be sex-linked, as there are no data on sexes of parents or progeny.

Analysis of even apparently simple one-gene systems can nonetheless become clouded. Steiner (*in* Immelmann 1965) examined the genetics of gape-markings in hybrids between two species of estrildids, Masked Finch (*Poephila personata*) and Long-tailed Finch (*P. acuticauda*). All F_1s were reported as having Masked Finch markings (thus behaving as controlled by a dominant single gene). F_2s, on the other hand, allegedly segregated into $\frac{1}{4}$ Masked, $\frac{1}{2}$ intermediate and $\frac{1}{4}$ Long-tailed, the alleles now showing no dominance. Either data were incorrectly taken (or reported), or this is a more complex situation (one mimicking single-gene inheritance, such as threshold polygenes; see page 15). In the absence of more complete data, we can only assume the former.

If in F_2 progeny one finds many more than the three phenotypes of single-gene inheritance with no dominance, then genetic control by two pairs of independently assorting autosomal genes is next to be suspected. This is true whether the two gene pairs control one character (comb in roosters in a classic example) or two (colour and surface texture in Mendel's peas). As gametes in both egg and sperm are normally produced in equal number and assort and recombine at random with each other, in the two-gene (= dihybrid) situation the four genetic combinations (AB, Ab, aB and ab) will, when simple dominance obtains, produce phenotypes in the familiar 9:3:3:1 ratio. Genotypes, on the other hand, will be in a 1:2:1:2:4:2:1:2:1 ratio; there is no dominance, so genotypic and phenotypic ratios will be identical. Identification of the double recessive (aa bb) is usually easy: this phenotype occurs in only $\frac{1}{16}$th (about 6%) of progeny. Test-crossing a dihybrid is done exactly as with monohybrids: a suspected heterozygote (Aa Bb) is mated to a known double recessive (aa bb): only the double heterozygote will give multiple phenotypes (in this case, four) in a ratio of 1:1:1:1. If the test animal is heterozygous at only one of the two loci (Aa BB or AA Bb), then only two phenotypes will appear, still in a 1:1 ratio.

Figure 1 illustrates dihybrid inheritance of comb type in Domestic Fowl (*Gallus gallus*) roosters. In this example the two parental comb types (rose: RR pp and pea: rr PP) are each homozygous dominant at one locus and homozygous recessive at the other, but their F_1 (Rr Pp) is heterozygous at both, so the F_2 yields the familiar 9:3:3:1 phenotype ratio. The Punnett square allows calculation of the genotype ratios (1:2:1:2:4:2:1:2:1). Note that even though the two genes are controlling one character, comb type, they are assorting and segregating independently—evidence that they are on different chromosomes (i.e. unlinked) or very far apart on the same chromosome. The same procedures may be followed in the case of three or even four pairs of alleles that are assorting and segregating independently, only the ratios will differ. Table 1 indicates the expected phenotypic ratios for an F_2 trihybrid, with all genes dominant. Were one to do a trihybrid test-cross, the heterozygote would, when crossed to the homozygous recessive, yield eight phenotypes in equal number.

A tetrahybrid situation occurs in Domestic Fowl, where four independently segregating genes control feather colour, comb type (yet a different set of genes from those described earlier), elaborate facial feathering called "muffs and beard", and skin colour. Testcrossing a suspected tetra-heterozygote yielded, as expected, 16 different phenotypes in equal numbers (Hutt 1964).

A quick examination of progeny data often gives a clue as to whether characters are under Mendelian or polygenic control. If one compares variability for the character in the F_1 and F_2 generations and finds it essentially the same in both, inheritance is likely polygenic; in Mendelian inheritance the F_2 is more variable than the F_1, after segregation has occurred.

There may also be more than two alleles (as few as three, sometimes hundreds) at one locus. This is known as multiple allelism, and while common in many organisms, is rarely reported in birds at other than biochemical loci (see chapter 4). The number of alleles in a multiple allele system determines the number of genotypes available. For example, in a

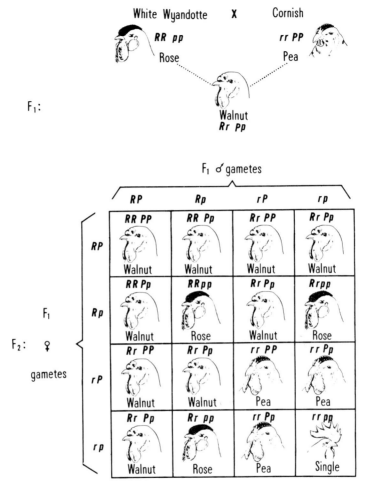

Fig. 1. Dihybrid control of rooster comb type in Domestic Fowl. Note that the F₁s are all RrPp even though the parental generation cross was not RRPP × rrpp. From "Animal Genetics" by F. B. Hutt (Ronald Press, Copyright, 1964).

hypothetical system with three co-dominant alleles, X^A, X^B and X^C (one of the conventional notation systems for multiple alleles), there would be six possible genotypes: $X^A X^A$, $X^B X^B$, $X^C X^C$, $X^A X^B$, $X^A X^C$ and $X^B X^C$, which if there were no dominance would probably mean six phenotypes as well. If one has n alleles, then $n(n + 1)/2$ genotypes are possible; of these n would be homozygous and $n(n - 1)/2$ would be heterozygous. At least two different multiple-allele series control body-wide plumage patterns in domesticated

Table 1. Phenotype ratios in a variety of non-sex-linked crosses with their likely responsible genetic bases

1:2:1	F$_2$ monohybrid, incomplete dominance
3:1	F$_2$ monohybrid, complete dominance
1:1:1:1	Dihybrid testcross
1:2:1:2:4:2:1:2:1	F$_2$ dihybrid, incomplete dominance
3:6:3:1:2:1	F$_2$ dihybrid, one of two pairs with complete dominance
9:3:3:1	F$_2$ dihybrid, both genes showing complete dominance
1:4:6:4:1	F$_2$ dihybrid, two additive genes, no dominance
3:7:5:1	F$_2$ dihybrid, two additive genes, one pair with dominance
9:3:4	F$_2$ dihybrid, recessive epistasis
9:7	F$_2$ dihybrid, epistasis, fully dominant, both dominants necessary ("duplicate recessive epistasis")
15:1	F$_2$ dihybrid, epistasis, fully dominant, either dominant ("duplicate dominant epistasis")
12:3:1	F$_2$ dihybrid, dominant epistasis, complete dominance necessary
9:6:1	F$_2$ dihybrid, additive duplicate dominance
13:3	F$_2$ dihybrid, epistatic dominance duplicate for a recessive
7:6:3	F$_2$ dihybrid, dominant epistasis, incomplete dominance
6:3:3:2:1:1	F$_2$ dihybrid, one fully dominant, other codominant
6:3:3:4	F$_2$ dihybrid, alternating dominant epistasis, incomplete dominance
7:4:3:2	F$_2$ dihybrid, partial additive interaction
11:5	F$_2$ dihybrid, alternating duplicate dominance
3:1:6:2: (4 missing)	F$_2$ dihybrid, simple dominance and lethality
1:2:1:2:4:2: (4 missing)	F$_2$ dihybrid, codominance and lethality
4:2:2:1: (7 missing)	F$_2$ dihybrid, incompletely recessive lethal
1:1:1:1:1:1:1:1	Trihybrid testcross
27:9:9:9:3:3:3:1	F$_2$ trihybrid, all three genes showing complete dominance
27:37	F$_2$ trihybrid, fully dominant, all three dominants necessary ("triplicate recessive epistasis")
81:27:27:9:27:9:9:3: 27:9:9:3:9:3:3:1	F$_2$ tetrahybrid, all four genes showing complete dominance

(and wild?) Mallards (*Anas platyrhynchos*). In the first, dark (Li) is dominant to light (li) and harlequin (li^h); in the second, restricted (M^R) and mallard (M) show no dominance to each other, but both are dominant to dusky (m^d) (Lancaster 1963). Other examples occur in Domestic Fowl (Hutt 1949), and domesticated Rock Doves (*Columba livia*) (Levi 1977).

2.1.2 Sex-linked genes

Well-known in wild and domesticated birds are genes located on sex chromosomes whose pattern of inheritance and methods of detection differ from those on autosomes. However, it is important to distinguish between sex-*influenced* (or sex-*limited*) genes and sex-*linked* genes. The former are genes on sex chromosomes or autosomes whose expression is influenced or limited by sex; an obvious example is egg size or production by female birds. Sex-linked genes are found only on Z chromosomes and their expression is therefore directly affected by the sex of the bird. Heterogametic female birds, being ZW, have only one allele for any genes located on the Z chromosome; genes there are hemizygous, so genotype and phenotype will be identical. (Only one (hemizygous) gene, for a histocompatibility function in Domestic Fowl, is believed to occur on the avian W-chromosome; see Bloom 1974 for a review.) Males have two Z chromosomes whose genes can be homozygous or heterozygous as on autosomes. It should be noted that genes affecting sexual characters are not necessarily located on sex chromosomes.

The first suggestion that a gene might be sex-linked would be the appearance of phenotypes in numbers differing from expected ratios, say the 3:1 for a dominant autosomal gene in the F_2, *and particularly if traits appear to occur in different ratios in the two sexes of progeny.* In a hypothetical example, assume reddish eye-ring is a single-gene dominant to white. A homozygous reddish-ringed male and a white-ringed female are bred, producing, as expected, all reddish-ringed progeny. When these are bred *inter se*, the F_2 appear in the expected 3:1 ratio of reddish- to white-ringed, *except* that all the males are reddish-ringed, while half the females are reddish, half white. In addition, the females breed true for their eye-ring colour, while the males appear to be of two kinds, one yielding only reddish-ringed males and females, the other producing reddish males but females equally divided between reddish and white-ringed. These results are clearly not expected under ordinary Mendelian inheritance.

They occur because if a gene is sex-linked and recessive in birds, males will express it only when they have it on both their Z chromosomes, that is, they are homozygous recessive. Hemizygous females, on the other hand, will always express every gene on their single Z chromosome. Dominance in sex-linkage can be discriminated from autosomal dominance by reciprocal-cross tests, where a male of type A is mated to a female of type B, and a male of type B to a female of type A (Figs. 2 and 3). With easily observable characters, identical F_1 progeny in both sexes from the two crosses suggest autosomal inheritance; different progeny indicate sex-linkage. If lethal sex-linked genes occur, one obtains reduced numbers of one expected phenotype in females, sometimes even no females at all. I am aware of no sex-linked

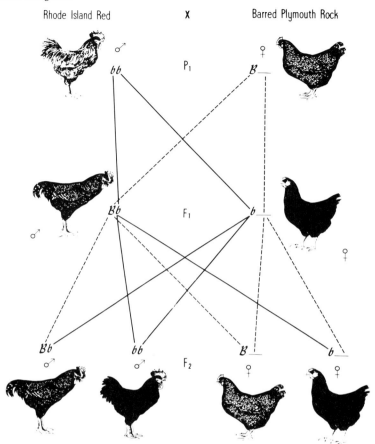

Rhode Island Red   X   Barred Plymouth Rock

Fig. 2. Sex-linked inheritance of barring in the cross Rhode Island Red male ×
Barred Plymouth Rock female. From "Animal Genetics" by F. B. Hutt (Ronald
Press, Copyright 1964).

lethals in wild birds, but they are not uncommon in inbred cage birds and
domesticated species (fowl; ducks; pigeons; Budgerigars [*Melopsittacus
undulatus*; Common Canaries [*Serinus canarius*], etc.).

Characters controlled by sex-linked recessives appear more frequently in
females, and do not appear in male progeny unless expressed by their female
parent. Traits inherited as sex-linked dominants, on the other hand, occur
more frequently in males, are not transmitted to female offspring unless the
male parent showed them, and appear in all male progeny whose female
parents exhibited them.

If a species' plumage permits easy external sexing, and a sex-linked

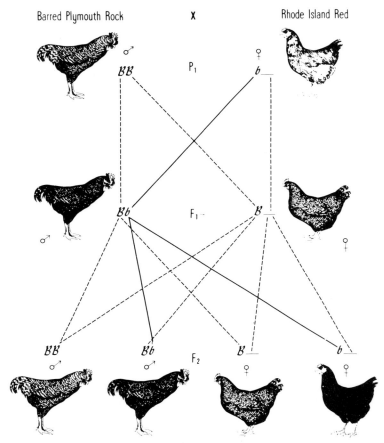

Fig. 3. Reciprocal cross to that in Fig. 2, yielding different results in both F₁ and F₂ generations. From "Animal Genetics" by F. B. Hutt (Ronald Press, Copyright 1964).

dominant is suspected, one can analyse results from a sex-linkage testcross, as Schmutz and Schmutz (1981) did with Ferruginous Hawks (*Buteo regalis*). They recorded the progeny from matings between light-phase males (presumed recessives) and dark-phase females (presumed (hemizygous) dominants), a cross which predicts only reciprocal offspring: dark males and light females, analogous to autosexing breeds of domestic birds (page 16). Finding darks and lights of both sexes, and knowing the allele for dark colour to be dominant, they rejected sex-linkage in favour of autosomal inheritance. Where in cases of suspected dominance parents are not easily sexed externally, examination of progeny sex:morph ratios is instructive, as

1:1 morph ratios effectively eliminate sex-linkage. If a sex-linked recessive is suspected, the same kind of sex-linked testcross can be made. Munro *et al.* (1968), knowing white Mute Swan (*Cygnus olor*) down colour to be recessive to grey, analysed the progeny from white (recessive) males and grey (dominant (hemizygous)) females. Finding only grey males and white females from these pairings, they accepted the sex-linked recessive hypothesis.

2.1.3 Epistasis

Yet another not uncommon genetic phenomenon the field worker might come across in dihybrid or more complex genetic situations is epistasis. It is, simply, the interference with the phenotypic expression of one pair of alleles by the presence of another pair, and may be considered a kind of dominance/recessivity relationship between loci, instead of the more usual kind, within one locus. It usually involves different genes controlling the same character, resulting in distortion of expected phenotype ratios—but fortunately in predictable patterns. Several kinds of epistatic interaction are common, and the ratios they produce in F_2 dihybrid crosses are noted in Table 1. Figure 4 indicates how the expected 9:3:3:1 F_2 ratio in a certain Domestic Fowl dihybrid cross is modified to a phenotypic ratio of 7 (pure white):6 (white with black flecking):3 (coloured), the ratio for incompletely dominant epistasis.

While few examples of epistatic interactions are known in wild birds, they are not uncommonly found in domesticated birds. A good example in a multiple-locus setting is discussed later concerning body colour inheritance in certain varieties of Japanese Quail, *Coturnix japonica* (page 34). Epistasis is known to operate in the inheritance of the complex of colour phases (morphs) on Gouldian Finch, *Poephila gouldiae* (see page 21) and Table 4 for details), and Mayr (1956) has proposed an as-yet untested genetic model involving epistasis for the inheritance of colour in Great Blue and "Great White" Herons (*Ardea herodias* and "*occidentalis*"). See page 33 for another untested model in Arctic Tern (*Sterna paradisaea*). Epistatic interactions can quickly become complex as the number of potentially interacting gene pairs increases. Table 1 lists some of the more common kinds of dihybrid epistatic ratios one might encounter, although there is no agreement on the names for all of them. The term epistasis has increasingly come to mean any intergenic interactions, including additive/complimentary genes as well as those strictly epistatic/hypostatic.

2.1.4 Linkage

In dihybrids, say Aa Bb, meiotic processes normally ensure that equal numbers of the four haploid gamete combinations (AB, Ab, aB, ab) will

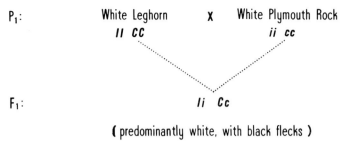

P₁: White Leghorn   X   White Plymouth Rock
              II CC   *ii cc*

F₁: *Ii Cc*

(predominantly white, with black flecks)

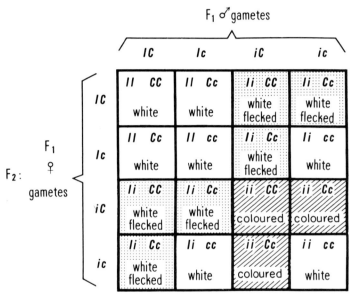

Fig. 4. Epistatic interactions producing unexpected combinations and deviations from usual dihybrid phenotype ratios when "dominant white" and "recessive white" fowl are crossed. From "Animal Genetics" by F. B. Hutt (Ronald Press, Copyright 1964).

occur. Sometimes, however, the expected proportions do not materialize, there being instead an excess of some classes and a deficiency of others. Assuming no inviability of gametes, this is usually an indication the gene pairs are occurring on the same chromosome, and thus are not assorting independently, a phenomenon called linkage. If suspected, its presence is confirmed by a testcross.

A good avian example involves Domestic Fowl white (dominant) versus coloured (recessive) plumage, and the peculiar feathering known as frizzling (dominant) versus normal (recessive). Testcrosses (data from Hutt 1949) revealed that frizzling and colour were not segregating. Of the 33 observed progeny in one such cross (Ff Ii × ff ii), instead of approximately one-quarter of each recombinant type, there were found 15 frizzled, white (Ff Ii); 12 normal, coloured (ff ii); 2 *frizzled, coloured* (Ff ii); and 4 *normal, white* (ff Ii). The latter two combinations were produced in much lower numbers than expected because F and I, and f and i, are linked alleles on the same chromosome. Linkage also occurs on sex chromosomes, where its detection is difficult. One method involves two genes (one not lethal), with crossing-over measured in the hemizygous females (cf. Cole 1961 for details).

2.1.5   Lethal genes

Sometimes one entire progeny genotype (and phenotype) class fails to appear. This is usually an indication of allelic segregation within a homozygous lethal gene. Lethals may not be uncommon, and, like most genes, can be recessive, dominant, show no dominance or even be polygenically inherited. Dominant lethals are understandably rare, being eliminated from populations quickly. One such example, included in the genetic analysis of plumage colours in Japanese Quail on page 34, is Manchurian Golden, where all dominant homozygotes die, recessives appear "wild-coloured", i.e. brown, and heterozygotes are golden-yellow (Kraszewska-Domanska and Pawluczuk 1977, Somes 1979). Some lethals are sex-linked and some autosomal. They vary in their expression, some killing before hatching, some at hatching, some for varying periods after hatching. They also vary in their penetrance, some being expressed only in males, and some not killing all carriers of the appropriate allelic combination (so-called semi-lethal, sub-lethal or subvital genes; see Somes 1979 for an example in Japanese Quail). Lethals are most easily revealed initially by deficiencies of expected classes of progeny, by abnormal sex ratios, or where detectable, by high pre-hatching mortality.

2.2   Confounding effects

Despite the array of phenomena, principles, ratios and expectations just enumerated, the real world of genetics is often not so simple. Other, fortunately well known, effects can complicate genetic analyses. Also it must be remembered that while hundreds or thousands of structural and/or major genes probably typify most avian genetic systems, avian karyotypes have a diploid range of 40–80 (chapter 3), so linkage must be the rule, not the exception. Dobzhansky (1961) expressed a view of the milieu in which genes operate, one that most geneticists would agree with: (1) probably almost every character is the product of the interaction of genes and the environments (genetic and biotic) in which their actions are expressed; (2) almost every trait is probably controlled, ultimately, by many genes; (3) many, if not most, genes have some effect on many characters; and (4) modifying genes control or change the phenotypic expression of most genes. In this section, I describe a few of these confounding effects, particularly those the field ecologist/geneticist is likely to encounter. Some are difficult or impossible to quantify or predict, others yield easily to analysis, especially mathematical manipulations. All are worth attention.

2.2.1 Penetrance and expressivity

Penetrance and expressivity are concepts often paired. Penetrance refers to the frequency with which a gene—dominant or recessive—manifests itself; expressivity denotes, once a gene or gene combination is expressed, the degree to which its expression varies. Put another way, penetrance indicates the *proportion* of the population showing the character, while expressivity notes *variation* in the character among those showing it. One good example of penetrance, coincidentally sex-limited, is the gene for cock-feathering (i.e. male-typical alternate plumage) in Domestic Fowl: it is an autosomal recessive but one that is penetrant only in recessive males. Thus all birds, male or female, and regardless of genotype (HH, Hh or hh) are hen-feathered except hh males. A good example of expressivity occurs in the "variegated" pattern in domestic canaries, where phenotypes heterozygous for a single gene (Vv) vary enormously (Fig. 5). Incomplete penetrance confuses genetic analyses. Similarly, expressivity warns against careless categorization of

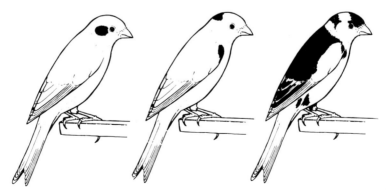

Fig. 5. The "variegated" pattern in canaries is due to the heterozygous condition of a single gene (Vv) which varies enormously in its expressivity. From "Coloured Canaries" by G. B. R. Walker (Arco, Publishing Company, Inc., New York, Copyright 1977).

phenotypes, especially when scoring in the field. It would be all too easy, in the absence of suitable testcrosses, to assume that polygenic inheritance was responsible for what could be merely monohybrid control with high expressivity (see also discussion on pp. 31 ff.).

2.2.2 Pleiotropy

Pleiotropy is the effect Dobzhansky was referring to in his third point —most genes seem to affect many characters—and is often detected by looking for characters that segregate with known single-gene effects. Pleiotropy has rarely been reported in birds, even in domesticated species. Two examples are at hand: (*a*) a melanism in Ring-necked Pheasants (*Phasianus colchicus*), controlled by an autosomal recessive, was associated with a severe neuromuscular tremor that proved to be neither lethal, nor subvital, at least under laboratory conditions. Azevedo *et al.* (1972) concluded that the mutational pleiotropic effect was likely due to inter-ference with neutral crest cells early in embryogenesis. (*b*) Murton *et al.* (1973) reasoned that melanism (again) was the pleiotropic effect of an allele in Rock Doves that alters photoperiod, hence influencing the time when pigeons carrying it will breed.

2.2.3 Threshold polygenes

Polygenic inheritance (chapter 2) normally expresses itself in continuously varying characters. However, some characters have segregation patterns that are discontinuous despite an underlying polygenic inheritance. These phenotypes can be of two kinds: all-or-nothing characteristics (presence or absence), or those falling into a relatively small number of discrete classes (say, 4 versus 5 toes). The phenomenon occurs when the genotypes have a continuity with some threshold point which imposes a discontinuity on the phenotypes: above that threshold, character state *a* appears; below it, character state *b*. Thus the terms threshold or quasi-continuous characters/ effects, and threshold polygenes are used. While I am aware of no cases even in domestic birds, the phenomenon is one that field workers should be aware of, especially because the resulting segregation ratios can mimic those of simple Mendelian characters. Dempster and Lerner (1950) and Edwards (1960) describe detection of threshold polygenes, and to my knowledge Rattray and Cooke's (1984) elimination of it as a possible explanation for the inheritance of colour in blue/white Lesser Snow Geese is its first application in avian genetic analyses, at least of wild birds.

Sewell Wright (1934) described a threshold polygene example in Guinea Pigs (*Cavia* cf. *cobaya*) that is instructive. Two strains differed in the number of toes on their hind legs: one had three (the usual number); the other four.

All F_1s were three-toed, and the F_2s were roughly in the ratio of 3:1 three-toed to four-toed, results almost everyone would accept as indicating simple dominance by the three-toed allele. Even a testcross of F_1s back to recessive homozygotes yielded equal numbers of three- and four-toed individuals. Unfortunately for this reasonable hypothesis, the presumed heterozygotes from the testcross, when mated back to the recessive homozygotes, yielded *four*-toed young and three-toed young in a 3:1 ratio—nowhere near single-gene complete dominance inheritance. Subsequent analysis revealed four genes, each with two alleles, controlling the inheritance of polydactyly in these guinea-pigs. Techniques such as probit analysis for detection and analysis of threshold effects are discussed in Falconer (1981) and Finney (1971).

2.3   Extra-chromosomal inheritance

Extra-chromosomal inheritance implies that genetic material is transmitted to progeny in some way other than by autosomes or sex chromosomes. This may be via cell organelles such as mitochondria (see chapter 5), Golgi bodies, cytoplasm, etc., or via extracellular routes ("maternal effects") such as across the mammalian placenta, or in milk; in birds this could include via egg yolk, or crop milk in pigeons and doves. At present, extra-chromosomal inheritance has been demonstrated by quantitative genetic techniques (as a maternal-effects variance component) in a number of wild birds, among them shorebirds (Väisänen *et al.* 1972), Great Tit, *Parus major* (Schifferli 1973, Ojanen *et al.* 1979, van Noordwijk *et al.* 1981, van Noordwijk 1984), Herring Gull, *Larus argentatus* (Parsons 1970), Laughing Gull, *L. atricilla* (Ricklefs *et al.* 1978) and Darwin's Finches, *Geospiza* spp. (Price and Grant 1985), as well as in Domestic Fowl and Japanese Quail. Detection of maternal effects is tedious. If not using ANOVA or ANCOVA, one looks for differences in reciprocal crosses not attributable to sex-linkage, for the absence of meiotic segregation, for character constancy after repeated backcrossing to parental types, for the failure to obtain evidence of linkage or of crossing over, or failure to map the gene relative to others, etc. For further information see Jinks (1964), Sager (1972) and Gillham (1977).

2.4   Two specialized Mendelian-gene techniques

2.4.1   Auto-sexing breeds

Taking advantage of sex-linkage, breeders of domestic birds have developed what are called auto-sexing breeds, where simple inspection of the down of newly hatched chicks or squabs consistently and unambiguously indicates the bearer's sex. As the basic principle is the same in all cases, one example suffices. Hollander (1942) discovered a sex-linked dominant gene in pigeons he called *faded*. Hemizygous dominant females (Z^F W) are light grey, as are heterozygous males ($Z^F Z^f$), whereas homozygous dominant males ($Z^F Z^F$) are white. Homozygous recessive males ($Z^f Z^f$) and hemizygous recessive females (Z^f W) are both blue. Selective breeding soon produced a strain where all males were homozygous dominant (white) and all females hemizygous dominant (light grey). From any such mating, all males resegregate as white on hatching and all females as light grey: a self-perpetuating auto-sexing strain. The same technique, sometimes with other sex-linked genes, those occasionally behaving epistatically or complimentarily, has been used to develop many other auto-sexing breeds of domestic pigeons and fowl. The auto-sexing principle is one that field workers should be aware of, as it might occur as a natural polymorphism, allowing sexing of chicks in species that are monomorphic as adults, and it would give insight into inheritance of the polymorphism.

2.4.2 Estimating the number of segregating polygenes

Although overlapping the province of quantitative genetics (chapter 2), estimation of the number of segregating polygenes giving rise to continuous variation should still be in the field worker's arsenal of analytical tools. Several techniques have been developed for this purpose, all but one relying on results from ANOVA to controlled breeding test results. Two examples will suffice.

Estimating genic variance
Inputting data on the total additive genetic variance for the F_2 generation (σ_A^2), and the genotypic difference between the two extreme phenotypes (D), one obtains n (or k; notation is variable)—the number of segregating units—via

$$n = D^2/8\sigma^2.$$

This model makes a number of assumptions, among them that the parental types are from true-breeding pure lines, that all genes contribute equally, that there is no dominance or epistasis, etc. However, as constituted it is conservative, underestimating the number of genes, but apparently not greatly, with deviations from these assumptions. It was modified by Lande (1981) for use with wild, natural populations, and he also provides means for calculating standard errors of the estimates. This general technique was used by Kovach (1980), for example, to conclude that between four and eight genes controlled Japanese Quail colour preferences when tested in an experimental apparatus.

Proportion of extreme F_2 phenotypes

A less mathematically rigorous but more field-amenable technique estimates the number of genes from the proportion of extreme phenotype classes in the F_2, even where variation is for all practical purposes continuous. A simple formula is used, namely $(\frac{1}{4})^n$, where n is the number of genes involved. One counts the actual number of individuals in *either* (but not both) of the extreme phenotype classes, calculates what fraction of the total number of observed phenotype classes *either* (but not both) extreme constitutes, and then compares the resulting fraction with various powers of $(\frac{1}{4})^n$ to determine the number of gene pairs. An avian example makes two points simultaneously. Punnett and Bailey (1914) recorded weights of roosters from two breeds of Domestic Fowl, Seabrights with a mean of about 550 g and Hamburgs with a mean of about 1300 g. F_1s ranged over 1100–1300, but F_2s from 600 to 1400 g. One individual out of the 112 progeny fell into the Seabright-type class, giving a fraction of $\frac{1}{112}$. The nearest power of $(\frac{1}{4})^n$ to $\frac{1}{112}$ is somewhere between $(\frac{1}{4})^3$, or $\frac{1}{64}$, and $(\frac{1}{4})^4$, or $\frac{1}{256}$. Thus they concluded that three to four genes were controlling weight in these breeds. But the distribution of phenotypes across classes in the F_2 was skewed greatly to the left, which led them to conclude further that dominance, at an unknown number of loci, was also involved in the inheritance of this character.

For additional discussion of these and other methods of estimating the numbers of genes controlling continuously varying characters, see Serra (1966), Mather and Jinks (1977), Spiess (1977), Falconer (1963, 1981) and Lande (1981).

3 INHERITANCE PATTERNS IN WILD BIRDS

Most data on the Mendelian inheritance of characteristics in wild birds concern plumage patterns (normal and abnormal) as well as plumage polymorphisms. There is also limited information on species-specific behaviour patterns, obtained through natural or captivity hybridization studies.

3.1 Plumage coloration

3.1.1 *Normal and abnormal pigmentation*

Avian pigments include the melanins (of the four known, blackish eumelanin and brownish phaemelanin are the most common); carotenoids (carotenes, basically red, and xanthophylls, basically yellow); and porphyrins (uncommon, but responsible for some bright greens, reds and yellows). Most avian colours are due to pairwise interactions between pigments (usually a melanin and a carotenoid) or between pigments and structural colours such as blues and whites, both produced by light scattering.

When one of the melanins is produced in abnormal amounts or replaces other pigments in areas not normally dark, the condition is known as melanism; the carotenoid equivalent is carotenism. Whole-body absence of colour is either albinism (accompanied by pinkish (pigment-free) eyes) or, far more commonly, leucism. Leucism is white plumage without pink eyes, can be partial or complete, and unlike albinism is usually bilaterally symmetrical. Less well known but quite common (and usually misidentified) is schizochroism: the absence of one of a pair of normally overlying pigments, allowing the remaining colour to dominate. It often involves eu- and phaeomelanin. When eumelanin is lost, the remaining phaeomelanin imparts a warm brown colour, producing what is known as a fawn schizochroic; loss of phaeomelanin produces a grey schizochroic. Similarly, most green colours in wild birds result from carotenoids overlying melanins. Thus, when the melanic component is lost through schizochroism, the yellow predominates, and such individuals are called lutinos (incorrectly, because lutein is not involved); when the carotenoid is lost, the feathers often appear blue when the remaining melanin is light scattered. Yet another plumage aberration is dilution, the even reduction in all pigments over the entire body. As might be imagined, correct identification of these various effects is difficult, and the literature abounds with errors. Moreover, more than one can occur in the same individual. For a fuller discussion of the terminology and occurrence of various plumage anomalies, see Buckley (1982).

How are these characteristics inherited? For many of them (melanins other than eu- and phaeomelanin; porphyrins; many carotenoids) we have no information whatsoever. Inheritance of abnormal plumage pigmentation is reasonably well known, although many of the data come from cage birds such as Zebra Finch (*Poephila guttata*), Budgerigar and Common Canary. Table 2 summarizes the distribution of inheritance patterns; although there is great diversity, some general patterns do emerge. Albinism is reasonably widespread, but I know of no example that is not fully recessive; autosomal and sex-linked versions are about equally frequent. All naturally occurring white species or morphs are leucistic, not albinistic. Leucism is probably slightly more frequently dominant than recessive, and probably more commonly autosomal than sex-linked. Melanism is more commonly dominant than recessive, and all cases I am aware of are autosomal. Curiously, melanism is apparently all but unknown in common cage birds (Canaries, Zebra Finches, Budgerigars) whose genetics have been reasonably well studied, while essentially nothing is known about the genetics of

Table 2. Incidence of various kinds of inheritance of commonly encountered plumage aberrations. Blanks indicate insufficient data or that the phenomenon has rarely been tested for; "never recorded" means consistently negative results despite search. Dilution is poorly known and often incorrectly reported

Phenomenon	Genetic control			
	Autosomal		Sex-linked	
	Dominant	Recessive	Dominant	Recessive
Melanism	×	×	Never recorded	
Leucism	×	×		×
Albinism	Never recorded	×		×
Dilution	×	×		
Schizochroisms:				
Fawn		×		×
Grey		×		
Lutino		×		×

carotenism. In domesticated birds (pigeon, Domestic Fowl, Japanese Quail) it is not uncommon to find that in various strains wholly different genotypes and inheritance control similar plumage characters such as leucism, and it is understandable that effects such as epistasis, complimentarity and multiple allelic systems are detected regularly, while they seem to be unknown or unrecognized by most cage bird breeders. Nonetheless, there is no reason to assume the genetic systems of cage birds (or of wild birds) differ in significant ways from those of domesticated species, inbreeding effects aside.

Anecdotal, non-breeding observations, especially of cage bird hybrids, give some insight into the probable differential inheritance of some plumage characteristics but not information on the mode of inheritance. For example, the carotenoid red crown of European Green Woodpecker (*Picus viridis*) is inherited apart from the rest of its plumage; the red face of *Agapornis personata lilianae* is unaffected when plumage melanins are lacking, although the maroon wing patches of Rose-ringed Parakeet (*Psittacula krameri*) become bright red in the same circumstances (a melanin-carotenoid schizochroism); the heads of melanin-carotenoid schizochroic Plum-headed Parakeets (*P. cyanicephala*) lose their plum colour, becoming pinkish-rose; the neck ring of Rose-ringed Parakeets remains in a lutino; and one kind of leucino African Grey Parrot (*Psittacus erithacus*) is all white, except for the normal scarlet tail (examples taken from Harrison 1963). These observations suggest future points for genetic analysis of plumage, and *Psittacula* seems a good genus to work with. Other curious inferences emerge from perusal of the plumage aberration literature; for example, there seem to be no cases of leucism occurring in areas normally pigmented by carotenoids, and melanism and erythrism (excessive erythromelanin, a third, chestnut-red melanin) often occur in the same individual.

Simple inheritance of plumage colour can be further compounded by the occurrence of epistatic modifiers. In Budgerigars an incompletely dominant gene called "dark inheritance" routinely alters the phenotype of most well-known colour patterns, giving no indication of linkage to any of them (Rogers 1975). In Domestic Fowl, a homozygous dominant suppresses the "frizzling" in most heterozygous frizzles, and in about 40% of homozygous dominant frizzles (Hutt 1936). In Japanese Quail, "defective feathers" is controlled by a dominant autosomal gene, lethal when homozygous, whose manifestation is permitted by a recessive epistatic gene at another locus, the combination resulting in females being more severely affected than males (Fulton *et al.* 1983).

3.1.2 Gouldian Finch plumage genetics

Doubtless the wild bird whose plumage genetics is best known is the Australian estrildid, Gouldian Finch, a naturally polymorphic species. Gouldian Finch exhibits three morphs differing largely in the colour of a conspicuous facial mask. Its genetics was first examined by Southern (1946), who determined that colour inheritance in the red-faced morph is sex-linked and dominant to that of the black-faced morph. Subsequent work by Murray (1963) extended Southern's original findings to yellow- (actually orange-) faced birds. While red and black faces are determined by alleles at the same sex-linked locus, yellow face is determined by an autosomal gene which produces its effect only when homozygous recessive and only on genetically red birds. This recessive epistasis is the only proven example, of which I am aware, of a polymorphism involving epistasis. When the double recessive yellow autosomal occurs with sex-linked recessive black the effect is yet again different: if the sex-linked black bird, which must be homozygous recessive in males or hemizygous recessive in females, bears the autosomal allele for yellow face as a homozygous dominant, the black individual will merely be black. And if the sex-linked black bird is heterozygous for yellow, it will still appear to be a normal black bird. But if the sex-linked black bird is homozygous recessive for the yellow gene, then it will still have a black face, but instead of the red-tipped bill typical of all other Gouldian finches, it will have a yellow-tipped bill. This is summarized in Table 3, which is constructed from several sources, notably Murray (1963), Immelmann (1965) and Heap (1972).

Fortunately the actual physiology and genetic control of pigmentation in the three facial colour phases is known. Völker (1964) suggested that yellow-faced homozygous recessives (yy) are unable to transform ingested yellow

Table 3. Summary of phenotypes and genotypes of the three face-colour phases of Gouldian Finch. From Buckley 1982: 73, reprinted with permission.

Males
$Z^R Z^R$ YY: Red-faced, red-tipped bill
$Z^R Z^R$ Yy: Red-faced, red-tipped bill but heterozygous for yellow face
$Z^R Z^r$ YY: Red-faced, red-tipped bill but heterozygous for black face
$Z^R Z^r$ Yy: Red-faced, red-tipped bill but heterozygous for black face and
                         yellow face
$Z^R Z^R$ yy: Yellow-faced
$Z^R Z^r$ yy: Yellow-faced, but heterozygous for black face
$Z^r Z^r$ YY: Black-faced, red-tipped bill
$Z^r Z^r$ Yy: Black-faced, red-tipped bill but heterozygous for yellow face
$Z^r Z^r$ yy: Black-faced, yellow-tipped bill

Females
Z^RW YY: Red-faced, red-tipped bill
Z^RW Yy: Red-faced, red-tipped bill but heterozygous for yellow face
Z^RW yy: Yellow-faced
Z^rW YY: Black-faced, red-tipped bill
Z^rW Yy: Black-faced, red-tipped bill but heterozygous for yellow face
Z^rW yy: Black-faced, yellow-tipped bill

R = dominant sex-linked red-face allele; r = recessive sex-linked black-face allele; Y = dominant autosomal nonyellow-face allele; y = recessive autosomal yellow-face allele; W = W-chromosome of females; Z = Z-chromosome of males and females.

carotenes into the red colour deposited either at the tip of the bill or on the feathers of the face. Thus, any individual with the yy genotype would have either a yellow face or a yellow-tipped bill, as we see in Table 3. Brush and Seifried (1968) pursued the chemical analysis further, and also looked at facial feather structure in the three morphs. They found that the feathers of the red- and yellow-faced morphs have a highly modified structure evolved presumably for the efficient display of the metabolically produced pigments. They also found that Völker was incorrect in his interpretation of the action of yy, finding rather that yy in some way suppressed the effect of the gene responsible for the red carotenoid, producing instead its own pigment, lutein epoxide, derived from lutein of body feathers, unlike the canthaxanthin of red-faces which is derived from beta-carotene. Black-faced birds totally lacked any beta-carotene in the face and presumably the mutation responsible for black face colour was one of low ability to metabolize beta-carotenes. Finally, they concluded that facial colour in Gouldian finch was under the control of several loci: one for the structures of the feathers (location/type unknown), one for the production of lutein epoxide in yellow-faced morphs (known to be autosomal), and yet a third for the production of red- and black-faced morphs (known to be sex-linked). This degree of knowledge of the inheritance and physiology of a complex colour pattern in a wild bird remains unique. It is surprising, therefore, that no studies have been done of the polymorphisms in wild populations.

3.2 Plumage polymorphisms

3.2.1 Definition

Genetic polymorphisms were brought to the attention of ornithologists by Huxley (1955), who coined the useful term "morph" for discrete plumage types unrelated to age and occurring in the same interbreeding population. The notion was developed and refined by Ford (1940, 1965, 1975), who postulated that it represented a class of variation distinct from "ordinary" inherited variation such as that produced by mutation, immigration or recombination. His definition of polymorphism—widely accepted until the demonstration of the great amount of hidden genetic variation in gene products detectable only by biochemical methods (chapter 4)—included in it the means of maintenance, namely only by heterozygote advantage, ignoring other possible mechanisms such as recurrent mutation, drift, etc. Modern genetics has abandoned Ford's definition for the objective criterion of simple occurrence at a frequency as low as 1% (chapters 4 and 10), recognizes that chromosomal polymorphisms also occur (chapter 3), and no longer places any restrictions on means of maintenance; see chapter 15 for additional discussion. Sexual dimorphism is a polymorphism, but by convention is regarded as *sui generis.*

A great deal of attention has been focused on avian plumage polymorphisms, so more than passing treatment in any avian genetics book is warranted. The colour phases (morphs) of Arctic Skua studied so extensively by O'Donald and colleagues, and the blue and white Lesser Snow Geese dissected by Cooke and colleagues, are now classic examples; they are discussed in this book in chapters 13 and 14, respectively. Notwithstanding these efforts, there has often been more heat than light generated by ornithologists about avian plumage polymorphisms; it is time for mid-course corrections.

3.2.2 Detection

Detection of plumage polymorphism is usually easy, although certain species' breeding biology, ecology or habitat requirements can complicate matters. Essentially, one must demonstrate that the variation is (*a*) discrete, not continuous; (*b*) not merely ordinary geographic, seasonal, age- or sex-related;

and (c) inherited, not ontogenetic. Clues are the occurrence of different morphs in the same brood and mixed-morph parents independent of sex. Breeding data are needed to posit testable hypotheses about the polymorphism's inheritance (dominant, recessive; autosomal, sex-linked), preferably obtained in one population and tested in another.

3.2.3 Classification

Despite overlap, several categories of external polymorphism can be distinguished in birds. Those of adult plumage are most frequently reported, and are widespread in certain taxa, notably shearwaters and gadfly petrels, herons, hawks, skuas, owls, cuckoos, muscicapids, larks, wheatears and shrikes. Polymorphisms in young birds are less well known, some examples being bill colour in geospizine fledglings (Grant *et al.* 1979) and Royal Tern (*Sterna maxima*) chicks (Buckley and Buckley 1970), as well as chick down colour in Snow (Rattray and Cooke 1984), and Ross's Geese (Cooke and Ryder 1971), and in Mute (Munro *et al.* 1968), Trumpeter (*Cygnus buccinator*) and Black (*C. atratus*) swans (Murton and Westwood 1977). Rarer still is polymorphism restricted to only one sex. Examples occur in *Cuculus* cuckoos and may be related to egg-parasitic behaviour (Voipio 1953), while three different morphs occur in male Chestnut-bellied Wattle-eyes (*Platysteira concreta*), a species in addition showing geographic variation in occurrence of morphs (Prigogine 1969).

Polymorphisms are frequently geographically distributed (e.g. in herons; see Hancock and Kushlan 1984), and are often clinal. Morph-ratio or diffusion clines have been described across wide taxonomic and geographic spectra. They are known in Common Murres (*Uria algae*) (Jefferies and Parslow 1976), Northern Fulmar (*Fulmarus glacialis*) (Fisher 1952), Lesser Snow Goose (Chapter 13), and Arctic Skua (O'Donald 1983 and Chapter 14). On a microgeographic scale, intra-island morph-ratio clines have been studied in Mascarene White-eyes (*Zosterops borbonica*) on Réunion by Gill (1973) and in Bananaquits (*Coereba flaveola*) on Grenada by Wunderle (1981).

The most complex situation yet described (Hall *et al.* 1966) involves eleven species of African *Malaconotus* shrikes which collectively exhibit probable mimicry and/or parallel evolution, geographic variation in morph-ratios, and restriction of some morphs to one sex—all intertwined.

3.2.4 Inheritance

Despite the long list of species for which various polymorphisms have been described, their genetics have seldom been ascertained. Possible genetic explanations have been advanced in many cases, but they remain, regrettably, only hypotheses awaiting testing. There are species whose morphs' inheritance is known, however. In Lesser Snow Geese, blue colour is incompletely dominant to white, the dimorphism appearing in downy chicks as well as adults (Cooke and Cooch 1968, Geramita *et al.* 1982). In closely related Ross's Goose where only chicks are dimorphic, Cooke and Ryder (1971) suggest that a modifier-suppressed expression of the blue phase in adult Ross' Geese. Recently, blue Ross' Geese have been reported in California-wintering flocks, presumably by introgression from Lesser Snow Geese through hybridization (Trauger *et al.* 1971). White down in Mute Swan chicks is a sex-linked recessive to (normal) grey (Munro *et al.* 1968). From his thorough studies of Arctic Skua morphs on Fair Isle, O'Donald (1983) suggests that light is an autosomal, incompletely dominant to dark. In some raptors, melanism is incompletely dominant to normal (light) colouration, as in Ferruginous Hawk (Schmutz and Schmutz 1981) and Eleonora's Falcon (*Falco eleonorae*) (Wink *et al.* 1978, Walter 1979), as black is to pied in New Zealand Fantails (*Rhipidura fuliginosa*) (Craig 1972). Black colour in Bananaquits is completely dominant to yellow (Wunderle 1981). On the other hand, white colour in Southern Giant Petrel (*Macronectes giganteus*) is inherited as an incompletely dominant autosomal recessive to dark colour (Shaughnessy 1970, Shaughnessy and Conroy 1977). "Ringing" or "bridling" in Common Murres is caused by an autosomal recessive allele that is apparently unknown in Pacific Ocean populations of the species, but reaches 70% in some North Atlantic colonies (Jefferies and Parslow 1976). Similar data on morph frequencies are available for Arctic Skua (O'Donald 1983) and Lesser Snow Goose (Geramita *et al.* 1982), but for almost no other species.

3.2.5 Maintenance

Theoretically, polymorphisms are only intrinsically self-perpetuating (when in Hardy–Weinberg equilibrium) in infinite populations and must otherwise be maintained by a variety of genetic mechanisms. While much theoretical genetic work has been done on this topic in recent years, convincing demonstration of what actually does maintain avian plumage polymorphism is restricted to possibly only three cases: Arctic Skua, Lesser Snow Goose and White-throated Sparrow (*Zonotrichia albicollis*). Many authors have advanced tentative explanations, often based on intuitively logical and empirical correlations between morph types and environmental variables or gradients. Nonetheless, despite many published assertions to the contrary *these remain merely testable hypotheses.* As such, though, they are fruitful grounds for future field work in the genetics of natural avian populations.

How would one test for mechanisms maintaining avian plumage polymorphisms? It is a tedious, time- and labour-intensive process that requires detailed data on gene frequencies, on mate preferences, on survival rates or reproductive success of different morphs and genotypes at different stages in the species' life cycle (arrival on breeding ground; clutch size; laying dates; hatching success; fledging success; survival over first and subsequent winters to first reproduction; morph mate-choice and where it occurs), and on measures of gene flow through the population. In certain cases, experimental cross-fostering of morphs can provide critical data. Then genetic and mathematical models can be empirically constructed, and successively eliminated, preferably tested in populations different from those wherein they were derived, if one hopes to derive globally applicable interpretations. In essence, one must quantify any differential fitnesses among morphs, and then systematically ascribe this to one best-fit model by iterative elimination. For examples of the process, cf. the only two species for which it has been done satisfactorily: Lesser Snow Goose (summarized in Geramita *et al.* 1982, and in chapter 13) and Arctic Skua (summarized in O'Donald 1983, and updated in chapter 14).

Geramita *et al.* (1982) concluded that spread of the blue morph through monomorphic white populations of Lesser Snow Goose was due to "*gene flow tempered by assortative mating based on familial colour*". Moreover, it was only when allowance was made for some 10–15% mistakes in assortative mating (known to happen at that rate) that the model fitted reality. O'Donald (1983) believed that, despite many years' work on Arctic Skua, there were still some uncertainties; nonetheless, that species' polymorphism appeared to be maintained by a combination of *sexual selection (favouring dark morphs) and natural selection (favouring lights), augmented by assortative mating and gene flow*, a complex situation. One interesting point arising from both of these studies is that none of the morphs in either species had higher overall fitnesses, notions in clear contrast to ideas of, say, twenty years ago, and to be viewed reflectively in the context of recent thinking on "selectively neutral" alleles (chapter 15).

Heterozygous advantage (heterosis) was initially envisaged (Ford 1965) as the sole means for maintaining polymorphisms. Yet, except for one not fully convincing case involving allozymes in Japanese Quail (Lucotte and Kaminski 1978), it has never been demonstrated in birds. It has, however, frequently been advocated as the mechanism of choice, rarely with even circumstantial evidence.

Assortative or disassortative mating will maintain polymorphisms, and to some degree is important in Lesser Snow Geese and Arctic Skuas, and in White-throated Sparrows (Lowther 1961, Thorneycroft 1966). This is probably also true for Eleonora's Falcon (Walther 1979) and feral Rock Doves (Murton *et al.* 1973).

Frequency-dependent selection has been proposed (apostatic selection) as important in hawk polymorphisms (Paulson 1973), in Arctic Skuas in Norway (Arnason 1978), as the means by which "predator" parasitic cuckoos are able to dump alien eggs on their "prey" host species (Payne 1967), and finally as the explanation for the complex polymorphism in African *Malacontus* shrikes (Hall *et al.* 1966). Obviously, two different interpretations of apostatic selection—multiple prey types to confuse predators and multiple predator types to confuse prey—would be involved, a fine area for future study. The only other kind of frequency-dependent selection proposed for birds is that suggested as maintaining the male-only, plumage-cum-behavioural "polymorphism" in Ruffs (*Philomachus pugnax*; see page 37).

Ecological mosaicism has been advocated more often than any other explanation for polymorphism in wild birds, and while good correlative evidence has been adduced in some cases, proof of polymorphism maintenance by these mechanisms is still lacking, attractive as this hypothesis might be. Examples of this genre include: Eastern Screech-Owl (*Otus asio*) colour phases (the ecological mosaic being cold-temperature resistance: Mosher and Henny 1976; but see Owen 1967); Common Murre bridling (cold-temperature survival of young birds in their first winter: Jefferies and Parslow 1976, Järvinen and Vepsäläinen 1973); black and pied morphs of New Zealand Fantail (differential use of vegetation habitat types: Craig 1972); white- and brown-breasted morphs of Eurasian Dipper (*Cinclus cinclus*) (forests versus steppes: Mayr and Stresemann 1950); grey and yellow morphs of Sooty-capped Bush-Tanager (crypticity in ash-covered forests after volcanic eruption: Johnson and Brush 1972); and black and yellow morphs of Bananaquits (shade-seeking preference of black morphs: Wunderle 1981).

3.2.6 Plumage-and-chromosomal polymorphism

So far unique among wild birds is the situation in the North American emberizid, White-throated Sparrow, which had the first chromosomal polymorphism reported from birds (Thorneycroft 1966, 1968, 1975) following Lowther's (1961, 1962) calling attention to the striking variation in the colour of the head stripes in this species. Previously thought by most workers to be age- or sex-related, headstriping was demonstrated by Lowther to be in fact a dimorphism, with birds clearly divisible into what he called tan-stripe (TS) and white-stripe (WS) morphs.

Thorneycroft suspected that there might be chromosomal variation which could be correlated with the headstripes, and indeed he found seven morphs involving chromosomes II and III. He was also able to demonstrate that the presence of a single chromosome type, II^m, even when heterozygous, invariably produced white headstripes in alternate (= breeding) plumage. The remaining six alleles did not appear to result in unique alternate plumages, but were hypothesized to affect expression of basic (= winter) plumages, at least in females.

Subsequent studies have revealed that (a) the presence of chromosome II^m is undetectable when birds are in basic (= winter) plumage (Vardy 1971); (b) the range of variation, overlapping both morphs, was greater in winter, presumably promoting flock cohesion (Atkinson and Ralph 1980); (c) the polymorphism is maintained by disassortative mating (WS birds of either sex usually pair with TS birds of the opposite sex: Lowther 1961, Thorneycroft 1966); (d) there are no consistent differences between the two main pair types (WS male × TS female; TS male × WS female) in success rates of nests, number of young fledged per nest, or growth rate and weight at fledging (Knapton, Cartar and Falls, in preparation); (e) there were differences in parental contribution among pair types, explained by different optimal strategies between morphs (Knapton and Falls 1983); (f) there were differences in choice of breeding territory habitat, with WS male × TS female pairs occupying a narrower range than the reciprocal cross (Knapton and Falls 1982); (g) there were morphometric differences between morphs, TSs having shorter legs, longer tails, longer, narrower bills and smaller sizes than WSs (Rising and Shields 1980); (h) WSs were aggressors significantly more often than expected by chance, irrespective of the recipient's type, the size of the group or the morphic composition of the group (Ficken et al. 1978). As all, and only, WSs possess the II^m chromosome, the authors concluded that the increased aggression was due to II^m, the first such case of simple control of aggressive levels in a bird; (i) morph types are apparently not related to certain physiological differences such as body weight, lipid deposits, molt, cloacal protuberances or Zugunruhe (Kuenzel and Helms 1974). Additional work on this most extraordinary avian example of a combined chromosomal and plumage polymorphism will surely shed important light on the maintenance and ramifications of polymorphisms.

In summary, even the most basic aspect of most avian polymorphisms—their genetics—remains to be demonstrated, and with a handful of exceptions, suggestions as to the means of maintaining those polymorphisms are premature. If we can extrapolate from Lesser Snow Geese, Arctic Skuas and White-throated Sparrows, polymorphism maintenance will prove to (a) be not simple; (b) reflect balances among mutation, migration and selection; (c) be tied strongly to gene flow patterns; (d) possibly not be globally applicable; and (e) perhaps be unrelated to traditional notions of natural selection.

3.3 Inheritance of behavioural traits

Some work has been done on the inheritance of behaviour in birds (e.g. Dilger 1962 a,b, Buckley 1969) and reviews are available in Buckley (1982), and particularly in Baptista (1981). Most studies have found behavioural differences to be inherited polygenically, but a few intimations of simple Mendelian inheritance have been found.

Among estrildids, Zebra Finches apparently never use their feet to hold down food items, while African Silverbills (*Eudice cantans*) usually do. Four hybrids between these species regularly manipulated grass seedling heads with their feet, suggesting inheritance of a simple dominant (see Baptista and Matsui, in Baptista 1981). Also in the Estrildidae, two tribes (grass finches: Poephilae, and mannikins: Lonchurae) are apparently distinguished by begging calls: bisyllabic in grass finches and monosyllabic in mannikins (Güttinger and Nicolai 1973, Zann 1975). Sonagrams of a hybrid *Spermestes* (grass finch) × *Lonchura* (mannikin) show only bisyllabic begging calls, again indicating inheritance of a simple dominant. Also in estrildids, a display known as Peering occurs (Immelmann 1965). In a number of crosses between species normally performing Peering and those not (including *Euodice*, *Lonchura* and *Poephila*), Peering was always performed by F_1 hybrids (see Baptista and Matsui, in Baptista 1981). Lastly, in a complex study of the male courtship behaviour of five species of doves, Davies (1970) found that in the Bow-coo display, hybrid males behaved as one parental species during that phase of the display when the head is held low, and as the other parental species during that phase when the head is held high. This finding suggests a simple genetic control of two separate components within the same display, and parallels similar results from detailed analyses of the complex courtship displays of waterfowl (cf. von de Wall 1963, Kaltenhäuser 1971).

3.4 Genetic effects of domestication

Predictably, domestication has selected for many traits not normally found in wild birds, often because they severely reduce fitness. Sossinka (1982) summarized his on-going studies on Zebra Finch, finding that while most characters are polygenically inherited, some—especially colour varieties— are inherited in simple Mendelian fashion. Various kinds of leucism, dilution, schizochroism and even albinism occur routinely, and the typical "wild-type", captivity-bred Zebra Finch itself is greyish, not brown as are wild individuals. Many similar plumage changes have been wrought in Canaries by domestication, the wild-type birds being rather ordinary, unadorned, greenish-yellow, streaked carduelines.

Extended inbreeding (chapter 6) leads to allelic fixation in various strains;

Table 4. Lethal mutants from Domestic Fowl:
D = dominants; S = sex-linked. From "Animal
Genetics" by F. B. Hutt (Roland Press, Copyright
1964)

	Domestic fowl	Symbol
D	Creeper	Cp
	Chondrodystrophy	ch
D	Cornish lethal, short limbs	Cl
	Amaxilla	mx
	Missing mandible	md
	Wingless, lungless syndrome	wg
	Diplopodia	dp
	Diplopodia 2	dp-2
	Splitfoot	sf
	Micromelia	—
	Short upper beak (semi-lethal)	sm
D	Apterylosis (semi-lethal)	Ap
S	Naked (semi-lethal)	n
	Dwarfism (thyrogenous)	td
	Stickiness	sy
	Talpid	t
	Talpid 2	t-2
	Congenital loco	lo
	Lethal with recessive white	l
	Crooked-neck dwarf	cn
	Blindness (semi-lethal)	—
	Congenital tremor	—
	Bilateral microphthalmia	mi
	Short mandible	sm
D	Atresia of oviduct	—
	Short neck, and beak	—
	Donald Duck (beaks curled)	dck
S	Sex-linked lethal	xl
S	Shaker	sh
S	Jittery	j
S	Paroxysm	px

cf. the situation described in Japanese Quail (page 34). It also allows the accumulation of different genes, on different chromosomes, that produce the same phenotypic effect. In Domestic Fowl at least four loci are known for leucism (Hutt 1949), and Lancaster (1963) detected four whiteness gene systems in domesticated Mallards: recessive, dominant, epistatic and albinistic. The array of lethals that has collected in Domestic Fowl (Hutt 1964; Table 4) would have been largely eliminated in a wild bird by natural selection; note that four are even dominant, as is Manchurian Golden colour in Japanese Quail (page 34). The detailed breeding regimens feasible with domestic species allow genetic analyses that are exceedingly difficult to perform in the wild, and have uncovered information of use to the avian geneticist in the field. For example, Lancaster (1963) examined the genetics of blue and brown "dilutions" (probably grey and fawn schizochroism, respectively) in waterfowl, finding the effect in both Mallards and Muscovies (*Cairina moschata*), but at completely different loci.

4 PERFORMING MENDELIAN GENETIC ANALYSES

4.1 Procedures

In their assay of the genetics of bridling in Common Murres, Jefferies and Parslow (1976) make three universal points relevant to any genetic analyses, namely, that they can only be done by (1) ringing and subsequent recovery in the field of young of known parentage; (2) breeding in captivity; or (3) rearing in captivity wild-born young of known parentage. In most field studies some approximation of the first technique is often the best one can hope for. Only in rare cases can one hope to have colour-marked individuals of known parentage spanning several generations, and even those cases are dependent on significant philopatry or sedentariness. Thus the average single-season field worker must rely on obtaining data, in many cases, covering only two generations. However, this apparent debility can be turned to advantage by careful assessment of large amounts of data (a good reason for choosing colonially breeding species).

Initially, consideration must be given to careful experimental design of the genetic and statistical requirements of the study. Once in the field, obtain as large a sample size as possible, spread across types according to design. Particularly careful attention should be paid to taking accurate parent–progeny data relative to numbers of both sexes, and especially to the phenotypes under study, splitting categories as finely as possible in the field. Whenever possible, record as many phenotypic characteristics of each individual. Remember that characters which appear at first sight to be discontinuous may be continuous when examined in closer detail. Even where it seems clear that characters are qualitative and apparently segregating as such, if at all possible, record data quantitatively as well, as if the characters were under polygenic control. That way, both reclassification of qualitative characters, as well as ANOVA testing for polygenic inheritance, can be done on the same set of data. During analysis, pay close attention to reductions in absolute sizes of any expected phenotypes, and to presence of expected segregation ratios, as well as deviation from them, especially when data are cast by sex of progeny. Be suspicious of unique, anomalous data points or outliers, and temporarily cast them aside during analysis: they may be genuinely spurious. Pool data when appropriate. In the actual genetic analysis, start with the simplest hypothesis, that of single-gene control. First, try to determine the dominance/recessivity relationship. Second, look for sex-linkage. Once the single-gene, autosomal/sex-linked explanation proves inadequate consider first multiple alleles, then threshold polygenes. If those test results are still inconclusive, and analysis of phenotype ratios is indicative, try two-gene and epistatic explanations. Remember to consider non-genetical explanations for anomalies, and be aware of such biological phenomena as extra-pair copulations, egg-dumping, polyandry, nest helpers and so forth.

After an apparent explanation for observed inheritance patterns has been worked out, alternative hypotheses need to be systematically eliminated in order to arrive at a final explanation that is both *sufficient and unique*. Optimally, this explanation should then be tested against field data in a population different from that used to derive the explanation. Only in this way will a globally valid explanation be achieved. Probably the best approach to this technique was used by Rattray and Cooke (1984) to validate the previous explanation (Cooke and Cooch 1968) of a single-gene two-locus model with incomplete dominance for morph colour in Lesser Snow Geese. Rattray and Cooke carefully tested that model, as well as a multi-allelic system, and a threshold polygenic system, against a variety of data sets, confirming the first and conclusively eliminating the second and third, in a paper that should serve as an example for these kinds of analyses.

When the analysis is complete, publication should include as much original data (in usable summary form), so that subsequent investigators can rework the original data, testing them against other hypotheses, or asking new questions of them. And always, it is instructive to remember Sewell Wright's (1934) analysis of polydactyly in guinea-pigs, lest it seem too easy.

4.2   Sample analyses

Examination of a few examples of actual genetic analyses (some more successful than others) is useful to impart the kinds of thinking and approaches that have been used, and to include a few cases more complex than I have so far considered.

Common Murre. Building on a good literature base on the bridling morph-ratio, Jefferies and Parslow (1976) worked with birds of known phenotype hand-reared in the laboratory, on the assumption (suggested by others) that bridling was an autosomal recessive. Their first conclusion was that co-dominance was unlikely owing to the rarity of intermediates (birds with

Table 5. Crossing protocol used to determine genetic control of bridling in Common Murres, based on the hypothesis that bridling is controlled by a single autosomal recessive; this example is peculiar in that different letters are used for the recessive (b) and for the dominant (N) alleles. From *J. Zool., Lond.* **179**, 411–420 (The Zoological Society of London, Copyright 1976)

Mating	Parents		Offspring	
	Genotype	Phenotype	Genotype	Phenotype
1	NN·NN	Normal·Normal	NN	Normal
2	bb·bb	Bridle·Bridle	bb	Bridle
3	NN·bb	Normal·Bridle	Nb	Normal
4	Nb·Nb	Normal·Normal	$\frac{1}{4}$NN·$\frac{1}{2}$Nb·$\frac{1}{4}$bb	$\frac{3}{4}$Normal·$\frac{1}{4}$Bridle
5	Nb·NN	Normal·Normal	$\frac{1}{2}$NN−$\frac{1}{2}$Nb	Normal
6	Nb·bb	Normal·Bridle	$\frac{1}{2}$bb−$\frac{1}{2}$Nb	$\frac{1}{2}$Bridle−$\frac{1}{2}$Normal

bridling on one side of the head and not on the other). As both males and females are bridled, they eliminated both hologynic and sex-limited inheritance, and owing to apparently equal numbers of bridled males and females, sex-linkage was an inadequate explanation. Finally, all six predictions in an autosomal recessive-based crossing protocol were realized (Table 5), ruling out everything but multiple alleles. This possibility they excluded on the grounds that the scant evidence of intermediates (explainable in ontogenetic ways) rendered a multiple allelic system highly improbable. (See chapter 8 for an analysis of selection coefficients in these birds.)

Ross' Goose. Cooke and Ryder (1971) used a different approach to analysis of inheritance of chick down colour in this species. Assuming the population to be in Hardy–Weinberg equilibrium, they calculated gene frequencies from four areas, ascertained they were not significantly different and pooled them. They then calculated expected frequencies of different morph mixtures in broods of sizes 1–5, and compared observed morph frequencies by brood size with those expected under the grey-dominant and yellow-dominant hypotheses, rejecting the latter decisively. Next, they made similar predictions for morph frequencies for females only, under three regimes: no sex-linkage, sex-linked grey dominant and sex-linked yellow dominant, firmly rejecting both sex-linked models but not the autosomal. Thus they concluded both that grey colour is determined by a completely dominant autosomal allele, and that mating between (monomorphic) adults is random relative to their natal down colour.

Arctic Tern. Lemmetyinen *et al.* (1974) considered chick colour "poly-morphism" in relation to substrate. They categorized chicks generally as brown or grey, following earlier authors, but then, subdividing, recognized four categories: pure brown, or with light mottling (B); predominantly brown with clear grey mottling (GB); predominantly grey with clear brown mottling (BG); and pure grey, or with very slight brown mottling (G). In two widely separated locations in Finland, they recorded frequencies of the four classes for 5–7 years in succession. To these data they fitted the following genetic model. Two gene pairs (A and B) determine chick colour: A, type of colour, and B, its distribution. They are unlinked, each with two alleles showing simple dominance. A- produces brown, aa grey colour; B- produces uniform colour, bb mottling. A is epistatic to bb. Thus, the four phenotypes would be genotypically:

Phenotype	B	GB	BG	G
Genotype	A- B-	A- bb	aa bb	aa B-

Then, assuming Hardy–Weinberg equilibrium, expected frequencies were calculated for each phenotype and compared with those observed. Thirteen of the sixteen matches were perfect, and in two cases there was a slight difference. In the remaining instance, a highly significant difference was explained as possibly due to misclassification. The authors concluded that the data confirmed their model. Aside from the fact that there was no examination of parent–offspring data (they readily admitted none were available), and that the fit of observed to expected results was extraordinarily good, a cautionary note is in order. Chaniot (1970) examined Caspian Tern (*Sterna caspia*) chicks for "polymorphism", as did Buckley and Buckley (1970) for Royal Terns. Both papers reported that apparently discontinuous variation was in fact continuous across several plumage variables, and was even greater when soft parts were included. Non-genetic analysis of Royal Tern character variation suggested polygenic control of several different components of chick body part/plumage colour. Similar variation (i.e. essentially continuous) characterizes Least (*S. antillarum*), Common (*S. hirundo*) and Roseate (*S. dougallii*) terns (pers. obs.), so one must wonder about the sharpness of class boundaries in the Arctic Tern chicks. Still, the good fit of the model lends support to the authors' interpretation. At any rate, this is another kind of genetic analysis, although one that properly only provides a solid hypothesis for subsequent field testing by known parent and young morph types.

Japanese Quail. Somes (1979) performed a series of crosses offering good insight into the process of genetic analysis, and even though he used domesticated birds, all crosses involved only F_1s or backcrosses—not out of line with opportunities available to the field investigator. He started with five varieties (Pharaoh (wild type), Manchurian Golden, British Range, English White and Tuxedo), and through a series of crosses was able to dissect their

Table 6. Results of five-way test breeding in Japanese Quail to determine inheritance of plumage patterns. From *J. Heredity* **70**, 206 210 by R. G. Somes (reproduced by kind permission of the publisher, Copyright 1979)

(a) Segregations from crosses between British Range (BR) and wild-type (WT) quail

Cross	Progeny phenotypes			χ^2	Ratio
	Brown	Shafted	Wild type		
BR × BR	All (all)[a]			0·00	All
BR × WT		All (all)		0·00	All
F₁ × BR	123 (112)	101 (112)		2·16	1:1
F₁ × WT		93 (87)	81 (87)	0·82	1:1
F₁ × F₁	45 (48·8)	102 (97·5)	48 (48·8)	0·51	1:2:1

[a] Expected numbers in parentheses.

(b) Segregations from crosses between English White (EW) and wild-type (WT) quail

Cross	Progeny phenotypes						χ^2	Ratio
	White	Shafted-tuxedo[a]	Wild type	Shafted	Tuxedo	Brown		
EW × EW	All (all)[b]						0·00	All
EW × WT		All (all)					0·00	All
F₁ × EW	32 (32)	16 (16)			16 (16)		0·00	2:1:1
F₁ × WT		116 (110·5)	197 (221)	129 (110·5)			5·98	1:2:1
F₁ × F₁	37 (32·3)	28 (32·3)	22 (24·2)	18 (16·1)	16 (16·1)	8 (8·1)	1·83	4:4:3:2:2:1

[a] The F₁ phenotype for these crosses.
[b] Expected numbers in parentheses.

Table 6—*contd.*

(c) Segregations from crosses between English White (EW), Tuxedo (TUX) and British Range (BR) quail

Cross	Progeny phenotypes			χ^2	Ratio
	Brown	Tuxedo	White		
TUX × TUX	65 (69·8)[a]	143 (139·5)	71 (69·8)	0·43	1:2:1
BR × EW		All (all)		0·00	All
TUX × BR	41 (44)	47 (44)		1·64	1:1
TUX × EW		46 (47)	48 (47)	0·04	1:1

[a] Expected numbers in parentheses.

(d) Segregations from crosses between Manchurian Golden (MG) and wild-type (WT) quail

Cross	Progeny phenotypes				χ^2	Ratio
	Yellow	Shafted	Wild type	Shafted-tuxedo		
MG × MG	133 (134)[a]		68 (67)		0·02	2:1
MG × WT	35 (33·5)		32 (33·5)		0·13	1:1
MG × BR		All (all)			0·00	All
MG × EW				All (all)	0·00	All

[a] Expected numbers in parentheses.

(e) Summary of colour genetics of five Japanese quail varieties

Variety	Gene	Symbol	Inheritance	Genotype
British Range	Brown extension	E	Autosomal incomplete dominant	E/E, Wh^+/Wh^+, y^+/y^+
English White	Recessive white	wh	Autosomal recessive	E/E, wh/wh, y^+/y^+
Manchurian Golden	Yellow	Y	Autosomal dominant	e^+/e^+, Wh^+/Wh^+, Y/y^+
Tuxedo	—	—	—	E/E, Wh^+/wh, y^+/y^+
Pharaoh (wild type)	—	—	—	e^+/e^+, Wh^+/Wh^+, y^+/y^+

rather complex genetics. When each of the five varieties was mated *inter se*, three breeds (Pharaoh (WT), British Range (BR) and English White (EW)) bred true, suggesting homozygosity, while Manchurian Golden (MG) and Tuxedo (TUX) segregated for several colour patterns, so were presumed heterozygous. Then, the four non-wild types were reciprocally crossed with wild type, in a (negative) test for sex-linkage.

The complex results are shown in Table 6. Table 6 (*a*) indicates that a single incompletely dominant gene (E) separated BR and WT, heterozygotes manifesting a condition known as "shafting" of ventral feathers. Table 6 (*b*) is more complex, revealing that EWs were homozygous for E, and for another gene epistatic to E causing white colour (wh). This was recessive as shown in the backcross to the wild type (half of the progeny would have been wild-type Tuxedo if it had been dominant). Table 6 (*c*) (crosses among EW, TUX and BR) shows that the TUX genotype must be EE Wh wh, and due to EE modification by wh heterozygosity. Table 6 (*d*) compares MG and WT, clarifying that the MG autosomal dominant (Y) was a homozygous lethal, and that colour genes in BR and EW were epistatic to it. Table 6 (*e*) summarizes the results of this detailed analysis; note that the TUX pattern is due to the complimentarity between EE and Wh wh (in heterozygous condition only), and that Pharaoh-type Japanese Quail are homozygous recessive for two of the three genes controlling these plumage characteristics.

4.3   Suggested research topics

Perusal of the growing literature on avian genetics reveals topics and examples where interesting work could be done on the genetics of major genes in wild birds.

Amassing basic genetic information for wild birds. The inheritance of carotenoids, of erythromelanin, of other than the two common schizochroisms, and of most dilutions, is unknown. The occurrence and incidence of epistasis and complimentarity are all but unknown in wild birds, and despite material presented in this chapter we still know little about the patterns of inheritance of plumages in wild birds, beyond that most are apparently inherited polygenically; even the evidence for that is inferential and anecdotal.

Polymorphism genetics. Unknown for most species, but particularly for the extraordinary situation in the *Malaconotus* shrikes (Hall *et al.* 1966), and in Ruff, a Eurasian shorebird where the males are highly variable and perform courtship on leks. Two males types, with white and with coloured heads, have been described as constituting a plumage dimorphism "linked" with a behavioural dimorphism (Hogan-Warburg 1966, van Rhijn 1973) but in fact nothing is known about plumage or behaviour inheritance in this unique shorebird.

Polygenic or threshold polygenic inheritance. Two cases well described in the literature are felt by their authors to be puzzling because certain genetic anomalies remained unexplained by their models. Baker (1973) reported essentially continuous variation in the Variable Oystercatcher (*Haematopus unicolor*) as controlled by a single gene. Birds' plumage when homozygous recessive is all black, pied when homozygous dominant, and variably intermediate when heterozygous. Smith (1969) suggested that foot-webbing in Semipalmated and Ringed Plovers (*Charadrius hiaticula* and *semipalmatus*) in a zone of sympatry in the Canadian Arctic was controlled by a single completely dominant gene. Unexpected segregation in two kinds of crossings suggest that a more complex control might be operating. In both these cases, reassessment, possibly assuming continuous variation and using quantitative genetics techniques, and especially consideration of threshold effects, is warranted.

Variability in assortative mating patterns. Suggestions that assortative mating is not geographically constant have been made for Eleonora's Falcon (Walter 1979) and Arctic Skua (Arnason 1978). This is a phenomenon as yet undemonstrated in wild birds, and if true, theoretical analysis of its effects on polymorphism maintenance is mandated.

Geographic variability in polymorphism, and its possible polygenic control. The strange situation in Eastern Screech-Owl, reddish in the northern and extreme southern parts of its range but grey in between, and described as having only two (red and grey) or up to six colour morphs controlled by a single gene, red dominant to grey (Hrubant 1955, Owen 1967), seems no closer to resolution today than 30 years ago.

Cuckoo gentes. Nothing whatever is known about the genetics of these "female races" of apparently host- and egg-specific Common (and other?) Cuckoos, and although hologynic inheritance has been suggested, it is not even known if heritable differences are involved.

Industrial melanism. Reported anecdotally in House Sparrows (*Passer domesticus*) in the British Isles (Hardy 1937, Rollin 1964), the phenomenon has not been documented, nor (if it occurs) are there any data on possible modes of inheritance.

"Artificial polymorphism". Feral polymorphic populations of Budgerigar, a normally monomorphic species in Australia, have become established in Florida and California. The species' genetics is reasonably well known from

captivity work, and it is also known that strong assortative mating occurs, based on colour of nest-mate siblings. This has been hypothesized as preventing the spread of alleles caused by the occasional non-green birds in Australia (Stamm and Blum 1971). The behavioural, ecological and genetic phenomena apparently permitting (?) polymorphism in the US population are worth study.

Modelling polymorphisms, morpho-ratio clines and gene flow. Once data are available, modelling population genetics and structure as have been done for Lesser Snow Geese and Arctic Skua must be extended to other species for detection of patterns and evolutionary significance. New data such as obtained by Wunderle (1981) for Bananaquits need to be applied to species like Mascarene White-eye (Gill 1973) once we have hard numbers on effective population sizes and dispersal distances. Only then will we be able to bridge the gaps between major genes and the evolutionary ecology of wild birds.

REFERENCES

Arnason, E. (1978). Apostatic selection and kleptoparasitism in the Parasitic Jaeger. *Auk* **95**, 377–381.

Atkinson, C. T. and Ralph, C. J. (1980). Acquisition of plumage polymorphism in White-throated Sparrows. *Auk* **97**, 245–252.

Ayala, F. (1982). "Population and Evolutionary Genetics: A Primer". Benjamin/Cummings, Menlo Park, California.

Azevedo, J., Hunt, E. and Woods, L. (1972). Melanistic mutant in Ringneck Pheasants. *Calif. Fish Game* **58**, 175–178.

Baker, A. J. (1973). Genetics of plumage variability in the Variable Oystercatcher (*Haematopus unicolor*). *Notornis* **20**, 330–345.

Baptista, L. (1981). Behaviour genetics studies with birds. *In* "Proc. First Int. Birds in Captivity Symposium, Seattle 1978" (eds A. Risser, L. Baptista, S. Wylie and N. Gale). Dvtl. Intl. Found. for Conserv. of Birds, Holywood, Calif., pp. 217–249.

Bloom, S. E. (1974). Current knowledge about the avian W chromosome. *Bioscience* **24**, 340–344.

Brush, A. H. and Seifried, H. (1968). Pigmentation and feather structure in genetic variants of Gouldian Finch, *Poephila gouldiae*. *Auk* **85**, 416–430.

Buckley, P. A. (1969). Disruption of species-typical behavior patterns in F_1 hybrid *Agapornis* parrots. *Z. Tierpsych.* **26**, 737–743.

Buckley, P. A. (1982). Avian genetics. *In* "Diseases of Cage and Aviary Birds", (ed. M. Petrak) 2nd edn, Chapter 4, pp. 21–110. Lea & Febiger, Philadelphia.

Buckley, P. A. and Buckley, F. G. (1970). Color variation in the soft parts and down of Royal Tern chicks. *Auk* **87**, 1–13.

Chaniot, G. (1970). Notes on color variation in downy Caspian Terns. *Condor* **72**, 460–465.

Cole, R. K. (1961). Paroxysm—sex-linked lethal of the fowl. *J. Heredity* **52**, 46–52.

Cooke, F. and Cooch, F. G. (1968). The genetics of polymorphism in the Snow Goose *Anser caerulescens*. *Evolution* **22**, 289–300.

Cooke, F. and Ryder, J. P. (1971). The genetics of polymorphism in the Ross' Goose (*Anser rossii*). *Evolution* **25**, 483–490.

Craig, J. L. (1972). Investigation of the mechanism maintaining polymorphism in the New Zealand Fantail, *Rhipidura fuliginosa*. *Notornis* **19**, 42–55.

Davies, S. J. J. F. (1970). Patterns of inheritance in the bowing display and associated behavior of some hybrid *Streptopelia* doves. *Behaviour* **36**, 187–214.

Dempster, E. R. and Lerner, I. M. (1950). Heritability of threshold characters. *Genetics* **35**, 212–236.

Dilger, W. C. (1962a). The behavior of lovebirds. *Scient. Am.* **206**, 88–98.

Dilger, W. C. (1962b). Behavior and Genetics. *In* "The Roots of Behavior". (ed. E. L. Bliss), pp. 35–77. Hoeber, New York.

Dobzhansky, T. (1961). Adaptation in Man and Animals. A synthesis. *In* "Genetic Perspectives in Disease Resistance and Susceptibility" (ed. R. H. Osborne). *Ann. N.Y. Acad. Sci.* **91**, 598–818.

Edwards, J. (1960). The simulation of mendelism. *Acta Genetica* **10**, 63–70.

Falconer, D. S. (1963). *In* "Methodology in Mammalian Genetics". (ed. W. Burdette), pp. 193 ff. Holden-Day, San Francisco.

Falconer, D. S. (1981). "Introduction to Quantitative Genetics", 2nd edn. Longmans, London.

Ficken, R., Ficken, M. and Hailman, J. (1978). Differential aggression in genetically different morphs of the White-throated Sparrow (*Zonotrichia albicollis*). *Z. Tierpsych.* **46**, 43–57.

Finney, D. J. (1971). "Probit Analysis". 3rd edn. Cambridge University Press, London.

Fisher, J. (1952). "The Fulmar". New Naturalist Series. Collins, London.

Fleiss, J. (1981). "Statistical Methods for Rates and Proportions." 2nd edn. Wiley, New York.

Ford, E. B. (1940). Polymorphism and taxonomy. *In* "The New Systematics" (ed. J. Huxley), pp. 493–513, Clarendon Press, Oxford.

Ford, E. B. (1965). "Genetic Polymorphism". Faber & Faber, London.

Ford, E. B. (1975). "Ecological Genetics", 4th edn. Chapman & Hall, London.

Fulton, J., Juriloff, D., Cheng, K. and Nichols, C. (1983). Defective feathers in Japanese Quail. *J. Heredity* **74**, 184–188.

Geramita, J. M., Cooke, F. and Rockwell, R. F. (1982). Assortative mating and gene flow in the Lesser Snow Goose: a modelling approach. *Theor. Pop. Biol.* **22**, 177–203.

Gill, F. B. (1973). Intra-island variation in the Mascarene White-eye, *Zosterops borbonica*. *Ornithological Monographs* **12**, 1–66.

Gillham, N. (1977). "Organelle Heredity". Raven Press, New York.

Grant, P. R., Boag, P. T. and Schluter, D. (1979). A bill color polymorphism in young Darwin's Finches. *Auk* **96**, 800–802.

Güttinger, H. and Nicolai, J. (1973). Struktur und Funktion der Rufe bei Praktfinken (Estrildidae). *Z. Tierpsych.* **33**, 319–334.

Hall, B. P., Moreau, R. E. and Galbraith, I. C. J. (1966). Polymorphism and parallelism in the African Bush-shrikes of the genus *Malaconotus* (including *Chlorophoneus*). *Ibis* **108**, 161–181.

Hancock, J. and Kushlan, J. (1984). "The Herons Handbook". Harper & Row, New York.

Hardy, E. (1937). Polluted wild life. *Country Life* **81**, 676.

Harrison, C. J. O. (1963). Non-melanic, carotenistic and allied variant plumages in birds. *Bull. Br. Orn. Club* **83**, 90–96.

Hartl, D. (1981). "A Primer of Population Genetics". Sinauer, Sunderland, Mass.

Heap, N. (1972). "Gouldian Finch Genetics & Colour Expectations". Australian Finch socoety, Bristol, England.

Hogan-Warburg, J. A. (1966). Social behavior of the Ruff, *Philomachus pugnax* (L.). *Ardea* **54**, 109–229.

Hollander, W. F. (1942). An auto-sexing breed in pigeons. *J. Heredity* **33**, 135–140.

Hrubant, H. (1955). An analysis of the color phases of the Eastern Screech Owl, *Otus asio*, by the gene frequency method. *Am. Natur.* **89**, 223–230.

Hutt, F. B. (1936). Genetics of the fowl: V. The modified frizzle. *J. Genetics* **32**, 277–285.

Hutt, F. B. (1949). "Genetics of the Fowl". McGraw-Hill, New York.

Hutt, F. B. (1964). "Animal Genetics". Ronald, New York.

Huxley, J. (1955). Morphism in birds. *Acta 6th Int. Ornith. Congress, Basel 1954*, pp. 309–322.

Immelmann, K. (1965). "Australian Finches in Bush and Aviary". Angus & Robertson, Sydney.

Järvinen, O. and Vepsäläinen, K. (1973). Intensity of selection in Bridled Guillemots (*Uria aalge*) on Bear Island. *Astarte* **6**, 35–41.

Jeffries, D. J. and Parslow, J. L. F. (1976). The genetics of bridling in guillemots from a study of hand-reared birds. *J. Zool., Lond.* **179**, 411–420.

Jinks, J. L. (1964). "Extrachromosomal Inheritance". Prentice-Hall, Englewood Cliffs, N.J.

Johnson, N. K. and Brush, A. H. (1972). Analysis of polymorphism in the Sooty-capped Bush Tanager. *Systematic Zool.* **21**, 245–262.

Kaltenhäuser, D. (1971). Über Evolutionsvorgänge in der Schwimmentenbalz. *Z. Tierpsych.* **20**, 349–367.

Kempthorne, O. (1957). "An Introduction to Genetic Statistics". Wiley, New York.

Knapton, R. W. and Falls, J. B. (1982). Polymorphism in the White-throated Sparrow: habitat occupancy and nest-site selection. *Can. J. Zool.* **60**, 452–459.

Knapton, R. W. and Falls, J. B. (1983). Differences in parental contribution among pair types in the polymorphic White-throated Sparrow. *Ibid.* **61**, 1288–1292.

Kovach, J. K. (1980). Mendelian units of inheritance control color preferences in quail chicks (*Coturnix coturnix japonica*). *Science* **207**, 549–551.

Kraszewska-Domanska, B. and Pawluczuk, B. (1977). The gene of golden plumage color linked with lower fertility in Mangurian (*sic*) golden quail. *Theor. Appl. Genet.* **51**, 19–20.

Kuenzel, W. J. and Helms, C. W. (1974). An annual cycle study of tan-striped and white-striped White-throated Sparrows. *Auk* **91**, 44–53.

Lancaster, F. M. (1963). The inheritance of plumage color in the common [= Mallard] duck (*Anas platyrhynchos*). *Bibliographica genetica* **29**, 317–404.

Lande, R. (1981). The minimum number of genes contributing to quantitative variation between and within populations. *Genetics* **99**, 541–553.

Lemmetyinen, R., Portin, P. and Vuolanto, S. (1971). Polymorphism in relation to the substrate in chicks of *Sterna paradisea*. *Ann. Zool. Fenn.* **11**, 265–270.

Levi, W. M. (1977). "The Pigeon", 3rd ed. Levi, Sumter, S.C.

Lowther, J. (1961). Polymorphism in the White-throated Sparrow *Zonotrichia albicollis* (Gmelin). *Can. J. Zool.* **39**, 281–292.

Lowther, J. (1962). Colour and behavioural polymorphism in the White-throated Sparrow, *Zonotrichia albicollis* (Gmelin). Ph.D. Thesis, University of Toronto, Toronto.

Lucotte, G. and Kaminski, M. (1978). Biochemical homeostasis of the heterozygote at the lysozyme locus in Japanese Quail. *Biochem. System.* **6**, 145–147.

Mather, K. and Jinks, J. L. (1977). "Introduction to Biometrical Genetics". Cornell University Press, Ithaca.

Mayr, E. (1956). Is the Great White Heron a good species? *Auk* **73**, 71–77.

Mayr, E. and Stresemann, E. (1950). Polymorphism in the chat genus *Oenanthe* (Aves). *Evolution* **4**, 291–300.

Mosher, J. A. and Henny, C. J. (1976). Thermal adaptiveness of plumage color in Screech Owls. *Auk* **93**, 614–619.

Munro, R. E., Smith, L. T. and Kupa, J. J. (1968). The genetic basis of color differences observed in the Mute Swan (*Cygnus olor*). *Auk* **85**, 504–505.

Murray, R. (1963). The genetics of the yellow-masked Gouldian Finch. *Avic. Mag.* **69**, 108–113.

Murton, R. K. and Westwood, N. J. (1977). "Avian Breeding Cycles". Clarendon Press, Oxford.

Murton, R., Westwood, N. and Thearle, R. J. (1973). Polymorphism and the evolution of a continuous breeding season in the pigeon *Columba livia. J. Reprod. Fert. Suppl.* **19**, 563–577.

O'Donald, P. (1983). "The Arctic Skua: A Study of the Ecology and Evolution of a Seabird". Cambridge University Press, Cambridge.

Ojanen, M., Orell, M. and Väisänen, R. A. (1979). Role of heredity in egg size variation in the great tit *Parus major* and the pied flycatcher *Ficedula hypoleuca. Ornis Scand.* **10**, 22–28.

Owen, D. (1967). Polymorphism in the Screech Owl in eastern North America. *Wilson Bull.* **75**, 183–190.

Parsons, J. (1970). Relationship between egg size and post hatching chick mortality in the herring gull (*Larus argentatus*). *Nature* **218**, 1221–1222.

Paulson, D. (1973). Predator polymorphism and apostatic selection. *Evolution* **27**, 269–277.

Payne, R. B. (1967). Interspecific communication signals in parasitic birds. *Am. Natur.* **101**, 363–375.

Price, T. and Grant, P. (1985). The evolution of ontogeny in Darwin's Finches: a quantitative genetic approach. *Am. Natur.* **125**, 169–188.

Prigogine, A. (1969). Polymorphism of the Chestnut-bellied Wattle-eye *Dyaphorophyia concreta. Ibis* **11**, 95–97.

Punnett, R. C. and Bailey, P. G. (1914). The inheritance of weight and poultry. *J. Genetics* **4**, 23–39.

Rattray, B. and Cooke, F. (1984). Genetic modelling: an analysis of a colour polymorphism in the Snow Goose. *Zool. J. Linn. Soc.* **80**, 437–445.

Ricklefs, R. E., Hahn, D. C. and Montevecchi, W. A. (1978). The relationship between egg size and chick size in the Laughing Gull and Japanese Quail. *Auk* **95**, 135–144.

Rising, J. and Shields, G. (1980). Chromosomal and morphological correlates in two New World sparrows (Emberizidae). *Evolution* **34**, 654–662.

Rogers, C. H. (1975). "Encyclopedia of Cage and Aviary Birds". Macmillan, New York.

Rollin, N. (1964). Non-hereditary and hereditary abnormal plumage. *Bird Res.* **2**, 1–44.

Sager, R. (1972). "Cytoplasmic Genes and Organelles". Academic Press, New York.

Schifferli, L. (1973). The effect of egg weight on the subsequent growth of nestling Great Tits *Parus major. Ibis* **115**, 549–558.

Schmutz, S. M. and Schmutz, J. K. (1981). Inheritance of color phases of Ferruginous Hawks. *Condor* **83**, 187–189.

Serra, J. A. (1966). "Modern Genetics", Vol. 2. Academic Press, New York.

Shaughnessy, P. D. (1970). The genetics of plumage phase dimorphism of the Southern Giant Petrel *Macronectes giganteus. Heredity* **25**, 501–506.

Shaughnessy, P. D. and Conroy, J. W. H. (1977). Further data on the inheritance of plumage phases of the Southern Giant Petrel *Macronectes giganteus. Br. Antarct. Surv. Bull.* No. 49, pp. 25–28.

Smith, N. G. (1969). Polymorphism in Ringed Plovers. *Ibis* **111**, 177–188.

Sokal, R. R. and Rohlf, F. J. (1981). "Biometry", 2nd ed. Freeman & Co., San Francisco.

Somes, R. G. (1979). Genetic bases for plumage color patterns in four varieties of Japanese Quail. *J. Heredity* **70**, 205–210.

Sossinka, R. (1982). Domestication in birds. *In* "Avian Biology" (eds D. Farner, J. King and K. Parkes). Vol. 6. Chapter 7, pp. 373–403. Academic Press, New York.

Southern, H. N. (1946). Polymorphism in *Poephila gouldiae* Gould. *J. Genetics* **47**, 51–57.

Spiess. E. (1977). "Genes in Populations". Wiley, New York.

Stamm, R. A. and Blum, U. (1971). Partnerwahl beim Wellensittich: die Faktor Körperfarbe (*Melopsittacus undulatus* [Shaw]; Aves, Psittacidae). *Rev. Suisse Zool.* **78**, 671–679.

Thorneycroft, H. B. (1966). Chromosomal polymorphism in the White-throated Sparrow, *Zonotrichia albicollis* (Gmelin). *Science* **154**, 1571–1572.

Thorneycroft, H. B. (1968). A cytogenetic study of the White-throated Sparrow, *Zonotrichia albicollis* (Gmelin). Ph.D. Thesis, University of Toronto.

Thorneycroft, H. B. (1975). A cytogenetic study of the White-throated Sparrow, *Zonotrichia albicollis* (Gmelin). *Evolution* **29**, 611–621.

Trauger, D., Dzubin, A. and Ryder, R. (1971). White geese intermediate between Ross' Geese and Lesser Snow Geese. *Auk* **88**, 856–875.

Väisänen, R., Hildén, O., Soikkeli, M. and Vouolanto, S. (1972). Egg dimension variation in five wader species: the role of heredity. *Ornis Fennica* **49**, 25–44.

van Noordwijk, A. J. (1984). Quantitative genetics in natural populations of birds illustrated with examples from the great tit, *Parus major. In* "Population Biology and Evolution" (eds K. Wohrmann and V. Loschcke), pp. 67–79. Springer-Verlag, New York.

van Noordwijk, A. J., Keizer, L. C. P., van Balen, J. H. and Scharloo, W. (1981). Genetic variation in egg dimensions in natural populations of the great tit. *Genetica* **55**, 221–232.

van Rhijn, J. G. (1973). Behavioural dimorphism in male Ruffs, *Philomachus pugnax* (L.). *Behaviour* **47**, 153–229.

Vardy, L. (1971). Color variation in the crown of the White-throated Sparrow, *Zonotrichia albicollis* (Gmelin). *Condor* **73**, 401–404.

Voipio, P. (1953). The *hepaticus* variety and the juvenile plumage types of the cuckoo. *Ornis Fenn.* 30, 97–117.

Völker, O. (1964). Die gelben Mutanten des Rotbauchwürgers (*Laniarius atrococcineus*) und der Gouldamadine (*Chloebia gouldiae*) in biochemischer Sicht. *J. Ornithol.* **105**, 186–189.

von de Wall, W. (1963). Bewegungsstudien an Anatiden. *J. Ornithol.* **104**, 1–43.

Walker, G. B. R. (1977). "Colored Canaries". Arco, New York.

Walter, H. (1979). "Eleonora's Falcon: Adaptation to Prey and Habitat in a Social Raptor". University of Chicago Press, Chicago.

Wilson, E. and Bossert, W. (1971). "A Primer of Population Biology". Sinauer, Stamford, Conn.

Wink, M., Wink, C. and Ristow, D. (1978). Biologie des Eleonorenfalken (*Falco eleonorae*): 2. Zur Vererbung der Gefiderphasen (hell-dunkel). *J. Ornithol.* **119**, 421–428.

Wright, S. (1934). The results of crosses between inbred strains of guinea pigs, differing in number of digits. *Genetics* **19**, 537–551.

Wunderle, J. (1981). An analysis of a morpho-ratio cline in the Bananaquit (*Coereba flaveola*) on Grenada, West Indies. *Evolution* **35**, 333–344.

Zann, R. (1975). Inter- and intraspecific variation in the calls of three species of Grassfinches of the subgenus *Poephila* (Gould) (Estrildidae). *Z. Tierpsych.* **39**, 85–125.

2

Quantitative Genetics

Peter T. Boag

Department of Biology, Queen's University, Kingston, Ontario, Canada K7L 3N6

and Arie J. van Noordwijk †

Department of Population and Evolutionary Biology, University of Utrecht, P.O. Box 80.005, 3508 TB Utrecht, The Netherlands

1 INTRODUCTION

The previous chapter emphasized avian phenotypic characters with a relatively simple genetic basis. By simple, we mean it has been possible to relate discrete phenotypes to genotypes on a more or less one-to-one basis. Such Mendelian characters form the basis of the rich theory of population genetics and dominate the literature on genetic variation. However, there are relatively few Mendelian polymorphisms in birds with obvious adaptive significance. Indeed, variation in most of the avian characters of traditional

† Present address: Zoologisches Institut der Universität Basel, Rheinsprung 9, CH-4051 Basel, Switzerland.

AVIAN GENETICS
ISBN 0-12-187570-9

evolutionary interest (e.g. clutch and beak size, migratory and courtship behaviour) does not have a simple genetic basis. Instead, most avian phenotypic variation is the sum of many different genes acting in concert, whose joint expression is further blurred by environmental variation introduced during development and growth. In this chapter we turn to the study of quantitative genetics, or of traits which display metric or continuous variation.

Our discussion is organized as follows. First, we introduce the basic statistical model used by quantitative geneticists to simulate the behaviour of genetic systems too complex for a locus by locus, allele by allele approach. Depending on the reader's background, this necessarily abbreviated section should be complemented by reading either an introductory textbook on the subject (e.g. Ayala 1982) or the excellent textbook on quantitative genetics by Falconer (1981). Next, we show how these techniques have been applied to natural populations of birds, reviewing repeatability and heritability data available for avian morphology, as well as for reproductive characters such as egg size, clutch size and laying date. Lastly, we underline some of the difficulties of the approach, discussing topics such as non-genetic resemblance, correlated characters, genotype–environment interactions, and the general question of how faithfully current models of polygenic inheritance reflect biological reality.

2 QUANTITATIVE GENETICS: AN EMPIRICAL APPROACH TO INHERITANCE

In many ways quantitative genetics is like a toolbox; it makes use of empirically derived experimental plans and statistical tools to deal with genetical problems that would be difficult to tackle otherwise. Words like "toolbox" and "plan" connote a "cookbook" approach to science. Whether this is true in a given application of quantitative genetics depends very much on the problem at hand. In theory, it is easy to connect most of the abstract statistical constructs used in quantitative genetics with real entities at lower levels, such as individual genes. However, in practice this is almost always impossible, and is not attempted. The onus falls on the individual researcher to decide what is the "domain of applicability" of these techniques in his or her study population.

2.1 Continuous phenotypic variation

It is not difficult to imagine genetic systems which might give rise to the type of continuously distributed phenotypic variation we associate with polygenic

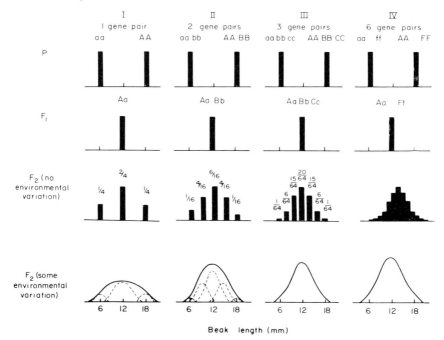

Fig. 1. Results of hypothetical crosses between two inbred lines of birds, differing at 1, 2, 3 or 6 loci controlling beak size. The parental generation (P) mates randomly, producing in turn an F_1 and F_2 generation. The bottom row shows the effect of adding environmental variation to the expression of the F_2 genotypes (see text). From "Population and Evolutionary Genetics: A Primer" by F. J. Ayala (Benjamin/Cummings Publishing Company, Copyright 1982).

inheritance. Figure 1 illustrates the progression from the phenotypic distribution displayed by two alleles at a single locus to that displayed by a continuously varying genetic trait such as bill size. In the case where variation (such as that in the plumage colour of Snow Goose (*Anser caerulescens*) see chapter 13) is controlled by two alleles at a single locus with incomplete dominance, three phenotypic classes are expected. Homozygotes are either blue or white, while heterozygotes display "blending inheritance", and turn out to be a mixture of blue and white.

If the expression of each genotype were blurred slightly by a random variation in the amount of pigment laid down during development (e.g., as a function of variations in incubation temperature), each genotype might produce a family of phenotypes distributed around some average genotype-specific value. Depending on the magnitude of the environmental variation, the resulting phenotypic distribution would lose the discreteness typical of single-locus genetics. If one adds additional loci, there are more genotypic classes to consider in the F_2, and if each produced a family of environmentally induced variants, it would be difficult to distinguish the resulting distribution from that of a trait such as bill size. The key concept is that a quantitative genetic trait involves two or more loci, at least some of which display incomplete dominance and environmentally sensitive phenotypic expression.

2.2   Shared genes are reflected in similar phenotypes

The statistical model used to summarize the type of phenotypic variation described above is by no means a recent invention; it was first produced by Galton (1889) and then extended by Fisher (1918). The key observation made by Galton was that relatives tended to resemble each other in a predictable fashion; for instance there existed a close, linear relationship between the stature of human parents and their children (Galton 1889; summarized by Roughgarden 1979, p. 135). It was assumed that the phenotypic value (P) of a trait (such as the length of a bird's bill in millimetres) was the sum of a predictable genotypic value (G), owing to the particular combination of genes possessed by an individual and some unpredictable deviation (E) from that value, caused primarily by random environmental influences acting during development. The concept of genotypic value is of limited use, because parents pass on genes, not genotypes, to their offspring. Thus the idea of *breeding value* (A) was introduced; an empirical measure of the tendency for parents to produce offspring with a mean phenotypic value similar to their own because of the genes they share.

When genes from two parents unite to form a new diploid genotype in a zygote, recombination may produce novel combinations of alleles at individual loci which affect the offspring phenotype in ways not seen in either parent; such genetic effects on the phenotype are not transmitted from parent to offspring and are referred to as the *dominance deviation* (D) of the offspring's genotypic value from its parent's breeding value. In the same way that interactions between alleles at a given locus can cause genotypic values to differ from breeding values, offspring phenotypes may be influenced by interactions between loci. This effect, again not transmitted from parent to offspring, is the *epistatic* or *interaction deviation* (I) of the offspring genotype from the breeding value. To sum up, the genotypic value of an offspring is $G = A + D + I$, where only A is inherited directly from the parents. As we shall see later, it is this breeding value (A) which determines the degree to which the phenotypes of offspring forming a new generation resemble the group of adults which natural selection chose to be their parents in the previous generation, i.e. the degree to which selection results in evolutionary change.

Unlike the physical presence of electromorph bands on a gel or summary statistics such as the observed heterozygosity of individuals (h_i; see Corbin 1983), there is no obvious way to assess either the genotypic or breeding value of an individual with respect to one or more polygenic traits. Values of G and E could be calculated for a population of genetically identical birds, generated by either inbreeding or cloning, but such populations under natural conditions are rare, to say the least. Hence one of the first devices in the toolbox of quantitative genetics is to focus on the phenotypic *variation* of characters within and between strategically selected samples of relatives. This approach has a number of significant consequences. By definition we express the phenotypic variance as the sum of several components (see equation (1) below). We use the methods of analysis of variance (ANOVA; see Sokal and Rohlf 1981) to estimate the magnitudes of these components, and hence must meet the statistical assumptions called for by ANOVA. Two important assumptions are that the components are derived from normal distributions and are additive. When these assumptions are violated, the data may have to be transformed, for instance by taking the cube root of characters such as weight, and using logarithms to make typically log-normally distributed morphological characters more normal. Or, when a component shows signs of non-additivity, we must define a new, additive variance component that comprises the non-additive parts of the old component.

Thus the simple model of an individual's phenotypic value described above can be made operational by rewriting it in terms of variance components. We define the total phenotypic variation in a population as being the sum of at least the following components:

$$V_P = V_A + V_D + V_I + V_E \tag{1}$$

Here V_P is the total phenotypic variance, V_A the additive genetic variance (or the variance of breeding values), V_D the non-additive genetic variance due to interactions within loci (dominance), V_I the non-additive genetic variance resulting from interactions between loci (epistasis) and V_E the environmental variance. As we shall see later in our discussion of genotype–environment interactions, the V_E component may sometimes include non-additive variance which must be allocated to additional components such as V_{GE}.

Having defined the model, the next step is to make it useful by indicating how the components can be measured. One must keep in mind that apart from V_P, these components are *totally artificial* and can be estimated only by indirect, statistical means. They are usually measured as differences in variances or covariances between groups of individuals of known genetic relatedness. It is also important to remember that even when these components have been measured, it will not always be possible to attach unambiguous interpretations to the results. The model described above and the specific techniques presented below all make assumptions; for instance that parents mate at random, that non-genetic causes of resemblance between relatives are not important, and that the V_E component is truly independent of the V_A component. Often, the utility of the quantitative genetic approach depends to a large extent on one's ingenuity in meeting such assumptions. Later in this chapter we return to this topic to see how well quantitative genetic studies of wild bird populations have fared.

2.3 Repeatability, heritability and artificial selection

2.3.1 Partitioning V_P. repeatability

The quantity and quality of data required to fully partition the phenotypic variation in an avian population into its causal components are often formidable; in many cases, impossible to obtain. However, one simple way to determine whether a full, pedigree-based quantitative genetic analysis will be profitable is to carry out a repeatability analysis. This technique uses repeated measurements of a character from the same individual, separated in space or time, to assess the magnitude of environmental variation resulting from measurement error or other temporary changes in character value between measurement periods. To understand repeatability fully, it is useful to think of the total environmental variance component (V_E) as being composed in turn of two subcomponents. These are V_{Es}, the special environmental variance, which includes the "within-individual variance arising from temporary or localized circumstances" (Falconer 1981). An example of this would be variation of the weight of successive eggs in a bird's clutch caused by a combination of measurement error and the hen's nutritional state on the day the egg was formed. The other subcomponent is V_{Eg}, or the general environmental variance, which Falconer (1981) again defines as the between-individual variance "arising from permanent or non-localized circumstances". The corresponding example here would be permanent, non-genetic differences between females in the average size of egg produced, caused perhaps by a physiological relic of nutritional conditions when they themselves were reared, such as an increased oviduct weight which in Starling (*Sturnus vulgaris*) leads to larger eggs (Ricklefs 1977). Ignoring the subcomponents of the genotypic variance (V_G), we can write $V_P = V_G + V_{Eg} + V_{Es}$. The formal definition of repeatability is $r = (V_G + V_{Eg})/V_P$, which measures the fraction of the phenotypic variance in a character resulting from "permanent, or nonlocalized, differences between individuals, both genetic and environmental" (Falconer 1981). The results of several repeatability analyses are given in Tables 1 and 2, and will be described in more detail later when we turn to the data from natural populations of birds.

In most cases, ANOVA is used to partition the total phenotypic variation in a group of organisms, each measured twice or more, into between- and within-individual variance components; the between-component divided by the sum of the within- and between-component estimates the intraclass correlation, which is equal to the repeatability (Sokal and Rohlf 1981). Given the formula for r shown above, one can see that in some situations, repeatability values can be used to set an upper limit to the ratio V_G/V_P or V_A/V_P, which as we shall see below refer to the coefficient of genetic determination and the heritability, respectively. They are also useful in determining how many times an individual should be measured to provide a reliable estimate of the "parametric value" of its phenotype (Falconer 1981). Obviously if repeatability values are low and temporary environmental variation alone explains most of the total phenotypic variation (i.e. the between-individual variation is negligible). there is little chance that more sophisticated analyses will turn up a significant genetic component to the variation.

Such a negative result might mean the end of the contemplated quantitative genetic investigation, but more often it leads one to examine the possible sources of environmental variation in more detail. If the variation is due primarily to measurement error, the character definition can often be altered slightly or the measurement technique improved. Sometimes idiosyncrasies in measurements made by different instruments or researchers have to be corrected. Often it may be possible to eliminate systematic sources of variation due to age or seasonal effects by reducing the data to homogeneous subsets, or by use of analysis of covariance. But some thought must be given to such manipulations in order to avoid biasing the outcome of a subsequent genetic analysis. For instance, when there is annual variation in the expression of a trait, this difference will always be present in the comparison of phenotypic values of the same individual, but will only partly contribute to the variance between individuals. This can produce negative repeatabilities in the absence of genetic variation or repeatabilities that are lower than a heritability based on parent–offspring regression.

The reverse can happen also. If, for example, there is sexual dimorphism in a metric trait, repeatabilities for seasonal variation in say wing length calculated over both sexes will be high because the between-individual variance component will be boosted by the dimorphism while the within-individual component remains more or less unaffected. In the case of a trait whose expression changes systematically within individuals (e.g. age-related clutch size changes), one alternative to statistical removal of the age effect is the redefinition of clutch size as two or more age-specific traits that are genetically correlated (Falconer 1981).

These are essentially questions of statistical design, and rapidly extend beyond the scope of this review. However there is one very important, general question one must answer in deciding how best to partition or adjust one's data set so as to minimize "extraneous" environmental variation. Assuming one wants to estimate the amount of additive genetic variance (V_A) in a population so as to predict how a trait will respond to selection, it is crucial to try to understand what state the environment and the population are likely to be in when the anticipated selective event occurs. In other words, how is selection going to "see" the phenotypic variation it will have to sift through, compared to how the researcher has measured it at some other time? Will selection act on variation within a single sex or across the sexes? Across several age classes or primarily within a single age class, perhaps in a single season? Will it consistently favour certain phenotypic rankings year in, year out, or will most of the selection occur as differentials seen between phenotypes only in good year–bad year contrasts? A complete answer to this question obviously demands an intimate understanding of the natural history of one's study species, so that at each stage of the life cycle the major correlates of fitness and the population composition are documented. There are few bird populations which have been studied thoroughly enough to allow us to partition a life cycle into its relevant stages, during each of which a given character may experience a distinct selective regime and display different levels of heritability (Arnold and Wade 1984 a,b, van Noordwijk *et al.* 1985, Price and Grant 1985).

2.3.2   Heritability

Like repeatability analysis, the estimation of heritabilities is based on phenotypic correlations among several measurements of homologous characters. However, in the former case the measurements were from a single individual, so it could be assumed that the repeatability reflected the extent to which largely post-developmental environmental variation contributed to phenotypic variation, with genotype held constant. Heritability analysis uses multiple measurements from different individuals of known genetic relatedness, so one can measure the effect of shared genes on phenotypic similarity.

In the case of sexually reproducing species (i.e. all known birds), every individual receives half of its genetic material from each parent, with the exception of genes on the sex chromosome, which we will ignore for the sake of simplicity. For the same reason we ignore mutation and individual fitness differences (i.e. number of offspring reaching reproductive age). Because

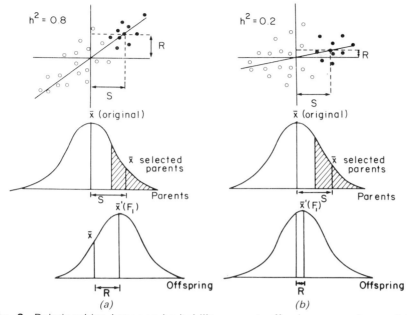

Fig. 2. Relationships between heritability, parent–offspring regression and the response to selection for a hypothetical avian body size trait. In (*a*) heritability is 0·8, while in (*b*) it is 0·2. *S* is the selection differential when the largest 25% of the parents are chosen to breed, while *R* is the predicted response in their offspring's generation.

offspring share half their genes with each parent, the midparent value of a trait (i.e. the mean of the parental values) is expected to equal the offspring value or mean value of all offspring, if the phenotypic variation reflects underlying additive genetic variation. If there is a significant environmental component to the phenotypic variation, the offspring value will (on average) drift away from the midparent value towards the population mean, with the magnitude of the drift proportional to the relative sizes of the genetic and environmental components of phenotypic variation. The key assumption here, mentioned earlier, is that the environmental variation component acts like a random normal deviate, independent of the breeding value.

The accuracy with which the phenotypic values of parents (or sibs) predict the phenotypic values of their offspring (or sibs) forms the basis of heritability analysis. There are several different ways to calculate heritabilities, of which the regression of mean offspring value on midparent value is perhaps easiest to illustrate. In Fig. 2 we show the hypothetical relationship between a passerine body size character measured in offspring and their parents, given low versus high heritability for the character. As discussed above, if parental values predict offspring values perfectly, there should be a one-to-one correspondence between parent (x) and offspring (y) data points, resulting in a straight line with a slope close to one passing through the bivariate mean. This corresponds to the linear equation $y = bx + a$, where b is the slope and a the y-intercept. Remember that the slope of a regression is estimated by $Cov_{x,y}/V_x$, so what we are saying is that if the covariance between parents and offspring is equal to the variance among midparents, the slope will equal one, whereas if there is no covariance between parents and offspring, the slope will equal zero. This index between 0·0 and 1·0 estimates the accuracy with which parental phenotypic values predict offspring phenotypic values, and is referred to as the *heritability* of a trait. It can be shown that the heritability (often abbreviated h^2) estimates the ratio V_A/V_P, i.e. the proportion of the total phenotypic variance V_P which can be attributed to additive genetic variance (V_A). This "narrow sense" heritability is a key parameter in quantitative genetics because the rate at which natural or artificial selection can produce evolutionary change is directly proportional to the additive component of polygenic variation (Falconer 1981). The coefficient of genetic determination shown earlier is sometimes referred to as the "broad sense" heritability, but is seldom used in applied quantitative genetics, being difficult to calculate and not useful in predicting the response to selection.

Types of pedigree data other than midparent–offspring pairs can be used to estimate heritabilities (Boag 1983). Single parent–offspring regressions are often required in cases where only one sex reliably returns to the natal colony to breed (e.g. Lesser Snow Goose; see Findlay and Cooke 1983), or when one is looking at an essentially sex-limited trait such as clutch size. Because a single parent contributes on average only half of its genome to its offspring, the expected phenotypic resemblance due to additive genetic effects is lower than in the midparent case, and regression slopes must be adjusted accordingly. Compared to the midparent analysis, disadvantages of single parent regressions include a sensitivity to assortative mating in the parents (Falconer 1981), a larger error in the estimation of regression slopes, and especially in the case of female–offspring regressions, the possibility of maternal effects increasing resemblance for non-genetic reasons. One can also calculate heritabilities based on the resemblance of full sibs, using ANOVA to partition variation within and between sibships in the same way that intraclass correlations were used to estimate repeatabilities earlier. The main problem with this approach is that it tends to overestimate heritabilities, because, like repeatability analysis, the between-family additive genetic variance component is augmented by part of the non-additive genetic variance and, probably more importantly, by the fact that the variation within families can be reduced because young birds share a common nest environment (e.g. Alatalo and Lundberg 1986).

As we shall see later, despite the fact that we expect variation in territory quality or parental care between breeding pairs, there is little evidence for either maternal or common nest environment effects in the avian studies carried out to date. There are also specific conditions under which the latter result may not even be expected. For instance Falconer (1981) points out that if one were interested in comparing growth rates of young within and between families, and food was limited, then competition between sibs might lead to the establishment of size/dominance hierarchies in each brood, which would in turn result in most of the variance in growth rates being within and not between families. van Noordwijk (1984 b and unpublished data) has collected data which indicate that this process may occur in Great Tit populations in years when food for nestlings is in short supply; the phenotypic variability among offspring is increased and heritabilities are reduced (e.g. Fig. 4 (c)).

More complex experimental designs are possible, many of which are difficult to implement in field situations. One approach that has been carried out successfully in natural avian populations is the experimental randomization of offspring among nests of the same species. One can then compare the resemblance among siblings within and between the parental and foster nests, or compare offspring with their foster parents as well as their biological parents. Such comparisons should provide a test for common environment effects. Smith and Dhondt (1980) carried out this type of experiment with the Song Sparrow (*Melospiza melodia*) population on Mandarte Island. Dhondt (1982) followed with a study of Blue Tits (*Parus caeruleus*) in Belgium, and then Alatalo and Lundberg (1986) cross-fostered young flycatchers in Sweden; in all cases there was no evidence for a non-genetic component to parent–offspring resemblances determining the heritabilities of morphological characters. On the other hand, James (1983) cross-fostered Red-winged Blackbird (*Agelaius phoeniceus*) young between nests at opposite ends of two geographical clines in body size. She found that fostered young tended to resemble the morphology of their foster parents, for reasons as yet unclear. One alternative to cross-fostering offspring among environments is to compare them with their relatives and also with the pheno-types of unrelated individuals known to share a common environment. This approach was recently suggested by van Noordwijk (1984 a) as one way to circumvent a "common nestbox environment" effect which seems to have been responsible for a spuriously high heritability of natal dispersal distance in Great Tit (Greenwood *et al.* 1979). Earlier, van Noordwijk *et al.* (1980) used a similar technique to validate their calculations of laying date heritability in Great Tit. In this case, the problem occurred because pairs of parents and offspring breed simultaneously in particularly early or late years, the effect of which is to increase laying date similarity within family groups. The solution was to regress offspring also on a parent other than their own but which was breeding in the same year, and take the difference between the "true-parent" and "control-parent" regressions.

Still other experimental designs are commonly used in laboratory-based quantitative genetic investigations, but have yet to be applied to natural populations of birds. For instance, half sib designs, in which one male is usually mated to several females, provide one way of estimating maternal and common nest environment effects. They are widely used in laboratory studies of mammalian inheritance where such effects are known to be important, particularly as a result of lactation and litter size variation (e.g. Atchley 1984). An obvious application of this design in wild bird populations might be to use a polygynous species to generate half sibships, although it might be argued that in cases such as marsh breeding Red-winged Blackbirds, a strong common territory effect would still exist (e.g. Menard 1986). Pied and Collared Flycatchers (*Ficedula hypoleuca* and *F. albicollis*) studied by R. V. Alatalo and his colleagues in Sweden may be more promising in this regard, as their "polyterritorial" polygyny means that females raise young on different territories. Unfortunately this situation is complicated by a high rate of uncertain paternity (Alatalo *et al.* 1984).

Even more elegant are designs such as diallel crosses, in which animals from several inbred lines are mated in all possible combinations; such an analysis permits one to partition phenotypic variation into components due to non-additive genetic variance, as well as separating out maternal effects and even the effects of epistasis (e.g. Lynch and Sulzbach 1984). Obviously such an experiment is virtually impossible to carry out under natural conditions or even with wild-derived outbred populations of birds. This illustrates a general weakness of quantitative genetic methodology, namely that the more thoroughly a technique can partition phenotypic variation, the more detached from nature it tends to become. Some compromise between realism and accuracy is necessary.

2.3.3 Artificial selection

Selection in birds is dealt with in detail in chapter 8. However we will briefly discuss a simple case of artificial selection here to underline the relevance of the concept of heritability. In Fig. 2 selection is shown acting on two populations, one where the heritability is 0·2 and another where it is 0·8. Unlike natural selection, most artificial selection involves truncation of the phenotypic distribution to form a breeding population of reduced numbers; if $h^2 = 0·8$, we expect the selected parents to produce offspring which on average exceed the phenotypic value where the truncation occurred, so that the offspring generation averages larger than the total population mean prior to selection. If $h^2 = 0.2$, then we expect offspring phenotypes to fall as a normal distribution around a point close to the original population mean, so that little detectable change in the mean of the F_1 generation has occurred as the result of selection. This is one of the key distinctions which must be made when one is dealing with polygenic traits. In the single-locus Mendelian situation, the close correspondence between phenotypes and genotypes means that changes in the frequencies of phenotypic classes almost always signals changes in gene frequencies, i.e. selection = evolution. But changes in the phenotypic distribution of a metric trait due to selection only results in evolutionary change to the extent that the heritability of the trait exceeds zero.

3 THE DATA AVAILABLE FROM NATURAL POPULATIONS OF BIRDS

3.1 Morphological characters

Much of the early history of quantitative genetics involved measurements of the external morphology of organisms. Animal breeders had observed for centuries the tendency for "like to beget like". Indeed, as pointed out earlier, Galton first illustrated linear regression using data comparing the stature of human fathers with that of their sons. He found that the imperfect ability of paternal size to predict filial size led to a "regression" of the filial measurements towards the population mean. The "regression" is obviously due to the fact that sons get only 50% of their genes from their fathers, in addition to a significant added environmental variance component, which explains about 35% of the phenotypic variation in human stature (Falconer 1981).

The external morphology of birds has been measured for some time, with several different goals in mind (James 1982). The initial reason was probably to refine classifications, the assumption being that phenotypic similarity reflected common descent. More recently such comparisons have been extended to the lower taxonomic units of populations and individuals. Often the goal has been to show that a plausible mechanism exists for natural selection to translate inherited differences between individuals into adaptive mean differences between groups of related individuals (Boag and Grant 1981).

Recent studies on the repeatability and heritability of external morphology in wild birds are summarized in Tables 1 and 3. Many other data are available for domestic birds (e.g. Falconer 1981), although the uncertain

Table 1. Repeatabilities of some avian morphological characters. Scale of repeated measurements indicates time period between successive measurements on an individual, which indicates whether measurement error alone is reducing repeatabilities, or whether there are added seasonal or annual components of variation. Italicized values are not significantly different from zero.

Species	Scale of repeated measurements	Characters						Citation
		Weight	Wing	Tarsus	Bill length	Bill depth	Bill width	
Geospiza fortis	Hours	1·00	0·98	0·96	0·99	1·00	1·00	Boag 1983
G. fuliginosa[1]	Hours	—	0·97	0·99	0·99	0·98	0·99	Grant *et al.* 1985
G. fortis	Years	0·73	0·75	0·91	0·96	0·94	0·98	*Ibid.*
G. scandens	Years	0·55	0·62	0·94	0·80	0·87	0·95	*Ibid.*
G. conirostris	Years	0·71	0·86	0·88	0·78	0·94	0·98	Grant 1983
Melospiza melodia[2]	Years	0·42	0·52	0·56	0·76	0·65	0·62	Smith and Zach 1979
Parus major	Months	—	0·99	0·96	—	—	—	Garnett 1976
P. major	Months	—	—	0·93	*0·25*	*0·33*	0·76	van Noordwijk and Klerks 1983
P. major	Years	0·70	—	0·85	—	—	—	van Noordwijk 1984 b; unpublished data
Ficedula hypoleuca[3]	Hours	—	—	0·89	—	—	—	Alatalo *et al.* 1984

[1] Museum skins.
[2] Averages of male and female values.
[3] Repeat measures by different researchers.

Table 2. Repeatabilities of some non-morphological avian characters. Estimates are for females unless indicated otherwise. The scale of repeated measurements includes: Eggs—repeatability of eggs within clutches, Clutches—eggs between clutches within a year, Years—eggs between years. Values not significantly different from zero are italicized.

Species	Scale of repeated measurements	Egg length	Egg breadth	Egg volume	Laying date	Clutch size	Citation
Sterna hirundo	Eggs	0·74	0·54	—	—	—	Preston 1974
Troglodytes aedon	Eggs	0·42	0·54	—	—	—	Kendeigh 1975
Parus major[1]	Clutches	0·74	0·67	0·62	—	—	van Noordwijk et al. 1980
P. major	Years	0·79	0·59	0·59	0·27	0·42	Ibid.
P. major[2]	Years	*0·08*	*0·19*	*0·12*	*0·06*	0·19	Ibid.
P. major	Years	—	—	0·72[3]	0·34	0·51	Jones 1973
P. major[4]	Eggs	0·72	0·71	0·72	—	—	Ojanen et al. 1979
P. major	Clutches	0·75	0·70	0·74	—	—	Ibid.
P. major	Years	0·68	0·54	0·56	—	—	Ibid.
Ficedula hypoleuca[4]	Eggs	0·74	0·73	0·76	—	—	Ibid.
F. hypoleuca	Years	0·68	0·76	0·75	—	—	Ibid.
Phoenicurus phoenicurus	Eggs	0·79	0·73	0·76	—	—	Ibid.
Sturnus vulgaris	Eggs	0·70	0·80	0·81	—	—	Ibid.
Geospiza conirostris	Clutches	0·81	0·72	0·72	—	—	Grant 1982
G. magnirostris[5]	Clutches	*0·18*	0·94	*0·67*	—	—	Ibid.
Melospiza melodia	Years	—	—	—	—	0·23[6,7]	Smith 1981
Anser caerulescens	Years	—	—	—	0·22	0·25[7]	Findlay and Cooke 1983; Hamann, unpub.
Branta canadensis	Years	—	—	0·80[3]	0·20	*0·05*	Lessells 1982
Accipiter nisus[7]	Years	—	—	—	0·23	—	Newton and Marquiss 1984
A. nisus[2,7]	Years	—	—	—	0·63	—	Ibid.
Lagopus lagopus	Eggs	—	—	0·62[8]	—	—	Moss and Watson 1982
L. lagopus	Years	—	—	0·75[8]	—	—	Ibid.

[1] Averages of 1st 2nd clutch values for 2 years.
[2] Values for males, not females.
[3] Egg weight.
[4] Mixed data including more than 1 clutch per female.
[5] Averages of 1st 2nd and 2nd 3rd clutch comparisons.
[6] Total number of eggs laid per year. Smith (1981) also gives estimates for number of nests per year, and number of young raised to 6 and 30 days of age.
[7] Values corrected from published version (see Lessells and Boag 1987).
[8] Averages for 2 sites over several years.

Table 3. Heritabilities of avian morphological characters. Methods used to calculate heritabilities include: M—offspring on midparent regression, S—offspring on sire, D—offspring on dam, F—full sib correlation, G—offspring on grandparent. Where more than one method was used in a study, the method used for the data presented here is italicized. Values not significantly different from zero are also italicized.

Species	Methodology	Weight	Wing	Tarsus	Bill length	Bill depth	Bill width	Citation
Geospiza fortis	M, S, D, F	0·91	0·84	0·71	0·65	0·79	0·90	Boag 1983
G. scandens	M, S, D, F	*0·58*	*0·12*	0·92	*0·32*	*0·14*	*0·34*	Ibid.
G. conirostris[1]	M, S, D	0·95	*−0·68*	0·87	0·48	0·66	0·74	Grant 1981
G. conirostris	M, S, D	1·08	*0·72*	0·79	1·09	0·71	0·82	Grant 1983
Melospiza melodia	M, S, D	*0·04*	*0·14*	0·32	0·33	0·51	0·50	Smith and Zach 1979
Melospiza melodia[2]	M, S, D	—	—	0·76	0·37	0·98	0·56	Smith and Dhondt 1980
Melospiza melodia[3]	M, S, D	—	—	*−0·06*	*−0·06*	*−0·18*	*−0·09*	Ibid.
Parus caeruleus[2]	M, S, D	—	—	0·64	—	—	—	Dhondt 1982
P. caeruleus[3]	M, S, D	—	—	*−0·32*	—	—	—	Ibid.
P. major	M	—	—	0·76	—	—	—	Garnett 1981
P. major	M, S, D	0·59[4]	—	0·52	—	—	—	van Noordwijk 1984 b; unpublished data
P. major	M, S, D	—	—	*−0·07*	0·49	0·71	0·68	van Noordwijk and Klerks 1983
P. major	S, D	—	—	0·80	—	—	—	Alatalo et al. 1984
Ficedula hypoleuca	S, D	—	—	0·57	—	—	—	Ibid.
F. albicollis	S, D	—	—	0·59	—	—	—	Ibid.
F. hypoleuca[2]	D, F	—	—	0·50	—	—	—	Alatalo and Lundberg 1986
F. hypoleuca[3]	D, F	—	—	0·04	*—*	—	—	Ibid.
Puffinus puffinus[1]	M	—	0·66	0·92	0·76	—	—	Brooke 1977
Branta canadensis	M, S, D	*0·15*	—	*0·11*	*0·46*	—	—	Lessells 1982
Anas platyrhynchos[4]	D	0·42	—	—	—	—	—	Prince et al. 1970
Lagopus lagopus	M, S, D	0·65	—	—	—	—	—	Moss and Watson 1982

[1] Offspring measured in nest and regressed on parents' adult measurements.
[2] Using true parents.
[3] Using foster parents.
[4] Mean of separate estimates of male- and female—offspring regressions.

histories of birds in such studies (i.e. degree of inbreeding or artificial selection) may mean that such heritabilities are not representative of wild birds (Rose 1982). Most field ornithologists have demonstrated that external morphological features are significantly and sometimes highly heritable. These results are probably biased to some extent, insofar as investigators seem to perceive low or non-significant heritability estimates as scientifically uninteresting and not worth publishing. The repeatability data in Table 1 show how the time scale of remeasurement affects the magnitude of the V_{Es} component; over a period of hours, only V_{Es} is expected, and it seems consistently small for most morphological characters (which is not entirely surprising given that part of the reason these characters have been used so often is their ease of measurement!). Over months or years between measurements, additional sources of variation creep in, but in most cases there remains a substantial amount of between-bird variation. Even characters such as weight or wing length, which one expects to show at least seasonal variation, are only 20% less repeatable than the other characters on average, and retain significant values in the range 60–70%.

There are few consistent patterns in the combined set of heritability data, i.e. certain characters do not seem to have consistently high or low values (Table 3). Most show heritability values of 60–70%. Note that this is only slightly lower than the repeatability values in Table 1. One of the main reasons it is difficult to find differences between characters is the large standard errors typical of most repeatability or heritability estimates, particularly when made from relatively small samples of field data. Often it is impossible to claim anything more specific about a given value than the fact it appears significantly greater than zero. It is also important to keep in mind that most of these characters have high phenotypic correlations between them (e.g. Boag 1984), and hence much of the variation they display probably stems from the same set of underlying, pleiotropic "body size genes". As shown by Table 3, several studies have calculated heritabilities using a variety of methods on more or less independent groups of relatives. In general, these have not shown dramatic differences in heritability estimates for the same population, i.e. female–offspring regressions and even full sib analyses have shown little sign of producing the inflated estimates one would expect if maternal or common nest environment effects were profoundly important. The field studies which have involved some experimental manipulations (e.g. Smith and Dhondt 1980, Dhondt 1982, Alatalo and Lundberg 1986) tend to support such a conclusion.

The most interesting exception to this consistency of estimates based on different sets of relatives involves male–offspring regressions. Boag (1983) noted that upon first examination, male–offspring regressions in one year's *Geospiza fortis* data appeared surprisingly low, contrary to other estimates

Table 4. Heritabilities of non-morphological avian characters. Conventions as in Table 3.

Species	Methodology	Characters					Citation
		Egg length	Egg breadth	Egg volume	Laying date	Clutch size	
Parus major	D, G	*0·53*	0·80	0·61	0·40	0·37	van Noordwijk *et al.* 1980
P. major	S, G	—	—	—	*0·04*	*0·05*	*Ibid.*
P. major	D, F	—	—	0·72[1]	*0·14*	0·48	Jones 1973, Perrins and Jones 1974
P. major	M	—	—	0·86	—	—	Ojanen *et al.* 1979
Melospiza melodia	D	—	—	—	—	−*0·31*[2]	Smith 1981
Anas platyrhynchos	D	—	—	0·55	—	0·46	Prince *et al.* 1970
Anser caerulescens	D	—	—	—	—	*0·21*[3]	Findlay and Cooke 1983
Sturnus vulgaris	D	—	—	—	—	0·34	Flux and Flux 1982
Lagopus lagopus	D, F	—	—	0·99[4]	—	—	Moss and Watson 1982

[1] Egg weight.
[2] Total number of eggs laid per year. Smith (1981) also gives estimates for number of nests per year, and number of young raised to 6 and 30 days of age.
[3] Value corrected from published version (see Lessells and Boag 1986).
[4] Average of several estimates.

the same year using other methods, and to male–offspring regressions in another year. The answer was that in that year, several females mated sequentially with different males; when the analysis was restricted to "faithful" pairs, the male–offspring regressions were as expected, indicating that some newly mated males had been cuckolded by their female's previous mate. Alatalo *et al.* (1984) found a similar effect in both Pied and Collared Flycatchers (*Ficedula hypoleuca* and *F. albicollis*), again related to cuckoldry. They were able to carry out an elegant analysis using the difference between male–offspring and female–offspring heritability regressions to actually estimate the rate of cuckoldry. Furthermore, using additional linear comparisons, they showed that neighbouring males were probably the real fathers of most cuckolded broods.

3.2   Characters other than morphology

Morphological variation is obviously only part of the evolutionarily important phenotypic variation displayed by birds. Other characters are of considerable ecological interest, but are often more difficult to measure and analyse using quantitative genetic techniques. Tables 2 and 4 summarize some of the repeatability and heritability studies conducted on non-morphological characters: more work has been done on egg size and shape than on measures of reproductive performance such as clutch size or laying date. One of the main problems with characters such as clutch size and laying date is that they can vary tremendously for the same female in different years, i.e. annual repeatability is often low. The repeatability of egg size and shape can be difficult to evaluate in some species because of predictable effects due to the position of an egg in the laying sequence (Kendeigh 1975). Also characters such as laying date may not be normally distributed and hence are difficult to analyse correctly using ANOVA. Transformation of data is always advisable in such cases.

Nevertheless, like the morphological traits discussed above, several studies present fairly convincing evidence for significant heritabilities of reproductive characters, on average in excess of 30–40%. One expects such characters to have lower heritability values than morphology, on both theoretical and empirical grounds (Falconer 1981, Gustafsson 1986). This expectation is, however, derived largely from quantitative genetic studies of captive animal populations, and there is now some question as to the applicability of those results to wild populations (Rose 1982). As with morphological data, there is often very good correspondence between h^2 estimates derived from mother–daughter regressions and repeatability analyses, e.g. clutch size inheritance in Great Tit and in Lesser Snow Goose. This once again argues for the absence of major maternal or common environment contributions to phenotypic resemblance between relatives.

Perhaps the least amount of attention has been paid to the heritability of behavioural characters in birds (Jacobs 1981). In Darwin's Finches territory size can be considered a behavioural character, one which is known to be a good predictor of mating success. Price (1984) found that the adult territory sizes of *Geospiza fortis* siblings were strongly correlated; even with the effect of body size removed (because it is known to be highly heritable (Boag 1983)), the intraclass correlation for territory size was 0·43, giving a "heritability" of 0·86. In an elegant series of experiments, Berthold and his colleagues have been able to show that the migratory behaviour (along with several morphological characters) of European Blackcap Warblers (*Sylvia atricapilla*) has a heritable component (Berthold and Querner 1981, 1982). Their study illustrates a completely different approach to the problem of demonstrating that a continuously variable trait has a genetic basis. They carry out hybridization experiments between groups of birds with different phenotypes, whose populations are known to be at least partly reproductively isolated in nature. If, as in Berthold's case, the F_1 hybrids are behaviourally intermediate when raised under controlled conditions, this suggests that some additive combining of distinct sets of alleles from the two populations is taking place (see also Gwinner and Neusser 1985).

Such hybridization experiments can in principle be used to estimate heritabilities (e.g. Biebach 1983) or even to generate crude estimates of the number of "genes" or independent segregating units responsible for additive genetic variation in a character (Lande 1981). Given the ease with which many genetically distinct avian taxa hybridize in the lab or even in nature (see Rising 1983), it is surprising how little attention has been paid to the possibilities of quantitative genetic analysis based on such crosses. Certainly Dilger's (1962) and Buckley's (1969) studies of hybridization between the lovebirds *Agapornis roseicollis* and *A. personata ficheri*, and the resulting intermediate and mixed expression of characters such as nest building behaviour warrant further investigation. Several other avian groups, notably the ducks (Lack 1974), quail (Johnsgard 1971), and doves (Davies 1970) show an equal proclivity to hybridize and produce intermediate, presumably polygenically inherited phenotypic variation. These and other examples of avian hybrids are reviewed more fully in Buckley (1982).

Yet another way to demonstrate that a trait has a heritable basis is to calculate realized heritabilities based on either artificial or natural selection. One of the few examples of such an approach applied to a natural population of birds was carried out by Flux and Flux (1982) in New Zealand (Fig. 3). They showed that by systematically destroying European Starling (*Sturnus vulgaris*) clutches smaller than the mean size for the population each year,

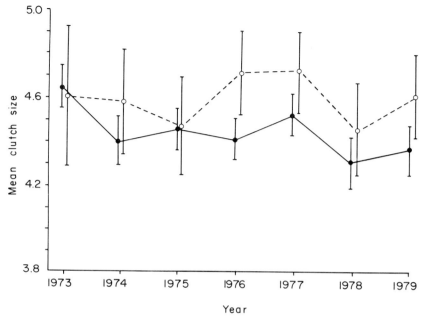

Fig. 3. Each year chicks from nests with less than the mean annual clutch size in a New Zealand starling colony were killed, while control nests were unmanipulated. Though there was year-to-year variation, F_1 starlings selected for high clutch size ($\bigcirc$) diverged from unselected controls ($\bullet$). The total response to selection (R) was 0·12, while the total selection differential (S) was 0·72. This is twice the required midparent value as the clutch size of fathers is unknown; thus $h^2 = 0·12/0·36 = 0·33 \pm 0·02$. This was similar to the heritability estimated from mother–daughter regression (see Table 4). From *Naturwissenschaften* **69**, 96–97 by J. E. C. Flux and M. M. Flux (Springer-Verlag, Copyright 1982).

they induced a response to selection comparable to that predicted by parent–offspring heritability regressions (Table 3). Boag (1983) showed that when the response to selection in young Darwin's Finches was compared to the selection differential imposed on their parents' morphology as a result of drought conditions (Boag and Grant 1981), the realized heritability values closely matched those predicted by parent–offspring regressions.

A final method to establish whether geographic variation in a metric trait has a genetic basis is to carry out transplant or explant experiments. James (1983) transplanted Blackbird young between either end of a cline in body size and shape, showing that a large environmental component of variation existed. Boag (1987) discusses explants, and notes the fact that such approaches have not been used to full advantage in the study of avian phenotypic variation.

4 PROBLEMS AND PROSPECTS

4.1 Statistical concerns

Throughout this chapter we have tried to instil a modicum of caution in the reader by pointing out limitations in the application of quantitative genetic techniques to natural populations. Whether or not results are meaningful depends very much on how carefully the data have been collected and the appropriateness of the analysis. Most regression techniques are highly sensitive to outliers; small numbers of misidentified parents or mistakes in data coding can have large effects on both the accuracy and precision of heritability estimates. All ANOVA procedures are sensitive to departures from normality in the data, and to unequal variances (heteroscedasticity) between data subsets. For instance, many field studies measure offspring and parents at different ages; environmental effects, such as those discussed later, may inflate V_P among young offspring, while selection may reduce variance in a cohort of birds as they mature. Several quantitative genetic analyses of wild bird populations have been published with serious errors (Preston 1975, van Noordwijk 1984a, Lessells and Boag 1987); one common difficulty is confusion over what constitutes an "intraclass correlation" in repeatability and full sib analyses (Sokal and Rohlf 1981). Hailman (1986) discusses the difficulties of field heritability studies; unfortunately the critique is itself flawed in logic and data interpretation.

To guard against such problems, a dataset must be carefully "cleaned" prior to analysis. Scatterplots are useful in detecting outliers, while histograms provide a quick check on normality. It is always a good idea to validate a new statistical procedure with a known dataset; this is particularly important when using non-standard family-size weighting techniques (Falconer 1963) or methods such as maximum likelihood estimation when confronted with the unbalanced designs all too typical of data from field studies. When the results of an analysis are published, all corrections and transformations applied to the data should be summarized, together with full details of ANOVAs and regressions, including F values and sample sizes, as well as standard errors for all estimates (Becker 1984). Because parameters such as h^2 are ratios, the actual level of phenotypic variation (V_P) for a character should always be provided, as either a standard deviation, variance or coefficient of variation (CV). A large CV is one of the simplest indications that a quantitative genetic analysis *may* be feasible, as it reduces the relative importance of extraneous measurement error, and reduces the sample sizes needed to demonstrate statistical differences. The unusually high CVs of *Geospiza fortis* morphology, due in part to hybridization (Grant and Price 1981, Grant *et al.* 1985), are one of the main reasons this species has consistently produced among the highest heritabilities in any field study of avian morphology.

A final technical point worth noting is that one should check for assortative mating with respect to the character in question. If present (and there are no conclusive examples of assortative mating with respect to a metric trait in birds, see Boag (1983); van Noordwijk *et al.* (1985)), heritability estimates based on some methods will be increased (Falconer 1981). Compared to the estimation errors typical of field data, the increase would be minor except for *very* strong correlations between mates. The commonly used midparent–offspring regression is not affected by assortative mating.

4.2   Environmental effects between populations

Ignoring the *caveat* voiced earlier, namely that the current literature is probably biased towards reporting "positive" results of quantitative genetics studies of birds, the main message which emerges from presently available data is that most of the phenotypic variation studied by avian ecologists can be shown to be "heritable" in nature. What does this mean? It should mean that variation in these characters is not only accessible to natural selection, but that when selection does occur, it should produce permanent changes in the frequencies of additively acting genes within the population in question. One thing it does *not* mean is that average differences in heritable characters *between* populations of the same species necessarily indicate genetic differences. This type of point has been made by many authors, particularly with reference to human populations (e.g. Feldman and Lewontin 1975). For instance, Boag (1983) found that in two years, independent sets of Darwin's Finch parents and their offspring displayed parallel midparent–offspring regressions, but had significantly different Y-intercepts (Fig. 4(*a*)). Thus adults of a given size produced different size offspring in the two years; this was due to differences in the food supplies and growth rates of young in the two years, not differences in genetic potential.

The cross-fostering experiments carried out by James (1983) with Blackbirds also suggest that environmental effects can be partly responsible for morphological differences between populations. Many ornithologists continue to assume that avian morphological growth is essentially determinate, or "target-seeking" (Atchley 1984). Although this may be true when compared to the type of growth displayed by many plants or fish, there has been remarkably little work done to establish how true it is for particular avian characters or populations. Thus Boag (1987) carried out an experiment in which three groups of captive Zebra Finches (*Poephila guttata*) were allowed to rear young on "normal", "high" and "low" protein diets. The results (Fig. 4(*b*)) were clear; not only were growth rates affected by the food

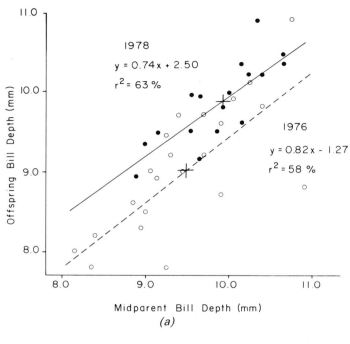

(a)

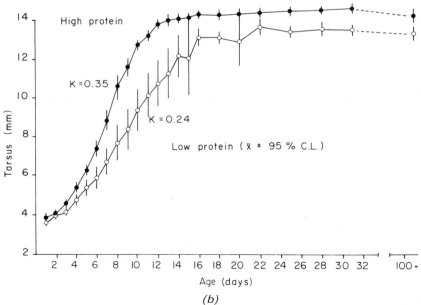

(b)

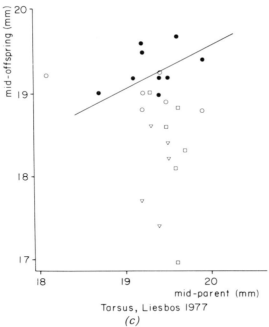

Tarsus, Liesbos 1977

(c)

Fig. 4. (*a*) Environmental effects can produce large size differences between *Geospiza fortis* offspring in two years, despite a high heritability for bill depth each year. From *Evolution* **37**, 877–894 by P. T. Boag (reproduced by kind permission of the publisher, Copyright 1983). (*b*) The protein level of Zebra finch nestling diets can influence the growth rates of the birds, and also their ultimate size. The tarsus lengths of adults raised on the two diets shown here were significantly different. (From Boag 1987.) (*c*) Environmental effects can reduce the heritability of Great Tit tarsus length in a poor year by increasing the phenotypic variation among offspring. Here some young hatched late, with either < 25% (●) or > 25% (○) nestling mortality. Others hatched early with < 25% (▽) or > 25% (□) mortality. Early hatching and high nestling mortality are associated with poor rearing conditions; when conditions are poor, young are variable and small in size, and parent–offspring resemblance is low. The best group here (●) has a regression slope of 0·51; this is close to the normal h^2 value (see Table 3). (From van Noordwijk *et al.* 1984 b; unpublished data.)

available, as has been shown in field studies (e.g. Bryant 1975), but there were significant, permanent morphological differences in the adult measurements of young raised on the three diets, which were not evident in either the parents or subsequent offspring of the experimental groups (Boag 1987). Similar effects have been documented in domestic animals, and even in human populations (e.g. Allee and Lutherman 1940, Fisher and Griminger 1963, Lister and McCance 1965, Hulse 1968, Johnson 1971). There would seem to be considerable scope for avian biologists to seek evidence not only of genetic but also for environmental effects on the phenotype (see also Alatalo and Lundberg 1986).

4.3   Environmental effects within populations

The major problem in applying the techniques of classical quantitative genetics to natural populations remains the difficulty of achieving the experimental control which forms the cornerstone of traditional laboratory-based studies. There, the possibility of non-genetic effects enhancing resemblance can often be controlled, and steps can be taken to ensure that genotype–environment interactions and correlations are minimized. Genotype–environment correlations occur when the environmental deviation is not independent of the genotypic value. For instance, big male birds might obtain the richest territories and produce environmentally big, as well as genetically big offspring. In statistical terms, the V_P term is increased by twice the covariance between V_G and V_E; this tends to increase the slope of a parent–offspring regression curve, and make young and their parents more highly correlated with each other. In most cases it is probably correct to include the covariance with V_G; the special environment a small or large bird might raise its young in is viewed as an extension of its phenotype. Genotype–environment interactions are non-linear associations between V_G and V_E. For example, there might be two types of food patch available; small birds did best in one, large birds best in another. In the former environment, small bird environmental deviations would be positive, while large bird deviations were negative, and vice versa. The statistical effect of such a situation is to add a V_{GE} term to V_P; thus a large interaction will usually reduce heritabilities.

Experimental control, for instance randomizing genotypes across environments, is much harder in the field than in the lab; indeed in much of behavioural ecology it is assumed that there is considerable variance in the "quality" of individuals, whether reflected in territory size, amount of food in the territory, dominance status, ability to attract a mate, the efficacy of parental care, and so on (Orians 1980). Such variance among parents, coupled with the often highly disproportionate contribution of a few breeders to future cohorts (van Noordwijk and Scharloo 1981), means that we should not be surprised to find some evidence for non-genetic factors either enhancing or masking the phenotypic similarity of related individuals. But as we saw earlier, the only clear case in which this has been shown to affect previously published data is in the heritability of natal dispersal in Great Tit (van Noordwijk 1984 a). The more typical finding is that seen in Fig. 4(a); here the parallel parent–offspring regressions, in the face of two very (environmentally) different years argues against the presence of an interaction term. Even in controlled studies, genotype–environment correlations and interactions seem hard to demonstrate except in combinations of very different genotypes and environments (Falconer 1981). Nonetheless, the evidence produced by van Noordwijk (1984 b) that heritabilities may be reduced by increased variation among offspring in poor years, suggests that more attention should be paid to the sensitivity of avian phenotypic characters to environmental variability, or in other words to examine what traditional quantitative geneticists describe as "norms of reaction" (Falconer 1981). Such work again requires experimentation, and some control over the environment in which the characters grow and are expressed.

Another area of interest at the moment is resemblance between relatives during growth, obviously a time when environmental effects are likely to be most active. The standard assumption in quantitative genetics is that a character is measured at a particular point in the life cycle, with reference to a particular population. Thus it assumes that the character *beak length in birds* means the deviation from the population mean of a bird's beak at, say, 100 days of age. This assumption is difficult to meet precisely in the field, and thus an attempt has been made to examine the resemblance among sibs and between parents and offspring while the young are growing and the parents are already adult size (Grant 1981, 1983, Atchley 1984, Price and Grant 1985). The results to date suggest that early environmental (e.g. maternal) effects fade relatively quickly, and that unless rearing conditions are poor, morphological characters are highly genetically correlated at various ages (Price and Grant 1985). There is little theoretical or empirical reason to suspect that age of measurement effects are significant sources of bias in existing field data. However, Ricklefs and Peters' (1981) and Ricklefs' (1984) studies with Starling nestlings indicate that important local environmental conditions can mask genetic components of variation; the latter work also provides a good introduction to the methods and difficulties of designing experiments to partition the phenotypic variation in a natural population of birds.

4.4   Correlated characters and multivariate evolution

When Darwin wrote *The Origin of Species* (1859), he used the analogy of artificial selection to argue for the plausibility of evolution by natural selection. In discussing the application of quantitative genetics to natural populations of birds, it is important to keep in mind that this *was* an analogy, and that there are some fundamental differences between the way natural and artificial selection operate. Thus quantitative genetic techniques were originally developed for use under controlled conditions, primarily for livestock improvement. When one moves out into a field situation, one encounters two major problems. First, it becomes difficult to assume or to ensure that genotypes are randomized across environments, which we have already discussed.

Second, in predicting the response of a character to selection, or in carrying out an *a posteriori* analysis of selection, it is difficult to know which character or combination of characters selection has acted on. For instance, measurements of most avian morphological characters are strongly correlated with each other and with overall size. Correlations among characters are less of a problem in the laboratory because in artificial selection, the target of selection can be explicitly defined.

In the theory of "antagonistic pleiotropy" (Rose 1982), different types of selection act on many different characters within a generation, each linked to fitness by its own causal pathway. Because of pleiotropy, many of these characters will be positively or negatively correlated with each other, so that selection acting on one character can be inhibited by opposing selection pressures impinging on correlated characters. Thus in natural populations one cannot always assume that because the heritability of a trait seems high, it will necessarily respond to natural selection as predicted. One must understand what the mechanism of selection is, and the correlations between characters which may each be the main target of a given type of selection. A corollary is that in an *a posteriori* analysis of selection, one cannot assume that the response of a single character to selection can be used to calculate an accurate measure of realized heritability for that trait. Its response may actually be caused by selection on some other, correlated trait (Lande and Arnold 1983). The topic of natural selection acting on correlated characters is dealt with in more detail in chapter 8, and is introduced here primarily to point out that ornithologists must be aware of possible relationships among the characters they are calculating heritabilities or repeatabilities for, and between this subset of characters and other aspects of the total phenotype. In the same way one can partition phenotypic variation in a single character into its genetic and environmental components, it is possible to partition phenotypic covariation between characters into genetic and environmental correlations using pedigree data (Falconer 1981). An increasing amount of attention is being paid to genetic covariance structure in natural populations by evolutionary biologists (e.g. Dingle and Hegmann 1982, Arnold 1983, Price and Grant 1985). It remains to be seen how generally or productively the approach can be applied to wild bird populations, because even in the laboratory it is much more difficult to accurately estimate genetic correlations (Boag 1983) than it is to measure heritabilities, which as we have shown is itself no trivial task.

5 CONCLUSIONS

The main points of this chapter can be summarized as follows:

(1) Quantitative genetics involves the study of traits involving two or more loci, most of which have small, additive effects on the phenotype, and display incomplete dominance and/or environmentally sensitive expression.

(2) The likelihood that phenotypic variation in a trait has an additive genetic basis, allowing it to respond to selection, is estimated using statistical tools such as repeatabilities and heritabilities. These tools must be used carefully to yield meaningful results.

(3) An increasing number of studies of natural bird populations suggest that most external morphological characters have heritabilities of 60–70%, while traits more closely related to reproductive performance have significant, but lower heritabilities in the range 30–40%.

(4) The main problem in applying quantitative genetic techniques to field studies is lack of experimental control, making it difficult to interpret phenotypic resemblance (or lack thereof) between relatives as unambiguous evidence for the presence (or absence) of an additive genetic basis to phenotypic variation.

(5) However, the limited empirical data available does not support the thesis that field estimates of heritability are hopelessly confounded by common environment or maternal effects or genotype–environment correlations and interactions.

(6) In addition to more experiments, much work remains to be done on the phenotypic plasticity or "norms of reaction" of avian characters, and on the correlations between traits subject to similar selection pressures.

We stress again that tools such as heritability analysis provide an entirely artificial partitioning of observed phenotypic variation into its causal components (see Jacquard 1983). Parameters such as V_A derived from such procedures do not provide the concrete measure of genetic variation that one associates with measures such as mean heterozygosity in electrophoretic studies. In fact it is surprising that no study has actually combined biochemical and quantitative genetic investigation of an avian population; this might be a very useful approach, with the biochemical techniques used to establish the recent selective history of the population, the evidence for population size bottlenecks or hybridization, or even the certainty of paternity in parent–offspring regressions. As long as these limitations are kept in mind and a continued effort is made to integrate quantitative genetic theory with evolutionary theory (e.g. Lande 1982, Arnold 1983), it will continue to be worth while to collect quantitative genetic data from long-term studies of marked birds. Simple documentation of whether or not relatives resemble each other for traits of ecological interest will eventually cease to be of as much empirical interest as it is currently, but the approach will have left a legacy of an entirely new, highly disciplined, critical and quantitative attitude towards the origins of phenotypic variation in avian populations, and is sure to stimulate further study of the reasons for such similarities. It may well turn out that in some cases non-genetical sources of covariance between relatives is of as much biological interest as genetic causes of similarity, but the key is that the variation will be the item subject to the most concerted scrutiny.

REFERENCES

Alatalo, R. V., Gustafsson, L. and Lundberg, A. (1984). High frequency of cuckoldry in pied and collared flycatchers. *Oikos* **42**, 41–47.

Alatalo, R. V. and Lundberg, A. (1986). Heritability and selection on tarsus length in the Pied Flycatcher (*Fidecula hypoleuca*). *Evolution* **405**, 574–583.

Allee, W. C. and Lutherman, C. Z. (1940). An experimental study of certain effects of temperature on differential growth of pullets. *Ecology* **21**, 29–33.

Arnold, S. J. (1983). Morphology, performance, and fitness. *Am. Zool.* **23**, 347–361.

Arnold, S. J. and Wade, M. J. (1984 a). On the measurement of natural and sexual selection: Theory. *Evolution* **38**, 709–719.

Arnold, S. J. and Wade, M. J. (1984 b). On the measurement of natural and sexual selection: Applications. *Ibid.* **38**, 720–734.

Atchley, W. R. (1984). Ontogeny, timing of development, and genetic variance–covariance structure. *Am. Natur.* **123**, 519–540.

Ayala, F. J. (1982). "Population and Evolutionary Genetics: A Primer". Benjamin/Cummings, Menlo Park, Calif.

Becker, W. A. (1984). "A Manual of Quantitative Genetics". Academic Enterprises, Pullman, Washington.

Berthold, P. and Querner, U. (1981). Genetic basis of migratory behavior in European warblers. *Science* **212**, 77–79.

Berthold, P. and Querner, U. (1982). Genetic basis of moult, wing length, and body weight in a migratory bird species, *Sylvia atricapilla. Experientia* **38**, 801–802.

Biebach, H. (1983). Genetic determination of partial migration in the European Robin (*Erithacus rubecula*). *Auk* **100**, 601–606.

Boag, P. T. (1983). The heritability of external morphology in Darwin's ground finches (*Geospiza*) on Isla Daphne Major, Galapagos. *Evolution* **37**, 877–894.

Boag, P. T. (1984). Growth and allometry of external morphology in Darwin's finches (*Geospiza*) on Isla Daphne Major, Galapagos. *J. Zool. Lond.* **204**, 413–441.

Boag, P. T. (1987). Effects of nestling diet protein on growth and adult size of Zebra finches (*Poephila guttata*). *Auk* **104**, 155–166.

Boag, P. T. and Grant, P. R. (1981). Intense natural selection on a population of Darwin's finches (Geospizinae) in the Galapagos. *Science* **214**, 82–85.

Bryant, D. M. (1975). Breeding biology of house martins *Delichon urbica* in relation to aerial insect abundance. *Ibis* **117**, 180–215.

Brooke, M. de L. (1977). The breeding biology of the Manx shearwater. D.Phil. Thesis, Oxford.

Buckley, P. A. (1969). Disruption of species-typical behavior patterns in F_1 hybrid *Agapornis* parrots. *Z. Tierpsych.* **26**, 737–743.

Buckley, P. A. (1982). Avian genetics. *In* "Disease of Cage and Aviary Birds", 2nd edn (ed. M. Petrak). Chapter 4. Lea and Febiger, Philadelphia.

Corbin, K. W. (1983). Genetic structure and avian systematics. *In* "Current Ornithology". (ed. R. F. Johnston). Vol. 1, pp. 211–244. Plenum Press, New York.

Darwin, C. (1859). "On the Origin of Species". Murray, London.

Davies, S. J. J. F. (1970). Patterns of inheritance in the bowing display and associated behaviour of some hybrid *Streptopelia* doves. *Behaviour* **36**, 187–214.

Dhondt, A. A. (1982). Heritability of blue tit tarsus length from normal and cross-fostered broods. *Evolution* **36**, 418–419.

Dilger, W. C. (1962). The behavior of lovebirds. *Scient. Am.* **206**, 88–98.

Dingle, H. and Hegmann, J. P. (Eds.) (1982). "Evolution and Genetics of Life Histories". Springer-Verlag, New York.

Falconer, D. S. (1963). Quantitative inheritance. *In* "Methodology in Mammalian Genetics". (ed. W. J. Burdette), pp. 193–216. Holden-Day, San Francisco.

Falconer, D. S. (1981). "Introduction to Quantitative Genetics", 2nd edn. Longman, London.

Feldman, M. W. and Lewontin, R. C. (1975). The heritability hang-up. *Science* **190**, 1163–1168.

Findlay, C. S. and Cooke, F. (1982). Breeding synchrony in the lesser snow goose (*Anser caerulescens caerulescens*). I. Genetic and environmental components of hatch date variability and their effects on hatch synchrony. *Evolution* **36**, 342–351.

Findlay, C. S. and Cooke, F. (1983). Genetic and environmental components of clutch size variance in a wild population of lesser snow geese (*Anser caerulescens caerulescens*). *Evolution* **37**, 724–734.

Fisher, R. A. (1918). The correlation between relatives on the supposition of Mendelian inheritance. *Trans. R. Soc. Edinburgh* **52**, 379–433.

Fisher, H. and Griminger, P. (1963). Aging and food restriction: changes in body composition and hydroxyproline content of selected tissues. *J. Nutr.* **80**, 350–354.

Flux, J. E. C. and Flux, M. M. (1982). Artificial selection and gene flow in wild starlings, *Sturnus vulgaris. Naturwissenschaften* **69**, 96–97.

Galton, F. (1889). "Natural Inheritance". Macmillan Publishing Co. Inc., New York.

Garnett, M. C. (1976). Some aspects of body size in the Great Tit. D.Phil. Thesis. Oxford.

Garnett, M. C. (1981). Body size, its heritability and influence on juvenile survival among great tits *Parus major. Ibis* **123**, 31–41.

Grant, P. R. (1981). Patterns of growth in Darwin's finches. *Proc. R. Soc. Lond.* B **212**, 403–432.

Grant, P. R. (1982). Variation in the size and shape of Darwin's finch eggs. *Auk* **99**, 15–23.

Grant, P. R. (1983). Inheritance of size and shape in a population of Darwin's finches, *Geospiza conirostris. Proc. R. Soc. Lond.* B **220**, 219–236.

Grant, P. R., Abbott, I., Schluter, D., Curry, R. L. and Abbott, L. K. (1985). Variation in the size and shape of Darwin's finches. *Biol. J. Linn. Soc.* **25**, 1–39.

Grant, P. R. and Price, T. D. (1981). Population variation in continuously varying traits as an ecological genetics problem. *Am. Zool.* **21**, 795–811.

Greenwood, P. J., Harvey, P. H. and Perrins, C. (1979). The role of dispersal in the Great Tit (*Parus major*): The causes, consequences and heritability of natal dispersal. *J. Anim. Ecol.* **48**, 123–142.

Gustafsson, L. (1986). Lifetime reproductive success and heritability: empirical support for Fisher's fundamental theorem. *Am. Natur.* **128**, 761–764.

Gwinner, E. and Neusser, V. (1985). Postjuvenile moult of European and African Stonechats (*Saxicola torquata rubicola* and *S. t. axillaris* and their F_1 hybrids. *J. Ornithol.* **126**, 219–220.

Hailman, J. P. (1986). The heritability concept applied to wild birds. *In* "Current Ornithology" (ed. R. F. Johnston), Vol. 4, pp. 71–95. Plenum Press, New York.

Hulse, F. S. (1968). The breakdown of isolates and hybrid vigor among the Italian Swiss. *Proc. 12th Int. Congr. Genet.* (ed. C. Oshima), 2, p. 117. Science Council of Japan, Tokyo.

Jacobs, J. (1981). How heritable is innate behavior? *Z. Tierpsych.* **55**, 1–18.

Jacquard, A. (1983). Heritability: One word, three concepts. *Biometrics* **39**, 465–477.

James, F. C. (1982). The ecological morphology of birds: a review. *Ann. Zool. Fennici* **19**, 265–275.

James, F. C. (1983). Environmental component of morphological variation in birds. *Science* **221**, 184–186.

Johnsgard, P. (1971). Experimental hybridization of the New World quail (*Odontophorinae*). *Auk* **88**, 264–275.

Johnson, N. F. (1971). Effects of levels of dietary protein on wood duck growth. *J. Wildl. Mgmt* **35**, 798–802.

Jones, P. J. (1973). Some aspects of the feeding ecology of the Great Tit *Parus major* L. D.Phil. Thesis, Oxford.

Kendeigh, S. C. (1975). Effects of parentage on egg characteristics. *Auk* **92**, 163–164.

Lack, D. (1974). "Evolution Illustrated by Water-fowl". Blackwell, Oxford.

Lande, R. (1981). The minimum number of genes contributing to quantitative variation between and within populations. *Genetics* **99**, 541–553.

Lande, R. (1982). A quantitative genetic theory of life history evolution. *Ecology* **63**, 607–615.

Lande, R. and Arnold, S. J. (1983). The measurement of selection on correlated characters. *Evolution* **37**, 1210–1226.

Lessells, C. M. (1982). Some causes and consequences of family size in the Canada goose *Branta canadensis*. D.Phil. Thesis, Oxford.

Lessells, C. M. and Boag, P. T. (1987). Unrepeatable repeatabilities: A common mistake. *Auk* **104** 116–121.

Lister, D. and McCance, R. A. (1965). The effects of two diets on the growth, reproduction and ultimate size of guinea pigs. *Br. J. Nutr.* **19**, 311.

Lynch, C. B. and Sulzbach, D. S. (1984). Quantitative genetic analysis of temperature regulation in *Mus musculus*. II. Diallel analysis of individual traits. *Evolution* **38**, 527–540.

Menard, G. (1986). A quantitative genetic approach to the study of morphological differences between marsh and upland Red-winged Blackbirds. Ph.D. Thesis, Queen's University, Canada.

Moss, R. and Watson, A. (1982). Heritability of egg size, hatch weight, body weight, and viability in red grouse (*Lagopus lagopus scoticus*). *Auk* **99**, 683–686.

Newton, I. and Marquiss, M. (1984). Seasonal trend in the breeding performance of Sparrowhawks. *J. Anim. Ecol.* **53**, 809–830.

Ojanen, M., Orell, M. and Väisänen, R. A. (1979). Role of heredity in egg size variation in the great tit *Parus major* and the pied flycatcher *Ficedula hypoleuca. Ornis Scand.* **10**, 22–28.

Orians, G. H. (1980). "Some Adaptations of Marsh-nesting Blackbirds". *Monogr. in Pop. Biol.* No 14, Princeton University Press.

Perrins, C. M. and Jones, P. J. (1974). The inheritance of clutch size in the great tit (*Parus major* L.). *Condor* **76**, 225–229.

Preston, F. W. (1974). Ancient error in a 1955 *Auk* paper. *Auk* **91**, 417–418.

Price, T. D. (1984). Sexual selection on body size, territory and plumage variables in a population of Darwin's finches. *Evolution* **38**, 327–341.

Price, T. D. and Grant, P. R. (1985). The evolution of ontogeny in Darwin's finches: A quantitative genetic approach. *Am. Natur.* **125**, 169–188.

Prince, H. H., Siegel, P. B. and Cornwell, G. W. (1970). Inheritance of egg production and juvenile growth in mallards. *Auk* **87**, 342–352.

Ricklefs, R. E. (1977). Variation in size and quality of the Starling egg. *Auk* **94**, 167–168.

Ricklefs, R. E. (1984). Components of variance in measurements of nestling European Starlings (*Sturnus vulgaris*) in southeastern Pennsylvania. *Auk* **101**, 319–333.

Ricklefs, R. E. and Peters, S. (1981). Parental components of variance in growth rate and body size of nestling European starlings (*Sturnus vulgaris*) in eastern Pennsylvania. *Auk* **98**, 39–48.

Rising, J. D. (1983). The Great Plains hybrid zones. *In* "Current Ornithology" (ed. R. F. Johnston), Vol. 1, pp. 131–157. Plenum Press, New York.

Rose, M. R. (1982). Antagonistic pleiotropy, dominance, and genetic variation. *Heredity* **48**, 63–78.

Roughgarden, J. (1979). "Theory of Population Genetics and Evolutionary Ecology". Macmillan, New York.

Smith, J. N. M. (1981). Does high fecundity reduce survival in Song Sparrows? *Evolution* **35**, 1142–1148.

Smith, J. N. M. and Dhondt, A. A. (1980). Experimental confirmation of heritable morphological variation in a natural population of song sparrows. *Evolution* **34**, 1155–1158.

Smith, J. N. M. and Zach, R. (1979). Heritability of some morphological characters in the song sparrow. *Evolution* **33**, 460–467.

Sokal, R. R. and Rohlf, F. J. (1981). "Biometry", 2nd edn. W. H. Freeman & Co., San Francisco.

van Noordwijk, A. J. (1984a). Problems in the analysis of dispersal and a critique on its "heritability" in the great tit. *J. Anim. Ecol.* **53**, 533–544.

van Noordwijk, A. J. (1984b). Quantitative genetics in natural populations of birds illustrated with examples from the Great Tit (*Parus major*). *In* "Population Biology and Evolution" (eds K. Wöhrman and V. Loeschke), pp. 67–79. Springer-Verlag, Berlin.

van Noordwijk, A. J., van Balen, J. H. and Scharloo, W. (1980). Heritability of ecologically important traits in the great tit. *Ardea* **68**, 193–203.

van Noordwijk, A. J., van Balen, J. H. and Scharloo, W. (1985). Heritability of body size in a natural population of the Great Tit and its relation to age and environmental conditions during growth (unpublished work).

van Noordwijk, A. J. and Klerks, P. L. M. (1983). Heritability of bill dimensions in the Great Tit. *Verh. Kon. Ned. Akad. Wetensch., Afd. Natuurk. 2e reeks 81 Prog. Rep. I.O.O. 7–12.*

van Noordwijk, A. J. and Scharloo, W. (1981). Inbreeding in an island population of the Great Tit. *Evolution* **35**, 674–688.

van Noordwijk, A. J., van Tienderen, P. H. and de Jong, G. (1985). Genealogical evidence for random mating in a natural population of the Great Tit (*Parus major*) *Naturwissenschaften* **72**, 104–106.

3
Chromosomal Variation

Gerald F. Shields

Institute of Arctic Biology and Department of Biology, Fisheries and Wildlife, University of Alaska, Fairbanks, Alaska 99775, USA

AVIAN GENETICS
ISBN 0-12-187570-9

1 INTRODUCTION

Mutations are either genic or chromosomal. The former involve changes at the level of the nucleotide and constitute the major theme of this book. The latter are the domain of the cytogeneticist, who studies form, function and evolution of chromosomes and the numerous variations of these properties as they relate to recombination, transmission and expression of genes.

Because birds, like humans, are largely diurnal and communicate by sight and sound, they have been attractive organisms on which to test hypotheses concerning evolution, behaviour and ecology. In many ways birds are among the best studied animals and many classic studies of them underlie important areas of biological theory. In contrast to the relatively complete description of avian natural history is the woeful lack of sound descriptive cytogenetics for birds. Only about 6% of the 8900 extant species of birds have been karyotyped and most of these have not been done in detail (Shields 1980, 1982, 1983 a). By comparison, about 40% of the 4200 species of mammals have been karyotyped, many in large numbers, and numerous studies of intraspecific variability in chromosomes have been reported using the new differential staining ("banding") techniques. Thus, we are faced with only a rudimentary understanding of the structural diversity and evolution of the chromosomes of birds.

The lack of detailed data upon which reliable interpretations can be made concerning the evolution of the chromosomes of birds is partially due to the fact that most bird chromosomes are minute, and their number and morphology are obscure. Further, the development of methods of chromosome preparation and analysis specific to birds has lagged behind those for other groups, particularly mammals. Despite these difficulties, the field of avian cytogenetics has recently experienced renewed interest; more than 70% of all species karyotyped have been studied in the past ten years. This may be due, in part, to the fact that many hypotheses concerning the mode of chromosome evolution in other taxa are untested for the class Aves.

We know nothing about the chromosomes of species in 61 avian families. It is hoped that this summary will provoke new excitement in this long neglected aspect of the biology of birds.

2 CYTOGENETICS

The initial goal of the cytogeneticist is to describe the chromosome complement of each individual under study in as much detail as possible. Enlarged photographs of chromosomes on microscope slides constitute the raw material of the karyotypic description. Chromosomes are counted and identified as homologous sets where traditionally the largest set of chromosomes is placed first in the karyotype and the smallest is last. In conventionally stained material, chromosomes are paired according to their total lengths as well as the location of their centromeres. Additionally, features such as secondary constrictions (the locations of nucleolar organizer regions), and dimorphic sex chromosomes (see below) are also used. Recent procedures which result in the longitudinal differential banding of chromosomes (see below) allow for even more detailed analyses.

A species is judged to be monomorphic in karyotype if all individuals studied possess both the same diploid, $2n$, chromosome number and sets of homologous chromosomes which appear to be identical. Variation in karyotype can be either numerical or structural; the former is relatively obvious, the latter may be more difficult to verify. In either case the population under study can possess fixed variation (no heterozygotes) or floating variation (the existence of three variant types including the two homozygotes as well as the heterozygote). If only homozygotes are found (and verification of this fact may require large sample sizes) then, presumably, hybrids between the two structural types are not successful. The presence of heterozygotes attests to the fact that hybridization has taken place and that at least some heterozygotes are successful. The presence of fixed variation in chromosomes is of interest to the cytogeneticist since it is present-day evidence for a viable chromosomal mutation which occurred in the phylogeny of the group under study. Floating polymorphisms are of equal interest since they indicate that heterozygotes are at least successful. Further, they provide individuals in which the effects of hybrid meiosis might be studied. Identification of chromosome variants and the study of their survival constitute a significant portion of classical cytogenetic theory. The reader is referred to Dobzhansky (1970) and White (1973, 1978) for more detail.

3 KARYOTYPES

3.1 Problems inherent in avian karyology

A prerequisite to comparative karyology, the study of the chromosomes of closely related species, is that each chromosome can be identified and counted. This is particularly difficult for birds since most species possess large numbers of minute microchromosomes which are barely visible by light microscopy. Methods of preparation involve either manual squashing or air drying of isolated cells, each of which can result in excessive spreading of chromosomes on slides and the resultant loss of microchromosomes.

Conversely, weak squashing or reduced air drying may result in spreads in which microchromosomes are overlapped by larger chromosomes and thus go undetected in analyses. Aside from the development of good spreading procedures in the laboratory, which may have to be perfected individually for each species, a partial solution to this problem lies in the accumulation of many metaphase nuclei for each individual studied. Again this is problematic since for the most part large sample sizes of spreads for each individual necessitate the establishment of cells in culture; this may require that birds be killed for tissue extraction. Further, many species of birds can be obtained only in remote areas where tissue culture facilities are not available. It is not surprising, then, that most birds which have been karyotyped are those which are most easily captured and maintained in captivity until cell cultures can be established from their tissues.

Given the difficulties associated with the analysis of microchromosomes, most researchers simply work with small sample sizes and report a range of variation in diploid numbers. It is rather amazing that no one has yet devoted the time and effort necessary to assess the extent of true variation in diploid number for any wild species of bird (Shields 1983 a).

When large sample sizes are available, several methods have been suggested (Shields 1983 a) to ensure accurate analysis. These include meiotic studies and differential chromosome banding procedures. Once a large number ($n \geqslant 100$) of metaphase spreads is obtained one attempts not only to count the chromosomes but to separate them into homologous pairs. This can be done relatively easily for the macrochromosomes but is very difficult with microchromosomes even if differential banding is performed. Thus, most researchers assess variability only in the macrochromosomes.

Homologous chromosomes are paired by identity in length, centromere location and differential banding pattern. No standardized nomenclature for the chromosomes of wild birds has been proposed, but most authors arrange the chromosomes in decreasing order of size rather than by centromeric index (Levan *et al.* 1964). Most studies of the chromosomes of birds report a range of variation in diploid number and thus precise assessment of variation for individuals and even for species is difficult.

Polymorphism within populations and differences in karyotypes between species are very difficult to identify because of the large number of microchromosomes and their similar appearance. Further, most macro-chromosomes are of similar length, thus only obvious changes such as large pericentric inversions can be detected readily by conventional staining.

Polymorphism in macrochromosomes has been reported in 15 species of birds (see section on intraspecific variation) but most of these studies are based on small sample sizes and are accompanied neither by meiotic analyses nor differential banding procedures. The best known cases of intraspecific chromosome polymorphism are those of the White-throated Sparrow (*Zonotrichia albicollis*) by Thorneycroft (1966, 1968, 1975) and species of junco (*Junco* spp.) by Shields (1973, 1976) and Rising and Shields (1980).

Comparisons of the karyotypes of closely related species of birds are infrequent, but progress is being made (de Lucca and de Aguiar 1978, de Boer 1976, Ryttman *et al.* 1979, Hobert *et al.* 1982, Stock and Bunch 1982, de Boer and van Brink 1982).

3.2 Methods

3.2.1 Cell culture

As stated earlier, a prerequisite to accurate analysis of the chromosomes of birds is a large number of metaphase spreads which can be analysed in detail. Of the various methods for obtaining chromosomes of birds, the culture of fibroblasts offers many advantages (Shields 1983 a). For example, kidneys or whole embryos can be established in culture and harvested when maximum growth rates have been reached. Subcultures of the originals can be maintained as the need arises. Embryonic fibroblasts in log-growth phase can be harvested and fixed, and their chromosomes dropped on to slides and air dried (Shields 1983 a). These procedures routinely provide hundreds of well-spread metaphase and prometaphase nuclei which can then be subjected to any of the currently employed differential banding procedures.

Analysis of chromosomes obtained from the pulp of growing feathers is almost always inferior because cells in division are few and difficult to squash. The culture of lymphocytes from whole blood is also less satisfactory since the culture is terminated with the harvest of cells. Neither of the above procedures allows the flexibility afforded by the culture of fibroblasts.

3.2.2 Differential banding procedures

(*a*) *Discovery*. In 1970 it was felt that most of the significant observations in the field of cytogenetics had already been made. Since that time, however, a revolution in methodology has occurred. Casperson *et al.* (1969) synthesized the alkylating agent, quinacrine mustard, attached it to a fluorochrome molecule and produced differential fluorescent crossbands along the length of plant chromosomes. It is now known that the patterns of crossbands are specific to high concentrations of A–T base pairs, thus the distribution of DNA along each chromosome is non-random and banding patterns for each chromosome are unique. This procedure, and the others that followed, revolutionized the field of cytogenetics. It was then possible to characterize

FOX SPARROW, ♂

G BANDS

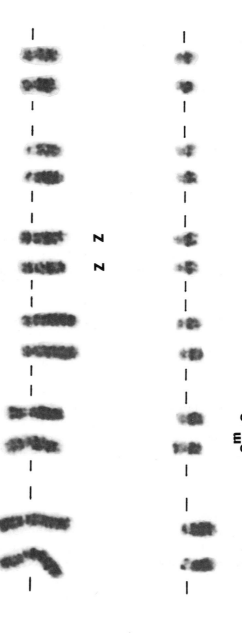

Fig. 1. Partial karyotype of a male Fox Sparrow demonstrating the extra piece of chromatin on the short arm of chromosome 8^m (m = metacentric). Only the largest twelve chromosomes are shown; z = sex chromosomes of the male.

and pair homologous chromosomes, and Casperson *et al.* (1970) soon described the quinacrine mustard (QM) band pattern for each human chromosome. Not only did these procedures allow proper characterization of homologous chromosomes, but they further advanced insight into the molecular basis of chromosome structure (Shields 1983 b). Q banding has not been widespread in the study of avian chromosomes but see de Boer and Belterman (1981).

(*b*) *Giemsa (G) banding.* Application of the quinacrine procedures was short-lived, probably because they required relatively expensive fluorescence microscopy (Hsu 1979) and because fluorescent banding patterns are unstable (Schweizer 1981). When air-dried chromosomes are treated with buffered trypsin and then exposed to Giemsa stain, crossbands result (Sumner *et al.* 1971, Patil *et al.* 1971, Drets and Shaw 1971). Positive (dark) G bands indicate high AT content, while negative (light) G bands indicate high GC content. These techniques have been widely used by cytogeneticists in general because they are diagnostic, inexpensive and relatively simple. Although only about 35 species of birds have been G banded, these procedures hold great promise not only in identifying homologous chromosomes but also in determining the bases of various chromosomal rearrangements (see Fig. 1; Shields 1983 a).

(*c*) *C banding.* Metaphase chromosomes treated with HCl and exposed to BaOH exhibit distinctive clusters of bands (Sumner 1972). Positive C bands are known to be areas of constitutive (permanently inert) heterochromatin. The W chromosome of female birds appears to be partially or even totally heterochromatic and thus exhibits extensive C band positive regions. Because of the small size of the W chromosome and its propensity to be C band positive in most birds, unequivocal identifications of W chromosomes can now be made. Application of C banding to autosomes will determine if modification of chromosome length and centromere position is based on additions or deletions of constitutive heterochromatin or whether it is caused by rearrangement in euchromatic areas. Rearrangement in chromosomes 2 and 5 of species of junco do not involve additions or deletions of heterochromatin (Shields 1983 a).

(*d*) *R banding.* Crossbanding opposite to G bands can be induced by exposing chromosomes to a hot phosphate buffer and staining in Giemsa (Dutrillaux and Lejeune 1971). When used in combination, G and R banding give complementary patterns. Moreover, telomeric (terminal) chromosome segments tend to be GC rich and are thus R band positive. R banding is essentially unexploited in chromosome studies of birds, but see Carlenius *et al.* (1981).

(*e*) *NOR banding.* When chromosome preparations are stained with borate buffer and aqueous silver nitrate, nucleolus organizer regions are stained with silver (Bloom and Goodpasture 1976). Nucleolus organizer regions (NORs) are templates of ribosomal RNA cistrons. Since NORs are achromatic, they are diagnostic chromosome markers. They are difficult to detect by conventional staining since they constitute only a secondary constriction which cannot be seen when terminal. Silver staining is specific for all NORs whether terminal or interstitial. Silver staining has not been widely exploited by avian cytogeneticists.

(*f*) *Silver staining of meiotic bivalents.* Pathak and Hsu (1979) have developed a methodology whereby synaptonemal complexes are stained with silver. Synaptonemal complexes are interchromosome layers of protein laid down before the pairing of homologous chromosomes. This procedure has great potential for avian cytogenetics in that it reveals the orientation of predivision meiotic chromatids, whether normal or rearranged, and in the latter case can indicate predisposition to both normal and abnormal divisions. Silver staining of meiotic chromosomes of male Cotton Rat (*Sigmodon fulviventes*) showed proper orientation of a paired trivalent despite the fact that the individual was heterozygous for a centric fusion (Elder and Pathak 1980). Proper orientation in this case suggests the potential for normal disjunction, which possibly accounts for high fertility despite the fusion. This technique has rarely been used for any group of organisms, but has great applicability, since information concerning division products of heterozygous bivalents will promote our understanding of the levels of selection that operate during meiosis.

Avian cytogeneticists have just begun to exploit the various differential banding procedures. When used extensively these methods will probably prove to be of even more value with birds than they have been with other groups, simply because the avian karyotype has proven so difficult to study through conventional means.

4   INTRASPECIFIC CHROMOSOME VARIANTS

4.1   White-throated Sparrow

4.1.1   Plumage polymorphism

The White-throated Sparrow is polymorphic in plumage (Lowther 1961), behaviour (Lowther 1962) and karyotype (Thorneycroft 1966, 1968, 1975). Lowther (1961) observed that the adult White-throated Sparrow in breeding plumage could be separated into two distinct phenotypes; no sex linkage was obvious. The colour of the median crown stripe (white or tan) was used to describe the morphs since this character alone was adequate to divide the species into two distinct classes. Some white-striped birds became tan in basic plumage, but they reverted to the white-striped condition during the following breeding season. Some tan-striped birds held in captivity over several years or recovered in the wild after being colour-banded and initially described as tan-striped never became white-striped. There were behavioural correlates of this plumage polymorphism. Lowther (1962) demonstrated that white-striped birds of either sex are more responsive to the playback of recorded song than are their tan-striped counterparts. He also observed non-random mating with white-striped birds of either sex mated with tan-striped birds of the opposite sex far more often than would be expected from their frequencies within the population; tan-striped × tan-striped and white-striped × white-striped matings were rare.

4.1.2 Chromosomal polymorphism

Thorneycroft (1966, 1968, 1975) described separate chromosomal poly-morphisms based on pericentric inversions in chromosomes 2 and 3. Chromosomes 2 and 3 were found to be ancestral and gave rise to chromosomes 2^m (m = metacentric) and 3^a (a = acrocentric) by separate pericentric inversions. All birds possessing at least a single 2^m chromosome were white-striped in alternate plumage (see Fig. 2); birds lacking this chromosome were tan-striped in both alternate and basic plumages. Phenotype (whether the bird was white or tan) was correlated with karyotype and the presence could be predicted without exception. No correlation was found between the presence of chromosome 3 and any obvious morphological character. Birds in first basic plumage and possessing the karyotypes 223^a3^a, $22^m3^a3^a$ and 22^m33^a were tan-striped. In most cases, the white-striped plumage is not acquired until after the first pre-alternate moult. This explains why samples taken in autumn are always composed of a higher percentage of tan-striped birds. Only the presence or absence of chromosome 2^m appears to be reflected in the bird's alternate plumage.

4.1.3 Population data and assortative mating

Nearly 400 white-throats were karyotyped in Thorneycroft's studies. Most males possessed the 22^m karyotype while most females possessed the 22 karyotype. Ninety-three per cent of all studied breeding pairs demonstrated negative assortative mating. Thus, selection for matings of opposite phenotype ensured that birds having chromosome 2 mated with birds lacking it; heterozygosity would be maintained in this way.

WHITE-THROATED SPARROW, WHITE MORPH, ♀

G BANDS

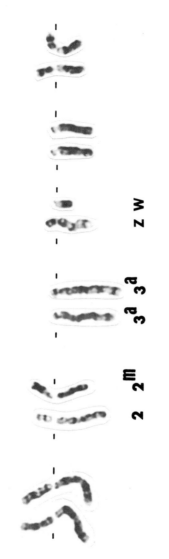
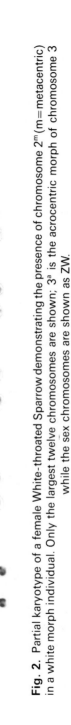

2   2ᵐ   3ᵃ 3ᵃ   Z W

Fig. 2. Partial karyotype of a female White-throated Sparrow demonstrating the presence of chromosome 2ᵐ (m=metacentric) in a white morph individual. Only the largest twelve chromosomes are shown; 3ᵃ is the acrocentric morph of chromosome 3 while the sex chromosomes are shown as ZW.

4.1.4 Transmission of chromosomes

Karyotypes of parents were compared with those of their offspring in an attempt to determine survivorship of the various chromosome morphs. Forty-two pairs of White-throats and their 108 offspring were studied. Birds with a single chromosome 2 transmitted this chromosome to about one-half (50 of 101) of their offspring, as expected. However, birds with a single chromosome 3 passed this chromosome on to only about one-fourth (11 of 41) of their offspring. This suggests selection against chromosome 3 at the gametic or zygotic level. These data suggest that chromosome 3 may be in the process of being eliminated from the population. There is, however, slight counter-selection for this chromosome in older birds ($s = 0.068$ and 0.060 in young males and females; $s = 0.074$ and 0.080 in migratory males and females). These data suggest that these birds may have a competitive advantage as juvenile or older birds, but more data are needed to resolve this issue.

4.2   Species of *Junco*

Polymorphism for chromosomes 2 and 5 occurs intraspecifically in Slate-coloured Junco (*Junco hyemalis hyemalis*), Oregon Junco (*J. h. oreganus*), Gray-headed Junco (*J. h. caniceps*) and in Mexican Junco (*J. p. phaeonotus*) (Shields 1973). With smaller samples, White-winged Junco (*J. h. aikeni*) is polymorphic only for chromosome 5 while Guadalupe Junco (*J. h. insularis*) and Volcán Junco (*J. vulcani*) possess only the standard karyotypes (2255).

Large samples, meiotic analyses (see below) and differential banding of chromosomes suggest that the basis of the polymorphisms in the juncos is two separate pericentric inversions. Comparisons with karyotypes of all species of the closely related genus *Zonotrichia* suggest that the polymorphisms in junco are unique and that chromosome 2 gave rise to chromosome 2^{sm} (sm = submetacentric) and that chromosome 5 gave rise to chromosome 5^{m} (m = metacentric).

Natural interbreeding occurs between Oregon Junco and Slate-coloured Junco and between Oregon and Gray-headed Juncos where their respective ranges overlap but White-winged Junco, Guadalupe Junco and Mexican Junco are geographically isolated and phenetically distinct. There are no recorded hybrids between northern Dark-eyed Juncos (*J. hyemalis*) and southern Yellow-eyed Juncos (*J. phaeonotus*) yet identical polymorphisms for chromosomes 2 and 5 occur in each. This suggests that the rearrangements occurred in the ancestor of these species and have been maintained subsequently in each group since divergence. Population genetic theory maintains that chromosomal rearrangements can become established only in

small populations through a random drift process (Lande 1979).
Rearrangements are generally deleterious when heterozygous, but have
normal fitness when homozygous. It is thus rather surprising that identical
polymorphisms for chromosomes 2 and 5 have been retained in species of
Junco. No obvious morphological character was correlated with the presence
of either chromosome 2 or 5 in the juncos (but see section on morphological
correlates below). Pairing appears normal in heterozygous bivalents for
chromosomes 2 and 5 in Slate-coloured Juncos but chiasma frequency is
reduced in these bivalents (Shields 1976). The inversion in chromosome 2 is
short, but the one in chromosome 5 must involve about one-half of the entire
chromosome. Either chiasmata do not normally occur or the birds have
evolved compensating mechanisms by which chiasmata do not occur within
the inversion (see section on meiotic studies).

4.3   Chromosomal and morphological correlates

Lowther (1961) hypothesized that white-striped White-throated Sparrows
may enjoy a selective advantage during nesting in areas where light-coloured
lichens are abundant; nesting females may be more cryptic than their tan-
striped counterparts. Tan-striped birds may have an advantage during
autumn migration when they might be less conspicuous to predators than
white-striped birds. No studies have tested these hypotheses, however. See
Chapter 1 for additional discussion of the White-throated Sparrow
polymorphism.

Rising and Shields (1980) correlated differences in bill size and appendage
size with karyotypic differences in both White-throated Sparrow and Slate-
coloured Junco. It was hypothesized that the variability maintained could
either be manifest in bill or foot size dimorphism associated with dominance
behaviour or with variability in structures used in foraging or food
manipulation. Differences such as these may facilitate habitat partitioning
and may well be of critical importance during winter when birds forage in
flocks and when food and perhaps roosting sites are limited, but these
hypotheses have yet to be tested in wintering flocks.

4.4   Other species

Approximately 600 species of birds have been karyotyped. Only about half of
these have been studied using advanced techniques. Of these, 16 species,
mainly passerines, have polymorphic chromosomes (see Fig. 3; Shields 1982).
Only the juncos and White-throated Sparrow have been studied in detail; the
majority of the others have been studied only at the so-called "alpha" level of

Tree Sparrow, a)7^m homozygote , b.)7^{m}7^a heterozygote, c.)G bands

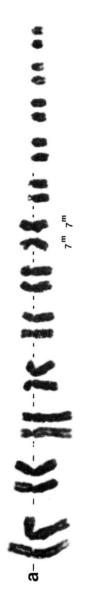

7^m 7^m

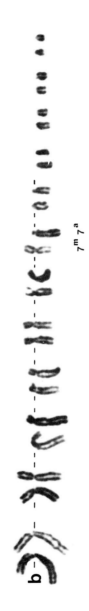

7^m 7^a

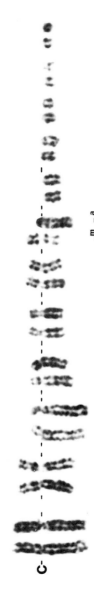

7^m 7^a

Fig. 3. Partial karyotypes of three male Tree Sparrows demonstrating the presence of the polymorphic chromosome 7. The m = metacentric and the a = acrocentric.

karyology (White 1978) in which chromosome numbers and approximate sizes of chromosomes only are determined. Twelve of the sixteen such species are passerines.

No populations of birds are known in which it has been shown that chromosomal rearrangements have become fixed.

5 MEIOTIC STUDIES

5.1 Introduction

Study of chromosomes during meiosis allows one to assess various cytological parameters relevant to chromosome behaviour, including orientation and extent of homologous pairing, chiasma frequency, behaviour at division and division products. Additionally, mutation in chromosomes can be verified or alternatively predicted from meiotic configurations (Sybenga 1975). Analysis of meiotic tissue has not been widespread in the study of the chromosomes of wild birds. This is probably because birds are meiotically active for a relatively short time and that in most cases extraction of tissue requires the birds to be killed. Ironically, Guyer's (1902) study of spermatogenesis in Rock Doves (*Columba livia*) was the first reference to bird chromosomes.

5.2 Methods

Males are preferred since large numbers of primary spermatocytes can be obtained from meiotically active birds. Some species can be induced to begin meiosis through controlled photoperiod (King *et al.* 1960) and hormonal stimulation (Thorneycroft 1968).

Methods of stimulation and extraction of meiotic tissue are given in Shields (1976). A general outline is given here. Testes are extracted and placed in distilled water at 40°C for 20 min. Tunics are broken and pieces of testis are dispersed in three changes of freshly prepared Carnoy fixative at 4°C. Dispersed tissue is then smeared on to albuminized slides, covered with a coverslip and then squashed. Coverslips can be removed in the fixative, and the slides can be air dried, stained and analysed.

5.3 White-throated Sparrow

Thorneycroft (1975) analysed meiotic tissue of male White-throated Sparrows in an attempt to verify the basis of polymorphism in chromosomes

2 and 3. In this study Thorneycroft compared standard (22, 33) males to heterozygotes for chromosomes 2 (22^m33) and 3 ($22\ 33^a$) as well as double heterozygotes (22^m33^a). Bivalents of standard males were properly oriented and possessed only terminal chiasmata in each arm. Pairing in heterozygous bivalents of (22^m33) and ($22\ 33^a$) individuals was end to end rather than throughout the length of the respective chromosomes. Chiasmata do not form between chromosome 2^m and the long arm of chromosome 2. Nor do they form between the long arms of chromosomes 3 and 3^a. Possibly the inversions in these chromosomes occur in regions where chiasma formation normally forms, or possibly they prevent pairing that would permit chiasma formation to occur in other regions of the long arms. In the latter case, recombination would be prohibited in some regions outside the limits of the inversion promoting the potential for increased divergence in genes within this linkage group. It is also of interest that both inversions, despite the considerable difference in their lengths, nonetheless result in an end-to-end pairing configuration. Chromosomes 2 and 3 constitute about 15% of the entire genome of the White-throat. In double heterozygotes a considerable portion of these uniquely paired bivalents is restricted from recombination. Double heterozygotes (22^m33^a) are rare in White-throated Sparrows (13% of males and only 4·0% of females); moreover, they cannot be identified phenotypically. Thus, nothing is known of the effects of reduced recombination in these birds.

No dicentric bridges and acentric fragments (indicative of either paracentric inversions or centric shifts) were observed by Thorneycroft. Thus, the meiotic analyses support the prediction, based on mitotic tissue, that pericentric inversions are at the basis of the chromosomal polymorphisms in the white-throat. G-band patterns of white-throats heterozygous for chromosome 2 support this conclusion (Fig. 2).

5.4 Juncos

Pairing in heterozygous bivalents ($22^{sm}5^m5^m$ and $2^{sm}2^{sm}55^m$) of juncos is normal (i.e. it is end to end) (Shields 1976). It is odd that different pairing processes occur in inverted chromosomes of such closely related sparrows. Chiasma frequencies in heterozygous bivalents of juncos are reduced. This suggests that the inversions in junco prevent pairing in regions which would normally undergo chiasma formation. Possibly the White-throats and juncos have evolved different mechanisms by which they can avoid the deleterious effects of duplication and deficient chromatids resulting from crossing over within the limits of pericentric inversions.

No bridges or fragments were observed in heterozygous bivalents of juncos

(Shields 1976) and thus pericentric inversions appear to be the basis for chromosomal polymorphism in juncos as well. Giemsa (G) banding patterns in heterozygous juncos support this conclusion (Shields, unpublished); moreover, C banding patterns in juncos (Shields 1983 a) do not suggest additions or deletions of constitutive heterochromatin in chromosomes 2 and 5.

5.5   Other species

Kaul and Ansari (1979) describe a chromosomal polymorphism in wild populations of Northern Green Barbet (*Megalaima zeylanica*) in India. A "chain" of four chromosomes in meiotic prophase tissue of a heterozygous male suggests that the polymorphism is based on an unequal translocation between the largest pair of macrochromosomes and one of the microchromosomes. These authors also suggest translocation heterozygosity in Black-headed Oriole (*Oriolus xanthornus*) (Ansari and Kaul 1979) and in Spotted Munia (*Lonchura striata*) (Ansari and Kaul 1978) but neither of these studies has been accompanied by differential chromosome banding.

5.6   Utility of technique

Aside from resolving uncertainties about chromosomal polymorphism based on mitotic tissue, meiotic studies can provide more accurate estimates of diploid numbers of birds (Shields 1983 a). Since bivalents are composed of paired chromosomes their structure is larger than individual chromosomes at metaphase of mitosis. Further, since their number is reduced by half they are easier to count. This is particularly important in species with high diploid numbers and many microchromosomes.

6   SEX CHROMOSOMES

6.1   Introduction

Ohno (1967) discusses female heterogamety and sex chromosome morphologies in birds based on the few species which had then been karyotyped by conventional methods at that time. Bloom (1973) comments on the evolution of the W chromosome in birds but no detailed review of sex chromosome evolution in birds has been attempted since the introduction of detailed differential banding techniques in 1970.

Early attempts were aimed at reconciling classical genetic results in Domestic Fowl (*Gallus domesticus*) with cytological data on chromosomes resulting from thin-sectioning (Guyer 1916). These results suggested female heterogamety (XX males and X0 female), but both monosomy for X in females and the identification of chromosome 1 as the sex chromosome were in error (Shiwago 1924).

Female heterogamety and the ZZ male, ZW female sex chromosome mechanism are now firmly established for birds. In the majority of birds, the Z chromosome is believed to be 4th or 5th in size and to comprise about 10% of the genome (Ohno 1970). Ohno (1967) has hypothesized a mechanism by which the W chromosome in female birds becomes specialized and reduced in size through inversions, chiasma formation within the inversions and consequent loss of DNA.

Exact identification of Z and W chromosomes in birds using traditional techniques is difficult, however. Since the W chromosome has been reduced in size in females of most species it consequently resembles any of the numerous microchromosomes which range from $1 \mu m$ or less in size. In some studies, the sex of the individual karyotyped is not known and the simple presence of an unpaired macrochromosome (Z?) is used to supposedly identify the individual as female.

It now seems clear that the C band procedure of Sumner (1972) can be used as a diagnostic test for the W chromosome in birds (Shields 1983 a). The C band procedure is specific for constitutive heterochromatin; a differential loss of DNA accompanies the treatment and the heterochromatic DNA of the W chromosome is preserved (Hsu 1979). This procedure results in darkly stained regions of heterochromatin and lightly stained regions of euchromatin, thus the W chromosome can be readily identified (Shields *et al.* 1982, Shields 1983 a).

6.2   Comparative studies

6.2.1   Woodpeckers

Ohno (1967, 1970) has proposed that the Z chromosome of birds has retained its original morphology and refers to it as the "original Z" to emphasize its conservative evolution. As more species are studied using current methodology, it appears that the morphology of the Z (and W) chromosomes has not remained constant in several lineages. Such observations are relevant to questions of phylogeny and whether major groups of birds have had monophyletic or polyphyletic origins.

All species of the order Piciformes which have been karyotyped have enlarged sex chromosomes (Shields *et al.* 1982). These include representatives of the families *Picidae* (Kaul and Ansari 1978, Shields *et al.* 1982), *Capitonidae* (Kaul and Ansari 1978, 1979) and *Ramphastidae* (Takagi and Sasaki 1980).

In each of the thirteen species that have been studied, the Z chromosome is the largest of the complement. The absence of extensive C banding on Z chromosomes of Lesser Spotted Woodpecker (*Dendrocopus minor*) suggests that the enlargement process was not accompanied by additions of large amounts of heterochromatin (Shields *et al.* 1982). Descriptions of the mechanism by which Z chromosomes in these species became enlarged must await detailed G- (Giemsa) and R- (reverse) banding studies.

Considerable controversy exists regarding the phylogenetic affinities of taxa within the Piciformes. Olson (1983) has consistently argued for a polyphyletic origin for the group, based on fossil remains. Simpson and Cracraft (1981) and Raikow and Cracraft (1983) support a monophyletic origin based on similarity of derived character states. The presence of enlarged Z chromosomes in representative species of three families within the Piciformes argues strongly for a monophyletic origin within the group; it is not likely that enlarged Z chromosomes arose independently at different times within this group.

6.2.2   Other taxa

Enlarged Z chromosomes are not unique to the Piciformes. Karyotypes of 20 species of the family *Accipitridae* (Falconiformes) have been described (Takagi and Sasaki 1974, de Boer 1976, Misra and Srivastava 1976, Williams and Benirschke 1976); each possesses enlarged Z and W chromosomes. Enlarged sex chromosomes have also been observed in three species of lark (*Alaudidae*) by Bulatova (pers. comm.) and in Black-legged Seriema (*Chunga burmeisteri*) (Takagi and Sasaki 1980). I know of no case for birds in which Z chromosomes are enlarged while W chromosomes are not. These preliminary data suggest that a coordinated mechanism of enlargement operates on both Z and W chromosomes of birds. The presence of enlarged Z chromosomes in four diverse orders of birds casts some doubt on the validity of Ohno's original hypothesis on the conservative nature of the Z chromosome.

6.2.3   The ratites

Takagi *et al.* (1972) were unable to differentiate Z and W chromosomes in female specimens of Ostrich (*Struthio camelus*), Australian Cassowary (*Casuarius casuarius*), Emu (*Dromicius novaehollandiae*) and Greater Rhea (*Rhea americana*). Slight, but consistent, length differences have been observed in homologues of chromosome 4 of females of these species (Takagi *et al.* 1972, Takagi and Sasaki 1974, de Boer 1980); homologues for chromosome 4 in males appear identical. It is possible that Z and W chromosomes of ratites have remained in an early stage of morphological differentiation.

It is difficult to describe evolutionary patterns of sex chromosome change in birds in general because modern differential banding techniques have been systematically used in only a few groups. Application of these new procedures over a broad range of taxa would certainly help to elucidate patterns of sex chromosome evolution in birds.

7 KARYOLOGY OF CLOSELY RELATED SPECIES

7.1 Introduction

White (1978) has used comparisons of karyotypes of closely related species of animals and plants to draw inferences about the mechanisms by which populations might become reproductively isolated from one another. Comparison of karyotypes of different species can be used to trace phylogenies. Correlation of extents of chromosome change with morphological variation within taxa have led to inferences concerning the way genes are regulated (Wilson *et al.* 1974). Finally, variation in chromosomes within lineages has been associated with the predicted age of these lineages based on fossil remains to compute rates of chromosome change through time. Birds have not been included in most of these analyses since reliable data for most groups of birds are lacking.

7.2 Chromosomal speciation

If the karyotypes of closely related species are different then one might infer that change in chromosomes might have been involved in the initial reproductive isolation of the groups. Such inferences are fraught with difficulties, however (Shields 1982). In an attempt to assess the degree to which chromosome change may have played a role in avian speciation karyotypes of congeneric bird species were compared in terms of differences in diploid numbers, relative chromosome lengths and centromeric indices. In conventionally stained material, these methods should be relatively sensitive to unequal translocations, Robertsonian fissions and fusions, centric transpositions and pericentric inversions. They are insensitive to paracentric inversions and equal translocations. The analysis (Shields 1982) included 140 species within 12 orders of birds. Nearly half of these species were passerines. All possible pairwise comparisons within a genus were made. Seventy-eight of the possible 177 species pairs had identical karyotypes. Tegelstrom *et al.* (1983) have arrived at a similar conclusion. Based on this relatively small sample it seems that most closely related bird species do not differ in these aspects of the karyotype. The conservative nature of evolution of bird chromosomes is also demonstrated by identical G-banded karyotypes of four species of gull (Ryttman *et al.* 1979). Biederman (personal communication) could find no variation in G-band patterns on chromosomes of four species of owls. Van Tuinen (personal communication) found identical G-band patterns of the 12 largest autosomes of five species of turaco (Musophagiformes). Only a few groups of closely related species have been studied through the use of G banding and it appears that chromosome change has not been involved in the promotion of reproductive isolation within these groups.

7.3   Rates of chromosome change

Shields (1980) used the methodology of Bush *et al.* (1977) to demonstrate that the rate of chromosome change among congeneric species of passerine birds was faster ($r = 0.144$) than that for non-passerines ($r = 0.026$). Prager and Wilson (1980) and Tegelstrom *et al.* (1983) have arrived at essentially the same conclusion. Rates of fixation of chromosomal rearrangement are most likely dependent, at least in part, on long-term effective deme sizes (Barrowclough and Shields 1984) and are discussed below.

7.4   Karyotypic comparisons at higher taxonomic levels

Virtually identical karyotypes can be found in distantly related taxa. Conversely, large karyotypic differences may exist in species of birds which are by other criteria considered to be closely related. It follows, then, that the degree of karyotypic resemblance or difference may or may not be a direct reflection of phylogenetic relationship. Among the 30 species of waterfowl studied by conventional staining the diploid numbers range from 80 to 84. Chromosome change was detected in only two species pairs (Shields 1982). No other reasonably well-studied group of birds exhibits such marked conservatism in rate of chromosome change. The relative ease by which waterfowl form interspecific hybrids may be based, in part, upon their extreme similarity in karyotype. Interestingly, species within the genus *Aix* are not known to hybridize. They also differ in karyotype.

On the other hand, de Boer (1976) noted extreme karyotypic dissimilarity between the Falconidae and the Accipitridae. Species of *Falco* have low (50–52) diploid numbers, and only chromosome 1 is biarmed. By contrast, 14 genera of the family Accipitridae have moderately high diploid numbers (60–80) while most of their chromosomes are biarmed. This extent of dissimilarity in karyotype between families within an order is unparalleled among birds. It may suggest a polyphyletic origin for the groups as proposed by Voous (1972) on anatomical grounds.

Stock and Bunch (1982) have used G and C banding on macro-chromosomes of eight species of Galliform birds belonging to four families. The significance of this study is that G-band patterns were determined from elongated prometaphase chromosomes whose bands are distinct. Chromosomes at midmetaphase are highly contracted and bands that otherwise appear discrete become fused into blocks of bands which then appear identical. Procedures for obtaining prometaphase material are discussed by Shields (1983 a). Stock and Bunch (1982) determined that the Galliform species differed largely by chromosome fusions and by pericentric inversions. Fissions and paracentric inversions were rare while translocations and centric transpositions were not detected. Significant additions and deletions of C-band heterochromatin were also detected. It is important that current methods be used on closely related species (Shields 1983 a) since conclusions based on conventional methods are so unreliable.

8   CHROMOSOME CHANGE AND POPULATION STRUCTURE

Recent observations based on demography (Barrowclough 1980), electrophoresis (Barrowclough 1983) and karyology (Shields 1982) suggest that the mechanisms by which species of birds become reproductively isolated from one another may be somewhat different from those of other vertebrate groups.

Barrowclough (1983) has summarized data on electrophoretic patterns in birds and concludes that, while the amount of genic variation within species examined is of the same order of magnitude as is that of other vertebrates, the among-population component of genetic variance is low. This suggests, for example, that conspecific populations of birds are more similar to one another genetically than are conspecific populations of mammals. Barrowclough (1983) suggests that the small among-population component of genetic variance may be due to gene flow as a consequence of the high vagility of birds (but see Wyles *et al.* 1983; Shields and Wilson 1987).

Templeton (1980 a,b) concludes that populations clustered in small demes and having large among-population components of genic variance will exhibit large genetic distances. Conversely, genetic distances will be small when populations are large and experience considerable gene flow. Barrowclough's (1983) data suggest that birds have large, panmictic populations. Templeton (1980 b) has associated the relative probabilities for various types of speciation with the particular type of population structure under consideration. The data for birds suggest that since their populations appear relatively large their speciation will be characterized by adaptive divergence and/or genetic transilience (Templeton 1980 b) which involves a strongly epistatic polygenic system in which changes in a few major genes occur. The latter process would seem to be supported by the low among-population component for genic variance in birds.

Estimates of long-term effective population sizes for birds can also be made from information on the rates of karyotypic change (Lande 1979). The assumptions of Lande's procedure are that individuals heterozygous for a chromosome change are at a selective disadvantage and that new mutations can become fixed only through a process of random genetic drift. One can use the rate of fixation of changes in chromosomes, then, to work backwards to estimate, N, the long-term effective population size of birds.

Using available data on chromosome variation in birds, primarily those of de Boer (1980), de Boer and van Brink (1982), Stock and Bunch (1982), Shields (1982) and Jo (1983), Barrowclough and Shields (1984) have estimated fixation rates, R, and used Lande's equations to estimate deme size. These estimates indicate that effective population sizes for species studied are about 100. Estimates for mammals and species of *Drosophila* (Lande 1979) are 30–200 and 200–800, respectively. Although more data are needed on fixation rates for birds, our data suggest that most populations of birds are not continuously small and prone to inbreeding. Thus, chromosomal speciation, whether stasipatric (White 1978) or otherwise, should not be common in birds.

9 SUMMARY

It is remarkable that our understanding of the structure and evolution of the chromosomes of birds is so limited. A full array of modern cytogenetic techniques is now available and while it will be impossible to study the chromosomes of birds in as detailed a fashion as, say, those of insects or mammals many important observations are yet to be made. For example, detailed population studies are needed in order that we might assess the true range of variability in chromosomes within species. The exceptional studies of Stock and Bunch (1982) have indicated that differential banding of chromosomes can be used to more accurately assess variation in chromosomes of closely related Galliform birds; similar studies are needed in other groups. We know very little about the evolution of sex chromosomes in birds; a survey of selected species of various orders using current banding techniques would certainly be rewarding. Finally, there is a need to coordinate studies of chromosomes with studies at the molecular level. Without the detail of molecular studies our observations at the chromosome level will be only superficial at best. It is hoped that this survey stimulates renewed interest.

REFERENCES

Ansari, H. A. and Kaul, D. (1978). Translocation heterozygosity in the bird (*Lonchura punctulata* (Linn.)) (Ploceidae: Aves). *Natl Acad. Sci. Lett.* **1**, 83–85.

Ansari, H. A. and Kaul, D. (1979). Somatic chromosomes of black-headed oriole (*Oriolus xanthornis*) (Linn.): A probable case of translocation heterozygosity. *Experientia* **35**, 740–741.

Barrowclough, G. F. (1980). Gene flow, effective population sizes, and genetic variance components in birds. *Evolution* **34**, 789–798.

Barrowclough, G. F. (1983). Biochemical studies of microevolutionary processes. *In* "Perspectives in Ornithology" (eds A. H. Brush and G. A. Clark Jr), pp. 223–261. Cambridge University Press, New York.

Barrowclough, G. F. and Shields, G. F. (1984). Karyotypic evolution and long-term effective population sizes of birds. *Auk* **101**, 99–102.

Bloom, S. E. (1973). Current knowledge about the W chromosome of birds. *Avian Chromo. Newsletter*, Vol. II, 1–15.

Bloom, S. E. and Goodpasture, C. (1976). An improved technique for selective silver staining of nucleolar organizer regions in human chromosomes. *H. Genetics* **34**, 199–206.

Bush, G. L., Case, S. M., Wilson, A. C. and Patton, J. L. (1977). Rapid speciation and chromosomal evolution in mammals. *Proc. Natl Acad. Sci. USA* **74**, 3942–3946.

Carlenius, C., Ryttman, H., Tegelstrom, H. and Jansson, H. (1981). R-, G-, and C-banded chromosomes of the domestic fowl (*Gallus domesticus*). *Hereditas* **94**, 61–66.

Casperson, T., Zech, L. and Johanson, C. (1970). Differential banding of alkylating fluorochromes in human chromosomes. *Exp. Cell Res.* **60**, 315–319.

Casperson, T., Zech, L., Modest, E. J., Foley, G. E. and Wagh, U. (1969). Chemical differentiation with fluorescent alkylating agents in *Vicia faba* metaphase chromosomes. *Exp. Cell Res.* **58**, 128–140.

de Boer, L. E. M. (1976). The somatic chromosome complements of 16 species of Falconiformes (Aves) and the karyological relationships of the order. *Genetica* **46**, 77–113.

de Boer, L. E. M. (1980). Do the chromosomes of the kiwi provide evidence for a monophyletic origin of the ratites? *Nature* **287**, 84–85.

de Boer, L. E. M. and van Brink, J. M. (1982). Cytotaxonomy of the Ciconiiformes (Aves), with karyotypes of eight species new to cytology. *Cytogenet. Cell Genet.* **34**, 19–34.

de Boer, L. E. M. and Belterman, R. H. R. (1981). Chromosome banding studies of the Razor-billed Curassow, *Crax mitu* (Aves, Galliformes: Cracidae). *Genetica* **54**, 225–232.

de Lucca, E. J. and de Aquiar, M. L. R. (1978). A karyosystematic study in Columbiformes (Aves). *Cytologia* **43**, 249–253.

Dobzhansky, Th. (1970). "Genetics of the Evolutionary Process". Columbia University Press, New York.

Drets, M. E. and Shaw, M. W. (1971). Specific banding patterns of human chromosomes. *Proc. Natl Acad. Sci. USA* **68**, 2073–2077.

Dutrillaux, B. and Lejeune, J. (1971). Sur une nouvelle technique d'analyse du caryotype humain. *C. R. Acad. Sci., Paris* **272**, 2638–2640.

Elder, F. F. B. and Pathak, S. (1980). Light microscopic observations of the behavior of silver-stained trivalents in pachytene cells of *Sigmodon fulviventer* (Rodentia, Muridae) heterozygous for centric fusion. *Cytogenet. Cell Genet.* **27**, 31–38.

Guyer, M. F. (1902). Spermatogenesis of normal and hybrid pigeons. *Univ. Cincinnati Bull.* **22**, 1–61.

Guyer, M. F. (1916). Studies on the chromosomes of the common fowl as seen in testes and in embryos. *Biol. Bull.* **31**, 221–268.

Hobart, H. H., Gunn, S. J. and Bickham, J. W. (1982). Karyotypes of six species of North American blackbirds (Icteridae: Passeriformes). *Auk* **99**, 514–518.

Hsu, T. C. (1979). "Human and Mammalian Cytogenetics: An Historical Perspective". Springer-Verlag, New York.

Jo, N. (1983). Karyotypic analysis of Darwin's finches. *In* "Patterns of Evolution in Gallapagos Organisms" (eds R. I. Bowman, M. Bersom and A. I. Leviton), pp. 201–217. American Association for the Advancement of Science, San Francisco.

Kaul, D. and Ansari, H. A. (1978). Chromosome studies in three species of Piciformes (Aves). *Genetica* **48**, 193–196.

Kaul, D. and Ansari, H. A. (1979). Chromosomal polymorphism in a natural population of the Northern Green Barbet, *Megalaima zeylancia caniceps* (Franklin) (Piciformes: Aves). *Genetica* **49**, 1–5.

King, J. R., Mewaldt, L. R. and Farner, D. S. (1960). The duration of postnuptial metabolic refractoriness in the White-crowned Sparrow. *Auk* **77**, 89–92.

Lande, R. (1979). Effective deme sizes during long-term evolution estimates from rates of chromosomal rearrangement. *Evolution* **33**, 234–251.

Levan, A., Fredga, K. and Sandberg, A. (1964). Nomenclature for centromeric position on chromosomes. *Hereditas* **52**, 201–220.

Lowther, J. K. (1961). Polymorphism in the White-throated Sparrow, *Zonotrichia albicollis* (Gmelin). *Can. J. Zool.* **39**, 281–292.

Lowther, J. K. (1962). Colour and behavioral polymorphism in the White-throated Sparrow, *Zonotrichia albicollis* (Gmelin). Ph.D. Diss., University of Toronto.

Misra, M. and Srivastava, M. D. L. (1976). The karyotypes of two species of Falconiformes. *Cytologia* **41**, 313–317.

Ohno, S. (1967). "Sex Chromosomes and Sex-linked Genes" (eds A. Labhart, T. Mann and L. T. Sammuels). Vol. I. Monographs of Endocrinology. Springer, Berlin–Heidelberg–New York.

Ohno, S. (1970). "Evolution by Gene Duplication". Springer, Berlin–Heidelberg–New York.

Olson, S. (1983). Evidence for a polyphyletic origin of the Piciformes. *Auk* **100**, 126–133.

Pathak, S. and Hsu, T. C. (1979). Silver-stained structure in mammalian meiotic prophase. *Chromosoma* **70**, 195–203.

Patil, S. R., Merrick, S. and Lubs, H. A. (1971). Identification of each human chromosome with a modified Giemsa stain. *Science* **173**, 821–822.

Prager, E. and Wilson, A. C. (1980). Phylogenetic relationships and rates of evolution in birds. *Proc. XVII Int. Ornithol. Congr.*, pp. 1209–1214. Verlag der Deutschen Ornithologen-Gesellschaft (Berlin).

Raikow, R. and Cracraft, J. (1983). Monophyly of the Piciformes: A reply to Olson. *Auk* **100**, 134–138.

Rising, J. D. and Shields, G. F. (1980). Chromosomal and morphological correlates in two new world sparrows (Emberizidae). *Evolution* **34**, 654–662.

Ryttman, H., Tegelstrom, H. and Jansson, H. (1979). G and C banding in four related *Larus* species (Aves). *Hereditas* **91**, 143–148.

Schweizer, D. (1981). Counterstain-enhanced chromosome banding. *Hum. Genet.* **57**, 1–14.

Shields, G. F. (1973). Chromosomal polymorphism common to several species of *Junco* (Aves). *Can. J. Genet. Cytol.* **15**, 461–471.

Shields, G. F. (1976). Meiotic evidence for pericentric inversion polymorphism in *Junco* (Aves). *Can. J. Genet. Cytol.* **18**, 747–751.

Shields, G. F. (1980). Avian cytogenetics: new methodology and comparative results. *Proc. XVII Int. Ornithol. Cong.* (1978), pp. 1226–1231. Verlag der Deutschen Ornithologen-Gessellschaft (Berlin).

Shields, G. F. (1982). Comparative avian cytogenetics: a review. *Condor* **84**, 45–58.

Shields, G. F. (1983 a). Bird chromosomes. *In* "Current Ornithology" (ed. R. F. Johnston), Vol. I, pp. 189–209. Plenum Press, New York.

Shields, G. F. (1983 b). Organization of the avian genome. *In* "Perspectives in Ornithology" (eds A. H. Brush and G. A. Clark Jr), pp. 271–290. Cambridge University Press, New York.

Shields, G. F., Jarrell, G. H. and Redrupp, E. (1982). Enlarged sex chromosomes of Woodpeckers (Piciformes). *Auk* **99**, 767–771.

Shields, G. F. and Wilson, A. C. (1987). Calibration of mitochondrial DNA evolution in geese. *J. Mol. Evol.* **24**, 212–217.

Shiwago, P. J. (1924). The chromosome complexes in the somatic cells of male and female of the domestic chicken. *Science* **60**, 45–46.

Simpson, S. F. and Cracraft, J. (1981). The phylogenetic relationships of the Piciformes (Class Aves). *Auk* **98**, 481–494.

Stock, A. D. and Bunch, T. D. (1982). The evolutionary implications of chromosome banding pattern homologies in the bird order Galliformes. *Cytogenet. Cell Genet.* **34**, 136–148.

Sumner, A. T. (1972). A simple technique for demonstrating centromeric heterochromatin. *Exp. Cell Res.* **75**, 304–306.

Sumner, A. T., Evans, H. J. and Buckland, R. A. (1971). A new technique for distinguishing between human chromosomes. *Nature New Biology* **232**, 31–32.

Sybenga, J. (1975). "Meiotic Configurations". Springer-Verlag, New York.

Takagi, N., Itoh, M. and Sasaki, M. (1972). Chromosome studies in four species of Ratitae (Aves). *Chromosoma* **36**, 281–291.

Takagi, N. and Sasaki, M. (1974). A phylogenetic study of bird karyotypes. *Chromosoma* **46**, 91–120.

Takagi, N. and Sasaki, M. (1980). Unexpected karyotypic resemblance between the Burmeister's seriema, *Chunga burmeisteri* (Gruiformes: Cariamidae) and the toucan, *Rhamphastos toco* (Piciformes: Rhamphastidae). *Chrom. Inf. Serv.* **28**, 10–11.

Tegelstrom, H., Ebenhard, T. and Ryttman, H. (1983). Rate of karyotype evolution and speciation in birds. *Hereditas* **98**, 235–239.

Templeton, A. R. (1980 a). The theory of speciation via the founder principle. *Genetics* **94**, 1011–1038.

Templeton, A. R. (1980 b). Modes of speciation and inferences based on genetic distances. *Evolution* **34**, 719–729.

Thorneycroft, H. B. (1966). Chromosomal polymorphism in the White-throated Sparrow (*Zonotrichia albicollis*) (Gmelin). *Science* **154**, 1571–1572.

Thorneycroft, H. B. (1968). A cytogenetic study of the White-throated Sparrow, *Zonotrichia albicollis* (Gmelin). Ph.D. Thesis, University of Toronto.

Thorneycroft, H. B. (1975). A cytogenetic study of the White-throated Sparrow, *Zonotrichia albicollis* (Gmelin). *Evolution* **29**, 611–621.

Voous, K. H. (1972). List of recent holarctic bird species, non-passerines. *Ibis* **115**, 612–638.

White, M. J. D. (1973). "Animal Cytology and Evolution". Cambridge University Press.

White, M. J. D. (1978). "Modes of Speciation". W. H. Freeman & Co., San Francisco.

Williams, R. M. and Benirschke, R. J. (1976). The chromosomes of four species of Falconiformes. *Experientia* **32**, 310–311.

Wilson, A. C., Sarich, V. M. and Maxson, L. R. (1974). The importance of gene rearrangement in evolution: evidence from studies on rates of chromosomal, protein and anatomical evolution. *Proc. Natl Acad. Sci. USA* **71**, 3028–3030.

Wyles, J. S., Kunkel, J. G. and Wilson, A. C. (1983). Birds, behavior, and anatomical evolution. *Proc. Natl Acad Sci. USA* **80**, 4394–4397.

4

Electrophoretic Variability of Gene Products

P. G. H. Evans

Edward Grey Institute, Zoology Department, Oxford University,
South Parks Road, Oxford OX1 3PS, UK

AVIAN GENETICS
ISBN 0-12-187570-9

1 INTRODUCTION

The last two decades have seen a plethora of studies on allozyme variation, but it is only very recently that much work has been carried out on birds. This may be illustrated by the fact that a review of allozyme variation amongst different classes of animals made by Nevo in 1978 listed only ten species of birds. Five years later this number had increased to seventy-one species (Corbin 1983) and many more were being examined at that time.

It is perhaps surprising that birds had received so little attention considering that much ecological and evolutionary theory has been based upon this class. Birds are relatively conspicuous and easy to observe, and many long-term studies involving marked populations have been undertaken (see Brown 1970, Perrins 1979, Dunnet and Ollason 1979, Watson and Moss, 1980, Cooke *et al.* 1982, Woolfenden and Fitzpatrick 1984, Coulson and Thomas 1985). In this chapter attention is drawn to ways in which allozyme analysis and long-term population studies might come together, to their mutual benefit. It is assumed the reader has little previous knowledge of allozyme research, so routine procedures (see the Appendix) and some commonly encountered pitfalls are briefly described. The results of major relevant studies are summarized and promising avenues for further study suggested.

Measuring genetic variation in quantitative terms is central to much of population genetics, and yet it presents many practical difficulties. Traditionally, variation has been examined using physical characters such as plumage or body dimensions, with breeding experiments carried out to reveal hidden variation present amongst heterozygotes. However, besides the labour often required for this procedure, it suffers in two important ways: (1) often the characters examined are not direct products of gene action but may involve the interactions of many genes; (2) by its very nature, this technique examines only variable gene loci—invariant genes are not detected, thus preventing an unbiased view of the genome. The solution (albeit partial) to this problem arose with the discovery in molecular genetics that the genetic information encoded in the nucleotide sequence of the DNA of a structural gene is translated directly into a sequence of amino acids that make up a polypeptide. This direct relationship between a protein and the genetic coding for it has allowed the measurement of genetic variation amongst individuals and populations in a *relatively* unbiased and unambiguous manner. The technique for doing this, gel electrophoresis, was developed in the late 1960s and is now widely used, being both relatively simple and cheap. Electrophoresis distinguishes different forms of the same enzyme, known as allozymes, the most common of proteins examined.

2 ANALYSIS OF ALLOZYME DATA

2.1 Identity and nomenclature of allozyme patterns

Bands in gels with different electrophoretic mobilities should by implication be coded by different alleles. A single band implies a gene with an identical pair of alleles (i.e. a homozygote). More than one band may imply a heterozygote (depending on the quaternary structure of the protein) or homozygotes at more than one locus. It is customary to represent the alleles coding for an enzyme by an abbreviation denoting that enzyme (e.g. "EST" or "Est" is Esterase) followed by a hyphenated number (if the enzyme possesses more than one locus) usually in order of mobility ("1" being anodal to "2"). Each allele is then given a superscript (also in order of mobility) which is often a letter (F, M, or S (fast, medium or slow) or a, b, or c ("a" is generally anodal to "b" although it may be used to denote the most common allele since this enables rare alleles found subsequently to be labelled in descending order)). Alternatively it may be a number, e.g. EST^{105} which denotes the distance (5 mm) that the allele is anodal of the most common allele (using the baseline 100).

The structure of an enzyme determines the zymogram (allozyme patterns on gels) obtained after electrophoresis. If the enzyme is monomeric, comprising two polypeptides, a homozygous individual will possess one band at that locus and a heterozygous individual will possess two bands, one corresponding to the position of one homozygote, and the other to the other homozygote. If the enzyme consists of three polypeptides (i.e. of dimeric structure, such as PGI), the heterozygote is represented by three bands with the central one usually being the strongest. A tetrameric enzyme has five bands in the homozygous state and eight bands in the heterozygous condition. However, the number of bands shown by an enzyme may vary depending on the tissue or organ from which it is derived, though usually it is constant across taxa. Commonly, one or more bands may be lost from an enzyme of complex structure. Thus, for example, LDH (a tetrameric enzyme) may stain up with only three or four bands in the homozygote, instead of the usual five. Table 1 lists 32 of the more common proteins/enzymes examined, together with details of their quaternary structure and supposed function.

A serious problem arises from different workers using different nomenclature for the enzymes they study. This applies at different levels. For example, Harris and Hopkinson (1976) use GDH to denote Glucose dehydrogenase (EC 1.1.1.47) whereas most workers use GDH to denote Glutamate dehydrogenase (EC 1.4.1.2). Some workers (e.g. Avise and Aquadro 1982, Ross 1983) refer to the Enzyme Commission number of

Table 1. Names, abbreviations, structure and function of proteins most commonly included in electrophoretic studies

Enzyme	Locus symbol[a]	E.C. No.[b]	Tissue distribution[c]	Quaternary structure[c]	Supposed physiological function[d]
1 Alcohol dehydrogenase	ADH	1.1.1.1	Mainly liver, also kidney	Dimeric	Controls branchpoint in fructose and fat metabolism
2 α-Glycerophosphate dehydrogenase* (glycerol-3-phosphate dehydrogenase)	GPD-1, -2 (GPDH, α-GPDH)	1.1.1.8	Mainly muscle, also kidney, heart, brain, testis	Dimeric	Links glycolysis and fat synthesis
3 Sorbitol dehydrogenase	SDH (SORDH)	1.1.1.14	Liver, kidney, muscle, brain, heart	Tetrameric	(Fructose metabolism)
4 Lactate dehydrogenase*	LDH-1, -2	1.1.1.27	Liver, kidney, muscle, brain, heart, rbc	Tetrameric	Control of NAD^+:NADH ratio
5 Malate dehydrogenase*	MDH-1 (soluble) MDH-2 (mitochondrial)	1.1.1.37	All tissues, rbc (soluble only)	Dimeric	Soluble (cytoplasm.): NAD^+/NADH shuttle; mitochond.: TCA cycle, gluconeogenesis
6 Malic enzyme*[e]	ME-1 (soluble) ME-2 (mitochondrial)	1.1.1.40	Liver, kidney, brain, heart (not in rbc)	Tetrameric	Soluble: produces NADP which limits rate of synthetic reactions; mitochond.: produces NADP limiting adrenal steroid synthesis
7 Isocitrate dehydrogenase*	ICD (IDH)-1 (soluble) ICD-2 (mitochondrial)	1.1.1.42	All tissues, rbc (soluble only)	Dimeric	Mitochond.: rate-limiting step in TCA cycle
8 6-Phosphogluconate dehydrogenase	6-PGD (PGD, PGDH)	1.1.1.44	All tissues, rbc	Dimeric	Pentose shunt
9 Glucose-6-phosphate dehydrogenase	G-6-PD (G-6-PDH)	1.1.1.49	All tissues, rbc	Dimeric/tetrameric	Modulates entry of hexoses into pentose metabolism
10 Xanthine dehydrogenase	XDH	1.2.1.37	All tissues (poss. not in rbc)	Dimeric	Uric acid formation
11 Glutamate dehydrogenase	GDH (GLUDH)	1.4.1.2	All tissues (not in rbc)	Dimeric	Nitrogen metabolism
12 Superoxide dismutase[f] (probably = indophenol oxidase)	SOD-1, -2 (IPO, TO)	1.15.1.1	All tissues, rbc (soluble only)	Dimeric/tetrameric	Removal of cytotoxic superoxide radical (O_2^-)
13 Nucleoside phosphorylase*	NP	2.4.2.1	All tissues (poss. not in rbc)	Trimeric	Purine salvage
14 Glutamate-oxaloacetate transaminase (aspartate aminotransferase)	GOT-1, -2 (AAT)	2.6.1.1	All tissues, rbc (soluble only)	Dimeric	Soluble: cytoplasmic transamination; mitochond.: glutamate metabolism

No.	Symbol[a]	EC number[b]	Tissue distribution[c]	Quaternary structure	Function
15 Creatine kinase*	CK-1, -2, -3	2.7.3.2	CK-1, -2 (brain, heart) CK-3 (muscle)	Dimeric	Catalyses reversible phosphorylation of creatine by ATP
16 Adenylate kinase	AK (ADKIN)	2.7.4.3	Most tissues, rbc	Monomeric	Modulates ATP/ADP ratio thus affecting metabolism generally
17 Phosphoglucomutase*	PGM-1, -2 (-3)	2.7.5.1	All tissues, rbc	Monomeric	Glycogen synthesis
18 Esterase*	EST-1, -2, -3 (-4, -5, -6)	3.1.1.1	All tissues, plasma/serum, rbc	Monomeric/dimeric	Various; primarily breakdown of ingested esters
19 Cholinesterase	E	3.1.1.8	Mainly plasma/serum	Prob. tetrameric	Non-specific ester hydrolysis
20 Acid phosphatase	ACP (ACPH)	3.1.3.2	Mainly rbc, plasma, also other tissues	Monomeric/dimeric	Non-specific dephosphorylation; Ca^{2+} metabolism in bone
21 Leucine aminopeptidase	LAP (PEP-E)	3.4.11/13	Mainly digestive system, plasma	Monomeric	Protein catabolism
22 Peptidase-A (leucyl-alanine or L-valyl-1-leucine substrate)	PEP-A	3.4.11/13	Mainly kidney, liver, muscle, brain, heart, also rbc	Dimeric	Protein catabolism
23 Peptidase-B (leucyl-glycyl-glycine)	PEP-B	3.4.11/13	Mainly rbc, skin, lungs	Monomeric	Protein catabolism
24 Peptidase-C (leucyl-alanine)	PEP-C	3.4.11/13	All tissues, rbc	Monomeric	Protein catabolism
25 Peptidase-D (phenyl-alanyl-proline)	PEP-D	3.4.11/13	All tissues, rbc	Dimeric	Protein catabolism
26 Adenosine deaminase*	ADA	3.5.4.4	All tissues, rbc	Monomeric	First step in adenosine purine salvage
27 Mannose phosphate isomerase*	MPI (PMI)$^{-1}$ ($^{-2}$, $^{-3}$)	5.3.1.8	All tissues (not in rbc)	Monomeric	Monosaccharide interconversion pathway
28 Glucose phosphate isomerase*	GPI (PGI)	5.3.1.9	All tissues, rbc	Dimeric	Glycolysis
29 Haemoglobin	Hb	—	Red blood cells	Monomeric	Oxygen transport in blood
30 Albumin	ALB	—	All tissues, plasma/serum, rbc	Dimeric	—
31 Transferrin	Tf (Trf)	—	All tissues, plasma/serum, rbc	Monomeric	—
32 Other non-enzymatic proteins	PT-1, -2	—	All tissues, plasma/serum, rbc	Monomeric/dimeric	—

* May be vulnerable to secondary modification.

[a] Recommended symbol with alternatives in parentheses, and locus number generally found in bird tissues. Note that different workers have used different locus numbers (see text) according to electrophoretic mobility and tissue.

[b] Enzyme commission number (International Union of Biochemistry (1979)).

[c] Tissue distribution and quaternary structure as found in birds.

[d] Sources: Dixon and Webb (1965), Harris and Hopkinson (1976), Jakoby (1980) and Johnson (1974).

[e] May appear on gels stained for CK or 6-PGD.

[f] May appear on gels stained for ADH or SDH.

Xanthine dehydrogenase (XDH) as 1.2.3.2 which should denote Xanthine oxidase; its recommended EC number is 1.2.1.37 (International Union of Biochemistry 1979). The other common confusion arises when possibly homologous loci are compared across species (and particularly between laboratories). Some workers use "1" to denote the more anodal locus of an enzyme, and others the more cathodal locus. This confusion also arises when different workers interpret which are the mitochondrial and soluble (supernatant) forms. Thus Harris and Hopkinson (1976), Nottebohm and Selander (1972), Smith and Zimmerman (1976) and Avise *et al.* (1980 a) refer to MDH-1 as the soluble form of Malate dehydrogenase, and this migrates anodally of MDH-2, whereas Ross (1983), among others, refers to the converse. Furthermore, Nottebohm and Selander (1972) refer to ICD-1 as the soluble and more cathodal form, whereas Ross (1983) refers to it as the mitochondrial form, and many others (e.g. Harris and Hopkinson 1976) as the soluble and more anodal form.

Finally, in addition to the above problems, there is an urgent need for different laboratories to co-operate in evaluating the possible homology of the loci they are examining. This will require the sharing of samples to obtain some common measure for different loci and alleles at these loci under the same electrophoretic conditions. It also requires use of the same tissue. At present, possibly different loci within an enzyme are treated as the same across tissues or they may be combined, with obscure results if workers homogenize a range of tissues together.

2.2   Problems of interpretation

Although there tends to be some homology in banding patterns for a particular enzyme across species, further caution is necessary. Post-translational modification of the enzyme molecule (usually during the freezing/thawing process) may produce spurious bands. The only way to test this is to obtain inheritance data from complete families and check that the putative genotypes are indeed passed on from parents to offspring in a typical Mendelian manner. Although this test is routinely performed by medical laboratories studying the genetics of humans and mice, it appears scarcely ever to have been carried out in avian studies. Exceptions are genetic studies of Snow Goose (*Anser caerulescens*) by Bargiello *et al.* (1977), Mute Swan (*Cygnus olor*) by Bacon (1979), European Starling (*Sturnus vulgaris*) by Evans (1980), and House Sparrow (*Passer domesticus*) by Burke (1984). Without such tests, "genotypes" derived from examination of zymograms should strictly be referred to as "phenotypes". Even under these conditions, one cannot be certain that a banding pattern has a genetic basis if the variation is

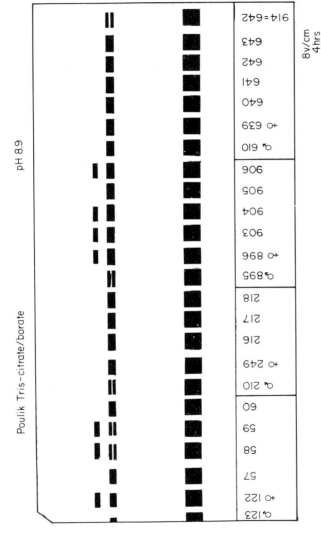

Poulik Tris-citrate/borate

pH 8.9

8v/cm
4hrs

♀123	♀122	57	58	59	60	♂210	♀249	216	217	218	♀895	♀896	903	904	905	906	♀610	♂639	640	641	642	643	914=642

Fig. 1. Lack of inheritance of a secondary A band for EST-1 locus in four complete families of European Starling. Note that the secondary band appears in two nestlings from the first family (numbered left to right) and one from the fourth family, but is absent from either parents of the respective broods, whilst in the other two families it is present in one parent but absent from all offspring.

caused by post-translational modification at other loci, so that normal segregation patterns occur. It is then necessary to map the variants and locate the loci involved.

The problem of misidentifying post-translational changes as inherited bands is a very real one, particularly for monomeric enzymes. With a dimeric enzyme, the strength of the bands in the heterozygote can be indicative of its genetic basis. For example, if the most cathodal band is the strongest and the next two bands become progressively weaker, it is likely that they are caused by modification of the protein molecule, since in dimeric enzymes it is generally the central of the three bands of the heterozygote that is the strongest (the strength of the three bands being approximately $1:2:1$). However, a monomeric enzyme may have many alleles at a particular locus, which are present as combinations of two bands in the heterozygote. An extra band with no genetic basis may thus be difficult to identify. This is illustrated in Fig. 1, where an extra band at an Esterase locus in European Starling was found not to be inherited, when otherwise it could have been interpreted as an extra allele. Commonly, this problem is tackled by calculating the gene frequencies in the sample and testing for deviation from a Hardy–Weinberg equilibrium (see below). This test is an insensitive one, however, which requires a large deviation in order to be statistically significant, and other factors such as selection inbreeding can cause a deviation.

These difficulties in interpretation should receive much greater attention than they are currently given by those using allozymes in their avian studies, which require the bulk of electrophoretic data to be taken on trust. Estimates of P, H, F_{ST}, the indices of genetic distance, and genetic comparisons between taxa are all based upon the premise that separate bands represent separate alleles. But in virtually all avian studies the only test of this is the insensitive one of deviation from a Hardy–Weinberg equilibrium. Table 2 presents a review of all studies known to the author in which a number of loci were examined: 86% (149/174) of these involved sample sizes of less than 50 individuals; 54% were samples of 15 individuals or less. When sample sizes are as small as this, rendering χ^2 tests of little value, the absence of an adequate test for the genetic basis of different phenotypes is all the more critical. One might expect secondary modification of a protein molecule, giving rise to spurious bands, to occur in only a few samples if the precautions described earlier are followed, so that if these were misidentified as new alleles, their frequencies would be near zero. Unfortunately this is the case in the great majority of avian electrophoretic studies, where many of the variable loci are due to 1–2 variants among small samples. Whilst this may truly reflect the situation (and argue in favour of alleles that are selectively effectively neutral—see later section), it lends little support for their genetic basis. Likewise some enzymes

Table 2. Summary of P, H and F_{ST} estimates for birds

Family/species	Number of Popns	Number of Indivs	Number of Loci	P	H_c	H_o	Number of Popns	Number of Loci	F_{ST}	Ref.
Procellariidae										
Thalassoica antarctica	?	8	16	0.250	0.114					11
Daption capense	?	8	16	0.313	0.143					11
Pagodroma nivea	?	11	16	0.438	0.175					11
Pachyptila desolata	?	8	16	0.313	0.134					11
$\bar{X}$				0.329	0.142					
Hydrobatidae										
Oceanites oceanicus	?	12	16	0.250	0.096					11
Ardeidae										
Ardea herodias	2	46	28	0.263		0.007				27
Anatidae										
Somateria mollissima		34	14	0.714	0.307		6	1	0.057	33
Tachyeres patachonicus		6	14	0.643	0.164					19
T. leucocephala			19	0.263						19
Cygnus buccinator	3	225				0.010				9
C. olor										5
$\bar{X}$				0.540	0.236					
Phasianidae										
Dendragapus obscurus	6	269	23	0.260		0.082	9	1	0.000	36
Lagopus lagopus	6	45	23	0.170		0.044				28
L. mutus	1	13	27	0.000	0.000	0.000				28
Tympanuchus pallidicinctus	1	13	27	0.111	0.031	0.026	4	1	0.006	26
Phasianus colchicus	1	30	27	0.197	0.075	0.062				26,40
Coturnix coturnix	1	47	36	0.542		0.065				26
C. pectoralis	2	12	27	0.148	0.052	0.052				8
Alectoris chukar	4	36	27	0.185	0.025	0.024				26
Lophortyx californicus	2	22	27	0.185	0.031	0.025				26
L. gambelii										26

(continued overleaf)

Table 2 (continued)

Family/species	Number of			P	H_c	H_o	Number of		F_{ST}	Ref.
	Popns	Indivs	Loci				Popns	Loci		
Callipepla squamata	3	29	27	0·130	0·037	0·032				26
Colinus virginianus	2	15	27	0·148	0·034	0·027				26
Oreortyx pictus	1	16	27	0·111	0·024	0·021				26
Cyrtonyx montezumae	2	31	27	0·204	0·039	0·031				26
$\bar{X}$				0·184	0·035	0·038				
Laridae										
Larus californicus	2	60	35	0·229	0·034	0·028	2	8	0·004	44
Columbidae										
Columba livia							2	1	0·030	23
C. palumbus							2	1	0·051	23
Picidae										
Sphyrapicus varius	1	7	39	0·128	0·032	0·022				31
S. nuchalis	3	34	39	0·171	0·048	0·043				31
S. ruber ruber	1	13	39	0·154	0·046	0·045				31
S. r. daggetti	2	15	39	0·154	0·044	0·041				31
S. thyroideus	3	18	39	0·077	0·015	0·016				31
$\bar{X}$				0·133	0·035	0·031				
Tyrannidae										
Nuttallornis (Contopus) borealis	1	8	38	0·282	0·079					43
Contopus virens	1	7	38	0·308	0·096					43
C. sordidulus	1	5	38	0·231	0·079					43
Empidonax flaviventris		19	38	0·282	0·084					43
E. virescens		10	38	0·308	0·091					43
E. traillii		20	38	0·282	0·088					43
E. alnorum		17	38	0·282	0·079					43
E. minimus		18	38	0·154	0·054					43
E. hammondii		13	38	0·154	0·060					43
E. oberholseri		17	38	0·231	0·073					43

E. wrightii		18	38	0·179	0·047		43
E. difficilis		16	38	0·154	0·054		43
E. flavescens	1	6	38	0·077	0·021		43
E. euleri		22	38	0·205	0·065		43
E. atriceps		18	38	0·128	0·043		43
X̄				0·217	0·068		
Alaudidae							
Eremophila alpestris		17	35		0·102		13
Hirundinidae							
Hirundo tahitica	1?	31	15	0·200		0·078	32
Petrochelidon ariel	1?	33	15	0·200		0·065	32
X̄				0·200		0·072	
Mimidae							
Dumetella carolinensis	?	8	24	0·208	0·028	0·034	1
D. carolinensis		24	23			0·018	4
Mimus polyglottos		8	23			0·010	4
Toxostoma rufum		7	23			0·048	4
X̄						0·028	
Motacillidae							
Motacilla flava							25
Muscicapidae							
Catharus ustulatus	?	17	27	0·296	0·065	0·053	1
C. ustulatus	?	5	18/26			0·032	3
C. guttatus	?	13	27	0·259	0·045	0·063	1
C. fuscescens	?	5	27	0·185	0·048	0·056	1
Hylocichla mustelina	?	5	27	0·148	0·060	0·104	1
Turdus migratorius	?	5	26	0·077	0·031	0·042	1
Sialia sialis	?	7	27	0·148	0·045	0·063	1
Pomastostomus temporalis	1	80	20	0·400		0·094	30
Regulus calendula	?	10	23	0·174	0·037	0·048	1
X̄				0·211	0·047	0·064	
Paridae							
Parus bicolor bicolor	2	12	36	0·278		0·060	14
P. b. atricristatus	1	12	36	0·306		0·060	14
X̄				0·292		0·060	

(continued overleaf)

Table 2 (continued)

Family/species	Number of Popns	Number of Indivs	Number of Loci	P	H_c	H_o	Number of Popns	Number of Loci	F_{ST}	Ref.
Emberizidae (Emberizinae)										
Melospiza melodia	?	7	20	0·050	0·007	0·019				2
M. melodia	?	14	39	0·179	0·038	0·042				42
M. georgiana	?	10	21	0·190	0·031	0·051				2
M. georgiana	?	16	39	0·231	0·040	0·042				42
M. lincolnii	?	8	39	0·179	0·054	0·054				42
Zonotrichia capensis	1	41	14	0·256	0·045	0·054				42
Z. capensis hypoleuca		195	14	0·428	0·099		5	6	0·015	29
Z. c. carabuyae		63	45	0·489	0·096					19
Z. leucophrys	?	19	39	0·231	0·032	0·036				42
Z. l. nuttalli		149	19	0·316	0·098		9	3	0·047	6
Z. l. nuttalli	4	64	46	0·246	0·085	0·048	8	12	0·032	18
Z. l. pugetensis	3	41	46	0·219	0·096	0·059				18
Z. l. oriantha		78	19	0·158	0·065					6
Z. albicollis	?	10	21	0·190	0·031	0·051				2
Z. albicollis	?	12	39	0·231	0·034	0·032				42
Z. atricapilla	?	15	39	0·154	0·041	0·039				42
Z. querula	?	18	39	0·128	0·019	0·020				42
Passerella iliaca	?	57	39	0·308	0·032	0·036	31	14	0·016	42
Junco hyemalis	2	48	39	0·179	0·029	0·029				42
J. hyemalis	?	10	21	0·143	0·045	0·058				2
J. hyemalis		33	25			0·061	6	9	0·008	13
Passerculus sandwichensis	?	10	20	0·250	0·042	0·049				2
Ammodramus savannarum	?	10	20	0·200	0·051	0·045				2
Spizella passerina	?	11	21	0·143	0·030	0·065				2
S. pusilla	?	6	21	0·143	0·054	0·083				2
Amphispiza bilineata	?	7	21	0·095	0·028	0·072				2
A. belli		20	43			0·047				11
Geospiza magnirostris	4	17	27	0·259		0·029	4	7	0·046	41
G. fortis	8	53	27	0·407		0·052	8	12	0·065	41

G. fuliginosa	10	80	27	0·444		0·065	10	12	0·054	41
G. difficilis	3	5	27	0·333		0·068	3	11	0·020	41
G. scandens	3	26	27	0·370		0·063				41
G. conirostris	2	21	27	0·222		0·056				41
Camarhynchus parvulus	4	21	27	0·074		0·034	4	8	0·057	41
C. (Platyspiza) crassirostris	4	8	27	0·148		0·044	4	8	0·125	41
Certhidea olivacea	4	15	27	0·296		0·027	6	1	0·229	41
Pipilo erythrophthalmus										38
P. fuscus	?	5	21	0·048	0·009	0·010				2
$\bar{x}$				0·221	0·040	0·047			0·061	
Parulidae										
Mniotilta varia	?	8	26	0·154	0·064					10
M. varia	?	6	18/26			0·026				3
Vermivora peregrina	?	13	30	0·333	0·158					10
V. peregrina	?	24	18/26			0·069				3
V. celata	?	8	31	0·355	0·130					10
V. celata	?	12	18/26			0·040				3
V. ruficapilla	?	22	31	0·335	0·123	0·042				10
Dendroica pensylvanica	?	10	18/26			0·014				3
D. caerulescens	?	6	18/26			0·040				3
D. discolor	?	8	18/26			0·012				3
D. tigrina	?	6	18/26			0·033				3
D. fusca	?	8	18/26			0·036				3
D. magnolia	?	12	18/26			0·004				3
D. coronata	?	35	31	0·419	0·121	0·039				10
D. coronata	?	10	18/26			0·005				3
D. c. coronata	1	48	32	0·156	0·031	0·036				12
D. c. auduboni	2	62	32	0·167	0·034					12
D. palmarum	?	12	31	0·290	0·126					10
D. striata	?	6	31	0·032	0·016					10
D. castanea	?	12	18/26			0·024				3
Setophaga ruticilla	?	12	30	0·200	0·069					10
S. ruticilla	?	16	18/26			0·031				3
Seiurus aurocapillus	?	10	31	0·032	0·016					10
S. aurocapillus	?	29	18/26			0·061				3

(continued overleaf)

Table 2 (continued)

Family/species	Number of			P	H_c	H_o	Number of		F_{ST}	Ref.
	Popns	Indivs	Loci				Popns	Loci		
S. noveboracensis	?	24	31	0.419	0.147	0.128				10
S. noveboracensis	?	7	18/26							3
Geothlypis trichas	?	16	30	0.233	0.084					10
G. trichas	?	32	18/26			0.037				3
G. formosa	?	16	18/26			0.056				3
G. philadelphia	?	16	30	0.222	0.081					10
Wilsonia citrina	?	6	18/26			0.015				3
Icteria virens	?	5	18/26			0.020				3
$\bar{X}$				0.262	0.080	0.035				
Vireonidae										
Vireo solitarius		20	42			0.045				11
V. solitarius		16	23			0.054				4
V. olivaceus		58	23			0.048				4
V. olivaceus	?	5	18/26			0.022				3
V. griseus		5	23			0.036				4
$\bar{X}$						0.040				
Icteridae										
Icterus galbula galbula	8	123	19	0.105	0.071	0.060	5	2	0.012	21
I. g. bullockii	8	66	19	0.105	0.073		8	2	0.018	21
Agelaius phoeniceus			15	0.533			3	1	0.037	15, 16, 39
Sturnella magna			15	0.600						39
S. neglecta			15	0.400						39
Quiscalus major			15	0.400						39
Q. quiscula			15	0.400						39
Euphagus cyanocephalus			15	0.333						39
Molothrus ater			15	0.533						39
$\bar{X}$				0.413					0.026	

	No. populations	N	No. loci	P	H_c	H_o	No. populations	No. loci	F_{ST}	Source
Ploceidae										
Passer domesticus	2	57	29	0·257	0·093	0·147	5		0·003	17,35
Passer domesticus				0·170			4		0·008	24
Sturnidae										
Aplonis cantoroides	4	94	18	0·125	0·016	0·026	4	2	0·127	20
A. m. metallica	9	186	18	0·118	0·054	} 0·055	6	2	0·029	20
A. m. nitida	7	139	18	0·111	0·046		4	2	0·040	20
A. m. purpuriceps	1	29	18	0·111	0·027					20
Sturnus vulgaris vulgaris (UK)	?	299	24	0·210	0·033	0·031	6	11	0·010	37
S. v. vulgaris (NZ)	?	298	24	0·250	0·043	0·038	6	11	0·032	37
S. v. vulgaris	15	1414	15	0·133		0·009				22
S. v. zetlandicus	3	178	15	0·130		0·021				22
S. v. faeroensis	1	70	15	0·200		0·002				22
$\bar{X}$				0·141	0·032	0·034			0·061	
Overall $\bar{X}$				0·240	0·065	0·044			0·048	
Number of species				103	79	86			23	

NOTES: Data with sample sizes of less than five individuals have been omitted. (?) Number of populations unknown, usually due to sampling wintering populations. Order and nomenclature of species follows Howard and Moore (1984, "A Complete Checklist of the Birds of the World". Macmillan, London).

P = Proportion of loci polymorphic (frequency of most common allele 0·99 or less) of all loci assayed for the total number of individuals noted, averaged across loci.

H_c = Mean heterozygosity calculated by $1 - \sum x_i^2$, where x_i is the frequency of the ith allele at locus x. These values are then averaged across loci.

H_o = Mean heterozygosity observed for all individuals at each locus separately, and then averaged across loci.

Overall mean values of P and H were obtained by averaging across species (an average value was obtained across sub-species/populations for those species sampled more than once).

F_{ST} = Wright's fixation coefficient which measures genetic differentiation of sub-populations within the total population.

KEY TO REFERENCE SOURCES: 1—Avise et al. (1980a); 2—Avise et al. (1980b); 3—Avise et al. (1980c); 4—Avise et al. (1982); 5—Bacon (1979); 6—Baker (1975); 7—Baker and Fox (1978); 8—Baker and Manwell (1975); 9—Barrett and Vyse (1982); 10—Barrowclough and Corbin (1978); 11—Barrowclough et al. (1981); 12—Barrowclough (1980); 13—Barrowclough (1983); 14—Braun et al. (1984); 15—Brush (1968); 16—Brush (1970); 17—Cole and Parkin (1979); 18—Corbin (1981); 19—Corbin (1983); 20—Corbin et al. (1974); 21—Corbin et al. (1979); 22—Evans (1980); 23—Ferguson (1971); 24—Fleischer (1983); 25—Gemeiner et al. (1982); 26—Gutierrez et al. (1983); 27—Guttman et al. (1980); 28—Gyllensten et al. (1979); 29—Handford and Nottebohm (1976); 30—Johnson and Brown (1980); 31—Johnson and Zink (1983); 32—Manwell and Baker (1975); 33—Milne and Robertson (1965); 34—Nottebohm and Selander (1972); 35—Parkin and Cole (1985); 36—Redfield et al. (1972); 37—Ross (1983); 38—Sibley and Corbin (1970); 39—Smith and Zimmerman (1976); 40—Vohs and Carr (1969); 41—Yang and Patton (1981); 42—Zink (1982); 43—Zink and Johnson (to be published); 44—Zink and Winkler (1983).

Table 3. Frequently investigated allozyme loci in birds showing distribution among taxa and the range of frequencies of commonest allele

Protein/enzyme locus	Number of taxa		Range of values
	Monomorphic	Polymorphic	
ADH	27	2	0·94
GPD-1	43	7	0·88–0·94
GPD-2	39	12	0·50–0·99
SDH	28	11	0·57–0·98
LDH-1	66	8	0·84–0·98
LDH-2	65	8	0·88–0·98
MDH-1	67	1	0·99
MDH-2	55	5	0·96–0·99
ME-1	8	5	0·59–0·96
ME-2	12	1	0·97
ICD-1	37	29	0·58–0·98
ICD-2	51	12	0·63–0·98
6-PGD	49	50	0·43–0·99
GDH	31	0	—
G-6-PD	18	2	0·68–0·93
XDH	12	5	0·70–0·97
SOD-1	30	1	0·90
SOD-2	31	0	—
NP	13	11	0·50–0·93
GOT-1	60	26	0·50–0·99
GOT-2	80	5	0·83–0·98
CK-1	40	4	0·95–0·98
CK-2	21	0	—
CK-3	42	1	0·92
AK	22	1	?
PGM-1	28	20	0·50–0·98
PGM-2	21	31	0·50–0·98
EST-1	33	44	0·32–0·99
EST-2	34	27	0·29–0·97
EST-3	22	12	0·44–0·98
EST-4	9	14	0·40–0·98
ACP	27	6	0·56–0·83
LAP	32	2	0·93–0·96
PEP-A	45	28	0·50–0·99
PEP-B	26	36	0·50–0·97
PEP-C	32	22	0·50–0·96
PEP-D	15	2	0·96
ADA	13	20	0·37–0·97
MPI	30	30	0·45–0·99
GPI	43	28	0·60–0·98
Hb	45	0	—
ALB	44	10	0·60–0·95
Tf	17	14	0·50–0·97
PT-1	42	7	0·70–0·97
PT-2	35	2	0·80–0·93

appear to be more frequently polymorphic than others (Table 3; Fig. 2). This may actually be the case, but it may also be due to differences between enzymes in their susceptibility to secondary modification. Attention to this problem is urged if confidence is to be placed in the published results.

2.3 Allele and genotype frequencies

Banding patterns visualized in gels represent phenotypes. However, if one knows the relationship between specific genotypes and the corresponding phenotypes (by genetic testing) we may transform the numbers of particular phenotypes in the sampled population into numbers of specific genotypes. These genotypic frequencies provide a measure of the genetic variation in the population. To be representative of the population, the sample must be random, i.e. unbiased. Genotypic frequencies are calculated by adding up the numbers of each genotype at a given locus and dividing each by the total number for all genotypes combined, i.e. the sample total. Having obtained genotypic frequencies, one can use them to calculate the frequencies of each allele at that locus. This is done simply by counting the number of times each allele is found and dividing this by the total number of alleles in the sample; the frequency of an allele calculated in this way is the frequency of individuals homozygous for that allele, plus half the frequency of heterozygotes for that allele. The frequency of each allele is calculated separately and when totalled should equal 1·0.

The allele frequency estimates from the sample may not accurately reflect the frequency in the population as a whole, particularly if the sample is small. It is therefore useful to calculate the variance of each allele frequency estimate as a measure of the accuracy of the estimate. Formulae for doing this for both a two-allele system and a multiple-allele system, together with an algebraic representation of the above method for estimating allele frequencies, are given in Table 4.

2.4 Hardy–Weinberg equilibria

The Hardy–Weinberg law states that in a randomly mating population, the expected distribution of genotypes is determined by the random combination of alleles, and this results in an equilibrium being set up amongst genotypic frequencies at any given locus that remains constant from one generation to the next.

The equilibrium genotypic frequencies are given by the square of the allele frequencies, so that with two alleles A and a, with frequencies p and q, the

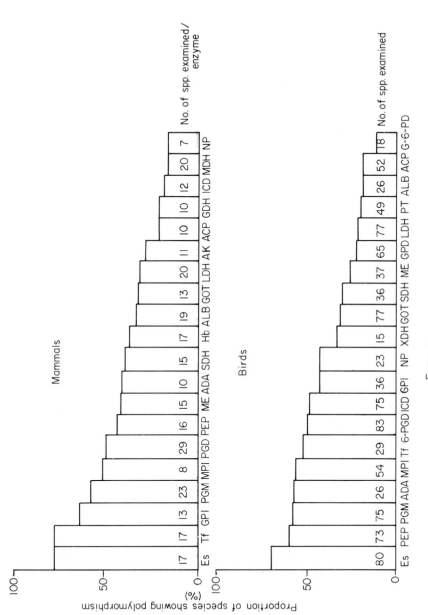

Fig. 2. The frequency of polymorphisms in specific enzymes in birds and mammals. Note that most of the species included in this analysis contained small sample sizes; studies were selected only when a fairly wide range of enzymes had been examined, to minimize biases due to some enzymes being tested more frequently within a taxonomic group than others. Note that data are used only from studies where a wide range of enzymes (comprising broadly similar sets) have been examined.

Table 4. Methods used to estimate allele frequencies and their variances from electrophoretic data

---

Two-allele genetic system

$$\hat{p} = \frac{N_{11} + \frac{1}{2}N_{12}}{N} \qquad \hat{q} = \frac{\frac{1}{2}N_{12} + N_{22}}{N}$$

$$V(p) = \frac{p(1-p)}{2N} \qquad V(q) = \frac{q(1-q)}{2N}$$

where N = total number of individuals; N_{11} = number of homozygotes of allele A_1; N_{22} = number of homozygotes of allele A_2; N_{12} = number of heterozygotes (of alleles A_1 and A_2); $\hat{p} = \bar{X}$ frequency of allele A_1; and $\hat{q} = \bar{X}$ frequency of allele A_2.

Multiple allele genetic system

$$\hat{p}_i = \frac{N_{ii} + \frac{1}{2}\sum_{i=1}^{n}N_{ij}}{N} \qquad \hat{q}_i = \frac{\frac{1}{2}\sum_{j=1}^{n}N_{ij} + N_{jj}}{N}$$

$$V(p_i) = \frac{P_i(1-p_i)}{2N} \qquad V(q_i) = \frac{Q_i(1-q_i)}{2N}$$

where N = total number of individuals in sample; N_{ii} = number of A_iA_i genotypes (i.e. homozygotes); N_{ij} = number of A_iA_j genotypes (i.e. heterozygotes); $\hat{p}_i$ = mean frequency of allele A_i; and $\hat{q}_j$ = mean frequency of allele A_j.

---

frequencies of the three possible genotypes are: $(p^2 + q)^2 = p^2 + 2pq + q^2$ (i.e. a binomial expansion). For three or more alleles, a polynomial expansion is used (i.e. n alleles with frequencies $p_1, p_2, \ldots p_n$ yield genotype frequencies $(p_1 + p_2 + \cdots + p_n)^2$). The expected frequency of each genotype is thus derived from the observed allele frequencies, and when multiplied by the number of individuals in the population sample, gives the expected Hardy–Weinberg equilibrium distribution.

There are four disruptive factors potentially affecting Hardy–Weinberg equilibria in natural populations. (1) The population must effectively be a randomly mating one, yet in nature, some individuals may have a greater or lesser probability of mating with others. (2) The law assumes the population is effectively infinite, but real populations obviously are not, and the frequency of an allele (particularly in small populations) may vary by chance. (3) All alleles should have an equal probability of making copies of themselves in order to enter the gene pool in the gametes. However, alleles may differ in their replacement rates by selection. (4) The law assumes no input of new copies of an allele to the population, either by migration of genes (gene flow) from another population with different gene frequencies, or by transformation of one allele into another (mutation). Mutation rates amongst vertebrates are probably very low (about 10^{-6} or 10^{-7}), but gene flow may vary considerably between populations, leading to significant substructuring. Sampling error may also contribute to the deviation from expected equilibrium values. For example, a deficiency of heterozygotes can result from combining within a single sample individuals from more than one genetically distinct population. This is known as the Wahlund effect. Assortative mating will also produce heterozygote deficiency in addition to the Wahlund effect. Finally, a marked deviation from Hardy–Weinberg equilibrium may also occur if the phenotype used to derive the genotype was not inherited (but is due to post-translational changes). These likely disturbing influences on the Hardy–Weinberg equilibrium represent some of the interesting questions commonly addressed by the evolutionary biologist or behavioural ecologist. It is therefore important to test whether or not a sampled population is in Hardy–Weinberg equilibrium at a given locus. This is done by calculating chi-squared values for each genotype and then summing over genotypes to obtain a total χ^2 value. This measures the deviation of the observed genotypic frequencies from the expected ones. The number of degrees of freedom equals $g - (a - 1)$, where g is the number of possible genotypes from the alleles, and a is the number of independent alleles (equal to the total number of alleles at the locus minus 1).

The expected distribution of genotypes holds among zygotes in the presence of disturbing factors, provided the zygotes are sampled before the disturbing factors have acted on the population. However even with disturbing factors, the equilibrium genotypic frequencies described above will hold before selection (Kimura 1983). In the case of sexual selection, when there is no assortative mating, the Hardy–Weinberg ratios always hold at equilibrium, regardless of the intensity of the selection so that at any stage in the life cycle, Hardy–Weinberg ratios will be found (O'Donald 1980).

2.5   Linkage and the effects of age and sex on allele frequencies

Sometimes gene loci may be linked so that alleles do not assort independently. Since the Hardy–Weinberg test is rather insensitive, sample populations may appear to be in equilibrium when in fact there is linkage or some other deviation from the assumptions of the model. The best test for autosomal linkage is to screen both parents and offspring and test for di-allelic segregation. Alternatively, an indirect test is a chi-square for non-random association of allele frequencies between loci (see Hill (1974) for computation of coefficients of linkage disequilibrium and tests of significance). Ideally, such tests should be carried out as early as possible in the life cycle of the bird, before selection has occurred.

The female is the heterogametic sex among birds, and thus a simple test for sex-linkage is to screen females for the presence of heterozygotes at each locus. If heterozygotes are present, it is unlikely that the locus is sex-linked. Some enzymes are generally known to be sex-linked, for example aconitase. An implicit assumption of the Hardy–Weinberg law is that males and females have the same genotypic frequencies. It is therefore important to test whether or not this is the case by carrying out the calculations and tests described in the two previous sections separately for each sex.

There may also be differences in allele frequencies between different age groups, and where information on age is available, comparisons may be made of genotypic and allele frequencies for those different groups. Any differences obtained may be the result of differential selection or dispersal, or when a population has not reached a stable age distribution (see Charlesworth 1980). These aspects are discussed below.

2.6   Heterozygosity and polymorphism

Two measures of the amount of genetic variation in a population are the amount of heterozygosity, and the proportion of loci that are polymorphic in the population. Both of these have been commonly used in the search for pattern in the genetic variation exhibited by populations, species and higher taxa (e.g. Powell 1975, Nevo 1978).

Cavalli-Sforza and Bodmer (1971) define a genetic polymorphism as the occurrence in the same population of two or more alleles at one locus, each with appreciable frequency. In practice, a locus is considered polymorphic when the frequency of the most common allele is less than 0·99 or alternatively less than 0·95. The former cut-off point is used most often, partly because a very rare allele may still be maintained in the population as a whole even though it is absent in some subpopulations or at a frequency of less than 5% (see Table 5).

To estimate the proportion of polymorphic loci (P) for a population where a number of loci have been examined, the number of polymorphic loci is counted and then divided by the total number of loci examined (remembering that there may be more than one locus per enzyme). The accuracy of this estimate depends upon the number of loci examined (a minimum of 14 loci is commonly taken, though at least 20 is recommended) and on the number of individuals (a minimum of 30 is recommended, and preferably at least 100, sampled over two or more regions). The variance of this estimate may be calculated as

$$V(\hat{P}) = \frac{\hat{P}(1 - \hat{P})}{m}$$

Table 5. *P* and *H* estimates for 19 populations of European Starling

Population	Number of individuals	Polymorphic loci per population (P)	Heterozygosity per locus per population (H)
Surrey	263	0·20	0·0140
Oxford	64	0·20	0·0172
Cambridge	92	0·20	0·0193
Slimbridge	57	0·00	0·0000
Brecon	44	0·13	0·0091
Aberdeen	322	0·20	0·0098
Orkney	64	0·13	0·0121
Fair Isle	65	0·13	0·0376
Shetland	57	0·13	0·0246
Lewis	56	0·13	0·0328
Faroes	70	0·20	0·0019
Norway	50	0·13	0·0093
Iceland	70	0·07	0·0076
Belgium	80	0·13	0·0100
Holland	33	0·13	0·0040
Germany	41	0·00	0·0000
Czechoslovakia	54	0·20	0·0062
Switzerland	138	0·20	0·0068
France	42	0·07	0·0079
Mean		0·136	0·0121
S.E.		0·014	0·0023

NOTE: *P* and *H* estimates based upon number of individuals noted above, assuming that total sample sizes of fifty was sufficient to determine if the enzyme was monomorphic.

where $\hat{P}$ is the proportion of polymorphic loci and m the number of sampled loci.

The polymorphism of a population is not an entirely satisfactory measure of genetic variation, being both arbitrary (dependent upon the criterion of polymorphism that is used) and imprecise (since a slightly polymorphic locus is treated in the same way as a very polymorphic one).

Probably the most widespread measure of genetic variation in a population is the amount of heterozygosity. The heterozygosity of a population is an estimate of the probability of two alleles from the same locus, taken at random from the population, being different. This may be calculated in a number of ways, depending on whether variation within individuals, populations or loci is being examined. The values may also be estimated as observed frequencies of heterozygotes, expected frequencies (assuming Hardy–Weinberg equilibria) or from allele frequency data. It is important to distinguish between these different heterozygosity estimates because they yield differences in the amount of variance associated with each parameter. The mean observed heterozygosity ($\hat{H}_0$) in a sampled population is usually calculated for a number of loci. This involves counting the number of individuals heterozygous at a particular locus and dividing by the total number of individuals examined. This is then repeated for other loci and a mean estimate obtained by averaging the values over all loci. Alternatively, the number of heterozygotes across all loci may be calculated for each individual, summed for all individuals, and then divided by the total number of individuals to give a mean heterozygosity estimate for the population as before. Both methods will provide the same estimates but the variance associated with each will differ (see Nei and Roychoudhury 1974, Corbin 1981, 1983). It will be larger in the first method of estimation because of the high diversity in the number of alleles per locus (with many loci being monomorphic); the variance may be reduced by increasing the number of loci sampled. In the second method, the variance is best reduced by increasing the number of individuals sampled.

If a population is not in Hardy–Weinberg equilibrium, the observed heterozygosity may not reflect well the amount of genetic variation in the population. This will occur, for example, if matings between relatives are common, even though allele frequencies may be identical to a population where mating is random. This difficulty can be overcome by calculating the expected heterozygosity from the allele frequencies *as if* they were mating at random, using the formula $1 - \sum_{i=1}^{n} \hat{p}_i^2$ where $\hat{p}_i$ is the frequency of the ith allele at a locus, with n alleles (Nei 1975), and averaging values over all loci. The expected heterozygosity may then be compared with the observed values, and chi-square tested.

2.7   Measures of genetic identity and genetic distance

Heterozygosities give one measure of genetic variation, but there are other methods which have the advantage that values may be directly compared between populations (demes, species, genera, etc.) and between differently sized groupings (i.e. between versus within species, or genera etc.), and thus used to measure genetic differentiation during the speciation process and possible phylogenetic relationships. Two commonly used methods are the indices of Nei (1972, 1978) and Rogers (1972).

Nei's genetic identity (I) estimates the normalized probability that two alleles, one taken from each population, are identical. Essentially it provides a measure of the similarity in frequency of each allele, summed over all alleles. It is given by $I = \sum I_{xy} / \sqrt{I_x I_y}$, where I_{xy}, I_x, I_y are the averages over all loci (including monomorphic ones) of $\sum x_i y_i$, $\sum x_i^2$ and $\sum y_i^2$, respectively, where x_i

and y_i are the frequencies of allele i for two populations X and Y. The genetic distance D between the two populations is then calculated by $D - \log_e I$. Nei (1978) has recently introduced a modification of the formula for I, to be used for small sample sizes.

Genetic identity may vary from zero (no alleles shared between the two populations) to one (where both populations have identical allele frequencies). Genetic distance varies from zero for populations with identical allele frequencies to infinity (in theory) for populations that do not share any alleles.

An alternative measure of genetic similarity is Roger's index S, which is expressed as follows:

$$S = 1 - \frac{1}{\sqrt{\sum_{i=1}^{n}(p_{ix}p_{iy})^2}}$$

where p_{ix} = frequency of allele i in population X, p_{iy} = frequency of allele i in population Y, and N = number of alleles at the locus. As above, the genetic distance $D = -\log_e S$.

The Nei and Roger indices of genetic similarity are highly correlated although Roger's index, S, gives slightly lower values than Nei's index, I. A third index of genetic identity/distance is that of Hedrick (1971). This makes use of observed genotypic frequencies, and is useful when populations are not in Hardy–Weinberg proportions for the loci examined.

Computer programs may then use these indices to reconstruct evolutionary relationships. The two most commonly used algorithms are those of Sneath and Sokal (1973), called UPGMA (unweighted pair groups) or WPGMA (weighted pair groups), which cluster taxa into hierarchical levels according to genetic similarity, and the Wagner tree algorithms of Farris (1972, 1973) which fit genetic distance values to the most parsimonious branching networks. A cladistic method similar to the latter is that of Fitch and Margoliash (1967), which constructs a number of trees by altering the branching structure and branch lengths.

Although Nei's indices tend to be more commonly used, Nei's D does not satisfy the conditions necessary for triangle inequality (i.e. when the distances between three taxa (A, B, C) are compared, distance (AC) must be equal to or less than distance (AB) plus distance (BC), and may thus result in negative branch lengths within a phylogeny (see Barrowclough and Corbin 1978, Farris 1981). However, Roger's indices may also not be appropriate since the common ancestor of three taxa cannot exist on any branch that connects any two of the three taxa (Farris 1981). One method to overcome these problems is to use actual characters (in this case, loci) retaining allelic data (as character states) in particulate form rather than as frequencies, and using shared characters/character states to infer phylogeny (Farris 1981; Mickevich and Mitter 1981, 1983, Wake 1981).

2.8 Testing for genetic heterogeneity

Populations may be genetically differentiated so that allele frequencies of two samples are significantly different. This may be tested using a chi-square test for heterogeneity over populations; alternatively a G-test may be used (Sokal and Rohlf 1981). A test for genetic heterogeneity (multiplying twice the tested sample size by the sum across alleles of the weighted variance of the allele frequency divided by the estimated mean allele frequency) has been commonly used in the literature following Workman and Niswander (1970) and Lewontin and Krakauer (1973). However, Ewens and Feldman (1976) have shown it to be invalid since it depends upon gene frequencies being normally distributed (whereas they are often rectangular or bimodal).

2.9 Wright's *F*-statistics

Genetic heterogeneity may also be examined using Wright's fixation coefficients F_{ST}, F_{IS}, and F_{IT} (Wright 1965, 1978). These have the advantage of allowing a simultaneous comparison of allele frequencies for a number of populations across many loci. They are, however, based upon the case for neutrality, applying to gene loci that are effectively neutral. F_{ST} is the most commonly used of the three coefficients and gives a measure of the extent to which a species is organized into demes with restricted gene flow. It represents the correlation between alleles of gametes sampled at random from two subdivisions of a population, with the distribution of alleles within the entire population sampled. It reflects the extent of local differentiation into subpopulations or demes.

F_{IS} is the average (over all subdivisions) of the correlations between alleles of uniting gametes (in practice, individuals) sampled at random within subdivisions relative to the distribution of alleles within those subdivisions. This indicates the degree of structuring (i.e. non-random mating) at a finer level within subpopulations, by measuring the deviation of genotypic frequencies from Hardy–Weinberg equilibrium.

F_{IT} is the correlation between alleles of uniting gametes sampled at random relative to the distribution of alleles in the entire population. It measures deviation from Hardy–Weinberg equilibrium within the total population, and combines the effects of both non-random mating and geographical subdivision of the total population. F_{ST} is always positive; F_{IS}

and F_{IT} may be positive, indicating a deficiency of heterozygotes; or negative, indicating an excess. The three coefficients are interrelated so that

$$F_{ST} = \frac{(F_{IT} - F_{IS})}{(1 - F_{IS})} \qquad \text{(Wright 1965)}$$

The value of F_{ST} is calculated for single loci comprising two alleles, using allele frequencies, $F_{ST} = V(q)/\hat{q}(1 - \hat{q})$ where $V(q)$ is the variance in the frequency of allele A_2, and $\hat{q} = \sum w_i q_i$ is the weighted frequency of A_2 in the total population. Generally, equal weight is given to each subpopulation (unless it is known that subpopulation sizes differ substantially) by $w_i = 1/k$, where k is the number of subpopulations. Subdivisions of the population (here termed "subpopulations") are usually made arbitrarily, primarily on the basis of practical sampling convenience, although they may represent geographically separated samples. Wright (1978) has also devised a method to allow for sampling error in the calculation of F_{ST}. A chi-square test is commonly used, where $\chi^2 = 2NF_{ST}$ ($2N =$ number of gametes in the sample), although it may be applied *only* if sample sizes are identical for all populations and only two alleles occur at the locus compared.

Nei (1977) has extended this analysis to multiple loci and loci with multiple alleles. The average F coefficients are calculated for multiple loci as

$$\hat{F}_{IS} = \frac{\bar{H}_S - \bar{H}_0}{\bar{H}_S}; \quad \hat{F}_{IT} = \frac{\bar{H}_T - \bar{H}_0}{\bar{H}_T}; \quad \hat{F}_{ST} = \frac{\bar{H}_T - \bar{H}_S}{\bar{H}_T}$$

where $\bar{H}_0$ is the average observed heterozygosity within a subpopulation over loci, $\bar{H}_S$ is the average expected heterozygosity within subpopulations over loci, and $\bar{H}_T$ is the average expected heterozygosity in the total population over loci.

Deviations from panmixia (random mating) within subpopulations ($\hat{F}_{IS} = 0$) can be tested for each locus by the non-parametric G-test (Sokal and Rohlf 1981) with one degree of freedom (following Cockerham 1973). The null hypothesis that there is no substructuring of the population (i.e. $\hat{F}_{ST} = 0$) may likewise be examined by testing for heterogeneity of allele frequencies between subpopulations using the G-test (with $M - 1$ degrees of freedom, where $M =$ number of populations). Since some alleles may be at very low frequencies, it is wise to combine these in contingency tables until all expected cell frequencies exceed $1 \cdot 0$ (and preferably most exceed $3 \cdot 0$). In those cases it is not possible to test for significant heterogeneity between subpopulations because of the lumping of different alleles. However, by combining cells containing alleles at low frequencies, the G-test may be used to determine the maximum number of cells that can be combined before heterogeneity reaches statistical significance. The means of F_{ST}, F_{IS} and F_{IT} estimated over all variable loci may be compared to zero by the t-test.

Finally, Corbin (1983) has shown that F_{ST} (corrected for sampling error) is nearly perfectly correlated in a linear fashion with Nei's indices (also corrected for sampling error). This may then be used to test the similarity between regression coefficients for different levels of taxonomic comparisons (e.g. comparisons between bird species versus comparisons between local populations within species) (see Corbin (1983) and chapter 10 for details).

3 PATTERNS OF GENETIC VARIATION

Before discussing avian genetic studies in the context of evolutionary theory, it may be useful to consider some of the limitations of the electrophoretic method of genetic analysis.

Most studies of genetic variation should ideally sample the entire genome in an unbiased manner. However, electrophoresis does not do this. Firstly, only structural genes code for enzymes and other proteins, and less than 10% of the DNA in eukaryotes comprises such structural genes (genes of regulatory or other function are inaccessible to this technique). Secondly, because of the redundancy of the genetic code, about 30% of the DNA base changes cause no modification in the amino acid sequence of proteins. Thirdly, because many kinds of amino acid substitution do not change the charge on a protein, the number of substitutions that can be detected by electrophoresis is reduced to about 25%. The band on the gel (often referred to as an electromorph) may comprise groups of alleles that appear alike. Recently, various techniques have been employed (termed "sequential electrophoresis") to reveal such hidden genetic variation, which previously had gone undetected (Coyne 1976, Singh *et al.* 1976, Johnson 1977). These include studies of thermostability or speed of denaturation by heat (Singh *et al.* 1976), gel sieving, and pH differentials (Johnson 1977, Ramshaw *et al.* 1979). These methods are not as easy to use as gel electrophoresis, requiring more time, effort and money so that they are not so widely used as perhaps they should be.

Although eukaryotes may synthesize many thousands of different kinds of protein, in practice less than 100 of these are readily used in electrophoresis. This is because the studied proteins are soluble, and are either enzymes for which a specific enzyme dye is available, or proteins with a high enough concentration to be detected with a general protein stain.

3.1 Amount of variation

Despite the above limitations, gel electrophoresis has revealed a great deal of genetic variation. Some classes of enzymes appear to have consistently higher heterozygosity across species than others (O'Brien *et al.* 1980). Gillespie and Kojima (1968) and Kojima *et al.* (1970) distinguished two general classes of protein according to their biochemical function in physiological processes: enzymes that metabolize glucose and non-specific enzymes. They found that the latter group showed higher levels of heterozygosity. Ward (1977) compared heterozygosity values for enzymes of different quaternary structure and found that monomeric enzymes were, as predicted, more variable than dimeric forms, which in turn were more variable than tetrameric forms. Johnson (1974) and Powell (1975) classified enzymes into three groups. Some enzymes use different substrates depending upon the external environment from which the substrates were derived. Others appear to be closely involved with metabolic pathways, regulating the flow of metabolites. These might be considered more susceptible to selection than those non-regulatory enzymes that do not play a limiting role in metabolism. The argument is that variable substrate enzymes might show greater genetic variability (higher heterozygosity) since they may need to adapt to a variety of environmental situations. Non-regulatory enzymes might be least variable (assuming selection is maintaining the presence of different alleles) since there would be less need for alternative forms of the enzyme. Both Johnson and Powell compared the heterozygosities of each enzyme group for different taxa, and both obtained broadly similar results (partly due to a similar data base): non-regulatory enzymes usually having the lowest, and variable substrate or regulatory enzymes the highest average heterozygosities. However, the pattern was not necessarily borne out across taxa; birds, for example, were most variable for non-regulatory enzymes. At the time of the studies, data were available from only five bird species, but a similar pattern is obtained with the broader data set summarized in Tables 2 and 3.

An alternative measure of variability amongst enzymes is, of course, the proportion of those examined that is polymorphic (*P*). If this is used on data sets of both birds and mammals (spanning a wide range of families), where at least fifteen enzymes have been examined, some enzymes are clearly more often polymorphic than others (Fig. 2). Eight out of ten of the most commonly polymorphic ones are shared by the two classes. There are a few differences between birds and mammals. For example, haemoglobin is more commonly polymorphic in mammals, as is malate dehydrogenase (see also Kitto and Wilson (1966) and Karig and Wilson (1971)), although Aquadro and Avise (1982) have uncovered some "hidden" variation among electromorphs of the latter enzyme. Of the twelve most common polymorphic enzymes whose metabolic function is known, seven of these are non-regulatory, three are regulatory and two have external substrates. Again, non-regulatory enzymes appear to be more commonly variable than other groups. However, it is difficult to know how to interpret these results and explain some of the observed differences between taxa. Such a classification of enzyme type may not be valid in this context, and it may be more profitable to examine specific enzymes and their function. Watt (1985) reviews the metabolic effects of different allozymes and the adaptive significance of such variants.

Whatever the significance, the results may be used to advantage when the need is to maximize the chances of finding an avian or mammalian polymorphism with the least expenditure of time and expense. This is particularly useful when genealogical analyses (e.g. paternity studies) are being carried out (see below). Calculations of P and H, however, should not be made on such data because of the obvious bias in this measure of genetic variability.

The extent of variation in allozyme loci for various classes of animals has been surveyed by Powell (1975), Selander (1976) and Nevo (1978). These showed that invertebrates are on average twice as polymorphic as vertebrates ($\hat{P} = 0.397$ versus 0.173), and nearly three times as heterozygous ($\hat{H} = 0.12$ versus 0.049). Values for birds were $\hat{P} = 0.150$ and $\hat{H} = 0.047$—figures that are comparable with mammals. At the time that these reviews were made, data from only seven bird species were available. A more recent survey by Barrowclough (1983) of 30 bird species each from a single breeding population (including between 17 and 269 individuals and 14–44 loci) gave a mean heterozygosity value of 0.053. A less restrictive survey by Corbin (1983) of 71 bird species (involving between 10 and 390 individuals and 14–45 loci), including most of those in Barrowclough's study, gave a comparable mean heterozygosity value of 0.0673, and $\hat{P}$ value of 0.222. Data from these two reviews, together with some further estimates of H and P, are given in Table 2. Generally the broader data base has increased the estimates of both H and P, to values slightly higher than those for mammals. This is probably the result of recent inclusion of estimates for Procellariiformes and Anseriformes which have had much higher values than most of the Passeriformes examined.

Although it is probably valid to draw some broad conclusions from the above results, there is need for caution. Neither $\hat{P}$ nor $\hat{H}$ should be regarded as species characteristics. In European Starling, for example, estimates of $\hat{P}$ for 19 populations vary from zero to 20%, and H varies from zero to 4% (Table 5). Forty per cent of the estimates in Table 3 involve single populations (using only those data where this information has been presented) and 80% involve samples of fewer than 50 individuals. Furthermore, studies by different laboratories have often come up with quite different estimates and their findings have differed with respect to whether a particular enzyme was monomorphic or polymorphic (see, for example, *Zonotrichia leucophrys* and *Dendroica coronata* in Table 2). These results suggest that, at present, comparisons of P and H between taxa are probably only useful above the level of the species. Nevo (1978) found significant correlations between P and H for animals, including birds. However, within a species this relationship may weaken. Comparisons of $\hat{P}$ and $\hat{H}$ values amongst populations for European Starling showed a low non-significant positive correlation (Table 5). Populations with high P values did not necessarily have high H values (for example, the Faeroese population) whereas some populations with intermediate values of P had high values of H (for example, offshore Scottish islands).

Notwithstanding the above remarks, there is no doubt that birds, like other animal classes examined, harbour a great deal of genetic variation as expressed by allozyme variation. Accounting for this variation forms the basis for many current population genetic studies, with some suggesting that the genome comprises primarily polymorphic lines maintained by selection and others that most lines are effectively neutral (Lewontin 1974, Nei 1975, Kimura 1983). It is not possible to test for neutrality, and so most studies search for evidence of selection. If they find it their case is strengthened: if they do not, neutrality is invoked, although they may simply not be looking at the appropriate parameter. Evidence for selection may be obtained in a number of ways, and this will be examined in the following sections.

3.2   Spatial and temporal variation

While differences in gene and genotype frequencies in allozyme loci are often found in different parts of a species range, it is seldom possible to provide unambiguous explanations for these differences. Extended studies by Baker and co-workers (Baker 1974, 1975, 1982 a,b, Baker and Mewaldt 1978, 1981; Baker *et al.* 1982) have shown correlations between allele frequency differences and song dialect distributions. Whether the genetic differentiation is caused by dialects or isolation by distance is not clear (Payne 1981, Petrinovich *et al.* 1981, Zink and Barrowclough 1984, Baker *et al.* 1984).

Spatial variation at individual loci has been detected and correlated with habitat or historical differences. Redfield (1973, 1974) showed a higher frequency of heterozygotes at the Ng locus in mature forests as opposed to early successional stages. Bacon (1979) found spatial variation in gene frequencies at the LDH locus in Mute Swan with high frequencies of the recessive allele in a local population of south-west England; this despite a considerable gene flow in other populations (Fig. 3). He concluded that differences in allele frequencies are maintained by local adaptation.

Several studies, for example of small rodents (Semeonoff and Robertson 1968, Gaines *et al.* 1978), have found a significant variation in gene frequencies over time (in rodents, usually between seasons) and where it has

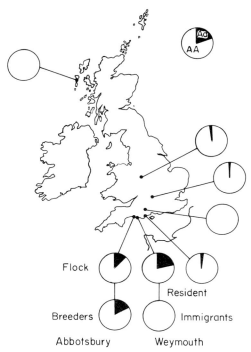

Fig. 3. Lactate dehydrogenase genotype frequencies in Mute Swan within Britain (from Bacon 1979). Note the differences in genotype frequencies between resident/breeding birds at Weymouth and Abbotsbury, and those from other localities in Britain.

occurred (for example, in rodents), there are indications that it simply reflects demographic changes in the age structure of the population (Charlesworth and Giesel 1972, Charlesworth, 1980). On the other hand, similar studies of birds have rarely detected such temporal variation (Redfield *et al.* 1972, Bacon 1979, Evans 1980). The maintenance of similar genotype frequencies from year to year, but differing from one another spatially, is illustrated for European Starling in Fig. 4.

Many of the above examples do little more than indicate that patterns exist for gene frequencies in space and time, at various allozyme loci, and in a number of avian species. In some cases the patterns may be linked with environmental heterogeneity, but rarely does this indicate the process by which the pattern is created. Natural populations of birds are not very amenable to experimental manipulation to demonstrate a cause–effect relationship between the environment and the frequency of electrophoretic alleles.

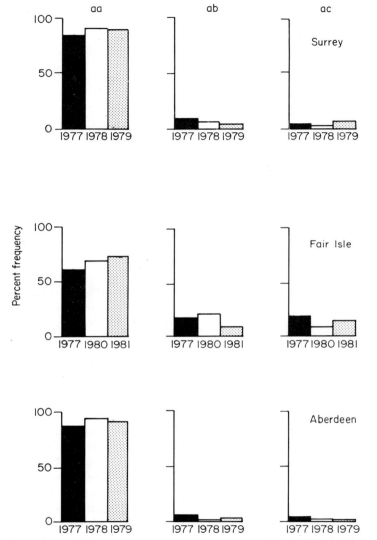

Fig. 4. Annual changes in Esterase genotype frequencies in European Starling for three sites in Britain. Two mainland sites maintain high frequencies (85% +) of the AA genotype over the years 1977–1979, whilst the isolated island population on Fair Isle maintains lower frequencies (60–70%) between the years 1977–1981.

3.3 Selection

Changes in the frequency of allozyme loci in the wild that could be ascribed to natural selection have seldom been demonstrated (Endler 1986). Two avian examples are discussed.

Among starling populations over most of Britain and north-west Europe, one genotype, AA at the EST-1 locus, is at frequencies of 85% or higher, whereas heterozygotes AB and AC are at very low frequencies (see, for example, Fig. 4); the homozygotes BB and CC are extremely rare and in a number of the populations sampled, have not yet been recorded (Evans 1980). Genotype frequencies for 19 localities showed significant spatial heterogeneity, with an excess of AC individuals north of latitude 57°, compared with populations sampled further south. On Fair Isle, an isolated island half-way between Shetland and Orkney, the gene frequencies are very different, with AA at only 70%, and AB and AC 10–20%. These frequencies remained stable over a period of six years. Comparisons of clutch sizes, laying dates, and subsequent breeding success indicated selection against the rarer genotypes in mainland Britain, with AB genotypes laying smaller clutches early in the breeding season and AC genotypes laying large clutches later. However, both of these genotypes have lower egg and nestling survival than AA genotypes, hence lower fecundity as measured by fledgling success. A breeding study on Fair Isle obtained differences in fecundity between genotypes comparable with those found for the two more southerly populations on the British mainland, but with some important differences. In a normal season, AB genotypes lay small clutches earlier, as in the more southerly populations, but AC genotypes lay no later and clutch size is not significantly larger; when the breeding season is late, AC genotypes were favoured. Thus we may have a balanced polymorphism where one genotype has the ability to lay relatively early but produces a smaller clutch, and another lays later but with a larger clutch size. The consequence of laying late within a season is that breeding success is lower (cf. most passerine breeding studies), but this is counterbalanced by the larger number of eggs laid so that fecundity is comparable. One genotype (AC) may be slightly favoured in years when breeding is later or in regions with later seasons, e.g. in the north of the European range; another genotype (AB) may be favoured when the converse conditions apply.

An interesting corollary to the above is Bacon's (1979) study on Mute Swan. Working on putatively the same EST-1 locus (it occupies the same anodal position behind the buffer front but comprises two alleles), he also found differences in clutch size and laying date between genotypes, although in his case significantly more females of one genotype (homozygous SS) laid *large* clutches early. This pattern was maintained between years. There was

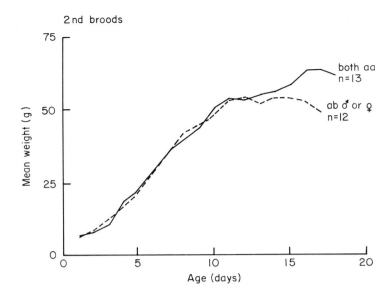

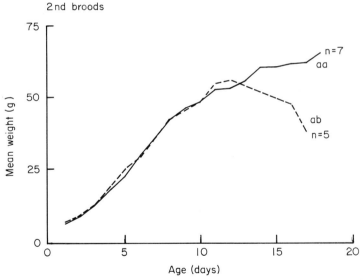

Fig. 5. (*a*) Differential growth rates of young starlings with parents of different EST-1 genotypes in Surrey. (*b*) Differential growth rates of young starlings of different genotypes with AB parent in Surrey. Note that nestlings from broods with an AB parent grew worse from day 12 than did those whose parents were AA genotype. In broods with an AB parent, those nestlings of AA genotype grew normally but those of AB genotype lost weight markedly after day 12. The differences in growth rates between offspring must therefore be a function of nestling genotypes rather than parental genotype.

also an effect of mate on clutch size and laying date such that the mates of heterozygous SF males laid larger than average clutches regardless of whether the females laid early or late. These genetic differences, which led to differences in productivity, were postulated to be mediated through habitat selection (Bacon 1979).

If there is a relationship between the timing of egg-laying and the number of eggs laid, for possibly the same Esterase locus, it would be useful to determine a biochemical/physiological basis for it. There is no reason, of course, why there should be such a basis, since if selection were operating, it might be doing so at another locus in linkage disequilibrium with that being examined. However, there is some indication of a direct physiological relationship in the following observation. The European Starling normally feeds its young on an invertebrate diet (particularly cranefly larvae), and in mainland Britain these are most abundant in May and June, usually coinciding with the nestling period (Evans 1980). Occasionally, if starlings have nested early, they have a second brood in late June, but by this time the food supply becomes unpredictable. Second broods are less successful than first broods, and in some years there may be high nestling mortality. In one such year this occurred, and although some young grew at a normal rate, others lost weight at a particular time and most of these died. Examination of the genotypes of these two groups revealed that the rare heterozygotes AB and AC grew poorly, whereas the common homozygotes AA grew normally (Fig. 5). This difference in growth rates between genotypes was further emphasized when a comparison was made (Fig. 5(*b*)) of the growth rates of offspring from mixed matings: within broods, AA genotypes grew normally whilst AB and AC genotypes did not, and indeed all of the latter died. At the time of the low growth rates, feeding observations indicated a failure in the food supply, with birds switching to a diet of poultry meal. Post-mortem analysis of those nestlings that died revealed that the poultry meal had not been digested. This suggested a genotypic difference in the ability to digest and assimilate this particular food. The functions of esterases are little known although they relate to the hydrolysis of fatty acids. It is possible that the rare genotypes are unable (at least as nestlings) to break down fatty acids, but this requires further work to be carried out in order to describe the biochemical properties of each genotype, and feeding experiments on captive starlings of different genotype.

3.4 Population structure

The subject of genetic differentiation in birds at different levels of classification has received intensive study. For excellent recent reviews, the

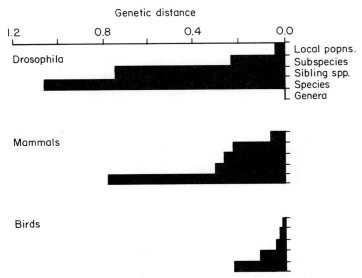

Genetic distance

Fig. 6. Genetic distances among and between different taxonomic levels using the method of Nei (1972). Birds show the least differentiation, with comparable genetic distances between genera as are found between subspecies of mammals and *Drosophila* fruit flies. (From Ayala (1976) for *Drosophila* and mammals; Corbin (1978) for birds.)

reader is referred to Avise and Aquadro (1982), Barrowclough (1983) and Corbin (1983). In this section I shall therefore summarize only those findings particularly relevant to this chapter.

The most striking result of many studies is that differentiation (as measured from allozyme variants) is far less pronounced among birds than is the case for other groups such as amphibians and reptiles. These results may reflect more recent speciation events amongst birds, or possibly slower rates of protein divergence due to their internal physiology (unusually high and stable body temperatures) (Avise and Aquadro 1982). Amphibian congeners are approximately 10–20 times more divergent in protein composition than are species of birds placed in the same genus. Even mammals are about three times as divergent (see Fig. 6).

3.5 Social behaviour and breeding systems

Genetic structuring of populations depends in part upon social structure and mating systems. Genetic heterogeneity between populations is enhanced (and hence effective population size reduced) if (i) some individuals obtain more matings than others, by promiscuity, polygyny or polyandry, or (ii) some mate monogamously but leave more offspring than others, and (iii) if there are overlapping generations so that offspring can mate with their parents. All of these are known to occur in birds, and form the basis for many of the interesting questions being asked by behavioural ecologists and evolutionary biologists. Social behaviour such as co-operative breeding, nest parasitism, infanticide, siblicide and nepotism may be explained by interdemic and kin selection, but studies using allozymes have rarely been carried out on birds.

One example of the use of allozyme variation to investigate the population structure of a bird species is provided by the work of Johnson and Brown (1980). They studied allozyme variation in a population of Australian Grey-crowned Babbler (*Pomastostomus temporalis*), which forms sedentary territorial social units, usually comprising one breeding pair and one to several non-breeding individuals who may act as helpers in raising the young. Johnson and Brown wanted to identify whether close inbreeding might account for possible altruistic behaviour. The results showed no deficiency of heterozygotes over expected values, and no substructuring at distances of up to 9 km, implying at least occasional long-distance dispersal from natal social groups. They concluded that there was no evidence for close inbreeding but recognized that the use of F statistics to assess inbreeding is not entirely reliable because of insensitivity of genotypic frequencies to departures from expectation (as I noted earlier).

Paternity is clearly something that is important to determine if a number of sociobiological questions are to be answered. Extra-pair copulations in apparently monogamous species, the dumping of eggs by females in the nests of others, and the degree of polygyny or polyandry exhibited by a species can be detected only by genetic evidence. Using allozymes, Evans (1980, in press) identified cases of nest parasitism in European Starling that would otherwise have gone undetected. Since then, similar methods have been used to detect multiple maternity and paternity in apparently monogamous Eastern Bluebirds (*Sialia sialis*) (Gowaty and Karlin 1984), multiple paternity in the territorial Bobolink (*Dolichonyx oryzivorus*) (Gavin and Bellinger 1985) and in the co-operatively breeding Acorn Woodpecker (*Melanerpes formicivorus*) (Joste *et al.* 1985).

Since putative and actual parents may share the same genotype, the probability of detecting parenthood is increased by combining data from a number of polymorphic loci using loci with multiple alleles, and examining species with large brood sizes. Both probabilistic models (Birdsall and Nash 1973, Merritt and Wu 1975) and maximum likelihood statistics (Thompson 1976, Foltz and Hoogland 1981) have been used for overall estimates but they are limited by the number of loci that are polymorphic and the distribution of the genotype frequencies. If alleles are close to fixation, the estimates will have high variances and this has been a common problem.

However, at least they allow the ranking of individuals according to the probabilities of their being the parent.

There is some scope for further use of allozyme studies in these contexts (Sherman 1983) though mainly to detect individual cases of multiple parentity; otherwise DNA techniques may be more favourable (chapter 5).

4 CONCLUSIONS AND FUTURE DIRECTIONS

Allozyme studies of birds indicate that they possess levels of variation at structural gene loci comparable to other vertebrate classes, with a mean corrected heterozygosity per individual per locus ($\hat{H}$) of 0·063 for 85 species examined, and a mean per cent polymorphism ($\hat{P}$) of 24% ($n = 109$ species). This large amount of genic variation may be maintained primarily by selection or, as more recent studies suggest, be mainly the consequences of recombination or mutation. Although we can probably never expect to determine the proportion of the genome that is one or the other, there are several ways that more substantive evidence could be obtained than we have at present. There are a number of examples of correlations between spatial genetic variation and environmental variation. Temporal correlates are less common although this may be due to the shortness of time that studies have been in progress. We need to progress beyond simply observing such correlations. There is a need to relate genotypes and their frequencies to components of fitness (see Christiansen and Frydenberg (1973) and Nadeau and Baccus (1981) for selection component analyses of natural populations). When one considers the wealth of ecological data collected from birds and the number of long-term studies of marked populations whose age structure is often known, it is surprising that so few studies have attempted this. A systematic examination of allozyme variants is required, testing for selection locus-by-locus. Absence of evidence for selection should be published along with positive evidence. When particular genotypes have higher fitness values, then is the time to examine the *in vitro* biochemical properties of these allozymes under different environmental conditions. Although there will be complicating factors such as pleiotropy and genetic interactions, if biochemical associations are found they will lend additional support to the selective importance of various allozymes, and may be further tested by perturbations of the environment or by modifying the genetic composition of the population. However, in most cases the latter methods may be beyond the reach of the experimental population geneticist working with birds, since such tests generally require massive sample sizes and replications to detect statistical significance.

The ways in which balanced polymorphism may be maintained need to be

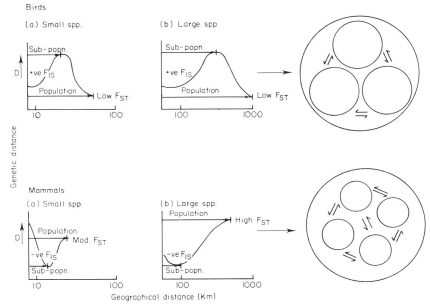

Fig. 7. Model of population structure in birds compared with mammals. *Birds.* Sub-populations show some sub-structuring, commonly yielding positive F_{IS} values. Moderate dispersal (mainly natal and usually female biased). Low F_{ST} values due to large population size and significant gene flow between sub-populations. Geographical area occupied by large species larger than for small species. *Mammals.* Systematic avoidance of inbreeding within sub-populations particularly among small mammals, with usually male-biased natal dispersal (and some breeding dispersal), commonly yielding negative F_{IS} values. F_{ST} values moderate (in small mammals) or large (in large mammals) due to semi-isolated sub-populations restricting gene flow. Geographical area occupied by large species larger than for small species. Notes: (1) Size of circles refers to relative size of *Ne*, not to land area occupied by population. (2) These models are generalized and do not take account of variation resulting from differences in demography, population history, mating system or territoriality. (3) Differences relating to large and small species will be modified if that species is migratory and shows low site fidelity (as may occur with some small passerine birds, for example).

examined in well-studied bird populations, taking account of the effects of population structure and population history. Allozyme studies lend themselves to such tests.

The role of genetic drift can only be determined by more realistic and more extensive estimates of effective population size. Although present F_{ST} values suggest high vagility and substantial gene flow, leading to substantially lower rates of genetic differentiation than other classes, there are few estimates of

F_{IS} or F_{IT} available. Furthermore, other forms of evidence (Greenwood *et al.* 1978, van Noordwijk and Scharloo 1981, Wunderle 1981) suggest high rates of inbreeding and significant substructuring of the population, at least at a local level. The balance between strong philopatry leading to genetic heterogeneity, and differential dispersal of the sexes providing outbreeding, needs to be carefully assessed. A possible scenario to account for seemingly conflicting observations (inbreeding versus vagility) is given in Fig. 7, and could readily be tested.

Genetic substructuring, measured by a combination of F statistics and genetic distance measures, should be studied in species with a range of behavioural–ecological attributes (territorial versus non-territorial; solitary versus colonial; island versus mainland; monogamous versus polygamous, etc.). Comparisons are required of different character sets (e.g. metric, plumage and genetic), using methods similar to those introduced by Evans (1980) and Barrowclough (1983) for evidence of concordance, and for samples at different levels of differentiation (populations, subspecies, sibling species and species).

Finally, the avian behavioural ecologist would do well to team up more frequently with the population geneticist studying allozymes, since together they could throw substantially more light on the roles (if any) of kin and interdemic selection in the evolution of altruistic behaviour, and in developing general theories of social behaviour.

APPENDIX: TECHNIQUES FOR THE COLLECTION OF ALLOZYME DATA

A1   Sample collection

Enzymes and other proteins are obtained from blood, tissues or organs. If the sample is to be collected without detriment to the bird, it is customary to take blood though sometimes breast muscle or fat biopsies have been used, e.g. Baker and Fox (1978); otherwise liver, kidney, heart, brain or gonads are commonly used. Recently electrophoresis has been carried out on proteins from feathers (Brush 1976, Knox 1980), feather pulp (Marsden and May 1984) and beaks (Frenkel and Gillespie 1979). Beaks appear to provide more protein loci than feathers but less than feather pulp. However, the latter comes from actively growing feathers and so can only be obtained from moulting birds (or individuals recaptured after one or two feathers have been plucked to stimulate re-growth). Furthermore, the study of small species may require use of two or more feathers. Marsden and May (1984) found that feather pulp yielded more loci than blood, though their results for blood were poorer than those obtained for birds elsewhere (Evans 1980).

Blood may be taken from brachial veins (under the wing), leg veins (in larger species) or by cardiac puncture. Birds are known to be able to tolerate greater blood loss than mammals (Kovack *et al.* 1969) and 50–70% of total blood volume has been taken from birds without long-term effects (Sturkie 1976). Total blood volume is estimated to be 6% of body weight and tests show that one can take up to 30% of the total volume (i.e. 0·18 ml per 10 g weight) without detriment to the bird (Evans 1980). Allowing a further 10% margin of error, it is recommended that 0·12 ml per 10 g weight be taken from an individual and, if this has to be repeated, that 24 hours elapse between sampling. If small passerines are being bled, it is best to draw the blood from the surface by syringe or pipette, having made a prick in the vessel (because it may easily collapse or become damaged). Since the blood may clot readily it should be mixed directly with an anti-coagulant (about 0·1 ml of sodium citrate or heparin). Sodium citrate is made up by adding 8·0 g disodium hydrogen citrate and 12·0 g glucose to 500 ml of distilled water; heparin solution is made up by adding 0·1 ml heparin to 250 ml 0·9% sodium chloride. Samples, whether blood, an organ or tissue, should be kept cool (4°C or less) from time of collection, but in the case of blood, not frozen until the red-cell fraction is separated from the plasma.

The advantage of using blood is that it should not affect survivorship of the bird. A disadvantage is that a number of enzymes are absent or at lower activity in blood than in an organ such as liver (see Table 4), and it is often not clear how or why the enzyme comes to be in the blood system.

A2 Sample preparation

Within 12 hours (preferably four) of collection, the sample should be prepared for storage in liquid nitrogen or a deep freeze. Blood is centrifuged at 1400–2000 g for about ten minutes, the supernatant plasma fraction removed to a separate tube for freezing, and the red cells re-centrifuged in the same manner but with 5–10 times the volume of 0·9% saline. After removal of the white cells, the red-cell walls are lysed with one-half to an equal volume of water (depending on enzyme activities typical of the species), and then stored deep-frozen. Red blood cells differ from those of mammals in being nucleated. This can lead to DNA from the cell nuclei obscuring band resolution, so it is important to have relatively "clean" cell lysates. The addition of detergent solutions such as an equal volume of 0·001% Triton X-100 in 0·9% saline may help to achieve this. For long-term storage of red blood cells, the lysate may be mixed with 2× volume of an ethylene glycol–citric acid mixture (60 g trisodium citrate . $2H_2O$ + 400 ml ethylene glycol, made up to 1 L, pH 8·4) (Vandeberg and Johnson 1977). This appears to improve significantly the enzyme activity (samples may be stored without lysis if kept at −15 to −25°C, and then applied directly to filter paper inserts).

Tissues or organs are homogenized in distilled water (1–2 ml g^{-1} of tissue) for about 30 seconds, then centrifuged at 35 000 g for 30 minutes (or 15–25 000 g for 45 minutes) at 4°C. For improved band resolution, a solution of 0·25 mg NADP and 0·8 µl β-mercaptoethanol per ml of distilled water may be added.

A3 Storage and degradation

Storage should be carried out at −20°C or below (−80°C is commonly used), either in a deep freeze or in liquid nitrogen. If they are to be transported, this is best done on dry ice in insulated containers. Samples are best stored in small aliquots. The faster the sample freezes and the fewer times it is thawed and re-frozen the better will be the activity and resolution of the enzymes. Post-translational modification of the protein molecule is a common problem for those undertaking electrophoresis and may lead to spurious bands being misidentified as different genotypes.

Considerable variation exists in storage capabilities of different enzymes in the same species and the same enzyme in different species (Evans 1980). For example, esterases are generally rather stable whereas some of the dehydrogenases are particularly susceptible to extremes of temperature, and even when stored deep-frozen they may lose their activity over time (2% of samples were inactive for GPI after 12 months and 21% inactive after two years (Evans 1980)). Corbin *et al.* (1974) found no activity in 6-PGDH within six months (and also in G-6-PGDH and PGM) in New Guinea starlings of the genus *Aplonis*, whereas Evans (1980) found inactivity in only 9% of samples in European Starling after 12 months. Since the former stored the blood and tissue samples at $-10°C$ in the field, then transferred them to a freezer at $-100°C$ and subsequently transported them to United States on dry ice, it seems unlikely that the loss of activity was due to a difference in technique. It may be that in tropical species these enzymes lose their activity much more quickly.

Various recipes have been devised to help retain the stability of samples, and these mixtures are commonly added immediately before electrophoresis. They include ethylene glycol and citric acid (made up as described above); a solution of 1·5% phenoxyethanol (15 ml), 0·25 M sucrose (85·6 g) and 0·1 M phosphate buffer (2·27 g KH_2PO_4 and 14·51 g K_2HPO_4), pH 7·5, made up to one litre with distilled water (Nakanishi *et al.* 1969); β-mercaptoethanol and NADP in water (see details above); or equal volumes of di-thio-threitol and 2% (v/v) phenoxyethanol (the latter in 0·4 M NaCl, 0·01 M Tris, 5×10^{-4} M $MgSO_4$, $1·5 \times 10^{-4}$ M $CaCl_2$ and bovine serum albumin (1 mg/ml) at pH 7·45 (Nolan and Nolan 1972)). The mixture used depends rather on personal preference, and it is recommended that each be tested first to determine which gives the best results for a particular enzyme and species.

A4   Electrophoresis

The principle of electrophoresis is that when a sample containing enzymes and other proteins is placed in a porous gel medium and that gel is subjected to a direct electric current, each protein will migrate in a direction and at a rate dependent upon the protein's net electric charge, molecular size and shape. Different individuals are compared by running samples side by side (27–41 samples if gel plates 32 cm long are used) in a gel for a certain time period, keeping conditions of charge, buffer concentration and pH constant so that the proteins migrate at a constant velocity. Better resolution is usually provided by including fewer samples in the gel (to reduce resistance across the gel) so it is best to initially run a 32 cm gel with 27 samples although many red-cell enzymes will give scorable results with 41 samples/gel.

After a suitable time the current is switched off and the positions of the proteins detected by applying stains specific for the protein under study. In the case of enzymes the stains contain a specific substrate and a dye. The enzyme catalyses the conversion of the substrate into an insoluble product, which then couples with the dye to give coloured bands at the points to which the enzyme has migrated. Because the primary sequence of amino acids in a protein is the product of a single gene, this enables one to estimate how many loci in the population have more than one allele and how many are electrophoretically invariant. If more than one enzyme may be resolved using a particular buffer, then the gel is sliced horizontally into the required number of sections and each is stained separately for that particular enzyme. This saves considerably on expense and time.

Electrophoretic methods vary between laboratories and one technique is not necessarily any better than another. The methods described below are those used by the author.

Samples (blood or tissue/organ homogenate) are soaked on small filter paper squares (4×4 mm or 4×3 mm), the thickness of which (and therefore enzyme concentration) may be varied according to the banding intensity required. Commonly, Whatman 3 MM thickness is used but if samples show low activity the thicker size 17 filter paper is advised. Fine forceps are used to ensure no direct handling since this may contaminate the sample with human proteins. Each square is placed carefully into a slot along the insert line (we use a metal comb applied in the centre of the gel if the enzymes to be stained migrate in both directions, but otherwise about 3 cm from the gel edge at either the anodal or cathodal end). Care must be taken to avoid cross-contamination of samples. This is achieved by placing the filter paper exactly into the slot, and by washing the forceps in distilled water between handling of each sample.

Gels are usually of hydrolysed starch because of its relative cheapness. However, the synthetic polymer acrylamide (e.g. Gemeiner *et al.* 1982) and cellulose acetate (e.g. Ferguson 1969) have also been used and may provide better resolutions and require smaller samples. Despite the advantages that the latter two media may possess, there is little evidence that their use has materially improved detection of electrophoretic variants, and they are relatively expensive. However, isoelectric focusing (where a protein moves to a position on a pH gradient such that it has a net charge of zero) is commonly used to provide much better resolution of small differences in the charge of variant proteins and in this case polyacrylamide is generally used. The main disadvantage of polyacrylamide is its cost, and this generally restricts the number of samples that one can test.

A variety of buffer solutions may be used both for the gel and to provide the electric field (termed box or electrode buffer). These may differ between enzymes and within enzymes between bird species, so that it is usually necessary to test a variety of recipes to determine the most suitable running conditions for optimum band resolution. Continuous buffer systems use the same constituents for both gel and electrode buffer; discontinuous systems (e.g. Poulik buffer) use different constituents. Details of recipes are provided by Shaw and Prasad (1970), Selander *et al.* (1971) and Harris and Hopkinson (1976) with useful modifications by Clayton and Tretiak (1972) and Barrowclough and Corbin (1978). A summary of the major gel and electrode buffer recipes is given in Table A1, and those found to be most useful in a variety of bird species are given for 26 of the more commonly assayed proteins in Table A2.

A5   Gel preparation

To prepare a gel, the gel solution (following the recipes in Table A1) is heated in a stoppered Buckner vacuum flask on a heated magnetic stirrer, with the hydrolysed starch (11–13% weight/volume) gently added at the start through a funnel, and mixed by the rotations of the magnet. Any starch adhering to the sides of the flask must be

Table A1. Electrode/gel buffer recipes

No.	Electrode buffer components (g/l)				pH adjust	Final pH	Gel buffer components (g/l)		pH adjust	Final pH
	1	2	3	4			1	2		
1	*Tris-HCl buffer* 0·3 M borate 18·55				1 N NaOH	8·2	0·01 M tris 1·21		1 N HCl	8·5
2	*Lithium hydroxide* 0·19 M borate LiOH · H_2O (0·03 M) 11·89	1·26			1 N NaOH	8·1	0·05 M tris-citrate (0·008 M) 6·2	1·6	1 N NaOH	8·4
3	*Discontinuous tris-citrate (Paulik)* 0·3 M borate 18·55				1 N NaOH	8·0–9·1 variable	0·076 M tris-citrate (0·0085 M) 9·21	1·79	1 N NaOH	8·6
4	*Continuous borate* 0·3 M borate 18·55				1 N NaOH	8·6	0·03 M borate		1 N NaOH	8·7
5	*Discontinuous tris-borate-citrate* 0·0546 M tris-borate (0·24 M) 6·61	15·17			1 N NaOH	8·6	0·076 M tris-citrate (0·005 M) 9·21	1·05	1 N NaOH	8·7
6	*Continuous tris-borate* 0·546 M tris-borate (0·245 M) 6·61	15·17			1 N NaOH	7·5–8·0 variable	0·001 M tris-borate (0·03 M) 0·12	1·79	1 N NaOH	7·5–8·0 variable
7	*Tris-versene-borate (TEB)* 0·9 M tris EDTA (0·02 M) borate (0·5 M) 108·99	7·44	30·92		dilute stock buffer 1 + 7H_2O 1 N NaOH	8·6	dil. stock buffer 1 + 9 H_2O		1 N NaOH	8·6

No.	Gel buffer		pH	Electrode buffer		pH
8	*Tris-versene-malate (TEM)*					
	0·1 M tris EDTA Malate (0·1 M) MgCl₂					
	12·1 3·72 11·6 2·03	1 N NaOH	7·4	dil. electrode buffer 1 + 9 H₂O	1 N NaOH	7·4
9	*Continuous tris-citrate*					
a	0·69 M tris-citrate (0·157 M)			0·02 M tris-citrate (0·005 M)		
	83·2 30·0	1 N NaOH	8·0	2·77 1·05	1 N NaOH	8·0
b	0·15 M tris-citrate (0·043 M)			dil. 66·7 ml electrode buffer to 1L		
	16·35 9·04	conc. HCl	$\overline{7}$·0		1 N HCl	7·0
c	0·233 M tris-citrate (0·086 M)			0·008 M tris-citrate (0·003 M)		
	27·0 18·06	1 N NaOH	6·0-6·3	0·97 0·63	1 N NaOH	6·4-6·7
10	*Tris-phosphate*					
	0·1 M tris NaH₂PO₄					
	12·1 15·6	Tris	8·6	dil. electrode buffer 1 + 9 H₂O	1 N NaOH	8·6
11	*Phosphate-citrate*					
	0·03 M citrate K₂HPO₄			0·001 M citrate K₂HPO₄		
	5·7 29·1	Either HCl or NaOH	6·7	0·254 1·06	Either HCl or NaOH	7·0
12	*Phosphate*					
	0·138 M KHPO₄ 0·062 M NaOH					
	18·78 2·48	1 N HCl (3-aminopropyl) -	6·7	dil. electrode buffer 1 + 19 H₂O	1 N HCl	6·7
13	*Amine-citrate*					
	0·04 M citrate					
a	8·4	N-morpholine	6·1	dil. electrode buffer 1 + 19 H₂O	1 N HCl	6·1
b	8·4	pH adjusted by addition of 1,3-Bis(dimethyl amino)-2-propanol to 13a	7·5	dil. electrode buffer 1 + 19 H₂O	1 N HCl	7·5

NOTES Borate = boric acid
       Citrate = citric acid

Table A2. Performance of different buffer systems for each protein/enzyme

Locus symbol	Electrophoretic mobility[a]	Buffer system															
		1	2	3	4	5	6	7	8	9a	9b	9c	10	11	12	13a	13b
ADH	Cathodal							G									
GPD	Cathodal							G		G		GG				G	
SDH	Cathodal							F								G	
LDH	Anodal/cathodal			G				G		G	G	G		G		G	G
MDH	-1 Anod. -2 cathod.								G	G	F	G			G	GG	G
ME	Anodal											GG			G	G	
ICD	-1 Anod. -2 cathod.					P											
6-PGD	Anodal	P	P	P				G	G	P	P	GG	P	G	G	G	GG
G-6-PD	Anodal				F				G	P	G	GG			G	G	G
XDH	Cathodal								G		P	F					
GDH	Anodal							G							G	G	
SOD	-1 Anod. -2 cathod.							G	G		P					G	
NP	Anodal																
GOT	-1 Anod. -2 cathod.			G						G		GG			G	G	G
CK	Anodal/cathodal											G				G	
AK	Anodal											G				G	
PGM	Anodal (cathodal)	F	F	G					P		G	GG	P		G	GG	GG
EST	Anodal/cathodal	G	G	G					G		G	G			G	GG	
E	Anodal	G	G	G						G		G					
ACP	Anodal		G				G			G		G					
LAP	Anodal	G	G								F	G				G	
PEP-A	Anodal	G	G	G								G					
PEP-B	Anodal	G	G	G		F					G	G/F	P				
PEP-C	Anodal	G	G	G		F					G	G/F	P				
PEP-D	Anodal	G	G	G								G					
ADA	Anodal							G									
MPI	Anodal							G									
GPI	Cathodal (anodal)			G				G	P			G		P	G	GG	
Hb	Cathodal							G			G	G	F		G	G	
ALB	Anodal	G	G	G								F					
Tf	Anodal	G	G	G								F					
PT	Anodal/cathodal	G	G	G								F					

[a] Electrophoretic mobility will vary according to buffer conditions, but locus "1" (e.g. ICD-1) will be anodal of locus "2" (e.g. ICD-2).
P = poor; F = fair; G = good; GG = good resolution across many species. (Note that some buffer systems have been used on only a few species so they may not reflect their performance. This should be used as a first guide only, and each worker is advised to experiment with different systems.)

quickly washed into the solution or it will form lumps in the gel when it sets. As the gel solution heats up, it thickens and the magnet rotates more slowly. If it stops, the flask should be agitated by hand and vigorous heating continued over a Bunsen flame until the solution is boiling. Otherwise the flask is retained on the stirrer until the contents have returned into solution and this starts to boil. At this point the flask is quickly attached to a vacuum water pump and degassed until the gel is bubbling vigorously and all small bubbles have disappeared. The vacuum is then terminated by gently removing the rubber tubing from the side-arm, and the gel poured in a sideways motion over a glass plate enclosed by side-formers of Perspex. Both the glass plate and Perspex formers are first cleaned with acetone and the formers then applied to the four glass edges with silicon vacuum grease. Sufficient gel solution is used so that the meniscus is slightly higher than the plate sides. A plastic sheet may then be unrolled over the surface whilst it is still molten, carefully ensuring that no air bubbles are trapped, and if necessary a glass plate may be placed on top with weights at each corner. This removes excess liquid which escapes from the edges, and leaves a constant volume free of air bubbles, with an even surface to the gel.

Different workers tend to use differently sized gel plates. We use two sizes: $21 \times 12\,cm \times 6\,mm$ for initial enzyme testing and $32 \times 12\,cm \times 6\,mm$ for subsequent routine screening. The former allows 16 samples to be run alongside each other, and requires about 200 ml of gel solution (allowing a small safety margin); the latter holds 27 or 41 (see above) samples and requires 300 ml of gel solution (with a similar safety margin). The side-formers are $10 \times 6\,mm \times$ length/width of the gel, and are made of Perspex. The gel is allowed to set at room temperature for about 30 minutes before it is held at $4\,°C$ until electrophoresis. It is best to run gels within about six hours of preparation; if they are left for much longer periods they are inclined to dry up, splitting may take place, and samples do not run so well. Each gel plate is individually numbered with a permanent marker, and the sequence of samples recorded.

A6   Gel running

The gel is placed horizontally between two Perspex tanks each filled with about one litre of the appropriate buffer solution (see Table A1). Contact with an electric current is established using two platinum electrodes (preferably each at least the length of the gel plate), one in each tank, and absorbing wicks (we use four thicknesses of J-cloths) previously soaked in the buffer and connecting the solution to the gel. The wicks should be exactly the width of the gels, overlap the anodal and cathodal edges of the glass plate by about 3 cm, and should be carefully aligned so that they are parallel with the length of the gel plate and to each other. After about 15 minutes, most of the enzyme will have diffused into the gel, and the samples can if necessary be removed with forceps (sometimes this improves band resolution and generally results in a straighter running buffer front).

Because of the voltages required in electrophoresis, the gels should be kept cool (usually $4\,°C$), for example by setting up in a refrigerator or refrigerated room. The power packs to supply a constant high-voltage DC current should be kept at room temperature, and switched on standby at least half an hour before the run. During the run, the surfaces of the gel and the wicks are best covered with a large piece of polythene film to prevent the gel from drying up, with a portion raised over the insert lines so that moisture does not result in contact between samples. Running

Table A3. Protein/enzyme stain recipes

(a) Agar overlays (30 ml volume)

Protein/enzyme	0.3 M Tris-HCl pH 7.1	0.3 M Tris-HCl pH 8.0	0.2 M Tris-HCl pH 8.2	0.2 M Tris pH 8.0	0.2 M Tris pH 9.0	0.2 M Tris pH 9.5	pH 8.8	Stain buffer (other) (ml)	Substrate	Special factors	G-6-PDH	MgCl₂[a] (µl mg ml)	NADP[b] 5 mg/ml	NAD[b] 5 mg/ml	MTT[c] 2 mg/ml	PMS[c] 2 mg/ml	2% Agar at 56°C
ADH								9.5 ml 0.5 M Phosphate[d] pH 7	0.5 ml 95% Ethanol					2	2	1	15
GPD					10				400 mg Na₃ DL-Glycerol-3-phosphate			30(0)		2	2	1	15
SDH						(10)			500 mg Sorbitol	50 mg Pyrazole, 50 mg Sod. pyruvate		30		2	2	1	15
LDH						(10)			2 ml 1 M Na-lactate pH 7.0					1	1	1	15
MDH-1				10					2 ml 1 M Na-L-malate pH 7.0					1	1	1	15
MDH-2				10					2 ml 2 M Na-DL-malate pH 7.0					1	1	1	15
ME				10					60 mg L-Malic acid				1		1	1	15
ICD			10						20 mg Na₃ Isocitric acid			30(0)	1		2	1	15
6-PGD		12							80 mg Na₃-6-Phosphogluconate	Can add NADP to gel		30(0)	2		1	1	15
G-6-PD		12							150 mg Na₂ Glucose-6-phosphate	Can add NADP to gel		30	1		1	1	15
XDH			10						1 ml Saturated hypoxanthine					2	2	1	15
GDH							12		30 mg Na-Glutamate	30 mg ADP				1	1	1	15
SOD						(10)	10		Appears on ADH/SDH gel			30		2	2	1	15
NP								13 ml 0.05 M Phosphate pH 7.5	5 mg Inosine	10 µl Xanthine oxidase					1	1	15
GOT								15 ml 0.1 M Phosphate pH 7.0	160 mg L-Aspartic acid	22 mg α-Ketoglutaric acid, 15 mg Pyridoxal phosphate, 60 mg Fast Violet B salt[g]							15
CK	12								72 mg Glucose, 20 mg Phosphocreatine (Na₂ · 6 H₂O)	30 mg ADP, 30 µl Hexokinase	30	30(0)	1		1	1	15
AK	12								80 mg Glucose	30 mg ADP, 30 µl Hexokinase	30	30(0)	1		1	1	15
PGM	12								300 mg Glucose-1-phosphate		15	30(0)	1		1	1	15
LAP								15 ml 0.2 M Phosphate pH 7.5	30 mg L-leucyl β-naphthylamide	30 mg Black K salt	30(0)						15
PEP-A								15 ml 0.2 M Phosphate pH 7.5	30 mg L-valyl-1-leucine	0.4 ml 0.5 M MnCl₂, 0.4 ml Snake venom, 5 mg Peroxidase	1 drop 3-amino-9-ethyl carbazole[f]						15
PEP-B								15 ml 0.2 M Phosphate pH 7.5	30 mg Leucyl-glycyl-glycine	0.2 ml 0.5 M MnCl₂, 0.2 ml Snake venom, 5 mg Peroxidase	1 drop 3-amino-9-ethyl carbazole[f]						15

PEP-C	15 ml 0.2 M Phosphate pH 7.5	30 mg Leucyl alanine	0.4 ml 0.5 M MnCl₂ 0.4 ml Snake venom, 5 mg Peroxidase	1 drop 3-amino-9-ethyl carbazole[f]	15
PEP-D	15 ml 0.2 M Phosphate pH 7.5	30 mg Phenyl-alanyl-proline	0.4 ml 0.5 M MnCl₂ 0.4 ml Snake venom, 5 mg Peroxidase	1 drop 3-amino-9-ethyl carbazole[f]	15
ADA	12 ml 0.05 M Phosphate pH 7.5	20 mg Adenosine	25 μl Xanthine oxidase, 25 μl NP	10 30(0) 1	2 1 15
MPI	12	50 mg Mannose-6-phosphate	5 μl PGIase	10 30(0) 1	1 1 15
GPI	12	100 mg Fructose-6-phosphate			1 1 15

(b) In solution (100 ml volume)

EST[h]	100 ml 0.1 M Phosphate pH 7.5 1 ml α-Naphthyl acetate[j] (0.186 g dissolved in 10 ml Acetone). 100 mg Fast Blue B.[g] Fix in Methanol:Acetic acid:H₂O (5:1:5).
E	Stain as above, but add 1 ml Eserine sulphate 10^{-5} M (inhibition of bands indicates cholinesterase). Fix as above.
ALB, Tf, PT	1 g Amido Black 10B[k] in 100 ml Methanol:Acetic acid:H₂O (5:1:5). Pour over gel, allow to stand for 30-60 s, pour off, washing off excess with tap water. Clear and fix with Methanol:Acetic acid:H₂O (5:1:5).
ACP	100 ml 0.05 M Sod. acetate pH 5.0, 100 mg Na α-Naphthyl acid phosphate, 100 mg Black K salt. Pour over gel, incubate until bands appear. Wash and fix with Methanol:Acetic acid:H₂O (5:1:5).

[a] Concentrations may be varied from 0.001–0.1 M. In some cases, MnCl₂ may alternatively be used, at comparable concs.

[b] NADP and NAD concentrations may need to be increased to 10 or 20 mg/ml. (NADP = Nicotinamide-adenine dinucleotide phosphate; NAD = Nicotinamide-adenine dinucleotide.)

[c] MTT and PMS concentrations may need to be increased to 5 mg/ml. (MTT = Methyl thiazolyl tetrazolium; PMS = Phenazine methosulphate.)

[d] Phosphate may be Na₂HPO₄, or KH₂PO₄ (esterase stain buffer, for example, commonly is made up by a mixture of 30 ml of Na₂HPO₄ (2.133 g per 100 ml) and 70 ml of KH₂PO₄ (2.044 g per 100 ml). Alternatively tris or tris-HCl may serve as a better stain buffer.

[e] Leucyl-alanine commonly used as alternative substrate.

[f] Prepared by dissolving 40 mg of 3-amino-9-ethyl carbazole in a few drops of N,N-Dimethyl formamide.

[g] Alternatively use Fast Blue B or Fast Blue RR or Fast Garnet BC.

[h] Alternative esterase stain is a fluorescent one in which 10 mg 4-Methylumbelliferyl acetate (or butyrate) is dissolved in a few drops of acetone and then mixed with 100 ml 0.1 M phosphate buffer, pH 6.5/7.5. Apply to gel on filter paper overlay, incubate at room temperature and inspect under long-wave UV lamp after a few minutes for fluorescent zones.

[j] Alternatively use β-Naphthyl acetate or a mixture of α- and β-Naphthyl acetate, or α(β)-Naphthyl butyrate.

[k] Alternatively Naphthalene Black, Fast Blue Black or Coomassie Blue.

NB Values in parentheses are alternative constituents/concentrations.

conditions should be kept constant and the voltage gradient (volts/cm) measured across the gel, bearing in mind that once the proteins within the sample start to migrate the voltage gradient may have altered from its initial value. The time of start and finish of the electrophoretic run, together with initial and final voltage and current from the power pack, as well as voltage gradient across the gel, should all be recorded for each gel.

Gels are usually run either for short periods (about four hours) at a high voltage gradient (usually 8 volts/cm on a gel of 32 cm length) or for much longer periods (usually 16 hours) at a lower voltage gradient (5 volts/cm). Sometimes one or other of these conditions gives better results (the former for esterases in high-pH buffers; the latter for dehydrogenases in relatively low-pH buffers) whilst convenience may also play a part in the choice (the latter conditions allow gels to be run overnight). Some workers use very high voltage gradients (10 or 20 volts/cm) for 4–5 hours, although one needs to be careful that the power packs used are capable of taking the high currents involved, and it is important the gels be kept sufficiently cool.

The time to end an electrophoretic run depends upon the mobility of the protein, which will vary between proteins, within proteins and between species. This can only be determined by trial and error, but once found it may be related to the distance moved by the buffer front (i.e. the point to which the proteins have moved) and this used as an index of when to terminate the run. In discontinuous buffer systems, this shows up as a line behind which the gel is of slightly different consistency. In continuous buffer systems, the addition of, for example, an albumin marker containing bromophenol blue run alongside the other samples, provides a measure of the rate of migration. Otherwise so long as all electrophoretic conditions are kept constant, the length of time for the run may be used to determine when to terminate it.

A7   Gel cutting and staining

Once the run is completed, the wicks and polythene films are removed, the gel is blotted and then sliced usually into two or three sections (but up to five sections for gels of 9 mm thickness). With all but the back formers removed and two glass/Perspex runners (2 mm thickness if three sections are required; 3 mm thickness for two sections) placed one on either side of the gel, sections may be cut using a wire gel-slicer (alternatively a broad knife with a thin even blade, such as an artist's palate knife). A glass plate may be placed so that the top surface is not raised upwards during gel cutting, leading to uneven slicing. The two or three equal horizontal sections of gel may then be gently peeled backwards on to a cloth, or directly floated off into a staining tray. The cut surface should be kept uppermost since it gives better resolution of stained bands, and so sections may need to be turned over from one cloth to another. Before the sections are transferred, a triangle should be cut out of one corner of the gel so that the sample order is known whatever surface of a gel section is uppermost. Each section is stained either in solution in a Perspex tray or by agar overlay directly on top of the plate.

Although each enzyme tends to have a specific stain, the quantities may be varied to minimize costs. Some substrates or co-factors such as MPI, 6-PGD and NADP are very expensive and continue to increase alarmingly in cost. Table 3 summarizes stain recipes developed to reduce these expenses, and these are designed for use as agar overlays. For gel plates of 32 × 12 cm, 30 ml of solution is required, with an equal volume of agar and staining solution. The agar is prepared as a 2% weight/volume solution in distilled water, boiled on a heated magnetic stirrer (being careful to prevent agar granules remaining on the side of the flask) and subsequently allowed to cool to 57°C in a water bath. The stain, substrate and any necessary co-factor are then added, thoroughly mixed and poured immediately over the gel surface to give an even coverage of the gel. The agar solution is retained by the Perspex side-formers and quickly sets (usually within one minute). It may then be covered with clear plastic sheeting to prevent desiccation, and placed in darkness in an incubator at 41°C until the bands have stained sufficiently for scoring (usually within one hour but occasionally up to six hours, ensuring the background does not overstain). The strength of bands and speed at which they appear may be increased by first placing the gels in a stain buffer solution before the stain, etc. are added (this is not so conveniently done with agar overlaps, however). A disadvantage of this method is that the resolution of the bands may be poorer.

Cheap stains (e.g. Amido Black for general protein, O-Dianisidine for esterases) may be made up in solution (see Table A3) and poured over gels in specially constructed Perspex trays. Gels stained in solution are cleared in a solution of glacial acetic acid:methanol:water (volumes 1:5:5) and then fixed in acetic acid:ethanol: glycerine:water (volumes 1:1:1:2). Exceptions are protein staining gels which are fixed in 7% acetic acid, and those stains soluble in methanol/ethanol. Gels may then be stored between moistened cloths at 4°C, ensuring that they do not dry out, and drawn directly or photographed. Agar overlays may be dried on to blotting paper in an incubator and stored flat.

REFERENCES

Aquadro, C. F. and Avise, J. C. (1982). Evolutionary Genetics of Birds. VI. A reexamination of protein divergence using varied electrophoretic conditions. *Evolution* **36**, 1003–1019.

Avise, J. C. and Aquadro, C. F. (1982). A comparative summary of genetic distances in the vertebrates. *In* "Evolutionary Biology" (eds M. K. Hecht, B. Wallace and G. T. Prance), pp. 151–185. Plenum Publ. Corp., New York.

Avise, J. C., Patton, J. C. and Aquadro, C. F. (1980 a). Evolutionary genetics of birds. I. Relationships among North American thrushes and allies. *Auk* **97**, 135–147.

Avise, J. C., Patton, J. C. and Aquadro, C. F. (1980 b). Evolutionary genetics of birds. II. Conservative protein evolution in North American sparrows and relatives. *Syst. Zool.* **29**, 323–334.

Avise, J. C., Patton, J. C. and Aquadro, C. F. (1980 c). Evolutionary genetics of birds. III. Comparative molecular evolution in New World warblers and rodents. *J. Hered.* **71**, 303–310.

Avise, J. C., Aquadro, C. F. and Patton, J. C. (1982). Evolutionary genetics of birds. V. Genetic distances within mimidae (Mimic Thrushes) and vireonidae (Vireos). *Biochem. Genet.* **20**, 95–104.

Ayala, F. J. (ed.) (1976). "Molecular Evolution". Sinauer Assoc. Inc., Sunderland, Mass.

Bacon, P. J. (1979). Population genetics of the Mute Swan *Cygnus olor*. D.Phil. Thesis, University of Oxford.

Baker, C. M. A. and Manwell, C. (1975). Molecular biology of avian proteins. XII. Protein polymorphism in the Stubble Quail *Coturnix pectoralis*—and a brief note on the induction of egg white protein synthesis in wild birds by hormones. *Comp. Biochem. Physiol.* **50B**, 471–477.

Baker, M. C. (1974). Genetic structure of two populations of White-crowned Sparrows with different song dialects. *Condor* **76**, 351–356.

Baker, M. C. (1975). Song dialects and genetic differences in White-crowned Sparrows (*Zonotrichia leucophrys*). *Evolution* **29**, 226–241.

Baker, M. C. (1982 a). Vocal dialect recognition and population genetic consequences. *Am. Zool.* **22**, 561–569.

Baker, M. C. (1982 b). Genetic population structure and vocal dialects in *Zonotrichia* (Emberizidae). *In* "Acoustic Communication in Birds" (eds D. E. Kroodsma and E. H. Miller), pp. 209–235. Academic Press, New York.

Baker, M. C., Baker, A. E. M., Cunningham, M. A., Thompson, D. B. and Tomback, D. F. (1984). Reply to "Allozymes and song dialects: A reassessment." *Evolution* **38**, 449–451.

Baker, M. C. and Fox, I. F. (1978). Dominance, survival, and enzyme polymorphism in Dark-eyed Juncos. *Junco hyemalis. Evolution* **32**, 697–711.

Baker, M. C. and Mewaldt, L. R. (1978). Song dialects as barriers to dispersal in White-crowned Sparrows (*Zonotrichia leuchophrys nuttalli*). *Evolution* **32**, 712–722.

Baker, M. C. and Mewaldt, L. R. (1981). Response to "Song dialects as barriers to dispersal: A re-evaluation." *Evolution* **35**, 189–190.

Baker, M. C., Thompson, D. B., Sherman, G. L., Cunningham, M. A. and Tomback, D. F. (1982). Allozyme frequencies in a linear series of song dialect populations. *Evolution* **36**, 1020–1029.

Bargiello, T. A., Grossfield, J., Steele, R. W. and Cooke, F. (1977). Isoenzyme status and genetic variability of serum esterases in the Lesser Snow Goose, *Anser caerulescens caerulescens. Biochem. Genet.* **15**, 741–763.

Barrett, V. A. and Vyse, E. R. (1982). Comparative genetics of three Trumpeter Swan populations. *Auk* **99**, 103–108.

Barrowclough, G. F. (1980). Genetic and phenotypic differentiation in a wood warbler (Genus *Dendroica*) hybrid zone. *Auk* **97**, 655–668.

Barrowclough, G. F. (1983). Biochemical studies of microevolutionary processes. *In* "Perspectives in Ornithology". (eds A. H. Brush and G. A. Clark, Jr.), pp. 223–261. Cambridge University Press, New York.

Barrowclough, G. F. and Corbin, K. W. (1978). Genetic variation and differentiation in the Parulidae. *Auk* **95**, 691–702.

Barrowclough, G. F., Corbin, K. W. and Zink, R. M. (1981). Genetic differentiation in the Procellariiformes. *Comp. Biochem. Physiol.* **69B**, 629–632.

Birdsall, D. A. and Nash, D. (1973). Occurrence of successful multiple insemination of females in natural populations of deer mice (*Peromyscus maniculatus*). *Evolution* **27**, 106–110.

Braun, D., Kitto, G. B. and Braun, M. J. (1984). Molecular population genetics in tufted and Black-crested forms of *Parus biocolor. Auk* **101**, 170–173.

Brown, J. L. (1970). Cooperative breeding and altruistic behaviour in the Mexican Jay *Aphelcoma ultramarina. Anim. Behav.* **18**, 366–378.

Brush, A. H. (1968). Conalbumin variation in populations of the Redwinged Blackbird, *Agelaius phoeniceus. Comp. Biochem. Physiol.* **25**, 159–168.

Brush, A. H. (1970). An electrophoretic study of egg whites from three blackbird species. *Univ. Conn. Occas. Pap.* **1**, 243–264.

Brush, A. H. (1976). Waterfowl feather proteins: Analysis of use in taxonomic studies. *J. Zool.* **179**, 467–498.

Burke, T. (1984). Population genetics of the House Sparrow *Passer domesticus.* Unpublished Ph.D. Thesis, University of Nottingham.

Cavalli-Sforza, L. L. and Bodmer, W. F. (1971). "The Genetics of Human Populations". W. H. Freeman, San Francisco.

Charlesworth, B. (1980). "Evolution in Age-structured Populations". Cambridge University Press, London.

Charlesworth, B. and Giesel, J. T. (1972). Selection in populations with overlapping generations. II. Relations between gene frequency and demographic variables. *Am. Natur.* **106**, 388–401.

Christiansen, F. B. and Frydenberg, O. (1973). Selection component analysis of natural polymorphisms using population samples including mother–offspring combinations. *Theoret. Pop. Biol.* **4**, 425–445.

Clayton, J. W. and Tretiak, D. N. (1972). Amine-citrate buffers for pH control in starch gel electrophoresis. *J. Fish. Res. Bd. Can.* **29**, 1162–1172.

Cockerham, C. C. (1973). Analyses of gene frequencies. *Genetics* **74**, 679–700.

Cole, S. R. and Parkin, D. T. (1981). Enzyme polymorphisms in the House Sparrow, *Passer domesticus. Biol. J. Linn. Soc.* **15**, 13–22.

Cooke, F., Abraham, K. F., Davies, J. C., Findlay, C. S., Healey, R. F., Sadura, A. and Seguin, R. J. (1982). The La Perouse Bay Snow Goose Project—A 13 year report. Queen's University, Ontario. 194 pp. (unpublished).

Corbin, K. W. (1978). Genetic diversity in avian populations. *In* "Endangered Birds": Management Techniques for preserving threatened species (ed. S. A. Temple), pp. 291–301. University of Wisconsin Press, Madison.

Corbin, K. W. (1981). Genic heterozygosity in the White-crowned Sparrow: a potential index to boundaries between subspecies. *Auk* **98**, 669–680.

Corbin, K. W. (1983). Genetic Structure and Avian Systematics. *In* "Current Ornithology" (ed. R. F. Johnston), Vol. 1, pp. 211–244. Plenum Press, New York, NY.

Corbin, K. W., Sibley, C. G. and Ferguson, A. (1979). Genic changes associated with the establishment of sympatry in orioles of the genus *Icterus. Evolution* **33**, 624–633.

Corbin, K. W., Sibley, C. G., Ferguson, A., Wilson, A. C., Brush, A. H. and Ahlquist, J. E. (1974). Genetic polymorphism in New Guinea starlings of the genus *Aplonis. Condor* **76**, 307–318.

Coulson, S. C. and Thomas, C. S. (1985). Changes in the biology of the Kittiwake *Rissa tridactyla*: A 31 year study of a breeding colony. *J. Anim. Ecol.* **54**, 9–26.

Coyne, J. A. (1976). Lack of genic similarity between two sibling species of *Drosophila* as revealed by varied techniques. *Genetics* **84**, 593–607.

Dixon, M. and Webb, E. C. (1965). "Enzymes". Longmans, London.

Dunnet, G. M. and Ollason, J. C. (1979). The Fulmar. *Biologist* **26**, 117–122.

Endler, J. (1986). "Natural Selection in the Wild". Princeton University Press.

Evans, P. G. H. (1980). Population genetics of the European Starling, *Sturnus vulgaris.* D. Phil. Thesis, University of Oxford.

Evans, P. G. H. Intraspecific nest parasitism in the European Starling. *Anim. Behav.* (in press).

Ewens, W. J. and Feldman, M. W. (1976). The theoretical assessment of selective neutrality. *In* "Population Genetics and Ecology". (eds S. Karlin and E. Nevo), pp. 303–337. Academic Press, New York.

Farris, J. S. (1972). Estimating phylogenetic trees from distance matrices. *Am. Natur.* **106**, 645–668.

Farris, J. S. (1973). A probability model for inferring evolutionary trees. *Syst. Zool.* **22**, 250–256.

Farris, J. S. (1981). Distance data in phylogenetic analysis. *In* "Advances in Distances". (eds V. A. Funk and D. R. Brooks), pp. 3–23. Academic Press, New York.

Ferguson, A. (1969). An electrophoretic study of the blood and egg white proteins of some Columbidae. Ph.D. Thesis, Queen's University, Belfast.

Ferguson, A. (1971). Geographic and species variation in transferrin and ovotransferrin polymorphism in the Columbidae. *Comp. Biochem. Physiol.* **38B**, 477–486.

Fleischer, R. C. (1983). A comparison of theoretical and electrophoretic assessments of genetic structure in populations of the House Sparrow (*Passer domesticus*). *Evolution* **37**, 1001–1009.

Fleischer, R. C., Johnston, R. F. and Klitz, W. J. (1983). Allozymic heterozygosity and morphological variation in House Sparrows. *Nature* **304**, 628–630.

Fitch, W. M. and Margoliash, E. (1967). Construction of phylogenetic trees. *Science* **155**, 279–284.

Foltz, D. W. and Hoogland, J. L. (1981). Analysis of the mating system in the black-tailed prairie dog (*Cynomys ludovicianus*) by likelihood of paternity. *J. Mammal.* **62**, 706–712.

Frenkel, N. J. and Gillespie, J. M. (1979). Proteins of beaks: possible use in taxonomy of birds. *Aust. J. Zool.* **27**, 443–452.

Gaines, M. S., McClenaghan, L. R. and Rose, R. K. (1978). Temporal patterns of allozymic variation in fluctuating populations of *Microtus ochrogaster*. *Evolution* **32**, 723–739.

Gavin, T. A. and Bollinger, E. K. (1985). Multiple paternity in a territorial passerine: the bobolink. *Auk* **102**, 550–555.

Gowaty, P. A. and Karlin, A. A. (1984). Multiple maternity and paternity in single broods of apparently monogamous eastern bluebirds (*Sialia Sialis*) *Behav. Ecol. Sociobiol.* **15**, 91–95.

Gemeiner, M., Miller, I. and Czikeli, H. (1982). Ultrathin-layer isoelectric focusing of enzymes in liver samples of wagtails (*Motacilla flava* ssp.). *Electrophoresis* **3**, 146–151.

Gillespie, J. H. and Kokima, K. (1968). The degree of polymorphism in enzymes involved in energy production compared to that in non-specific enzymes in two *Drosophila ananassae* populations. *Proc. Natl Acad. Sci. USA* **61**, 582–585.

Greenwood, P. J., Harvey, P. H. and Perrins, C. M. (1978). Inbreeding and dispersal in the great tit. *Nature* **271**, 52–54.

Gutierrez, R. J., Zink, R. M. and Yang, S. Y. (1983). Genic variation, and systematic and biogeographic relationships of some galliform birds. *Auk* **100**, 33–47.

Guttman, S. I., Grau, G. A. and Karlin, A. A. (1980). Genetic variation in Lake Erie Great Blue Herons (*Ardea herodias*). *Comp. Biochem. Physiol.* **66B**, 167–169.

Gyllensten, U., Reuterwall, C. and Rymann, N. (1979). Genetic variability in Scandinavian populations of willow grouse (*Lagopus lagopus* L.) and rock ptarmigan (*Lagopus mutus* L.). *Hereditas* **91**, 301.

Handford, P. and Nottebohm, F. (1976). Allozymic and morphological variation in population samples of Rufous-collared Sparrow, *Zonotrichia capensis*, in relation to vocal dialects. *Evolution* **30**, 802–817.

Harris, H. and Hopkinson, D. A. (1976). "Handbook of Enzyme Electrophoresis in Human Genetics". North Holland, Oxford.

Hedrick, P. W. (1971). A new approach to measuring genetic similarity. *Evolution* **25**, 276–280.

Hill, W. G. (1974). Estimation of linkage disequilibrium in randomly mating populations. *Heredity* **33**, 229–239.

International Union of Biochemistry. (1979). "Enzyme Nomenclature, 1978". Academic Press, London, New York.

Jakoby, W. B. (ed.) (1980). "Enzymatic Basis of Detoxication". Vol. 1. Academic Press, London, New York.

Johnson, G. B. (1974). Enzyme polymorphism and metabolism. *Sciences* **184**, 29–37.

Johnson, G. B. (1977). Hidden heterogeneity among electrophoretic alleles. *In* "Measuring Selection in Natural Populations" (eds F. B. Christiansen and T. M. Fenchel), pp. 223–244. Springer-Verlag, New York.

Johnson, M. C. and Brown, J. L. (1980). Genetic variation among trait groups and apparent absence of close inbreeding in Grey-crowned Babblers. *Behav. Ecol. Sociobiol.* **7**, 93–98.

Johnson, N. K. and Zink, R. M. (1983). Speciation in sapsuckers (*Sphyrapicus*). I. Genetic differentiation. *Auk* **100**, 871–884.

Joste, N., Ligon, J. D. and Stacey, P. B. (1985). Shared paternity in the acorn woodpecker (*Melanerpes formicivorus*). *Behav. Ecol. Sociobiol.* **17**, 39–41.

Karig, L. M. and Wilson, A. C. (1971). Genetic variation in supernatant malate dehydrogenase of birds and reptiles. *Biochem. Genet.* **5**, 211–221.

Kimura, M. (1983). "The Neutral Theory of Molecular Evolution". Cambridge University Press.

Kitto, G. B. and Wilson, A. C. (1966). Evolution of malate dehydrogenase in birds. *Science* **153**, 1408–1410.

Knox, A. G. (1980). Feather protein as a source of avian taxonomic information. *Comp. Biochem. Physiol.* **65B**, 45–54.

Kojima, K., Gillespie, J. and Tobari, Y. N. (1970). A profile of *Drosophila* species enzymes assayed by electrophoresis. I. Number of alleles, heterozygosities and linkage disequilibrium in glucose-metabolizing systems and some other enzymes. *Biochem. Genet.* **4**, 627–637.

Kovack, A. G. B., Szasz, E. and Pilayer, N. (1969). The mortality of various avian and mammalian species following blood loss. *Acta. Physiol. Acad. Sci. Hung.* **35**, 109–126.

Lewontin, R. C. (1974). "The Genetic Basis of Evolutionary Change". Columbia University Press, New York.

Lewontin, R. C. and Krakauer, J. (1973). Distribution of gene frequency as a test of the theory of the selective neutrality of polymorphisms. *Genetics* **74**, 175–195.

Manwell, C. L. C. and Baker, M. A. (1975). Molecular genetics of avian proteins. XIII. Protein polymorphism in three species of Australian passerines. *Aust. J. Biol. Sci.* **28**, 546–557.

Marsden, J. E. and May, B. (1984). Feather pulp: A non-destructive sampling technique for electrophoretic studies of birds. *Auk* **101**, 173–175.

Merritt, R. B. and Wu, B. J. (1975). On the quantification of promiscuity (or "*Promyscus maniculatus*?"). *Evolution* **29**, 575–578.

Mickevich, M. F. and Mitter, C. (1981). Treating polymorphic characters in systematics: a phylogenetic treatment of electrophoretic data. *In* "Advances in Cladistics". (eds V. A. Funk and D. R. Brooks) Vol. 1, pp. 45–48. New York Botanical Garden, New York.

Mickevich, M. F. and Mitter, C. (1983). Evolutionary patterns in allozyme data:

systematic approach. *In* "Advances in Cladistics". (eds N. I. Platnick and V. A. Funk), Vol. 2, pp. 169–176. Columbia University Press, New York.

Milne, H. H. and Robertson, F. W. (1965). Polymorphisms in egg albumin proteins and behaviour in the Eider duck. *Nature* **205**, 367–369.

Nadeau, J. H. and Baccus, R. (1981). Selection components of four allozymes in natural populations of *Peromyscus maniculatus*. *Evolution* **35**, 11–20.

Nakanishi, M., Nolan, R. A., Gorman, G. C. and Bailey, G. S. (1969). Phenoxyethanol: Protein preservative for taxonomists. *Science* **163**, 681–683.

Nei, M. (1972). Genetic distance between populations. *Am. Natur.* **106**, 283–292.

Nei, M. (1975). "Molecular Population Genetics and Evolution". North-Holland, Amsterdam.

Nei, M. (1977). *F*-statistics and analysis of gene diversity in subdivided populations. *Ann. Hum. Genet.* **41**, 225–233.

Nei, M. (1978). Estimation of average heterozygosity and genetic distance from a small number of individuals. *Genetics* **89**, 583–590.

Nei, M. and Roychoudhury, A. K. (1974). Sampling variances of heterozygosity and genetic distance. *Genetics* **76**, 379–390.

Nevo, E. (1978). Genetic variation in natural populations: patterns and theory. *Theoret. Pop. Biol.* **13**, 121–177.

Nolan, R. A. and Nolan, W. G. (1972). Phenoxyethanol as a fungal enzyme extractant and preservative. *Mycologia* **64**, 1344.

Nottebohm, F. and Selander, R. K. (1972). Vocal dialects and gene frequencies in the Chingolo Sparrow (*Zonotrichia capensis*). *Condor* **74**, 137–143.

O'Brien, S. J., Gail, M. H. and Levin, D. L. (1980). Correlative genetic variation in natural populations of cats, mice and men. *Nature* **288**, 580–583.

O'Donald, P. (1980). "Genetic Models of Sexual Selection". Cambridge University Press.

Parkin, D. T. and Cole, S. R. (1985). Genetic differentiation and rates of evolution in some introduced populations of the House Sparrow, *Passer domesticus* in Australia and New Zealand. *Heredity* **54**, 15–23.

Patton, J. L. and Avise, J. C. (1983). Evolutionary genetics of birds. IV. Rates of protein divergence in waterfowl (Anatidae).

Payne, R. B. (1981). Population structure and social behavior: Models for testing the ecological significance of song dialects in birds. *In* "Natural Selection and Social Behavior". (eds R. D. Alexander and D. W. Tinkle). Chiron Press, New York.

Perrins, C. M. (1979). "British Tits'. W. Collins and Sons Ltd, Glasgow.

Petrinovich, L., Patterson, T. L. and Baptista, L. F. (1981). Song dialects as barriers to dispersal: A re-evaluation. *Evolution* **35**, 180–188.

Powell, J. R. (1975). Protein variation in natural populations of animals. *Evol. Biol.* **8**, 79–119.

Ramshaw, J. A. M., Coyne, J. A. and Lewontin, R. C. (1979). The sensitivity of gel electrophoresis as a detector of genetic variation. *Genetics* **93**, 1019–1037.

Redfield, J. (1973). Demography and genetics in colonizing populations of Blue Grouse. *Evolution* **27**, 576–592.

Redfield, J. (1974). Genetics and selection at the Ng locus in the Blue Grouse (*Dendragapus obscurus*). *Heredity* **31**, 35–42.

Redfield, J., Zwickel, F. C., Bendell, J. F. and Bergerud, A. T. (1972). Temporal and spatial patterns of allele and genotype frequencies at the Ng locus in blue grouse (*Dendragapus obscurus*). *Can. J. Zool.* **50**, 1657–1662.

Rogers, J. S. (1972). Measures of genetic similarity and genetic distance. *Stud. Genet.* **7**, 145–153.

Ross, H. A. (1983). Genetic differentiation of starling (*Sturnus vulgaris:* Aves) populations in New Zealand and Great Britain. *J. Zool., Lond.* **201**, 351–362.

Selander, R. K. (1976). Genic variation in natural populations. *In* "Molecular Evolution" (ed. F. Ayala), pp. 21–45. Sinauer Assoc. Inc., Sunderland, Mass.

Selander, R. K., Smith, M. H., Yang, S. Y., Johnson, W. E. and Gentry, J. B. (1971). Biochemical polymorphism and systematics in the genus *Peromyscus*. I. Variation in the old-field mouse (*Peromyscus polionotus*). *Studies in Genetics VI. Univ. Texas Publ.* **7103**, 49–90.

Semeonoff, R. and Robertson, F. W. (1968). A biochemical and ecological study of plasma esterase polymorphism in natural populations in the field vole, *Microtus agrestis* L. *Biochem. Genet.* **1**, 205–227.

Shaw, C. R. and Prasad, R. (1970). Starch gel electrophoresis of enzymes: a compilation of recipes. *Biochem. Genet.* **4**, 297–320.

Sherman, P. W. (1983). Electrophoresis and avian genealogical analysis. *Auk* **98**, 419–422.

Sibley, C. G. and Corbin, K. W. (1970). Ornithological field studies in the Great Plains and Nova Scotia. *Discovery* **6**, 3–6.

Singh, R. C., Lewontin, R. C. and Felton, A. (1976). Genetic heterogeneity within electrophoretic "alleles" of xanthine dehydrogenase in *Drosophila pseudoobscura*. *Genetics* **64**, 609–629.

Smith, J. K. and Zimmerman, E. G. (1976). Biochemical genetics and evolution of North American blackbirds, family Icteridae. *Comp. Biochem. Physiol.* **53B**, 319–324.

Sneath, P. H. A. and Sokal, R. R. (1973). "Numerical Taxonomy". W. H. Freeman, San Francisco.

Sokal, R. R. and Rohlf, F. J. (1981). "Biometry". 2nd edn. W. H. Freeman, San Francisco.

Sturkie, P. D. (ed.) (1976). "Avian Physiology". Springer-Verlag, New York.

Thompson, E. A. (1976). Inference of genealogical structure. *Soc. Sci. Int.* **15**, 477–526.

Vandeberg, J. L. and Johnson, P. G. (1977). A simple technique for long term storage of erythrocytes for enzyme electrophoresis. *Biochem. Genet.* **15**, 213–214.

van Noordwijk, A. and Scharloo, W. (1981). Inbreeding in an island population of the great tit. *Evolution* **35**, 674–688.

Vohs, P. A., Jr. and Carr, L. R. (1969). Genetic and population studies of transferrin polymorphisms in Ring-necked Pheasants. *Condor* **71**, 413–417.

Wake, D. B. (1981). The application of allozyme evidence to problems in the evolution of morphology. *In* "Evolution Today". (eds G. G. E. Scudder and J. L. Reveal) Proc. 2nd Int. Congr. Syst. Evol. Biol., pp. 257–270. Carnegie-Mellon University Press, Pittsburgh, PA.

Ward, R. D. (1977). Relationship between enzyme heterozygosity and quaternary structure. *Biochem. Genet.* **15**, 123–135.

Watson, A. and Moss, R. (1980). Advances in our understanding of the population dynamics of Red Grouse from a recent fluctuation in numbers. *Ardea* **68**, 103–111.

Watt, W. B. (1985). Bioenergetics and evolutionary genetics: opportunities for new synthesis. *Am. Nat.* **125**, 118–143.

Whitehouse, D. B. (1979). Population genetics of the Manx Shearwater, *Puffinus puffinus*. Ph.D. Thesis, University of Nottingham.

Woolfenden, G. E. and Fitzpatrick, J. (1984). "The Florida Scrub Jay". Princeton University Press.

Workman, P. L. and Niswander, J. D. (1970). Population studies on Southwestern

Indian tribes. II. Local genetic differentiation in the Papago. *Am. J. Hum. Genet.* **22**, 24–49.

Wright, S. (1965). The interpretation of population structure by *F*-statistics with special regard to systems of mating. *Evolution* **19**, 395–420.

Wright, S. (1978). "Evolution and the Genetics of Populations". Vol. 4. "Variability Within and Among Natural Populations". University of Chicago Press.

Wunderle, J. M. (1981). An analysis of a morph ratio cline in the bananaquit (*Coereba flaveola*) on Grenada, West Indies. *Evolution* **35**, 333–344.

Yang, S. Y. and Patton, J. L. (1981). Genic variability and differentiation in the Galapagos finches. *Auk* **98**, 230–242.

Zink, R. M. (1982). Patterns of genic and morphological variation among sparrows in the genera *Zonotrichia, Melospiza, Junco,* and *Passerella. Auk* **99**, 632–649.

Zink, R. M. and Barrowclough, G. F. (1984). Allozymes and song dialects: a reassessment. *Evolution* **38**, 444–448.

Zink, R. M. and Johnson, N. K. (1984). Evolutionary genetics of flycatchers. I. Sibling species in the genera *Empidonax* and *Contopus. Syst. Zool.*, **33**, 205–216.

Zink, R. M. and Winkler, D. W. (1983). Genetic and morphological similarity of two California gull populations with different life history traits. *Biochem. Syst. Ecol.* **11**, 397–403.

5

Analysis of DNA Sequence Variation

Thomas W. Quinn and Bradley N. White

*Biology Department, Queen's University, Kingston, Ontario,
Canada K7L 3N6*

1   INTRODUCTION

Recent advances in recombinant DNA technology allow the direct analysis of DNA sequence variation by electrophoretic methods analogous to those used for protein and enzyme polymorphisms. Previous work on DNA variation in birds (see Sibley and Ahlquist 1983) has made extensive use of DNA hybridization studies to clarify taxonomic relationships among various groups but has been of little value in the study of intraspecific variation. The new recombinant DNA technology allows the study of DNA sequence

AVIAN GENETICS
ISBN 0-12-187570-9

variation within and between populations at a high level of resolution. The purpose of this chapter is to describe this analysis and to encourage avian population biologists to take advantage of it. Birds are ideally suited to these studies because their nucleated erythrocytes provide an accessible and abundant supply of nuclear DNA. A small blood sample which can be taken in the field and frozen later without significant damage to the DNA, is sufficient for large numbers of analyses.

We briefly review the information presently available on avian DNA variation and emphasize the new techniques used at the population level. Methods available for analysing the information from both nuclear and mtDNA studies are presented and compared. Where appropriate, we draw on our data and experience with Lesser Snow Goose (*Anser c. caerulescens*) populations to illustrate the application of the techniques. Since little is currently published on birds, we also present results that have been published on mammalian populations in order to illustrate the types of information that can be derived from these new techniques.

Before the advent of recombinant DNA procedures, DNA could be analysed only through the gene products, the proteins or by the examination of the hybridization of the total unique DNA of two species. Analysis of protein products has primarily been carried out by electrophoresis or, more recently, iso-electric focusing and heat stability studies on serum proteins and enzymes (see chapter 4 and Barrowclough 1983). Unfortunately, these procedures analyse less than 10% of the nuclear DNA (the fraction that codes for amino acid sequence), and only the small percentage of DNA changes which bring about size, charge or stability differences in the proteins can be detected. This procedure may be complicated by post-translational changes of proteins and by the shortage of polymorphic enzymes within the study population. In some cases, primarily for interspecies comparisons, complete amino acid sequences have been determined. This allows a more thorough analysis of the sequence differences but, owing to the technical difficulties in protein isolation and sequencing, cannot be applied on a routine basis to the large numbers of individuals needed for population comparisons.

The discovery and commercial availability of bacterial enzymes which cleave DNA at specific sequences (restriction endonucleases) have opened the way to the analysis of DNA sequence variation within a species. These enzymes evolved as a defence mechanism against invading foreign DNA molecules such as bacterial viruses. In the laboratory, they can be used in conjunction with recombinant DNA molecules to sample segments of the DNA and detect differences between individuals. Most of this chapter will be directed at the use of these enzymes in analysing mitochondrial and genomic DNA sequences. Only a small percentage of any DNA segment is analysed, and a complete analysis would require DNA sequencing of all the alleles present in a population. A technique for direct genomic DNA sequencing has been described (Church and Gilbert 1984). The information derived from nuclear DNA comparisons can be used to answer questions at a higher level of resolution than has been possible using protein polymorphisms. These would include studies on genetic differentiation and maternity/paternity. The ability to analyse mtDNA adds a new powerful tool to the population geneticist's arsenal. As the mtDNA is of maternal origin, it can be used as a molecular "tag" to ask questions about bird movement and migration. It will be particularly informative for those species where the female returns to the natal breeding area.

2 NUCLEAR DNA

2.1 Content and genetic information

For several aspects of DNA analysis it is useful to know the haploid DNA content of the study species. In birds the DNA content appears relatively constant at about 1·3 picograms per haploid genome (Bachman *et al.* 1972). This is about one-third of that in mammals and represents about 1×10^9 base pairs (b.p.) of genetic information.

Only 5–10% of the DNA codes for proteins. This is based on various estimates of higher eukaryotes having 50 000 to 100 000 genes and an average gene of 1000 b.p. long. Thus, of the 1×10^9 b.p., no more than 1×10^8 b.p. codes for the amino acid sequence found in proteins and in Aves only 20–60 different proteins can be easily analysed for polymorphisms (chapter 4 and Corbin 1983). Within a single species only a few of these proteins are likely to be polymorphic. Direct analysis of DNA therefore allows an examination of sequences not previously accessible by studies on protein polymorphism.

2.2 Classes of genomic DNA and their sequence organization

Eukaryotes contain both single copy (unique) DNA sequences and repeated sequences (Britten and Kohne 1968). The repeated DNA is divided into highly repetitive (HR) sequences with greater than 10^5 copies and moderately repetitive (MR) sequences with less than 10^5 copies. The HR sequences are usually associated with heterochromatin and are probably never transcribed. The avian genome appears to contain less repeated DNA than mammals and, surprisingly, it is arranged in a long-period interspersion pattern (Shields and Straus 1975, Shields 1983, Arthur and Straus 1978, Eden and Hendrick 1978, Epplen *et al.* 1978). With few exceptions, mammals have the so called

"Xenopus" pattern of genome organization, which means that about 60% of their DNA consists of single-copy sequences of about 1000 b.p. (1 kb) alternating with MR sequences of about 300 b.p. In the most widely studied bird, Domestic Fowl (*Gallus gallus*), the MR sequences are 2–4 kb long while the interspersed unique sequences are 5 kb or more. This pattern is found in about 40% of the genome, while in the remainder there are longer stretches of unique DNA. The evolutionary significance of the short-period interspersion found in most animals versus the long-period interspersion found in most birds and a few other organisms is still unknown. The long-period interspersion does appear to be correlated with a small genome size and may be correlated with ecotypic specialists (Shields 1983). This type of genome organization facilitates the isolation of the recombinant DNA probes for the new analyses (see later).

2.3   Analysis of genomic DNA variation

There has been a considerable amount of work done using DNA–DNA hybridization studies to examine taxonomic relationships among various avian species (see Sibley and Ahlquist 1983). The first such study was directed at measuring the relatedness of species in the genus *Junco* (Shields and Straus 1975). Comparisons of entire genomic DNA complements are not usually sensitive enough to analyse differences between individuals within a species, but see Britten *et al.* (1978) for a non-avian example. However, it is extremely valuable for genetic distance estimates of species which have already diverged considerably. DNA–DNA hybridization studies can only detect differences greater than one change in every 100 b.p. (Bonner *et al.* 1973). Intraspecific nuclear DNA sequence variation is probably about one difference in 100–1000 b.p. In order to examine this level of variation, a detailed comparison of the same DNA segment between individuals is required.

The advent of recombinant DNA technology made it possible to isolate specific genes or random DNA segments and use these as probes to look at the level of DNA sequence variation at the locus of the probe. The availability of large numbers of different restriction endonucleases makes routine analysis of DNA from many individuals straightforward. The basic procedure uses the Southern blot (Southern 1975), and is described in Fig. 1. High molecular weight DNA is first isolated from blood or other tissue such as the liver. This DNA is subjected to cleavage by a restriction enzyme and the resultant fragments are separated by electrophoresis on an agarose gel. When a restriction enzyme is used that recognizes a sequence of 4 b.p. it will cleave the DNA on average every $(4)^4$ or 256 b.p. If the restriction enzyme has to recognize a 6 b.p. sequence, it will cleave on average every $(4)^6$ or

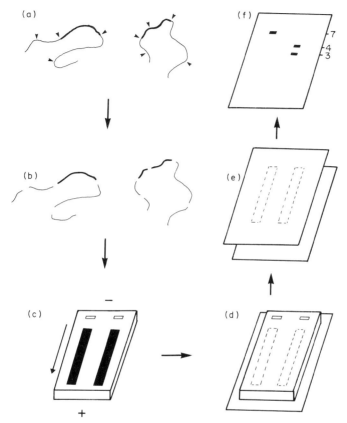

Fig. 1. Southern blot analysis of nuclear RFLPs. (*a*) Digestion with a restriction endonuclease cleaves genomic DNA at specific recognition sites. (*b*) A variant recognition site in the area of DNA with homology to the probe (heavy line) is shown. (*c*) After cleavage, the DNA is electrophoresed on an agarose gel, creating a "smear" of fragments of various lengths. (*d*) The DNA is denatured into single strands and transferred to a sheet of nitrocellulose. This sheet is incubated with a radioactively labelled single-stranded probe which hybridizes to homologous fragments on the nitrocellulose. (*e*) After washing off unbound probe DNA the nitrocellulose is placed against a sheet of X-ray film to detect radioactivity. (*f*) After development of the X-ray, areas of hybridization are seen as dark bands. In this example, one individual was homozygous for the 7 kb allele, and one was homozygous for the 4 kb and 3 kb allele. A heterozygote (not shown) would have all three bands.

4096 b.p. In either case an avian genome of 1×10^9 b.p. will yield more than 10^5 fragments of varying sizes, which appear as a smear on the electrophoretic gel (Fig. 1(c)). In order to examine differences between individuals, specific sequences must be analysed using a radioactively labelled DNA probe. Firstly one transfers the DNA from the agarose gel to a blot matrix, which is usually some derivative of nitrocellulose or nylon. Some nylon-based transfer membranes allow repeated use of the same blot. The DNA is denatured into single strands within the gel and blotted from the gel to the matrix, which has a high affinity for single-stranded DNA (Fig. 1(d)). The DNA is then immobilized by drying, baking or U.V. cross-linking. This blot is them hybridized with a single-stranded ^{32}P-labelled probe DNA. The probe is a cloned DNA sequence, usually, but not necessarily, from the same species as the DNA being analysed; its preparation will be described more fully later. The probe DNA is made radioactive by either replacing non-radioactive nucleotides with radioactive ones, using a procedure termed "nick translation" (Rigby *et al.* 1977) or by adding radioactive nucleotides to a primer (Feinberg and Vogelstein 1983). During hybridization the probe will hybridize to complementary DNA sequences on the blot. After removal of non-hybridized material, the blot is placed next to an X-ray film (Fig. 1(e)) and an enhancer (amplifying) screen which converts the β-emissions of the isotope to light, which is then detected by the film. When the X-ray is developed, black bands appear at the positions where the radioactive probe DNA was hybridized to the DNA blotted from the agarose gel (Fig. 1(f)).

2.4   DNA markers and restriction fragment length polymorphisms (RFLPs)

The DNA fragments resulting from the cleavage by a restriction enzyme may be of different lengths in different individuals. These restriction fragment length variants (RFLVs) can be used as Mendelian markers in the same way as electrophoretic variants of proteins or enzymes. When the frequency of the most common variant is less than 99%, the term "restriction fragment length polymorphism" (RFLP) is used. The detection of a polymorphic DNA segment is illustrated in Fig. 2. There is a sequence difference such that a base-pair change has taken place in the sequence GAATTC, which is recognized and cleaved by the restriction enzyme *Eco*RI (derived from the bacteria *Escherichia coli*). This region of the DNA is detected using a cloned probe DNA sequence which spans the *Eco*RI site in question. When the DNAs are cleaved with *Eco*RI, and the fragments separated by agarose gel electrophoresis and hybridized with ^{32}P-labelled probe, the autoradiograph

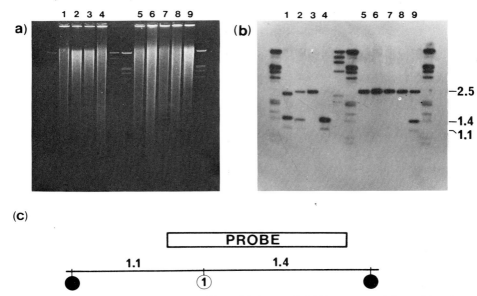

Fig. 2. Detection of a nuclear RFLP. (*a*) 5 μg of DNA extracted from blood samples of adult Lesser Snow Geese were digested with *Eco*RI, electrophoresed on a 1% agaraose gel, and stained with ethidium bromide. (*b*) Autoradiograph of a Southern blot prepared from *(a)* and probed with a radioactively labelled unique sequence DNA fragment. Unnumbered tracks are molecular size markers. Samples 3 and 5–8 are homozygous for the 2·5 kb allele. Sample 4 is homozygous for the 1·4, 1·1 kb allele. Samples 1, 2 and 9 are heterozygotes. (*c*) A map showing the relationship between probe and nuclear DNA. Solid circles are invariant *Eco*RI sites. Open circle is a variant *Eco*RI site which may be present or absent in different chromosomes.

shown in Fig. 2 (*b*) is produced. Five individuals homozygous for one sequence, one homozygous for the other sequence and three heterozygotes are illustrated. When the *Eco*RI recognition site is present, two restriction fragments of 1·4 and 1·1 kb are present while, when it is absent, one 2·5 kb fragment is observed. Thus, homozygotes have either a 2·5 kb or 1·4 and 1·1 kb bands, while the heterozygote has 2·5, 1·4 and 1·1 kb fragments, each with roughly half the intensity of those of the homozygotes.

Studies of RFLPs and RFLVs in man are well advanced, and we suggest adopting a similar nomenclature for alleles and random probe sequences in birds (see Skolnick *et al.* 1984). The alleles detected by a given probe are given letter and number designations such that the *Eco*RI variants described above would be allele A-1 (1·4 and 1·1 kb fragments) and allele A-2 (2·5 kb fragment). If another RFLP were found with the same probe, using a different restriction enzyme such as *Hind*III, the alleles would be termed B-1 and B-2. The frequencies of these various alleles can then be determined using large numbers of individuals in a population. The alleles represent sequence variation of an arbitrary DNA segment which may have no genetic function; they are alleles of a locus which is not necessarily a gene.

The major difficulty with this work is to obtain a suitable probe sequence that identifies the locus. The sequence should be unique or single-copy in order to allow interpretation of variation in the same locus in different individuals. Two approaches are possible: (1) utilize previously cloned genes, mainly from chickens, in order to detect homologous sequences in the bird species under study; (2) select random unique DNA segments from a recombinant DNA library prepared from DNA of the study species. Use of a combination of the above probes allows the comparative analysis of coding DNA sequences against other random unique DNA sequences.

2.5   Cloned avian genes

About 50 avian genes (primarily chicken) have been isolated, analysed and in some cases sequenced. The first eukaryotic gene characterized was the chicken ovalbumin gene (Lai *et al.* 1978). This came under intensive study because of the interest in hormonal gene regulation. The basic structure of avian genes is similar to those of mammals and other eukaryotes which have been studied. The fowl insulin gene is shown in Fig. 3. It has been used to examine the rate of evolution of eukaryotic genes in vertebrates. As expected, the exons (coding regions) are evolving much more slowly than the introns or

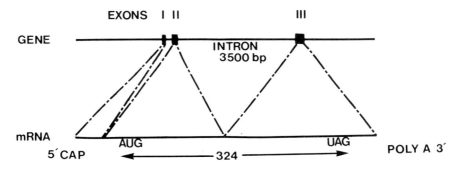

Fig. 3. The Chicken Preproinsulin gene. The gene structure is taken from Perler *et al.* (1980). The three exons (I, 37 b.p.; II, 203 b.p.; III, 218 b.p.) and the large intron are indicated. The small intron between exon I and II has a length of 119 b.p. The positions of the AUG start codon and UAG stop codon delineate the region (324 nucleotides) coding for the preproinsulin polypeptide. The mRNA has the characteristic 5' CAP and 3' poly(A) tail.

flanking sequences of the genes. Within the exons, changes in DNA sequence that leave the amino acid sequence unchanged, or changes that replace one amino acid with a similar one (conservative change), are the most frequent. As the time of the fish radiation, separation of birds from mammals and the mammal radiation are known from the fossil record, it is possible to establish a molecular clock of evolutionary change (Efstratiadis *et al.* 1980, Perler *et al.* 1980). The clock can then be used to examine other evolutionary changes for which there is no good fossil record. This sequence comparison of the same gene in a number of species complements the information derived from DNA hybridization studies (Sibley and Ahlquist 1983).

Most of the available cloned genes are from Domestic Fowl, but, because many coding sequences are evolving relatively slowly, they can likely be used on broadly divergent species. A fowl gene can therefore be used as a probe to detect appropriate restriction fragments on an electrophoretic gel of DNA of another species, so long as there is sufficient homology to allow hybridization and thereby yield a detectable signal on the autoradiograph. This approach has been used to examine the tempo of genomic evolution in seven species of the pheasant super family, *Phasianoidea* (Helm-Bychowski and Wilson 1986). As stated earlier, exons are evolving slowly and RFLPs are found less often than in non-coding unique sequences. In order to examine the non-coding regions, it is usually necessary to obtain or prepare a recombinant DNA library from the study species.

2.6   Recombinant genomic DNA libraries

A complete genomic library is one in which the DNA complement of an organism is present in small DNA segments recombined with bacterial vector DNAs (plasmids or phage DNAs), which are capable of autonomously replicating within bacterial hosts. For experimental details of library construction, the reader is referred to Maniatis *et al.* (1978, 1982). The easiest libraries to manipulate are those that are constructed in vectors derived from the *E. coli* bacteriophage lambda. A general outline of library construction is shown in Fig. 4. The first step is to isolate high molecular weight genomic DNA, cut it and isolate 10–20 kb segments. The present method of choice is to digest the DNA with an enzyme such as *Sau*3a that recognizes 4 b.p. pairs. This enzyme cleaves the DNA on average every 256 base pairs, but can be manipulated such that it only partially cuts the DNA to yield fragments of about 20 kb. These fragments have staggered single-stranded ends that are complementary to ends produced by another restriction enzyme *Bam*H1 that recognizes 6 b.p. pairs. There are a number of genetically engineered lambda phage vectors that contain *Bam*H1 sites in positions that allow the removal

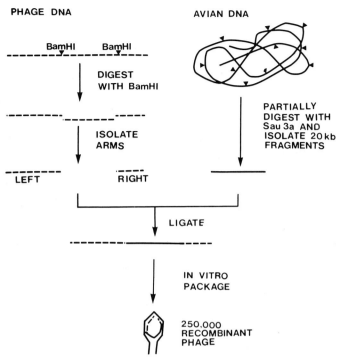

Fig. 4. Construction of an avian genomic library in phage. An outline of one approach to the construction of a genomic library in a phage vector is shown. The phage DNA is digested with the restriction enzyme *Bam*HI and the left and right arms isolated. The high molecular weight genomic DNA is partially digested with *Sau*3a and 20 kb fragments isolated. The *Sau*3a genomic DNA fragments have complementary single-stranded ends to the *Bam*HI digested phage arms and are ligated to them. The recombinant DNAs are packaged into phage particles *in vitro* to give more than 250 000 independent particles. These can then be amplified in *Escherichia coli* hosts.

of a segment of the λ DNA. The ends of the remaining phage arms are compatible with the 20 kb genomic DNA fragments, and can be spliced to them by means of the enzyme ligase. These recombinant DNAs can be packaged *in vitro* into phage coats, and then multiplied in *E. coli* hosts. In order to achieve a 99% probability of having a given DNA sequence in the library, about five genome equivalents of DNA must be present in the independently derived recombinant molecules. Therefore, the complete avian library consists of at least 250 000 different recombinant phage particles, containing about 18 kb of avian DNA each, which have been amplified 10^5–10^6 times.

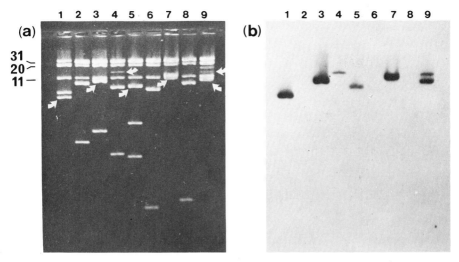

Fig. 5. Identification of unique and repetitive fragments within lambda clones chosen from a Lesser Snow Goose library. (*a*) One μg of DNA isolated from various lambda clones was digested with *Eco*RI, electrophoresed on a 1% agarose gel, and stained with ethidium bromide. Three fragments (31, 20, 11 kb) originate from the lambda-vector arms. All other fragments originate from goose DNA. Arrows indicate those fragments which are repetitive. *(b)* Autoradiograph of a Southern blot prepared from (*a*) and probed with radioactively labelled total goose DNA. Goose DNA fragments visualized in (*a*) but not in (*b*) represent unique DNA.

In order to obtain useful probes from the library, unique sequences must be isolated. This can be achieved by screening the recombinant phage DNA with ^{32}P-labelled total genomic DNA. A small portion of the library is spread out on a lawn of bacteria and the resultant plaques (areas of bacterial lysis resulting from phage infection) transferred to nitrocellulose (Benton and Davis 1977). The phage are broken and the single-stranded DNA blotted and fixed on to the nitrocellulose paper like a Southern blot. This blot is hybridized to total ^{32}P-labelled genomic DNA in which the only sequences present at sufficient concentration to hybridize in a short period of time are the repetitive ones. Thus, any recombinant phage that gives a signal, contains MR or HR DNA sequences, which have to be removed if this DNA is to be used as a probe. It is possible to select phage that do not give a signal, and use the isolated DNA as a probe directly (for example, the probe used in Fig. 6, see section 2.10). Because of the long interspersion pattern in birds, the number of recombinant phages containing 10–20 kb of unique DNA is much higher than that in mammals. Long probes allow the simultaneous examination of more restriction sites in the genomic DNA and so may be preferable to shorter ones. In order to obtain a unique sequence from a recombinant phage that contains repetitive segments, the DNA is digested with a variety of restriction enzymes, electrophoresed and a Southern blot prepared. This blot is probed with ^{32}P-labelled total genomic DNA to distinguish unique from repetitive restriction fragments (Fig. 5). Unique fragments can be isolated from agarose gels and used directly as probes or cloned into bacterial plasmid vectors and amplified (Maniatis *et al.* 1982). The latter approach is more time-consuming but allows the easy preparation of large amounts of pure probe DNA and facilitates transport of probes to other laboratories. This type of probe was used to detect the polymorphism shown in Fig. 2.

2.7   Labelling the probe, hybridization and autoradiography

There are a number of techniques for labelling DNA that yield satisfactory results, but the primer extension method of Feinberg and Vogelstein (1983) gives the most consistent results, and produces a randomly labelled probe. Using 50 μCi of one ^{32}P-labelled nucleoside triphosphate of specific activity 3000 Ci/mmol, 50 ng of DNA can be labelled up to specific activities as high as 1×10^9 cpm/μg. There is a wide variety of hybridization protocols, the details of which often depend on the blotting membrane. We presently prefer Gene Screen Plus™ membrane (New England Nuclear Corporation) and aqueous hybridization conditions at 68°C. For a complete review of hybridization protocols refer to Maniatis *et al.* (1982). Specific procedures are available from the individual manufacturers. After the blot has been hybridized and washed, it is placed next to an X-ray film with intensifying screens (Swanstrom and Shank 1978); the best intensifying screens are calcium–tungstate–phosphor (Dupont Cronex Lightning-Plus). The enhancement of film exposed at $-70°C$ with two intensifying screens, for ^{32}P, is about tenfold.

2.8   Strategies for identifying RFLPs

Three components need to be considered in the identification of RFLPs: (1) the individuals in the study population, (2) the probe sequences and (3) the restriction enzymes. For studies where several genetic markers are required, the first step is to identify a group of individuals that will maximize the likelihood of finding RFLPs, for example, by examining the most divergent individuals. In Lesser Snow Geese we chose to look at males, which because they are less philopatric than females, are potentially more genetically variable when collected at a single breeding colony. Thus analysis of males should maximize the likelihood of finding RFLPs. Skolnick and White (1982) chose to screen nine individuals when analysing a single human population. They have estimated that four is too few and 19 identifies rare RFLVs that may not be useful. We have routinely screened about 13 birds.

The choice of probe can be influenced by what is available from other research groups and the feasibility of constructing genomic libraries for the study species. Arbitrary DNA segments are, in the main, non-coding and therefore probably under less selection pressure than coding regions examined by cloned genes. This is important when interpreting RFLP data. Among arbitrary segments, longer sequences have the advantage of covering more restriction enzyme sites, but can produce Southern blots with complex hybridization patterns, especially when restriction enzymes with 4 b.p. recognition sequences are used. Long probes, however, are also more likely to detect insertions or deletions. There is some indication in mammals that unique probe sequences adjacent to repetitive regions identify RFLPs more frequently.

We have found that the nuclear DNA of Lesser Snow Goose is more polymorphic than that of man, and as a result it is easy to find randomly chosen probes that detect RFLPs (Quinn and White, 1987). Using 10–20 kb unique DNA segments cloned into a λ-vector (from the library), and screening these probes for detection of polymorphic sites of four restriction enzymes (*Eco*RI, *Hin*dIII, *Msp*I and *Taq*I) in nuclear DNA, we have found that all 17 probes tested detected polymorphisms with at least one of those enzymes.

A major issue considered in the search for RFLPs in human DNA is the number and type of restriction enzymes to be used (Skolnick and White 1982, Bastie-Sigeac and Lucotte 1983, Barker *et al.* 1984). RFLPs result from either base-pair changes at a restriction enzyme site, or insertion or deletion of large DNA sequences between restriction sites. The screen for base-pair changes is markedly affected by the number of bases in the recognition site, r, which directly influences the mean length of the resultant fragments, M. The length of the probe P dictates the number of sites that will be analysed, such that the number of bases screened for changes is $r(2 + P/M)$. This relationship suggests that enzymes recognizing 4 b.p. should be the best; however, these often generate many fragments below 200 b.p. which are not as easily analysed electrophoretically as the larger ones. In addition, restriction enzyme sites in human DNA containing the CpG dimer show a high frequency of polymorphism. For this reason the enzymes *Msp*I (C CGG) and *Taq*I (T CGA) have been the most extensively used. The cytosines in the CpG sequence are known to be frequently methylated and have been implicated as a hotspot for $C \rightarrow T$ transition mutations. These are the transition mutations detected by restriction enzymes which contain a CpG at their recognition site. The preliminary data we have on Snow Geese suggest that this may not be as pronounced a trend in birds, and we have found a considerable number of RFLPs with enzymes such as *Eco*RI and *Hin*dIII.

The rationale for detecting insertion/deletion changes depends on the magnitude of the size change of the restriction fragment in question. In theory, enzymes that cut infrequently such *Kpn*I are likely to be most informative. However it is difficult to detect small changes in large restriction fragments and there is always a problem in transferring large fragments during Southern blotting. In practice, then, the best approach is probably to use the more economical 6 b.p. recognizing enzymes.

2.9   Interpretation of RFLP data

The nature of the probes used influences the interpretation of the data. If DNA segments from known genes are used, they do not represent a random sample of the genome and will be under the evolutionary constraints of the product they code for. If arbitrary DNA segments are used, their relationship to coding sequences will be unknown. Most will not be coding and will likely be under less selective constraint than the coding regions. It seems probable that RFLP frequency differences between gene pools will represent predominantly neutral differences. If so, the magnitude of such differences between populations should represent the genetic distance between the populations. This is in contrast to interpretations of protein electrophoretic data which are likely to be confounded by selective effects. The validity of such an assumption of neutrality could be tested by comparing genetic distance estimates made using expressed versus non-coding DNA probes.

Once RFLPs have been identified, allele frequencies can be determined. These data can then be used to quantify genetic similarities between populations using the Nei (1972) or Rogers (1972) indices of genetic similarity. Both measures compare the interpopulational differences in allele frequencies at each locus, and combine these values in a final figure. In order to apply these indices to nuclear RFLPs (Nei and Tajima 1981), the alleles are first defined by the number and sizes of bands detected by a particular probe (for example, allele A-1 2·5 kb and allele A-2 1·4 kb and 1·1 kb). The index of genetic similiarity used by Nei (1972) for allozymes is

$$I_N = \sum_{i=1}^{m} (P_{ix}P_{iy}) \bigg/ \left[\left(\sum_{i=1}^{m} P_{ix} \right)^2 \left(\sum_{i=1}^{m} P_{iy}^2 \right) \right]^{1/2}$$

When applied to RFLP studies, P_{ix} represents the frequency of allele i in population x, and P_{iy} its frequency in population y. The number of alleles at that locus detected with a particular probe is represented by m. Nei and Tajima (1981) think that more information can be included if the number of restriction site differences between the various alleles are known. If they are, the mean number of restriction site differences between two randomly chosen alleles from the two populations can be calculated using the formula

$$\hat{v}_{xy} = \sum x_i y_j v_{ij}$$

where x_i is the frequency of the ith allele in population x, y_j is the frequency of the jth allele and v_{ij} is the number of restriction site differences between the ith and jth alleles. The summation is taken over all combinations of alleles between populations (when $i = j$, $v_{ij} = 0$). Taking into account the mean number of restriction site differences between two randomly chosen alleles within each population, the number of net restriction site differences between the two populations can be calculated by

$$\hat{d} = \hat{v}_{xy} - (\hat{v}_x + \hat{v}_y)/2$$

where

$$\hat{v}_x = (n/(n + 1))\left(\sum_{ij} x_i x_j v_{ij} \right)$$

that is, comparisons are now made between alleles within each population in order to account for intrapopulation diversity.

The Nei–Tajima theory (1981) has not been tested for nuclear DNA owing to paucity of data. Perhaps its weakest feature is the inability to account for insertions and deletions. However, our work with Snow Goose populations suggests that insertion/deletion changes are much less common than substitutional changes.

2.10   Opportunities for nuclear DNA analysis

In addition to general studies of genetic structuring in populations, RFLP analysis can be applied to pedigrees. Such assays are important in clarifying the effects which rape, cuckoldry or egg dumping may have on the inclusive fitness of individuals. The implications of such behaviours have been summarized by Sherman (1981). Protein polymorphism analysis is limited by the paucity of polymorphic proteins. RFLP analysis allows many more genetic markers to be simultaneously studied for paternity/maternity determinations. Some of these markers are exceptionally informative owing to the number of haplotypes detected. We have isolated a probe from the Snow Goose library that detects four variant EcoRI sites along a single 11 kb stretch of DNA (Fig. 6). The number of haplotypes that are detectable with this probe is $2^4 = 16$. A few probes such as this would be all that is required

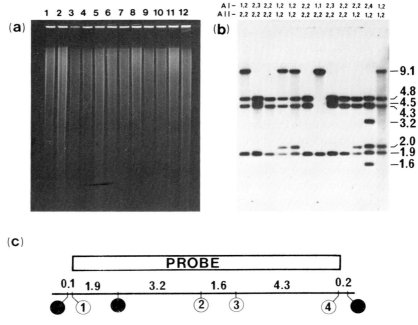

Fig. 6. Detection of a highly variable locus. (a) 5 μg of DNA extracted from blood samples of adult Lesser Snow Geese were digested with *Eco*RI and electrophoresed on a 1% agarose gel. (b) Autoradiograph of a Southern blot prepared from (a) and probed with a radioactively labelled fragment of unique DNA. (c) A map showing the relationship between probe and nuclear DNA. Solid circles are invariant *Eco*RI sites. Open circles are variant *Eco*RI sites which may be present or absent in various patterns to give the genotypes shown in (b).

for accurate paternity/maternity determinations. Among the random sample of 12 birds from La Perouse Bay shown in Fig. 6, seven different genotypes were detected. We have used a number of these DNA markers to detect the occurrence of intraspecific brood parasitism in the Snow Goose (Quinn *et al.* 1987).

Jeffreys *et al.* (1985 a,b,c) have isolated human DNA probes that identify many copies of a sequence of DNA ("mini-satellite") which may be involved in recombination events in human DNA. These probes have been shown to detect highly polymorphic DNA region in the human genome with levels of heterozygosity approaching 100%! The power of such probes for pedigree analysis is enormous, as the probability of two unrelated individuals sharing a common banding pattern for a single probe is 3×10^{-11} (Jeffreys *et al.* 1985 b). Such probes would be of obvious value in avian pedigree studies.

How applicable these human DNA probes will be to other animals is as yet undetermined, and will depend on how evolutionarily conserved the "mini-satellite" sequence is.

Our study of Snow Geese illustrates the considerable advantages that the approach to genetic analysis using RFLPs has over that of enzyme and protein polymorphism studies. Bargiello *et al.* (1977) tested four esterase isozymes of Lesser Snow Goose. They postulated that a minimum of seven structural gene loci were involved in the biosynthesis of those enzymes, and only one locus was polymorphic with allele frequencies of 0·95 and 0·05. We have tested 17 random DNA fragments and found all to be polymorphic at 1 to 13 restriction enzyme sites each. Altogether, we have identified over 70 individual polymorphic restriction enzyme sites. The levels of polymorphism allow a finer resolution of genetic differences (or distances) between populations of birds, and provide a more effective method for determining paternity or maternity of specific birds than was previously available.

3 MITOCHONDRIAL DNA

3.1 Content and genetic information

The avian mitochondrial genome, like that of most eukaryotes, is circular (Fig. 7) and is approximately 16 kb long (Glaus *et al.* 1980, Bangti *et al.* 1983). Mitochondria are maternally inherited (Lansman *et al.* 1983 b) and undergo rapid evolutionary change in nucleotide sequence compared to nuclear DNA (Avise *et al.* 1979 b, Brown and Simpson 1981, Brown *et al.* 1982, Lansman *et al.* 1981, and others). This rapid rate of change makes mtDNA restriction enzyme site analysis particularly appropriate for the comparison of conspecific populations and of recently divergent species. The interpretation of differences in restriction enzyme sites is simplified since mitochondria are usually monoclonal within individuals (Avise *et al.* 1979 b, Hayashi *et al.* 1979; but see Hauswirth and Laipis 1982, Harrison *et al.* 1985) and do not seem to undergo recombination in vertebrates (De Francesco *et al.* 1980). Once a variant is established in a female, all descendants of that individual carry it and, therefore, the inheritance pattern is clonal through the matriarchal lineage.

Kessler and Avise (1984, 1985) have made interspecific mtDNA comparisons of avian congeners and found that (1) phylogenetic trees and dendrograms constructed from their data by a variety of methods were highly concordant with each other and with phylogenies derived from independent sources of information using more traditional data bases; and (2) genetic distances derived from mtDNA RFLP data follow a similar trend

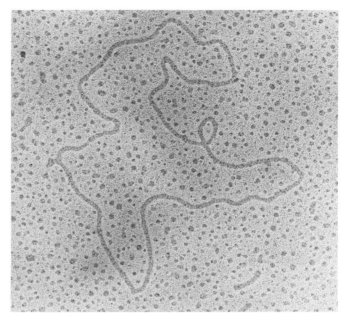

Fig. 7. An electron micrograph of mitochondrial DNA isolated from liver tissue of the Lesser Snow Goose.

to distances derived from protein electrophoretic data, and avian species tend to have lower interspecific genetic distance than their non-avian counterparts. While population studies of conspecific mtDNA variation in birds are at a preliminary stage (Shields and Wilson 1987), studies of mammals, insects and plants have all revealed populations of geographic-specific mtDNA variants. Avise *et al.* (1979 a) have compared allozyme against mtDNA variation patterns detected over a large geographic range of Pocket Gopher (*Geomys pinetis*). In a study of proteins at 25 loci in 171 samples, only two "macrogeographic assemblages" could be discerned. The concurrent study of mtDNA restriction site variation made use of six different restriction endonucleases on 87 samples in order to identify 23 different clones, including both widespread and more localized variants. The two macrogeographic assemblages were resolved in terms of "matriarchal phylogenies".

A later study of mtDNA restriction site variation of *Peromyscus maniculatus* by Lansman *et al.* (1983 a) again showed that an mtDNA study is superior to an allozyme study in resolution. In their study 135 samples were collected from areas across North America. Analysis of the mtDNA with eight restriction endonucleases (*Hinc*II, *Bgl*II, *Hind*III, *Bst*EII, *Eco*RI,

*Bam*HI, *Xba*I and *Hpa*II) generated data on 80 restriction sites. Only 29% of these sites were common to all samples, and many "restriction morphs" (defining all sites for an individual) were related by the loss or gain of a single site. Five geographic assemblages of mice were identified, including Southern California, Central States, Texas–Mexico, Northern Michigan and Eastern States. Within each assemblage, clones of restriction morphs differed by one to three mutation steps only (changes in restriction sites), while between assemblages from eight to twenty mutational steps were involved.

3.2   Isolation of mitochondrial DNA

Mitochondrial DNA can be visualized in one of two ways, dependent on the availability of various tissues. Where possible, the simplest approach is to purify mtDNA directly from a tissue such as heart or liver. Purified mtDNA can then be cleaved with restriction endonucleases, electrophoresed on agarose or acrylamide gels, and the restriction fragments visualized by ethidium bromide staining. If the amounts of mtDNA are limited, the sensitivity can be increased by radioactively labelling the fragments with ^{32}P (see Maniatis *et al.* 1982). Procedures for purification of mtDNA from liver, brain and kidney tissue are presented by Lansman *et al.* (1981). While Kessler and Avise (1984) reported that fresh heart tissue yielded the cleanest mtDNA preparations, we have found liver and brain tissue to give better results with our protocols. The tissue is homogenized in such a way that cells are ruptured to release intact organelles. Nuclei are pelleted by centrifugation under conditions in which most mitochondria remain suspended. The supernatant is decanted, pelleted and resuspended, and the mitochondria are lysed to release the mtDNA. An isopycnic CsCl–ethidium bromide centrifugation is used to isolate mtDNA from any remaining nuclear DNA and other cellular debris. This separates linear nuclear DNA from supercoiled circular mtDNA on the basis of a density difference resulting from differential binding of ethidium bromide. Two discrete bands of DNA result, the denser being mtDNA. In order to obtain mtDNA free from nuclear DNA, a second centrifugation is often required. The greatest difficulty in this approach is that it requires either a partial hepatectomy (removal of a portion of the liver) or, more frequently, sacrificing the bird.

The other approach is to analyse the mtDNA present as a "contaminant" in the DNA isolated from blood. White blood cells are the main source of this mtDNA. In order to identify the mtDNA sequences against the background "smear" of nuclear DNA fragments, cloned mtDNA segments or purified total mtDNA obtained from a single bird are used to probe Southern blots. We have analysed DNA extracted from Lesser Snow Goose blood samples in

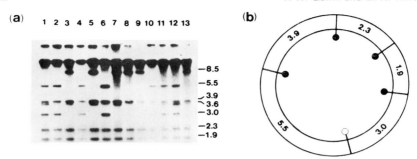

Fig. 8. A mitochondrial DNA polymorphism in the Lesser Snow Goose. (*a*) DNA samples extracted from liver were electrophoresed on a 1% agarose gel, blotted and probed with a partially purified mtDNA. In addition to the mtDNA restriction fragments, a 3·6 kb band of nuclear homology to the mitochondrial probe can be seen (also see Fig. 9). The high molecular weight hybridization is a result of nuclear contamination in the partially purified probe. (*b*) Map of the mitochondrial genome showing a variant *Hind*III site (open circle) which accounts for the two variants observed in *(a)*. Closed circles represent invariate *Hind*III sites.

this way, using both purified total mtDNA (Fig. 8) and cloned mtDNA segments (Fig. 9). Some mtDNA probes detect homologous sequences in the nuclear DNA in addition to those of the mtDNA (Fig. 9). The occurrence of mitochondrial sequences in nuclear DNA has been reported in several species, including maize (Kemble *et al.* 1983), sea urchins (Jacobs *et al.* 1983), locusts (Gellissen *et al.* 1983) and fungi (Farreliy and Butow 1983, Wright and Cummings 1983, van den Boogaart *et al.* 1982). This nuclear homology makes it more difficult to interpret results, as the origin of each band (nuclear or mitochondrial) must be ascertained for each probe/enzyme combination used. We have established band origins by comparing DNA extracted from liver and blood. The ratio of mtDNA to nuclear DNA is much greater in DNA extracted from liver, and this ratio is further increased if a crude mitochondrial preparation is made prior to DNA extraction. By electrophoresing restriction enzyme-digested samples of these three DNA preparations and probing Southern blots with the various mtDNA probes, the mtDNA bands can be identified by the change in band intensities of the three DNA samples. Figure 9 shows such an analysis performed with a 5·5 kb mtDNA probe and various restriction enzymes. As expected, when the DNA is digested with *Hind*III, the 5·5 kb band increases in relative intensity from blood to liver to enriched mtDNA, indicating that it is of mitochondrial origin. The 3·6 kb band changes in the opposite direction, indicating a nuclear origin. Another way of overcoming the probem of nuclear homology to mitochondrial DNA sequences is to use as probes those regions of the

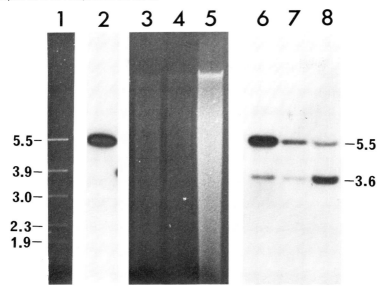

Fig. 9. The homologies within nuclear and mitochondrial DNA of a DNA fragment isolated from the mitochondrial genome of a Lesser Snow Goose. Track 1:0·2 μg of purified mtDNA was digested with *Hind*III and electrophoresed on a 1% agarose gel. When this gel is blotted and hybridized with the radioactively labelled clone of the 5·5 kb fragment, the 5·5 kb fragment shows hybridization on an autoradiograph (track 2). Tracks 3–5: DNA was isolated from a mitochondrial enriched fraction of liver (3), from liver (4) and from blood (5) and electrophoresed on a 1% agarose gel. When this gel was blotted and hybridized with the radioactively labelled clone of the 5·5 kb mitochondrial fragment, there was a relative decrease in the amount of hybridization to the 5·5 band (mitochondrial origin) and increase in hybrization to the 3·6 kb band (nuclear origin) with relatively increased proportions of nuclear DNA (moving from left to right).

mtDNA that have little or no homology with nuclear DNA. Such an approach may give a biased estimate of the average divergence between molecules, as Aquadro and Greenberg (1983) have shown that different regions of the molecule may diverge at different rates. Such a bias will be of significance when comparing molecules between studies in which different regions are analysed, but is acceptable within a study if the same regions in all molecules are inspected. In general, there is a relatively random distribution of variant sites in the mtDNA molecule (Brown and Simpson 1981, Lansman *et al.* 1983 a; but see Adams and Rothman 1982) with the exception of the D-loop region (Aquadro and Greenberg 1983) and certain blocks within the rRNA genes (Lansman *et al.* 1983 a).

When Southern blot analysis is used, difficulties may be encountered in detecting very small restriction enzyme fragments (<0.5 kb). If higher-percentage agarose gels are made with 50% formamide, fragments smaller than 300 b.p. can be clearly resolved (Sun *et al.* 1982). Very small fragments can be separated on acrylamide gels, transferred electrophoretically to nylon membrane and stabilized on the membrane by U.V. cross-linking (Church and Gilbert 1984). This allows detection of fragments in the range 26–516 b.p. using a 6% polyacrylamide gel. Such procedures will be particularly useful when restriction enzymes with 4 b.p. recognition sequences are used. In general, the Southern blot approach requires considerably more effort and expense than obtaining purified mtDNA from organs, but it does allow for simple non-destructive sampling in the field.

3.3   Analysis of mtDNA data: restriction morphs

When purified mtDNA is obtained, the products of restriction enzyme cleavage are a series of bands whose combined molecular weight should be about 16–17 kb (16·6 in Lesser Snow Goose; Figs. 8 and 9). If the Southern blot analysis is done using cloned mtDNA sequences as probes, a smaller subset of these bands is studied, corresponding to the region of mtDNA with homology to the probe DNA. Differences in the patterns between individuals result from the gain or loss of restriction enzyme recognition sites (Fig. 8). RFLPs due to major insertions or deletions have not been found in the animals studied to date, although DNA sequencing and high-resolution restriction mapping has revealed that small additions and deletions do occur (Upholt and Dawid 1977, Cann and Wilson 1983, Aquadro and Greenberg 1983, and others).

In this section, we use the term "restriction morph" as defined by Brown and Simpson (1981) to be a restriction fragment pattern produced by gel electrophoresis of mtDNA from an individual after digestion with a single restriction endonuclease. The term "composite restriction morph", following the usage of Lansman *et al.* (1983 a), is employed to mean the set of restriction fragment patterns produced by gel electrophoresis of mtDNA from an individual animal after digestion of aliquots with each of the various restriction enzymes used in a particular study. In the case of individuals sharing the same composite restriction morph, they can be considered to belong to the same mtDNA "clone" for the purposes of the study.

Several statistical procedures that estimate the nucleotide divergence among two samples or populations have been proposed, including those of Engels (1981), Nei and Tajima (1981), Upholt (1977), Templeton (1983), Kimura (1981), Kaplan and Risko (1982) and Nei and Li (1979). The most frequently cited method is that of Nei and Li (1979). Their estimation improves on that proposed by Upholt (1977) since it takes the heterogeneity of DNA sequences within populations into account; this is particularly important when the two populations compared are closely related. Nei and Li (1979) provide two approaches to the estimation of the mean minimum number of nucleotide substitutions per nucleotide site (δ) separating two populations: the "fragment" method and the "site" method. The fragment method involves pairwise comparisons of banding patterns read directly from a gel or autoradiograph. The fewer shared bands there are between two samples, the less closely related they are. This is the simplest approach in terms of the effort involved in data collection and interpretation, but can be used only where the compared populations are not very divergent, as for example with intraspecific comparisons. The site method requires mapping the locations of restriction sites along the mtDNA molecule. Comparison of shared versus unshared sites is then used to estimate differences between samples. While the site method is laborious, in some studies it is preferred because of the additional qualitative analyses which mapping allows (see below) and because of the additional information which can be gained on the nature of the substitutions that are occurring (see Lansman *et al.* 1983 a). In cases where more divergent populations are compared, the site method should be used. Both methods were used by Brown and Simpson (1981) for inter- and intraspecific comparisons of two rat species, and they obtained phenograms with the same taxonomic relationships, using both site and fragment comparisons.

3.3.1   The fragment method

In order to illustrate the analysis of data, we present the fragment method of Nei and Li (1979), using the hypothetical set of restriction morphs illustrated in Fig. 10. Two populations, A and B, are shown each to have three different mtDNA composite restriction morphs: 1, 2 and 3, and 4, 5 and 6, respectively. Although for this illustration only three restriction enzymes (each with a 6 b.p. recognition sequence) have been used to define the composite restriction morphs, in a population study it is important to use as many different restriction enzymes as possible in order to reduce the stochastic error of estimation. The frequencies of the six different composite restriction morphs in the two populations have been assigned arbitrarily. Initially, the proportion of shared bands between pairs of restriction morphs is calculated for all pairs (within and between populations), using the formula

$$\hat{F} = 2n_{xy}/(n_x + n_y)$$

where n_x and n_y represent the number of fragments in the composite

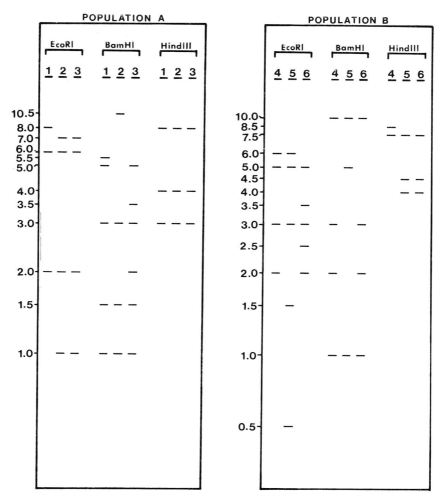

Fig. 10. A comparison of the hypothetical mtDNA restriction patterns of two populations. Using three restriction enzymes, three composite restriction morphs are defined for each of two populations (1–6). Band sizes are shown in kb. In the example (see text), it is assumed that in population A there are 35 individuals of composite restriction morph 1, 15 of morph 2, and 50 of morph 3. In population B there are 75 of morph 4, 5 of morph 5, and 20 of morph 6.

Table 1. Values of n_x, n_y and n_{xy} derived from Fig. 10. Matrix values represent n_{xy}, the number of bands common to both composite restriction morphs

							n_x	n_y
1	—							
2	8	—					$n_1 = 11$	$n_4 = 10$
							$n_2 = 11$	$n_5 = 11$
3	9	10	—				$n_3 = 13$	$n_6 = 12$
4	4	4	5	—				
5	4	3	4	6	—			
6	4	4	5	8	7	—		
	1	2	3	4	5	6		

restriction morphs x and y, respectively, and n_{xy} is the number of fragments common (in size) to both morphs. The values of n_x and n_y are given in Table 1, and the values of n_{xy} for all possible pairwise comparisons are also shown as they were derived directly from Fig. 10. Notice that in counting these numbers, the fragments from all the various enzyme digests (*Eco*R1, *Bam*H1 and *Hin*dIII) are combined for each composite restriction morph. This should be done where the enzymes used have the same number of b.p. in the recognition sequences (six in this case). If enzymes with 4 b.p. recognition sequences had been included, they would have been analysed separately. The upper-right corner of Table 2 gives the calculated $\hat{F}$ values for the pairwise comparisons.

The $\hat{F}$ values can then be used to estimate the average number of nucleotide substitutions per site ($\hat{\delta}$) for each pair. While Nei and Li (1979) provide a formula for this conversion using the "site method", they provide

Table 2. F values calculated from Table 1. F values are given in the upper-right matrix, $\hat{\delta}$ values in the lower-left

	1	2	3	4	5	6
1	—	0·73	0·75	0·38	0·36	0·35
2	0·0179	—	0·83	0·38	0·27	0·35
3	0·0163	0·0105	—	0·43	0·33	0·40
4	0·0572	0·0572	0·0496	—	0·57	0·73
5	0·0606	0·0785	0·0660	0·0325	—	0·61
6	0·0623	0·0623	0·0540	0·0179	0·0285	—

only a graph (Fig. 1 in their paper) for the conversion using the "fragment method", which was derived from the relationship

$$F = (e^{-r\delta/2})^4/(3 - 2e^{-r\delta/2})$$

where r denotes the number of base pairs in the enzyme recognition sequences ($r = 6$). It is easier to calculate $\hat{\delta}$ using Upholt's (1977) formula:

$$\hat{\delta} = 1 - [(-\hat{F} + (\hat{F}^2 + 8\hat{F})^{1/2})/2]^{1/r}$$

which gives a value identical to that of Nei and Li (1979). The conversion of $\hat{F}$ to $\hat{\delta}$ is given in Table 2.

The $\hat{\delta}$ matrix can be used to compare nucleotide differences within versus between populations. Nei and Li use the average number of nucleotide differences per site between two randomly chosen DNA sequences as an index of nucleotide diversity. Within each population $\hat{\delta}$ values are determined for all possible pairs of the different composite restriction morphs. Using these values, the mean and variance of $\hat{\delta}$ are calculated, taking the frequencies of each composite restriction morph into account. If, for example, 100 individuals from each population had been analysed, and in population A, 35 individuals were of composite restriction morph 1, 15 individuals were of composite restriction morph 2, and 50 individuals were of composite restriction morph 3, then the relative frequencies would be 0·35, 0·15 and 0·50 respectively. The average $\hat{\delta}$ value for that population ($\hat{\Pi}_A$) can be estimated from

$$\hat{\Pi}_A = \sum_{ij} A_i A_j \hat{\delta}_{ij}$$

where A_i is the frequency of the ith composite restriction morph in population A, and $\hat{\delta}$ is the number of nucleotide differences per nucleotide site between the ith and the jth composite restriction morphs (Table 2, lower-left). $\hat{\Pi}_A$ and $\hat{\Pi}_B$ are calculated in this fashion as given in Table 3. Similarly, the average $\hat{\delta}$ value between the two populations can be estimated using the formula $\Pi_{AB} = \sum_{ij} A_i B_j \hat{\delta}_{ij}$ as given in Table 4. If the sample sizes used in estimating the $\hat{\Pi}$ values are small, the final $\hat{\Pi}$ values should be multiplied by $n/(n-1)$, where n is the sample size (Nei and Tajima 1981). Finally, the net nucleotide difference between the two populations (correcting for the effects of intrapopulational variation) is given by $\hat{\delta}_{net} = \hat{\Pi}_{AB} - (\hat{\Pi}_A + \hat{\Pi}_B)/2$ as shown in Table 4. The sampling variances for these formulae can be estimated by referring to the Nei–Tajima (1981) formula [11] (also see page 153 in their paper) for within-population variance, and formula [26] for between-population variance, and formulae [25] to [28] for the $\hat{\delta}_{net}$ variance. The variance calculations are extensive and best done by computer.

The $\hat{\delta}_A$, $\hat{\delta}_B$ and $\hat{\delta}_{AB}$ values can also be compared statistically without calculating $\hat{\delta}_{net}$ by comparing the three using t-tests. If a t-test between $\hat{\delta}_A$ and

Table 3. Nucleotide diversity (Π). Calculated from Table 2

Population A

$$\hat{\Pi}_A = \sum_{ij} A_i A_j \hat{\delta}_{ij}$$

i	j	$\hat{\delta}_{ij}$	A_i	A_j	$\hat{\delta}_{ij}A_iA_j$
1	1	—	—	—	—
1	2	0·0179	0·35	0·15	0·000 94
1	3	0·0163	0·35	0·50	0·002 85
2	1	0·0179	0·15	0·35	0·000 94
2	2	—	—	—	—
2	3	0·0105	0·15	0·50	0·000 79
3	1	0·0163	0·50	0·35	0·002 85
3	2	0·0105	0·50	0·15	0·000 79
3	3	—	—	—	—
					0·009 16 = $\hat{\Pi}_A$

Population B

$$\hat{\Pi}_B = \sum_{ij} B_i B_j \hat{\delta}_{ij}$$

i	j	$\hat{\delta}_{ij}$	B_i	B_j	$\hat{\delta}_{ij}B_iB_j$
4	4	—	—	—	—
4	5	0·0325	0·75	0·05	0·001 22
4	6	0·0179	0·75	0·20	0·002 69
5	4	0·0325	0·05	0·75	0·001 22
5	5	—	—	—	—
5	6	0·0285	0·05	0·20	0·000 29
6	4	0·0179	0·20	0·75	0·002 69
6	5	0·0285	0·20	0·05	0·000 29
6	6	—	—	—	—
					0·008 40 = $\hat{\Pi}_B$

$\hat{\delta}_B$ shows no significant difference and their means and an F-test shows their variances to be similar, these two can be pooled and a t-test performed against $\hat{\delta}_{AB}$ to determine whether or not the two populations have diverged significantly. Nei and Tajima (1981) warn that their variance estimates account for sampling standard error only, and that the stochastic standard error may be quite large if a large number of restriction enzymes are not used.

If the site method is used, the proportion of shared (mapped) sites between two molecules is estimated by $\hat{S} = 2n_{xy}/(n_x + n_y)$ and from $\hat{\delta} = -(\ln \hat{S})/r$.

Table 4. $\hat{\Pi}_{AB}$ calculation

Populations A and B

$$\hat{\Pi}_{AB} = \sum_{ij} A_i B_j \hat{\delta}_{ij}$$

i	j	$\hat{\delta}_{ij}$	A_i	B_j	$\hat{\delta}_{ij} A_i B_j$
1	4	0·057 2	0·35	0·75	0·015 01
1	5	0·060 6	0·35	0·05	0·001 06
1	6	0·062 3	0·35	0·20	0·004 36
2	4	0·057 2	0·15	0·75	0·006 44
2	5	0·078 5	0·15	0·05	0·000 59
2	6	0·062 3	0·15	0·20	0·001 87
3	4	0·049 6	0·30	0·75	0·018 60
3	5	0·066 0	0·30	0·05	0·001 65
3	6	0·054 0	0·30	0·20	0·005 40

$$0·054\,98 = \hat{\Pi}_{AB}$$

Net nucleotide difference between A and B:

$$\hat{\delta}_{net} = \hat{\Pi}_{AB} - (\hat{\Pi}_A + \hat{\Pi}_B)/2$$
$$= 0·054\,98 - (0·009\,16 + 0·008\,4)/2$$
$$= 0·046\,2$$

Once the $\hat{\delta}$ value is calculated by either method, the subsequent computations (above) are similar; but refer to Nei and Tajima (1981) for the variance estimates.

The similarity matrix of $\hat{\delta}$ values (Table 2) is amenable to other sorts of analysis in addition to the averaging approach. Avise et al. (1979 a), in a study of Pocket Gopher, made such a matrix (for all sample pairs, not just the different composite restriction morphs) and subjected it to cluster analyses (following Sneath and Sokal 1973). This is especially useful in detection of genetic substructuring in species with continuous geographic distribution. Brown and Simpson (1981) used $\hat{\delta}$ matrix values to construct phenograms of taxonomic relationships between and within two species of rat.

Sequencing studies have shown that the Nei–Li (1979) model makes a reasonable prediction of the average sequence divergence between closely related mtDNAs where at least 40 restriction sites per sample are examined using several different restriction enzymes (Brown et al. 1982, Aquadro and Greenberg 1983). Avise and Lansman (1983) and Avise et al. (1983), however, point out that the high sampling variances associated with the Nei–Li model make it necessary to interpret results with caution when using numbers of restriction enzymes which are typical for such studies (5 to 10).

3.3.2 Cautions

The Nei–Li (1979) model makes some assumptions that are not upheld by "real" data, but the consequences of these violations are generally small when closely related mtDNAs are being compared. Such assumptions include the following.

(1) common restriction sites originate from one original ancestor. Intuitively, this seems realistic for closely related populations, as the likelihood of "back" mutations would be low if each mutation event occurred randomly throughout the genome. However, Lansman *et al.* (1983 a) have noted the existence of hypervariable sites which tend to mutate more frequently than other sites and switch back and forth between being "on" and "off" with respect to enzyme recognition. Since the rate of transitions is very high compared to transversion in closely related species (Lansman *et al.* 1983 a; Brown *et al.* 1982. Aquadro *et al.* 1984), such sites usually alternate between two nucleotides. Some consequences of the bias to sequencing studies are discussed by Brown *et al.* (1982). For restriction site studies, the consequences may not be as great, especially with qualitative analyses (see Lansman *et al.* 1983 a) and where the mtDNAs are closely related ($\delta < 5\%$) (Ferris *et al.* 1983). There is also strong evidence that substitutions in the coding regions occur at a relatively high rate in third-codon positions (Brown *et al.* 1982). Saturation of these sites would cause the rate of sequence divergence of distantly related mtDNAs to eventually decrease (see Fig. 5 of Ferris *et al.* 1981).

(2) Nucleotides are randomly distributed over DNA sequences with a given $G + C$ content. This assumption is also violated (Adams and Rothman 1982) but Nei and Li (1979) claim that the distribution would have to be extremely different from random to affect their model.

(3) All restriction fragments are detected. Very small fragments may not be detected. The use of restriction enzymes with four base-pair recognition sequences will accentuate the problem since on average, smaller fragments will be generated. While Lansman *et al.* (1981) recommend the use of enzymes with recognition sequences of 5 or 6 b.p., Ferris *et al.* (1981), in a study of chimpanzees found that the use of enzymes recognizing 4 b.p. sequences improved resolution. Nei and Tajima (1981) state that "the effect of elimination of small fragments is generally unimportant".

3.3.3 The mimimum-length phylogeny approach

An alternative approach to the analysis of mtDNA variation uses a qualitative comparison between restriction morphs to construct a minimum-length phylogenetic network. This has the advantage over more quantitative analyses in that information is not submerged in a single summary statistic. Avise *et al.* (1979 a,b) and Lansman *et al.* (1983 a) have used this procedure extensively on both mapped (site) and unmapped (fragment) data. A given restriction endonuclease will often generate more than one banding pattern when a number of geographically distinct samples are analysed. Avise *et al.* (1979 a,b) and Lansman *et al.* (1983 a) also assigned a unique letter designation to each pattern detected with a particular enzyme. A number of enzymes was used, so the composite restriction morph of a particular sample could be described by a series of letters, the order of which identified the enzyme each letter referred to. The various single-enzyme restriction morphs could often be related to another morph or morphs by a single or a few restriction site changes. A minimum-length phylogenetic network was built up by lining up the various morphs into a network showing the minimum number of stepwise changes required to interconvert adjacent morphs. Information on the networks generated with various enzymes was combined to generate a composite minimum-length phylogenetic network (see Lansman *et al.* 1983 a, Avise and Lansman 1983, Avise *et al.* 1983). Such a network readily depicts the phylogenetic relationships of composite restriction morphs that are inferred from the data set. Problems with convergent appearance or disappearance of certain restriction sites (see earlier discussion) in otherwise distantly related mtDNA genomes, encountered by Lansman and Avise in constructing their networks could usually be resolved. Templeton (1983) has proposed a method for the construction of phylogenetic trees from restriction maps which explicitly takes the possibility of convergent evolution into account. His model also accounts for the non-random distribution of restriction sites shown by Adams and Rothman (1982) and provides non-parametric statistical tests to choose the best fit between different hypothesized phylogenies.

3.3.4   Cautions

An area of major concern affecting studies using mtDNA polymorphisms to infer phylogenetic relationships is the interspecific transfer of mtDNA in hybrid zones. Such transfers have been noted to occur between species within the genera *Drosophila* (Powell 1983), *Mus* (Ferris *et al.* 1983) and *Rana* (Spolsky and Uzzell 1984). In all of these cases, individuals of one of the two species involved were found to possess a mtDNA restriction morph more closely resembling the mtDNA of the other species than that of other intraspecific individuals further away from the zones of hybridization. Such introgression of mtDNA into a population can occur in the absence of detectable nuclear DNA introgression and is crucial to an assessment of mtDNA studies for phylogenetic studies. The studies mentioned were specifically carried out near well-studied hybrid zones. The risks of such events depends on the location of the study and on the history of the species being studied. Avise and Saunders (1984) found no evidence of introgression of mtDNA into parent populations of Sunfish (*Lepomis*) even though much opportunity for hybridization exists. While F_1 individuals could be found, they were of low fertility. As previously mentioned, a mtDNA study of Anatidae by Kessler and Avise (1984) generated phylogenies that conformed closely to those derived from protein electrophoretic and classical systematic methods. Such agreement suggests that, at least for the two taxa studied, such interspecific mtDNA transfer has not been common.

3.4 Opportunities for mtDNA analysis

From the few population comparisons to date it appears that mtDNA analysis will provide a powerful tool for evolutionary biologists in the study of genetic structuring and phylogenetic relationships within species and between closely related species. Such studies will "provide otherwise inaccessible information on complex evolutionary histories of closely related species" (Spolsky and Uzzell 1984). Intraspecific mtDNA variation is present in Aves, as preliminary investigations have uncovered variation in mtDNA enzyme restriction sites of some pheasants and turkeys (Glaus *et al.* 1980), in sparrows (S. Cole, 1984, personal communication), and in geese (T. Quinn, F. Cooke and B. N. White, unpublished work), and in some species of *Anas* and *Aythya* (Kessler and Avise 1984). Ornithology stands to gain from these new techniques, especially for those species in which females are philopatric. If, as for mammals, intraspecific assemblages of restriction morphs exist (for colonial breeders assemblages could represent colonies) it should be possible to characterize each assemblage, and subsequently identify the natal origins of captured birds by their mtDNA composite restriction morphs. The implications of this for migratory studies would be profound. Similarly, the maternal natal origins of the founding members of recently established colonial breeders could be determined. In addition to studies of bird movement and migration, studies of gene flow and genetic differentiation can now be made at a higher level of resolution than has been possible previously. As a result of the maternal inheritance and lack of recombination, variants between different clones are not mixed during subsequent generations as they are between allozymic and nuclear DNA variants. In effect, new mutations in mtDNA provide molecular "tags" which are preserved over generations and can be used to trace maternal phylogenetic relationships intraspecifically or interspecifically where species are closely related.

REFERENCES

Adams, J. and Rothman, E. D. (1982). Estimation of phylogenetic relationships from DNA restriction patterns and selection of endonuclease cleavage sites. *Proc. Natl Acad. Sci. USA* **79**, 3560–3564.

Aquadro, C. F. and Greenberg, B. D. (1983). Human mitochondrial DNA variation and evolution: Analysis of nucleotide sequences from seven individuals. *Genetics* **103**, 287–312.

Aquadro, C. F., Kaplan, N. and Risko, K. J. (1984). An analysis of the dynamics of mammalian mitochondrial DNA sequence evolution. *Molec. Biol. Evol.* **1**, 423–434.

Arthur, R. R. and Straus, N. A. (1978). DNA-sequence organization in the genome of the domestic chicken (*Gallus domesticus*). *Can. J. Biochem.* **56**, 257–263.

Avise, J. C., Giblin-Davidson, C., Laerm, J., Patton, J. C. and Lansman, R. A. (1979 a). Mitochondrial DNA clones and matriarchal phylogeny within and among geographic populations of the pocket gopher, *Geomys pinetis*. *Proc. Natl Acad. Sci. USA* **76**, 6694–6698.

Avise, J. C., Lansman, R. A. and Shade, R. O. (1979 b). The use of restriction endonucleases to measure mitochondrial DNA sequence relatedness in natural populations. I. Population structure and evolution in the genus *Peromyscus*. *Genetics* **92**, 279–295.

Avise, J. C. and Lansman, R. A. (1983). Polymorphism of mitochondrial DNA in populations of higher animals. *In* "Evolution of Genes and Proteins" (eds M. Nei and R. K. Koehn), pp. 147–164. Sinauer Associates Inc. Massachusetts.

Avise, J. C. and Saunders, N. C. (1984). Hybridization and introgression among species of sunfish (*Lepomis*): Analysis by mitochondrial DNA and allozyme markers. *Genetics* **108**, 237–255.

Avise, J. C., Shapira, J. F., Daniel, S. W., Aquadro, C. F. and Lansman, R. A. (1983). Mitochondrial DNA differentiation during the speciation process in *Persomyscus*. *Molec. Biol. Evol.* **1**, 38–56.

Bachmann, K., Harrington, B. A. and Craig, J. P. (1972). Genome size in birds. *Chromosoma* **37**, 405–416.

Bangti, Z., Hongji, X., Shuyi, M., Lingyuan, L. and Tong, S. (1983). Restriction endonuclease cleavage map of mitochondrial DNA from Peking Duck liver. *Scientia Sinica* **26**, 1143–1154.

Barker, D., Schafer, M. and White, R. (1984). Restriction sites containing CpG show a higher frequency of polymorphism in human DNA. *Cell* **36**, 131–138.

Bargiello, T. A., Grossfield, J., Steele, R. W. and Cooke, F. (1977). Isoenzyme status and genetic variability of serum esterases in the Lesser Snow Goose, *Anser caerulescens caerulescens*. *Biochem. Genet.* **15**, 741–763.

Barrowclough, G. F. (1983). Biochemical studies of microevolutionary processes. *In* "Perspectives in Ornithology" (eds A. H. Brush and G. A. Clark, Jr.), pp. 223–261. Cambridge University Press, New York.

Bastié-Sigeac, F. and Lucotte, G. (1983). Optimal use of restriction enzymes in the analysis of human DNA polymorphism. *Human Genet.* **63**, 162–165.

Benton, W. D. and Davis, R. W. (1977). Screening λgt recombinant clones by hybridization to single plaques *in situ*. *Science* **196**, 180–182.

Bonner, T. I., Brenner, D. J., Neufeld, B. R. and Britten, R. J. (1973). Reduction in the rate of DNA reassociation by sequence divergence. *J. Molec. Biol.* **81**, 123–135.

Britten, R. J., Cetta, A. and Davidson, E. H. (1978). The single-copy DNA sequence polymorphism of the sea urchin *Strongylocentrotus purpuratus*. *Cell* **15**, 1175–1186.

Britten, R. J. and Kohne, D. E. (1968). Repeated sequences in DNA. *Science* **161**, 529–540.

Brown, W. M., Prager, E. M., Wang, A. and Wilson, A. C. (1982). Mitochondrial DNA sequences of primates: tempo and mode of evolution. *J. Molec. Evol.* **18**, 225–239.

Brown, G. G. and Simpson, M. V. (1981). Intra- and interspecific variation of the mitochondrial genome in *Rattus norvegicus* and *Rattus rattus*: Restriction enzymes analysis of variant mitochondrial DNA molecules and their evolutionary relationships. *Genetics* **97**, 125–143.

Cann, R. L. and Wilson, A. C. (1983). Length mutations in human mitochondrial DNA. *Genetics* **104**, 699–711.

Church, G. M. and Gilbert, W. (1984). Genomic Sequencing. *Proc. Natl Acad. Sci. USA* **81**, 1991–1995.

Corbin, K. W. (1983). Genetic structure and avian systematics. *In* "Current Ornithology" (ed. R. F. Johnston), Vol. 1, pp. 211–244. Plenum Press, New York.

De Francesco, L., Attardi, G. and Croce, C. M. (1980). Uniparental propagation of mitochondrial DNA in mouse-human cell hybrids. *Proc. Natl Acad. Sci. USA* **77**, 4079–4083.

Eden, F. C. and Hendrick, J. P. (1978). Unusual organisation of DNA sequences in the chicken. *Biochemistry* **17**, 5838–5844.

Efstratiadis, A., Posakony, J. W., Maniatis, T., Lawn, R. M., O'Connell, C., Spritz, R. A., DeRiel, J. K., Forget, B. G., Weissman, S. M., Slightom, J. L., Blechl, A. F., Smithies, O., Baralle, F. E., Shoulders, C. C. and Proudfoot, N. J. (1980). The structure and evolution of the human β-globin gene family. *Cell* **21**, 653–668.

Engels, W. R. (1981). Estimating genetic divergence and genetic variability with restriction endonucleases. *Proc. Natl Acad. Sci. USA* **78**, 6329–6333.

Epplen, J. T., Leipoldt, M., Engel, W. and Schmidtke, J. (1978). DNA sequence organisation in avian genomes. *Chromosoma* **69**, 307–321.

Farrelly, F. and Butow, R. A. (1983). Rearranged mitochondrial genes in the yeast nuclear genome. *Nature* **301**, 296–301.

Feinberg, A. P. and Vogelstein, B. (1983). A technique for radiolabeling DNA restriction endonuclease fragments to high specific activity. *Anal. Biochem.* **132**, 6–13.

Ferris, S. D., Brown, W. M., Davidson, W. S. and Wilson, A. C. (1981). Extensive polymorphism in the mitochondrial DNA of apes. *Proc. Natl Acad. Sci. USA* **78**, 6319–6323.

Ferris, S. D., Sage, R. D. Huang, C., Nielsen, J. T., Ritte, U. and Wilson, A. C. (1983). Flow of mitochondrial DNA across a species boundary. *Proc. Natl Acad. Sci. USA* **80**, 2290–2294.

Gellissen, G., Bradfield, J. Y., White, B. N. and Wyatt, G. R. (1983). Mitochondrial DNA sequences in the nuclear genome of a locust. *Nature* **301**, 631–634.

Glaus, K. R., Zassenhaus, H. P., Fechheimer, N. S. and Perlman, P. S. (1980). Avian mtDNA: structure, organization and evolution. *In* "The Organization and Expression of the Mitochondrial Genome" (eds A. M. Kroon and C. Saccone), pp. 131–135. Elsevier/North-Holland Biomedical Press, Amsterdam.

Harrison, R. G., Rand, D. M. and Wheeler, W. C. (1985). Mitochondrial DNA size variation within individual crickets. *Science* **228**, 1446–1448.

Hauswirth, W. W. and Laipis, P. J. (1982). Mitochondrial DNA polymorphism in a maternal lineage of Holstein cows. *Proc. Natl Acad. Sci. USA* **79**, 4686–4690.

Hayashi, J.-I., Yonekawa, H., Gotoh, O., Tagashira, Y., Moriwak, K. and Yosida, T. H. (1979). Evolutionary aspects of variant types of rat mitochondrial DNAs. *Biochim. Biophys. Acta* **564**, 202–211.

Helm-Bychowski, K. M. and Wilson, A. C. (1986). Rates of nuclear DNA evolution in pheasant-like birds: Evidence from restriction maps. *Proc. Natl Acad. Sci. USA* **83**, 688–692.

Jacobs, H. T., Posakony, J. W., Grula, J. W., Roberts, J. W., Xin, J. H., Britten, R. J. and Davidson, E. H. (1983). Mitochondrial DNA sequences in the nuclear genome of *Strongylocentrotus purpuratus. J. Molec. Biol.* **165**, 609–632.

Jeffreys, A. J., Brookfield, J. F. Y. and Semenoff, R. (1985 c). Positive identification of an immigration test-case using human DNA fingerprints. *Nature* **317**, 818–819.

Jeffreys, A. J., Wilson, V. and Thein, S. L. (1985 a). Hypervariable "minisatellite" regions in human DNA. *Nature* **314**, 67–73.

Jeffreys, A. J., Wilson, V. and Thein, S. L. (1985 b). Individual-specific "fingerprints" of human DNA. *Nature* **316**, 76–79.

Kaplan, N. and Risko, K. (1982). A method for estimating rates of nucleotide substitution using DNA sequence data. *Theor. Pop. Biol.* **21**, 318–328.

Kemble, R. J., Mans, R. J., Gabay-Laughnan, S. and Laughnan, J. R. (1983). Sequences homologous to episomal mitochondrial DNAs in the maize nuclear genome. *Nature* **304**, 744–747.

Kessler, L. G. and Avise, J. C. (1984). Systematic relationships among waterfowl (Anatidae) inferred from restriction endonuclease analysis of mitochondrial DNA. *Syst. Zool.* **33**, 370–380.

Kessler, L. G. and Avise, J. C. (1985). A comparative description of mitochondrial DNA differentiation in selected avian and other vertebrate genera. *Molec. Biol. Evol.* **2**, 109–125.

Kimura, M. (1981). Estimation of evolutionary distances between homologous nucleotide sequences. *Proc. Natl Acad. Sci. USA* **78**, 454–458.

Lai, E. C., Woo, S. L. C., Dugaiczyk, A., Catterall, J. F. and O'Malley, B. W. (1978). The ovalbumin gene: Structural sequences in native chicken DNA are not contiguous. *Proc. Natl Acad. Sci. USA* **75**, 2205–2209.

Lansman, R. A., Avise, J. C., Aquadro, C. F., Shapira, J. F. and Daniel, S. W. (1983 a). Extensive genetic variation in mitochondrial DNAs among geographical populations of the deermouse, *Peromyscus maniculatus. Evolution* **37**, 1–16.

Lansman, R. A., Avise, J. C. and Huettel, M. D. (1983 b). Critical experimental test of the possibility of "paternal leakage" of mitochondrial DNA. *Proc. Natl Acad. Sci. USA* **80**, 1969–1971.

Lansman, R. A., Shade, R. O., Shapira, J. F. and Avise, J. C. (1981). The use of restriction endonucleases to measure mitochondrial DNA sequence relatedness in natural populations. III: Techniques and potential applications. *J. Molec. Evol.* **17**, 214–226.

Maniatis, T., Fritsch, E. F. and Sambrook, J. (1982). "Molecular Cloning. A Laboratory Manual." Cold Spring Harbor Publications, New York.

Maniatis, T., Hardison, R. C., Lacy, E., Lauer, J., O'Connell, C., Quon, D., Sim, G. K. and Efstratiadis, A. (1978). The isolation of structural genes from libraries of eukaryotic DNA. *Cell* **15**, 687–701.

Nei, M. (1972). Genetic distance between populations. *Am. Natur.* **106**, 283–292.

Nei, M. and Li, W. (1979). Mathematical model for studying genetic variation in terms of restriction endonucleases. *Proc. Natl Acad. Sci. USA* **76**, 5269–5273.

Nei, M. and Tajima, F. (1981). DNA polymorphism detectable by restriction endonucleases. *Genetics* **97**, 145–163.

Perler, F., Efstratiadis, A., Lomedico, P., Gilbert, W., Kolodner, R. and Dodgson, J. (1980). The evolution of genes: the chicken preproinsulin gene. *Cell* **20**, 555–566.

Powell, J. R. (1983). Interspecific cytoplasmic gene flow in the absence of nuclear gene flow: evidence from *Drosophila. Proc. Natl Acad. Sci. USA* **80**, 492–495.

Quinn, T. W. and White, B. N. (1987). Identification of restriction fragment length polymorphisms in genomic DNA of the lesser snow goose. *Molec. Biol. Evol.* **4**, 126–143.

Quinn, T. W., Quinn, J. S., Cooke, F. and White, B. N. (1987). DNA marker analysis detects multiple maternity and paternity in single broods of the Lesser Snow Goose (*Anser caerulescens caerulescens*). *Nature* (in press).

Rigby, P. W. J., Dieckmann, M., Rhodes, C. and Berg, P. (1977). Labeling deoxyribonucleic acid to high specific activity *in vitro* by nick translation with DNA polymerase I. *J. Molec. Biol.* **113**, 237–251.

Rogers, J. S. (1972). "Measures of Genetic Similarity and Genetic Distance". Univ. Texas Publ. No. 7213, pp. 145–153.

Sherman, P. W. (1981). Electrophoresis and avian genealogical analyses. *Auk* **98**, 419–422.

Shields, G. F. (1983). Organization of the avian genome. *In* "Perspectives in Ornithology". (eds A. H. Brush and G. A. Clark, Jr.), pp. 271–290. Cambridge University Press.

Shields, G. F. and Straus, N. A. (1975). DNA–DNA hybridization studies of birds. *Evolution* **29**, 159–166.

Shields, G. F. and Wilson, A. C. (1987). Subspecies of Canada Goose (*Branta canadensis*) have distinct mitochondrial DNAs. *Evolution* (in press).

Sibley, C. G. and Ahlquist, J. E. (1983). Phylogeny and classification of birds based on the data of DNA–DNA hybridization. *In* "Current Ornithology" (ed. R. F. Johnston), Vol. 1, pp. 245–292. Plenum Press, New York.

Skolnick, M. H. and White, R. (1982). Strategies for detecting and characterizing resitriction fragment length polymorphisms (RFLP's). *Cytogenet. Cell Genet*, **32**, 58–67.

Skolnick, M. H., Willard, H. F. and Menlove, L. A. (1984). Report of the committee on human gene mapping by recombinant DNA techniques. *In* "Human Gene Mapping 7: Seventh International Workshop on Human Gene Mapping". *Cytogenet. Cell Genet.* **37**, 210–273.

Sneath, P. H. A. and Sokal, R. R. (1973). "Numerical Taxonomy". W. H. Freeman, San Francisco.

Southern, E. M. (1975). Detection of specific sequences among DNA fragments separated by gel electrophoresis. *J. Molec. Biol.* **98**, 503–517.

Spolsky, C. and Uzzell, T. (1984). Natural interspecies transfer of mitochondrial DNA in amphibians. *Proc. Natl Acad. Sci. USA* **81**, 5802–5805.

Sun, Y. L., Xu, Y. Z. and Chambon, P. (1982). A simple and efficient method for the separation and detection of small DNA fragments by electrophoresis in formamide containing agarose gels and Southern blotting to DBM-paper. *Nucleic Acids Res.* **10**, 5753–5763.

Swanstrom, R. and Shank, P. R. (1978). X-ray intensifying screens greatly enhance the detection by autoradiography of the radioactive isotopes ^{32}P and ^{125}I. *Anal. Biochem.* **86**, 184–192.

Templeton, A. R. (1983). Phylogenetic inference from restriction endonuclease cleavage site maps with particular reference to the evolution of humans and the apes. *Evolution* **37**, 221–244.

Upholt, W. B. (1977). Estimation of DNA sequence divergence from comparison of restriction endonuclease digests. *Nucleic Acids Res.* **4**, 1257–1265.

Upholt, W. B. and Dawid, I. B. (1977). Mapping of mitochondrial DNA of individual sheep and goats: rapid evolution in the D loop region. *Cell* **11**, 571–583.

Van den Boogaart, P., Samallo, J. and Agsteribbe, E. (1982). Similar genes for a mitochondrial ATPase subunit in the nuclear and mitochondrial genomes of *Neurospora crassa*. *Nature* **298**, 187–189.

Wright, R. M. and Cummings, D. J. (1983). Integration of mitochondrial gene sequences within the nuclear genome during senescence in a fungus. *Nature* **302**, 86–88.

Synthesis I—Assaying Genetic Variation

F. COOKE

The preceding five chapters have shown us both the diversity of ways in which genetic variation can be studied in natural populations, and how much genetic variability exists in most such populations. Whereas ornithologists in the past, particularly systematists, have emphasized variation between species or geographic entities below the species level, geneticists investigate variation within as well as between populations. Moreover, they have the techniques for partitioning such variation into its genetic and non-genetic components and, in so doing, can draw our attention to that variation of evolutionary significance.

In this book we have concentrated on intrapopulation variation although we have by no means neglected interpopulation differences and similarities. Some genetic techniques such as allozyme and recombinant DNA analyses are useful for exploring both inter- and intrapopulation variation; others such as DNA–DNA hybridization are useful mainly for between-species comparisons, while yet others such as the partitioning of variance used to measure heritability can only be used at the intrapopulation level. By stressing intraspecific variation in this book, we may have given insufficient credit to the role played by genetic techniques in avian systematics, particularly the pioneering work by Sibley and his associates, but our major aim has been to collect into one volume the techniques available to investigate genetic variation below the species level, and to document what has been discovered about birds from such techniques.

Some of the techniques for studying genetic variation have been available to us since the early years of this century, and even earlier. The theoretical basis for quantitative variation analysis was established by Francis Galton before the rediscovery of Mendel's laws, as Boag and van Noordwijk point out in chapter 2. Other techniques however are more recent and have arisen largely from the amazing advances that have come from molecular genetics. The realization that variation in the gene products, usually enzymes, could be used to examine underlying genetic variation, led to a burst of research activity in the 1960s and 1970s. The study of allozyme variation caused biologists to realize that genetic variation in natural populations was much more widespread than evolutionary theory had originally predicted. Peter

Evans, in chapter 4, documents the ways in which allozyme variation can be investigated. He points out, however, that few studies have confirmed that the variability of the gene product actually reflects the variability of the underlying gene itself. Post-translational changes can occasionally modify a gene product and lead the researcher to conclude that allelic differences occur when differences lie only in the gene products. Breeding studies are needed to confirm that the phenotypic patterns shown by electrophoresis reflect an underlying genetic variation. Conclusions about genetic variation, based upon allozymic studies, must always be treated with a little caution.

The more recent methodology described by Quinn and White overcomes this difficulty. Recombinant DNA techniques allow the direct examination of DNA itself. In this case the gene, rather than gene product, is being investigated for variation. As they point out, much of the genetic variation may be associated with non-coding regions of the genetic material and thus has no impact on the phenotypic expression of variability, nor is it subject to natural selection, which acts at the level of the gene product. Nevertheless, for inter- and intrapopulation studies, the technique for examining nuclear DNA, once mastered, offers several advantages over that involved in uncovering allozymic variation. First, the technique leaves no doubt that there is variability of the DNA itself. Second, it is not restricted to those parts of the genome with chemically detectable gene products. As such, it provides a more obviously random sample of the genome for investigating such questions as "how much polymorphism and heterozygosity is present in the population?" Third, it appears from early studies to yield more regions of variability and more alleles per locus. Fourth, in birds at least, DNA obtained from the nucleated erythrocytes appears to be more stable than many enzyme preparations. On the negative side, it is a more expensive and elaborate technique, which may take considerable investment of time and money to set up.

Despite these exciting new techniques, there have been many new developments in some of the older and more traditional ones. Shields, in chapter 3, documents the value of using various staining methods that highlight the banding patterns of chromosomes. This not only allows the identification of homologous chromosomes but allows chromosomal rearrangements to be detected. In this way inter- and intrapopulation chromosomal variability can be detected although, as yet, surprisingly few studies have been reported which investigate this type of variability.

The striking, and so far unique, avian chromosomal and plumage polymorphism in White-throated Sparrow discussed by Buckley in chapter 1 and by Shields in chapter 3 demands further study. Maintained by one of the few proven examples of disassortative mating in birds, it would profit by examination of morph mate-choices, of gene frequencies, of inbreeding and outbreeding rates, to name but a few topics now receiving the attention of theoretical population geneticists. This sparrow should prove to be a particularly amenable experimental subject—one easily raised in captivity.

Perhaps there have been few theoretical advances when it comes to heritability studies, but Boag and Price show that it is only recently that ornithologists have applied the techniques of quantitative genetics to field studies of wild populations of birds. Traditionally, heritability measures have been used mainly when environmental conditions can be carefully controlled, which of course does not apply to wild populations in the field. However, even though some of the assumptions of the theory do not strictly apply, population biologists are turning increasingly to these techniques to investigate quantitative phenotypic characters of potential evolutionary importance.

But what have the various techniques described in the previous five chapters told us about the genetics of birds? In many cases it is still too early to make generalizations. As several authors indicate, there is still much research to be carried out. Inheritance of colours or patterns in most normal and abnormal plumages is known in only a handful of cases. Sixty-one families of birds are as yet uninvestigated in terms of chromosomes, so the analysis of chromosomal evolution remains very tentative. Although recombinant DNA technology offers much promise, it is too early to say how valuable it will be for avian studies.

Nonetheless, genetic investigations have added much to our understanding of birds. The work of Sibley and associates has given us a much clearer picture of the evolutionary relationships in the class Aves. F_{ST} values have revealed that, in general, there is less genetic differentiation among birds than among other classes of vertebrates, suggesting perhaps a more recent evolutionary divergence of the group or a slower rate of evolutionary change. Here again, recombinant DNA techniques may help us clarify this issue, but only after many more species have been examined.

From chromosomal studies, we see that birds have two unusual features: heterogametic females and microchromosomes. It is difficult to point to any obvious functional explanation for these, but they do suggest that the class Aves has a unique and monophyletic evolutionary history. Quinn and White point out in their chapter that the organization of DNA in birds is generally quite different from that of mammals in having less repeated DNA and longer stretches of unique DNA. Whether this is typical of birds or is a generalization based on too small a sample size remains to be seen. From a practical point of view, this feature makes it easier to detect genetic variation in birds.

At the intrapopulation and intraspecific levels, it is surprising that no bird population has been investigated by all the techniques described in the previous chapters. There is no avian equivalent to *Drosophila melanogaster*. Birds, however, are not the ideal group for the geneticist interested in genetic mechanisms themselves. Genetic studies of birds are valuable, as Buckley points out in chapter 1, to build upon and to clarify the detailed ecological and behavioural studies which can be carried out on wild populations of birds. If evolutionary conclusions are to be drawn from such studies, it is essential that as much as possible be known about the genetic architecture of the populations. In view of this, it is a little disappointing that so few genetic studies have been carried out on bird species whose ecology and behaviour are well known.

One of the main generalizations which can be made from genetic studies of wild populations of birds is that genetic variability is widespread if not universal. All the different techniques suggest that, as with other groups of organisms, populations of birds contain a wide store of genetic variation on which natural selection could act. This applied not only to characters which may be neutral, but also to those such as clutch size which may be assumed to be subject to selection. One of the challenges to the evolutionary biologist is to explain why so much genetic variability remains in wild populations in the face of genetic drift, normalizing and stabilizing selection.

Buckley points out in chapter 1 that documented changes in gene frequency due to selection are relatively rare. In terms of the conspicuous polymorphisms that he discusses, in those cases where the genetic bases for the polymorphism are established, there is one case (Snow Goose) where gene frequency change occurs, but no evidence that the change is due to selection, and one case (Arctic Skua) where there is evidence of selection but no evidence of gene frequency change. He also points out that, despite widespread interest among ornithologists in plumage polymorphisms, evidence of the genetic basis for most of these is sadly lacking.

There are cases of selection in action from both allozyme studies and from quantitative genetics but, as in the case of plumage polymorphisms, these are infrequent in the literature. Again, the pattern which emerges is that populations of birds do not change much in their genetic composition over short periods of time, but the long-term studies necessary to document this have just not been carried out.

Genetic variation in space within species is also less than it is among other well-studied groups of organisms. Although the genetic variability within populations is relatively high according to allozyme studies, there is less differentiation among populations intraspecifically. This may simply reflect the greater vagility of birds with their high rates of dispersal and consequent potential for gene flow. It must be remembered, however, that these generalizations have emerged from studies of allozymic variation and, in one interesting study, Zink (1982) who examined variation in Fox Sparrows

(*Passerella iliaca*) showed that, whereas morphological variation conformed to geographic variation, allozymic variation did not.

Evans, and Quinn and White, point out an important use of genetic techniques for sociobiological studies. Often, the only way to discover the parentage of certain types of offspring is through genetic analysis. This is important in studies of mating systems, particularly cases where multiple mating or parentage is suspected. The use of genetic markers to investigate cases of disputed parentage is well known in man but is equally valuable in avian biology.

Mumme *et al.* (1985) have used allozyme variants to investigate paternity in Acorn Woodpeckers (*Melanerpes formicivorus*). The small number of usable gametic variants among allozymes restricts the usefulness of this technique, however, and the greater genetic variability which has been discovered at the level of nuclear DNA offers much more promise of success. Quinn's discovery of a segment of DNA in Snow Geese with at least six different variants is most encouraging.

Another biological phenomenon in birds that could be studied using these techniques is intraspecific nest parasitism or "dumping". Occasionally, two or more females lay eggs in the same nest; the maternal origins of such eggs could be examined (Quinn *et al.* 1987). In this case, in addition to allozyme and nuclear DNA variants, mitochondrial DNA variants may also be useful since mitochondria are transmitted matrilineally. Early evidence for birds, however, suggests that mitochondrial DNA is much less variable than nuclear DNA.

Just a few of the interesting general features mentioned in the first five chapters of this book have been covered. We have shown how genetic variation can be examined and have documented evidence for the patterns of variation found in birds. In the next five chapters, we consider the various ways in which genetic material is moulded by biological processes. We deal with stochastic processes such as genetic drift, as well as potentially directional processes such as selection and gene flow. We show how the behaviour of birds in their choice of mates can influence the genetic composition of a population. Although, as in the first section, we concentrate on intrapopulation effects, we also examine the consequences of these processes at an interpopulation level.

It is important to keep in mind that in natural populations all the various phenomena described in the following chapters may be occurring contemporaneously. A population may not be changing only in gene frequencies because of selection, but individuals may be entering or leaving the population, allowing for the possibility of gene flow. Members of the population may not be choosing their mates randomly and, in fact, are most likely not doing so. In addition, various stochastic processes will inevitably be occurring. Thus, in the real world, it becomes extremely difficult to disentangle all the various factors that modify gene frequencies. It is only in the relatively structured world of the book that we can focus on one phenomenon at a time.

REFERENCES

Mumme, R. L., Koenig, W. D., Zink, R. M. and Marten, J. A. (1985). Genetic variation and parentage in a California population of Acorn Woodpeckers. *Auk* **102**, 305–312.
Quinn, T. W., Quinn, J. S., Cooke, F. and White, B. N. (1987). DNA marker analysis detects multiple maternity and paternity in single broods of the Lesser Snow Goose, *Nature* **327**, 392–394.
Zink, R. M. (1982). Patterns of genic and morphologic variation among sparrows in the genera *Zonotrichia, Melospiza, Junco* and *Passerella. Auk* **99**, 632–649.

Part II

Moulding Genetic Variation

6

Inbreeding, Philopatry and Optimal Outbreeding in Birds

Paul J. Greenwood

Department of Adult and Continuing Education, University of Durham, Durham DH1 3JB, UK

1   INTRODUCTION

Individuals of many species of animals breed close to their birth site. Subsequently they may retain that breeding locality for the rest of their lives. Such philopatry is a feature of probably the majority of both migratory and resident birds (Baker 1978, Greenwood 1980, Greenwood and Harvey 1982).

AVIAN GENETICS
ISBN 0-12-187570-9

The term philopatry is not, as is sometimes assumed, a bastard term from the Latin for "father" and the Greek for "faithful". It is purely a Greek derivation meaning faithfulness to a homeland or country. It was probably first used in a biological context by Mayr (1963) who defined it as "the drive (tendency) of an individual to return to (or stay in) its home area (birthplace or adopted locality)." More recently, Shields (1982, 1983) has suggested that species should be described as philopatric if the median value of dispersal of the most dispersive group of individuals (usually young females in birds) is less than 10 territories (or equivalent spatial dispersion) from the natal area. Clearly this is a specialized definition so that, for the moment, philopatry should be regarded only as a qualitative and not as a quantitative term with any specific genetic connotations. Nevertheless, philopatry does have important genetic implications, most noticeably the likelihood that it will increase the probability of interactions between related individuals, including that of inbreeding. It is the purpose of this chapter to review the relationship between inbreeding and philopatry and to examine the effects of both on birds.

One of the perennial problems in evolutionary biology is to disentangle cause from effect. The potential difficulties that can arise in terms of the links between philopatry and inbreeding are dealt with in the first section of the chapter when discussing the three general models for the evolution of philopatry. The middle section of this review is concerned with the difficulties in measuring the frequency of inbreeding and the genetic and reproductive consequence of inbreeding in wild and laboratory populations. The final part of the chapter is concerned with the question of whether or not there is any causal link between inbreeding avoidance and dispersal, and then with the concept of optimal outbreeding. This motion suggests that in order to maximize fitness, an individual will preferentially avoid mating with others that are not only too closely related but also members of the same species which are too distantly related.

2   AVIAN PATTERNS OF DISPERSAL

2.1   Nomadism and sexual differences in dispersal

The level of inbreeding within a population will be influenced to a large extent by the overall pattern of effective dispersal. For example, nomadic species of birds respond periodically to major fluctuations in food availability (Nutcrackers, Crossbills, Sandgrouse). All age and sex categories within a species are usually highly dispersive. There may be limited potential for close inbreeding unless the population integrity of groups is maintained during the dispersal phase. Similarly, amongst the Anatidae the degree of dispersal of both young and adults males are high. For example, in Lesser Snow Goose (*Anser caerulescens*), the male returns to the female's colony of birth to breed (Cooke *et al.* 1975). Such extensive movements coupled with winter-ground pair formation may preclude the possibility of other than exceptionally rare cases of inbreeding.

2.2 Philopatry

Amongst the philopatric species there are a number of different types of dispersal. It is probably a feature of all such species that adults are much more faithful to a breeding territory or colony than young birds seeking their first opportunity to breed. In many cases the majority of adults will re-occupy or retain their previous year's site. When dispersal of breeders does occur, usually as a result of a poor reproductive performance or a loss or divorce of mate (e.g. Eurasian Sparrowhawk, *Accipiter nisus* (Newton and Marquiss 1982); Semipalmated Sandpiper, *Calidris pusilla* (Gratto *et al.* 1985), it is often to an area in the vicinity. Natal dispersal, on the other hand, is more widespread although a median dispersal of less than 10 territories from the birth site, and often considerably less, may be characteristic of many species of birds (see Shields 1982).

2.3 Communal breeding

Some of the most extreme cases of philopatry occur amongst the cooperatively breeding species (e.g. Florida Scrub Jay, *Aphelocoma caerulescens*). Established breeders usually remain on one territory throughout their life. Young males either inherit the natal territory from their father or sequester a portion of it. Young females usually leave their natal group and join one which is normally close-by (Woolfenden and Fitzpatrick 1978). It is in these socially structured species where the potential for close inbreeding is probably the greatest.

3   CONCEPTUAL MODELS OF THE EVOLUTION OF PHILOPATRY

3.1   Ecological

There are a number of models for the evolution of philopatry. They fall broadly into three groups: ecological, eco-genetic and genetic (Shields 1982).

Ecological explanations emphasize either the somatic advantages of staying at home or the somatic costs of dispersal. Animals that disperse may increase their risk of mortality from predation or food shortage. Those that stay at home may have the advantage of familiarity with local food supplies and potential predators and may be more successful at obtaining a territory in their natal area than elsewhere. Under these circumstances any genetic differentiation of populations would initially be a consequence of philopatry and not a cause. Despite the fact that ecological hypotheses have been proposed many times over the years (e.g. Burt 1940, Lack 1954, Hinde 1956, Baker 1978) we still do not know their relative importance in promoting philopatry in birds because the survivorship or reproductive consequences of dispersal have rarely been measured.

3.2 Eco-genetic

The eco-genetic models provide explanations for philopatry based on the spatial heterogeneity of the environment. If ecological conditions vary across the geographical range of a species then those individuals better adapted to their local area will be selected for. It would also be advantageous for their offspring to settle and breed with similar individuals in the vicinity because elsewhere, under different environmental conditions, a different genotype might be selectively favoured. This will be the case in coarse-grained environments where separate patches have different selective properties (Levins 1968). The eco-genetic models for philopatry are the ones most favoured by biologists both on theoretical and empirical grounds (Fisher 1930, Mayr 1963, Dobzhansky 1970, Ford 1964, Wilson 1975). As populations differentiate genetically in response to variation in ecological conditions, there may be additional effects on philopatry if the genotypes of different populations become incompatible. In other words, positive assortative mating by genotype (Shields 1983, Bateson 1983) should be selected for and lead to increased philopatry and reduced gene flow between populations.

3.3 Genetic

Recently a third, qualitative genetic model has been proposed by Shields (1982, 1983). He draws attention to the fact that the highest levels of philopatry often occur in species apparently living in spatially homogeneous environments, where on theoretical grounds we might expect widespread dispersal (Levins 1968). One example he puts forward is Laysan Albatross

(*Diomedea immutabilis*) which breeds in colonies on a series of extremely similar islands in the Pacific. Birds do not begin breeding until they are eight or nine years old, and there appears to be no shortage of nest sites. Nonetheless, males breeding for the first time nest on average only 19 m from their birth site, and females 24 m (Fisher 1976). To account for this type of philopatry, Shields proposes that if the same adaptation arises independently in different individuals but from different types of mutations and the resulting gene complexes are incompatible between those individuals, then selection will favour inbreeding and philopatry, in spite of ecological homogeneity. In other words, in these cases he considers inbreeding to be the primary function, not merely a consequence, of philopatry. Whatever the cause of philopatry, whether directly or indirectly, most agree it will increase the chances of inbreeding.

4 MEASURING INBREEDING

4.1 By genealogies

There are many incidental reports in the literature of inbreeding of birds normally assumed to outbreed (e.g. Nice 1937, 1943, Rowley 1981, Koenig and Pitelka 1979), but there are very few comprehensive studies. Two involve long-term European studies of Great Tit (*Parus major*). One major advantage of studying this particular species is that the birds use artificial nest boxes in preference to natural holes. A Dutch study was started by G. Wolda in 1912 and another at Oxford by D. Lack in 1947. As far as possible all breeding birds and nestlings in the study areas have been numbered and colour banded. With individually recognizable birds it is possible to construct detailed genealogies. Obviously, this pedigree method is the most direct way of measuring the level of inbreeding. For the population in Oxford an attempt was made to identify cases of inbreeding to the level of grandparent and grandchild (Greenwood *et al.* 1978), while the more detailed Dutch investigation checked for common ancestors to the level of greatgrandparent (van Noordwijk and Scharloo 1981).

Whilst this approach has probably produced the most accurate estimates to date of inbreeding in natural populations, there are a number of limitations. It is labour-intensive and takes a considerable number of years to collect sufficient data. Inevitably, not all genealogies are complete, but fortunately the consequence of a broken pedigree tends to reduce the likelihood of detecting cases of breeding between distant rather than close relatives, so that its effect on estimating the coefficient of inbreeding is minimized (Greenwood *et al.* 1978). In addition, certain assumptions have to be made. First, one assumes that new individuals in the study areas are genuine immigrants and that subsequent pairings between immigrants are unrelated ones. The second assumption is that the male feeding the young is the actual father. The possibility that this is not the case is likely to be much less of a problem for a relatively asocial monogamous species which defends a feeding territory, like Great Tit, than for other types of mating system. Inaccurate pedigrees could be constructed in polygamous species where a female may mate with several males, in communal species where more than one adult male is resident, and in colonial species where opportunities for cuckoldry may be high. If, in the future, there are to be accurate measures of inbreeding for such mating systems, then it is likely that studies will have to involve a genealogical analysis in conjunction with a biochemical one.

4.2   Biochemical approaches

Separating allozymes of different alleles at the same locus by electrophoresis has been a technique used in ornithology to date mainly for taxonomic studies and investigations of population differentiation (chapter 4). But, as Sherman (1981) has stressed, the method has successfully been used with other organisms (e.g. mammals, see Hanken and Sherman 1981, Hoogland 1982) to gain more fine-grained information on population structure, inbreeding avoidance and kin relations. It should be extended to birds. (See chapters 4 and 5 for additional discussion of these and similar approaches.)

In the absence of genealogical data, electrophoretic analyses of the genetic variation within a population can give only an indirect estimate of the intensity of inbreeding (but see chapter 5), and so should be treated with some caution. Alternatively, where a population is not closely observed but reproductive and dispersal data are available on marked individuals, it is possible to calculate a theoretical value for the effective population size which can provide, again, an estimate of inbreeding. Some of the theoretical difficulties and assumptions underlying the electrophoretic and demographic approaches in relation to estimating coefficients of inbreeding are discussed in Wright (1965, 1977, 1978), Shields (1982) and chapters 3 and 7.

4.3   The coefficient of inbreeding

When a population has been studied in sufficient detail that an accurate assessment can be made of the number of cases of inbreeding relative to those of outbreeding, a coefficient of inbreeding, F, can be calculated. The mathematical basis for the coefficient has been developed mainly by Wright

(1921, 1922, 1965) and is an indication of the common ancestry of a population. More precisely, if a diploid individual has two alleles at a single locus and which are identical by descent, that individual is referred to as autozygous. In the case of an offspring of a mother–son mating, the probability that two such alles are identical (coefficient of kinship) is 0·25. The coefficient of inbreeding for the population is thus defined as the probability that an average individual is autozygous. The coefficient F can range from 0, in the unlikely event of completely random mating, to 1, where all alleles in the population are identical by descent.

Coefficients of inbreeding based on pedigree have been calculated for only two species of birds, Yellow-eyed Penguins (*Megadyptes antipodes*), studied by Richdale (1957), and three independent populations of Great Tit (Bulmer 1973, Greenwood *et al.* 1978, van Noordwijk and Scharloo 1981). The coefficient of inbreeding is defined as: the probability of the pair of alleles carried by the gametes that produced it being identical by descent (Falconer 1960) and can be calculated as:

$$F = (na_1 + na_2 + na_3 \ldots)/N$$

where a_1, a_2, a_3 are measures of the coefficient of kinship. For example, the coefficient of kinship for brother–sister, mother–son and father–daughter is in each case 0·25, and for aunt–nephew and uncle–niece is 0·125; n is the number of inbred pairs of each coefficient of kinship, and N the total number of pairs in the study. For a detailed discussion of methods for calculating the coefficient of inbreeding see Falconer (1960).

In Yellow-eyed Penguins there were 244 pairings with seven cases of inbreeding: three brother–sister, one half-brother–half-sister and three second cousin cases of inbreeding. The coefficient of inbreeding in this instance was

$$F = ([3 \times 0·25] + [1 \times 0·125] + [3 \times 0·0156])/244 = 0·0037.$$

For the Oxford Great Tit population there were 13 inbreeding pairs (coefficient of kinship 0·125) out of 885 pairs nesting between 1964 and 1975. These consisted of five mother–son, seven brother–sister and one aunt–nephew pairings, giving

$$F = ([5 \times 0·25] + [7 \times 0·25] + [1 \times 0·125])/885 = 0·0035.$$

In the Dutch study one of the Great Tit populations was at a mainland site, the other on an island. On the mainland, coefficients of inbreeding ranged from 0·0011 to 0·0063, depending upon assumptions made about the status of certain individuals in the population; while on the island, the coefficients ranged from 0·015 to 0·036. Within this population van Noordwijk and Scharloo (1981) found a common ancestor in 19% of the clutches where both parents were identified and in 47% of the clutches where the genealogies were completely known up to the grandparents of the pair. There is limited scope for generalizations from so few studies, but it seems worth noting the overall similarity and relatively low levels of inbreeding in the mainland populations of Great Tits and in Yellow-eyed Penguins, contrasted with much higher coefficients for the island Great Tits.

5 THE EFFECTS OF INBREEDING

5.1 Genetic

Inbreeding in a population which normally outbreeds may have effects on the genetic structure of a population and on its fitness (Wright 1921, 1922, 1977, Haldane 1936, Lerner 1954, Falconer 1960, Crow and Kimura 1970, Jacquard 1974). Inbreeding can increase the frequency of homozygotes in the population. For example, in the extreme case of self-fertilization of a heterozygote, the frequency of heterozygotes will halve each generation if this intensity of inbreeding is maintained. In addition, if a population consists of subsets of inbreeding groups, then as the homozygosity of each set or deme increases, the genetic similarity of individuals within a group will also increase. But, as each group will become homozygous for a different suite of alleles, the genetic similarity between groups will decrease. These random fixations of alleles constitute genetic drift. Similar effects can occur if new colonies are founded initially by very few individuals, or when a population suffers a catastrophic decline in numbers. Initially the degree of heterozygosity will be similar to the original or source population but if isolation persists, heterozygosity should go down with inbreeding and the lack of immigrants from other populations.

5.2 Fitness

Inbreeding has been shown to have a number of detrimental effects on the reproductive success of domesticated and laboratory species of birds. These derive from two sources, although the relative importance of each for different species is unknown. First, if there is heterozygote advantage, then the inheritance of the homozygous state will decrease an individual's fitness. Second, an increase in homozygosity will also increase the chances of the expression of homozygous recessives which may be deleterious (see chapter 1).

The effects of inbreeding on reproductive performance can be very marked. In a laboratory study of Japanese Quail (*Coturnix japonicus*) by Sittman *et al.* (1966) several different consequences were recorded. Maternal inbreeding

Table 1. The effect of inbreeding on the fertility of Japanese Quail (from Sittman *et al.* 1966)

	Proportion of non-layers among survivors			
Inbreeding (F, in per cent)	0	0	25	37·5
≤ 12 weeks old				
Total survivors	836	146	376	77
Per cent infertile	9·0	8·4	17·0	26·4
≤ 16 weeks old				
Total survivors	793	128	350	61
Per cent infertile	5·0	5·0	8·7	14·6

caused a decline in hatchability of the eggs of about 3% for each 10% increase in F. In addition, hatchability decreased by about 7% for each 10% increment in inbreeding. And for inbreeding pairs, fertility was also depressed by approximately 11%, of which about 4% was due to complete male infertility (Table 1).

The Great Tit is the only bird for which any estimate of the effects of inbreeding has been calculated for a natural population. For the Oxford population, reproductive performance of outbreeding and inbreeding pairs was compared for a number of variables: timing of egg laying, number of eggs, number of fledglings, and the number recovered breeding in the same woodlot (Greenwood *et al.* 1978). Two significant differences were found. (1) Females paired with close relatives began egg-laying earlier in the breeding season than other females; the reason for this is unknown. (2) Nestling mortality was higher among inbreeding than among outbreeding pairs, although this study did not distinguish between eggs which failed to hatch and offspring which died after hatching.

Overall, mortality was, on average, 27·7% among inbreeders and 16·2% among outbreeders. For the larger sample in the Dutch study there was a parallel increase in mortality at the nestling stage (van Noordwijk and Scharloo 1981), results remarkably similar to those reported for Japanese Quail. They were also able to show that for every 10% increase in the coefficient of inbreeding there was a 7·5% decrease in the viability of eggs. After fledging there was a higher recruitment of inbred than outbred Great Tits into the population, but the data at present are too sparse to know the extent to which this counteracted the effects of inbreeding prior to fledging. In general these results from wild-bird populations reinforce the findings from domesticated species where inbreeding effects also tend to occur, or to be expressed, early in development.

6 INBREEDING AND DISPERSAL

The farther a philopatric bird moves from its natal area, the less likely it is to encounter a close relative as a potential mate. Most of the inbreeding pairs of Great Tits at Oxford occupied territories close to their birth site (Greenwood *et al.* 1978). Assuming that mating with a close relative could result in inbreeding depression, one must question the extent to which patterns of dispersal are the product of selection to reduce the level of inbreeding. Once most adults have begun breeding, they usually retain or re-occupy former nest sites so that the avoidance of inbreeding will mainly be achieved by the movement of young birds away from the natal area (Greenwood and Harvey 1982). But dispersal has many causes, among them intra-specific competition, lack of available nest sites, and choice of a better quality territory. If one of these variables is the major cause of dispersal, then the absence of inbreeding may be merely a byproduct.

Recently, Moore and Ali (1984) have presented the view that there is little if any justification for linking inbreeding avoidance and dispersal. But in making that suggestion they present a misleading picture of the literature on the subject. For example, they claim that inbreeding avoidance is responsible for all types of dispersal; they ignore more plausible alternative hypotheses advanced for dispersal in most species (e.g. Baker 1978, Greenwood 1980, Greenwood and Harvey 1982), and they also ignore certain limited conditions under which inbreeding avoidance might reasonably be linked to dispersal (e.g. Greenwood 1983). Furthermore, it is misleading for them to suggest that when inbreeding avoidance does occur, it will be through a behavioural mechanism rather than through dispersal. This assumes, incorrectly, that the two are alternatives, whereas dispersal can be merely a geographic process with no requirement that individuals be able to recognize their relatives. However, when behavioural interactions do occur and animals recognize (and avoid mating with) close relatives, such interactions will frequently be the prelude to dispersal (e.g. Hoogland 1982). Dispersal from a group or site would then be mediated through the behavioural mechanism.

At present we know very little about the interaction between inbreeding and dispersal in birds. Only limited information can be gleaned from simple patterns of dispersal. If we again use the Oxford Great Tits as an example, young males have a median dispersal of 4·4 territories, from their natal territories, while the comparable value for females is 6·9 territories (Greenwood *et al.* 1979). This sex difference in dispersal is a feature of most species of birds (Baker 1978, Greenwood 1980) and one possible interpretation is that it is caused by females moving farther to avoid inbreeding. However, as the frequency of inbreeding is approximately what one would expect given the known pattern of dispersal (Bulmer 1973), an alternative hypothesis is that the sex difference is caused by other factors and the birds in fact do not avoid inbreeding at all. The issue will not be resolved until more detailed behavioural studies have been made, similar to those on mammals (e.g. Hoogland 1982), and especially involving highly socially structured species.

At any rate, it is amongst kin-associated groups we might expect either higher levels of inbreeding or clearer indications of inbreeding avoidance. At this stage in our knowledge it is perhaps worth mentioning three species.

Acorn Woodpecker (*Melanerpes formicivorus*) is a communal species living in territorial family groups, which may contain several breeding individuals and a number of offspring serving as helpers (MacRoberts and MacRoberts 1976, Koenig *et al.* 1984). If the father of a young male dies, the son does not usually achieve mating status within his natal territory unless his mother has been replaced by an immigrant female; he disperses. Similarly, a female will usually transfer to another group when there is a breeding vacancy on her home territory and her father is still alive. Koenig and Pitelka (1979) conclude that these conditional transfers indicate the existence of a behavioural mechanism for inbreeding avoidance resulting in dispersal. Even so, cases of close inbreeding have been recorded (Koenig and Pitelka 1979).

Florida Scrub Jay also has a communal breeding system. Recently Moore and Ali (1984) have claimed that it is one species which shows clear inbreeding avoidance when females leave their natal territory to go elsewhere. However, the study by Woolfenden and Fitzpatrick (1978) provides no evidence for the presence or absence of such a mechanism. The impetus for female dispersal may merely be the opportunity to breed on another territory at a younger age than on the natal one (see Greenwood 1983).

Finally and conversely, estimates of low coefficients of inbreeding from electrophoretic studies of genetic variation do not necessarily indicate that close inbreeding is being avoided. This is especially true in the absence of detailed pedigrees, as in Grey-crowned Babblers (*Pomatostomus temporalis*) studied by Johnson and Brown (1980). In such cases, confidence limits for these estimates are extremely large, and the estimates themselves can be misleading as they may be confounded by selection or low levels of effective dispersal.

7 OPTIMAL OUTBREEDING

When an animal disperses it decreases its chances of mating with an individual of similar genotype and, conversely, increases the possibility of breeding with an animal of dissimilar genotype. The possible break-up

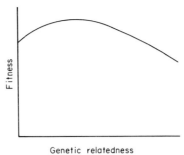

Fitness

Genetic relatedness

Fig. 1. Hypothetical illustration of optimal outbreeding. Inbreeding results in a reduction in fitness compared to mating with an individual less closely related. Fitness declines further as relatedness and outbreeding depression sets in.

of gene complexes or genetic incompatibility through mating with an
individual of different genotype might cause what has been termed outbreeding depression. The proposal that there is some intermediate level of
genetic similarity between mates where fitness would be maximized, avoiding
both close inbreeding and distant outbreeding, underlies the hypothesis of
optimal outbreeding. It has been developed independently in recent years by
Bateson (1978, 1980, 1982, 1983), Price and Waser (1979) and Shields (1979,
1982, 1983)—the latter confusingly referring to it as optimal inbreeding (see
Fig. 1).

The only reproductive data available so far (which in fact support the
optimal outbreeding model), are for the plant *Delphinium nelsoni* (Price and
Waser 1979). Selfed plants showed inbreeding depression (fewer seeds per
flower) when compared with plants pollinated by others a few metres away,
while pollen from flowers 100 metres away led to outbreeding depression. It is
presumed that the metric distance is correlated with genetic differences.

Analogous and suggestive data for birds are found in Bateson's elegant
experiments, involving imprinting by Japanese Quail. He tested a range
of phenotypes of differing degrees of similarity to that on which the test
animals were imprinted. The quail avoided both too similar and too dissimilar
types, preferentially choosing those of intermediate novelty. The preference is
finely tuned to the equivalent of cousins (Bateson 1982, 1983). It is assumed,
but awaits confirmation, that such behaviour in a natural population would
result in the avoidance of both inbreeding and outbreeding depression if it
involved a direct genetic basis.

If we accept that the optimal outbreeding model is substantially correct for
philopatric species, then we might naïvely assume that under ideal
conditions, the optimum distance of dispersal, as a reflection of genetic
difference, would be that predicted by the model. But to do so ignores one

crucial variable—the cost of dispersal. It seems reasonable to expect that costs will be an increasing function of the distance that an animal travels from its natal site. For example, dispersing male Eurasian Blackbirds (*Turdus merula*) have a higher mortality than philopatric individuals (Greenwood and Harvey 1976). Under these circumstances, the optimal dispersal distance would be less than that expected under simple optimal outbreeding. Moreover, if the cost of dispersal is a sufficient selective force, it may affect the mating preferences of individuals. Preferentially choosing to mate with a relative nearby might not result in an optimal mix of genotypes, but philopatry might improve an individual's chances of survival, and ultimately its fitness (Bengtsson 1978).

8 SUMMARY AND CONCLUSIONS

Evolutionary interest in inbreeding and its avoidance in higher vertebrates can be traced at least as far back as Darwin (1871). And from early in this century models for estimating the coefficients of inbreeding and various other components of population structure had become established and fundamental features of theoretical population genetics. Given the long-standing and widespread popularity of birds as research animals and the ease with which known individuals can be monitored in the field, it is remarkable how little empirical research has been done on inbreeding and related problems such as philopatry. There is a plethora of hypotheses but no avian examples which bear directly on the three general models for the evolution of philopatry. Currently there are only two species of wild birds whose frequencies of inbreeding have been calculated and only one where the effects of inbreeding have been determined in a natural population. The major disagreements over the role of dispersal in the avoidance of inbreeding stem mainly from a paucity of field data. It is also unrealistic to expect theoreticians to improve their models in the absence of relevant biological information. However, there are three areas of current research that may yet provide both stimuli and a more comprehensive picture. First, detailed and long-term studies will continue on many species of birds, which should eventually give us a better understanding of fine-grained aspects of population and social structure. Second, biologists are increasingly using biochemical techniques (allozymes, DNA) alongside the collection of demographic and behavioural data, particularly in studies of communal birds. Third, the recent upsurge of interest in optimal outbreeding may prompt theoretical population geneticists to produce some quantitative models that field biologists can test with field data. Birds seem to be ideal candidates for such an approach.

REFERENCES

Baker, R. R. (1978). "The Evolutionary Ecology of Animal Migration." Hodder & Stoughton, London.

Bateson, P. P. G. (1978). Sexual imprinting and optimal outbreeding. *Nature* **273**, 659–660.

Bateson, P. P. G. (1980). Optimal outbreeding and the development of sexual preferences in Japanese Quail. *Z. Tierpsych.* **53**, 231–244.

Bateson, P. P. G. (1982). Preferences for cousins in Japanese Quail. *Nature* **295**, 236–237.

Bateson, P. P. G. (1983). Optimal outbreeding. *In* "Mate Choice" (ed. P. Bateson), pp. 257–277. Cambridge University Press.

Bengtsson, P. O. (1978). Avoiding inbreeding: at what cost? *J. Theor. Biol.* **18**, 439–444.

Bulmer, M. G. (1973). Inbreeding in the great tit. *Heredity* **30**, 313–325.

Burt, W. H. (1940). Territorial behaviour and populations of some small mammals in southern Michigan. *Misc. Publ. Mus. Zool. Univ. Mich.* **45**, 1–58.

Cooke, F., MacInnes, C. D. and Prevett, J. P. (1975). Gene flow between breeding populations of the lesser snow goose. *Auk* **92**, 493–519.

Crow, J. F. and Kimura, M. (1970). "An Introduction to Population Genetics Theory." Harper & Row, New York.

Darwin, C. (1871). "The Descent of Man and Selection in Relation to Sex". J. Murray, London.

Dobzhansky, T. (1970). "Genetics of the Evolutionary Process". Columbia University Press, New York.

Falconer, D. S. (1960). "Introduction to Quantitative Genetics". Oliver & Boyd, London.

Fisher, H. I. (1976). Some dynamics of a breeding colony of Laysan Albatrosses. *Wilson Bull.* **88**, 121–142.

Fisher, R. A. (1930). "The Genetical Theory of Natural Selection". Clarendon Press, Oxford.

Ford, E. B. (1964). "Ecological Genetics". Methuen, London.

Gratto, C., Morrison, R. I. G. and Cooke, F. (1985). Philopatry, site tenacity and mate fidelity in the Semipalmated Sandpiper. *Auk* **102**, 16–24.

Greenwood, P. J. (1980). Mating systems, philopatry and dispersal in birds and mammals. *Anim. Behav.* **28**, 1140–1162.

Greenwood, P. J. (1983). Mating systems and the evolutionary consequences of dispersal. *In* "The Ecology of Animal Movement" (eds I. R. Swingland and P. J. Greenwood), pp. 116–131. Oxford University Press.

Greenwood, P. J. and Harvey, P. H. (1976). The adaptive significance of variation in breeding area fidelity of the Blackbird (*Turdus merula* L.) *J. Anim. Ecol.* **45**, 887–898.

Greenwood, P. J. and Harvey, P. H. (1982). The natal and breeding dispersal of birds. *Ann. Rev. Ecol. Syst.* **13**, 1–21.

Greenwood, P. J., Harvey, P. H. and Perrins, C. M. (1978). Inbreeding and dispersal in the Great Tit. *Nature* **271**, 52–54.

Greenwood, P. J., Harvey, P. H. and Perrins, C. M. (1979). The role of dispersal in the Great Tit (*Parus major*): the causes, consequences and heritability of natal dispersal. *J. Anim. Ecol.* **48**, 123–142.

Haldane, J. B. S. (1936). The amount of heterozygosis to be expected in an approximately pure line. *J. Genet.* **32**, 375–391.

Hanken, J. and Sherman, P. W. (1981). Multiple paternity in Belding's ground squirrel litters. *Science* **212**, 351–353.

Hinde, R. A. (1956). The biological significance of the territories of birds. *Ibis* **98**, 340–369.

Hoogland, J. L. (1982). Prairie dogs avoid extreme inbreeding. *Science* **215**, 1639–1641.

Jacquard, A. (1974). "Genetic Structure of Populations". Springer, Berlin.

Johnson, M. S. and Brown, J. L. (1980). Genetic variation among trait groups and apparent absence of close inbreeding in Grey-crowned Babblers. *Behav. Ecol. Sociobiol.* **7**, 93–98.

Koenig, W. D., Mumme, R. L. and Pitelka, F. A. (1984). The breeding system of the Acorn Woodpecker in central coastal California. *Z. Tierpsych.* **65**, 289–308.

Koenig, W. D. and Pitelka, F. A. (1979). Relatedness and inbreeding avoidance: counterploys in the communally nesting Acorn Woodpecker. *Science* **206**, 1103–1105.

Lack, D. (1954). "The Natural Regulation of Animal Numbers". Clarendon Press, Oxford.

Lerner, I. M. (1954). "Genetic Homeostasis". Oliver & Boyd, Edinburgh.

Levins, R. (1968). "Evolution in Changing Environments". Princeton University Press.

MacRoberts, M. H. and MacRoberts, B. R. (1976). Social organization and behaviour of the Acorn Woodpecker in central coastal California. *Ornithol. Monogr.* **21**, 1–115.

Mayr, E. (1963). "Animal Species and Evolution". Belknap Press of Harvard University Press, Cambridge, Mass.

Moore, J. and Ali, R. (1984). Are dispersal and inbreeding avoidance related? *Anim. Behav.* **32**, 94–112.

Newton, I. and Marquiss, M. 1982. Fidelity to breeding area in the Sparrowhawk *Accipiter nisus. J. Anim. Ecol.* **52**, 327–341.

Nice, M. M. (1937). Studies in the life history of the Song Sparrow. Part 1. *Trans. Linn. Soc. N.Y.* **4**, 1–247.

Nice, M. M. (1943). Studies in the life history of the Song Sparrow. Part 2. *Trans. Linn. Soc. N.Y.* **6**, 1–328.

Price, M. W. and Waser, N. M. (1979). Pollen dispersal and optimal out-crossing in *Delphinium nelsoni. Nature* **277**, 294–297.

Richdale, L. E. (1957). "A Population Study of Penguins". Clarendon Press, Oxford.

Rowley, I. (1981). The communal way of life in the Splendid Wren, *Malurus splendens. Z. Tierpsych.* **55**, 228–267.

Sherman, P. W. (1981). Electrophoresis and avian genealogical analyses. *Auk* **98**, 419–422.

Shields, W. M. (1979). "Philopatry, inbreeding, and the adaptive advantages of sex". Ph.D. Thesis, Ohio State University, Columbus.

Shields, W. M. (1982). "Philopatry, Inbreeding, and the Evolution of Sex". State University of New York Press, Albany.

Shields, W. M. (1983). Optimal inbreeding and the evolution of philopatry. *In* "The Ecology of Animal Movement" (eds I. R. Swingland and P. J. Greenwood), pp. 132–159. Oxford University Press.

Sittman, K., Abplanalp, B. and Fraser, R. A. (1966). Inbreeding depression in Japanese Quail. *Genetics* **54**, 371–379.

van Noordwijk, A. J. and Scharloo, W. (1981). Inbreeding in an island population of the Great Tit. *Evolution* **35**, 674–688.

Wilson, E. O. (1975). "Sociobiology: The New Synthesis". Harvard University Press, Cambridge, Mass.

Woolfenden, G. E. and Fitzpatrick, J. W. (1978). The inheritance of territory in group-breeding birds. *Bioscience* **28**, 104–108.

Wright, S. (1921). Systems of mating. *Genetics* **6**, 111–178.

Wright, S. (1922). Coefficients of inbreeding and relationship. *Am. Natur.* **56**, 330–338.

Wright, S. (1965). The interpretation of population structure by *F*-statistics, with special regard to systems of mating. *Evolution* **19**, 395–420.

Wright, S. (1977). "Evolution and the Genetics of Populations". Vol. 3. "Experimental Results and Evolutionary Deductions". University of Chicago Press.

Wright, S. (1978). "Evolution and the Genetics of Populations". Vol. 4. "Variability within and among Natural Populations". University of Chicago Press.

7
Gene Flow and the Genetic Structure of Populations

Robert F. Rockwell

Department of Biology, The City College of New York 10031, USA and
Department of Ornithology, American Museum of Natural History,
Central Park West at 79th Street, New York 10024

and George F. Barrowclough

Department of Ornithology, American Museum of Natural History,
Central Park West at 79th Street, New York 10024, U.S.A.

1   INTRODUCTION

The capacity to move from one location to another is a characteristic shared by almost all animal species at some stage in their life history. It is a property that is central to animal evolution in general and one on which many animal adaptations are based. Animal movements are often stimulated by deterioration of the local environment or by changes in proximate cues portending such deteriorations. Historically these movements have been

AVIAN GENETICS
ISBN 0-12-187570-9

categorized as dispersal and migration, with immigration and emigration indicating direction with respect to some local population.

The precise meaning of these terms has varied over time and with respect to the group of organisms being considered (e.g. Johnson 1969). Endler (1977) has provided a lucid comparison of the two terms with respect to a number of ecological characteristics. He defines *migration* as "the relatively long-distance movements made by large numbers of individuals in approximately the same direction at approximately the same time, and is usually followed by a regular return migration". This definition is certainly consistent with general ornithological usage. Endler defines *dispersal* as "the roughly random and non-directional small-scale movements made by individuals rather than by groups, continuously rather than periodically, as a result of their daily activities". For many vertebrate ecologists, dispersal is defined from a more reproductive slant, as in Howard's (1960) definition: "the permanent movement an individual makes from its birth site to the place where it reproduces or would have reproduced if it had survived and found a mate" (see also Merrell 1981). Greenwood and Harvey (1982) have suggested that this definition, which focuses on pre-reproductive individuals, be applied to the term *natal dispersal*, and that *breeding dispersal* refers to any subsequent movements from one breeding site (or group) to another. Further, when a successful breeding attempt follows either type of dispersal, then the dispersal is said by them to be *effective*. They state that effective dispersal is similar to migration as used in genetics. This assertion is unfortunately not entirely correct.

Migration has been used historically by geneticists to indicate the movements *and* incorporation of alleles, rather than individuals, among local populations. This is because the focus of population genetics is the genetic structure and differentiation within and among local populations. As such, the physical presence of an individual immigrant (or even a breeding pair of immigrants) does not necessarily result in the genetic alteration of the local population's gene pool (Endler 1977, Rockwell and Cooke 1977). That is, migration in the *genetic* sense is evidenced by the presence in a population of an individual that has only one parent from that local population (Ehrlich and Raven 1969). Thus, effective dispersal indicates migration in the population genetic sense only if the successful mating described by Greenwood and Harvey (1982) involves a dispersing individual, or its offspring, being coupled with a member of the local population.

The historical usage of the word "migration" in genetics is unfortunate because it has led to confusion in the application of population genetic theory to field situations. It is also unfortunate because, as pointed out by Endler (1977) and Merrell (1981), migration in the genetic sense is more likely to result from dispersal than from migration in the ecological sense. For these reasons, and in keeping with a recent shift in terminology among population geneticists (e.g. Spiess 1977), we use the term *gene flow* to indicate migration in the genetic sense. Formally, gene flow is the movement and incorporation of alleles between local populations.

Having defined gene flow and related it to dispersal and migration—in both the ecological and genetic senses—this chapter proceeds in the following way. Section 2 covers a simple model of gene flow and examines the underlying assumptions and the potential effects of violating these assumptions. Section 3 considers the potential evolutionary impact of gene flow and examines evidence concerning its relative importance. The closely related concept of the genetic structure of populations is introduced. Precise quantification of gene flow and genetic structure is needed; for the latter, the use of Wright's *F*-statistics is urged. In section 4 various approaches to measuring gene flow and the genetic structure of actual populations are discussed. Several applications using avian data are given. Section 5 contains a brief summary of the chapter.

It is stressed, finally, that gene flow in animals depends primarily on their capacity to move (Rockwell and Levine 1987). This is a sufficient but not a necessary mechanism for gene flow. For lucid reviews of gene flow in plants, the reader should consult Jain (1976) and Levin and Kerster (1974).

2 BASIC MATHEMATICS AND ASSUMPTIONS

At the simplest level, gene flow can be viewed as the unidirectional movement and incorporation of alleles at a locus between two populations (Fig. 1). Assume there are two alleles (A, a) with the frequency of a being q_t in population 1 and Q_t in population 2. Let I be a random sample of individuals from population 2 that moves into the range of population 1 during a specified time-interval and mates randomly with its members. Let N be the size of population 1 before the immigration. Define m, the rate of immigration, as $m = I/(I + N)$. Assuming reproduction is discrete with non-overlapping generations, that there is no selection or mutation, and that population 1 is sufficiently large to preclude random drift, the frequency of a among the progeny of population 1 is

$$q_{t+1} = q_t (1 - m) + Q_t m$$

The change in population 1 due to gene flow is then

$$\Delta q = q_{t+1} - q_t$$

Thus,

$$\Delta q = m(Q_t - q_t)$$

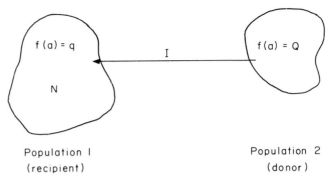

Fig. 1. A simple model of gene flow. A number of immigrants (I) join and randomly mate with the endemic members (N) of population 1. The immigrants are a random sample of the gene pool of population 2 in which the frequency of the allele *a* is *Q*. The frequency of that same allele in population 1, before immigration, is *q*.

The effect of gene flow on the genetic structure is clearly a function of the rate of immigration and the genetic difference between the recipient population and the immigrants.

It is important to stress that in this simple model we have assumed that the genetic contribution of the immigrants was randomly incorporated into the endemic gene pool. This need not always be the case. For example, suppose that immigrants do not have the same probability of mating with the endemics as the endemics do with each other. In such cases the variable m should be adjusted to take into account any departure from a one-to-one relation between "physical immigration" and genetic incorporation. In accordance with the change in terminology applied to adjusted population sizes (e.g. Crow and Kimura 1970), the adjusted variable could be considered m_e, the effective rate of immigration. For more complex models of gene flow, the reader should consult Wright (1951), Crow and Kimura (1970), Kimura and Ohta (1971), Jacquard (1974) and Karlin (1976). For the most part, however, these complex models assume that immigrants' genes are randomly incorporated.

There are two general classes of proximate causes that operate against the random incorporation of immigrants' genes. These encompass problems involving *movement* and *mating* and are not mutually exclusive. Problems involving movement include both those associated with moving between populations and those related to patterns of movement within the range of a recipient population, once immigration has occurred. Affecting both levels of movement is the tendency for dispersal to be leptokurtic rather than normal (Bateman 1951, Endler 1977). That is, many more individuals move short distances than would be expected if movement were random. Movement within the range of the recipient may be further restricted by a patchy or clumped distribution of suitable habitat. In fact, all those factors that determine the pattern of dispersion of the recipient population (e.g. clumped, uniform) may affect local movements of the immigrants (Merrell 1981). Slight differences in microhabitat preferences or tolerances may also make it less likely for the immigrants to obtain a random distribution within the range of the recipient population. If it persists through the period of mate selection, a non-random distribution of immigrants may lead to the non-random incorporation of immigrants' genes, even if mate choice is random.

Non-random mating behaviour may also complicate the random incorporation of immigrants' genes. For example, if mating preferences are related to some phenotypic trait that differs between immigrants and endemics, positive assortative mating will reduce the rate of incorporation of immigrant genes into the local gene pool. This mechanism may operate in cases involving secondary contact and hybrid zones (see chapter 10). On the other hand, if mating preference includes a strong negative assortative element deriving, perhaps, from a system related to the avoidance of inbreeding (Greenwood *et al.* 1978, Bateson 1983), then the rate of incorporation of immigrants' genes could be substantially higher than that expected from the observed level of immigration. In a similar fashion, an inverse frequency-dependent mating system, such as the "rare male" advantage (Ehrman 1972), would drastically inflate the effective rate of immigration. The effects of any departure from random mating on the incorporation of immigrants' genes will be further modulated by the mating system of the species being considered. For example, the impact of the "rare male" advantage on effective immigration would be smaller in a monogamous species than in a polygynous one.

Aside from studies centred primarily on interspecific hybridization, especially along zones of secondary contact, few studies have examined the relative success of immigrants in obtaining mates. One notable (and extreme) exception is the work by Cooke and associates on Lesser Snow Goose (*Anser c. caerulescens*). At the La Perouse Bay colony in northern Manitoba, virtually all of the breeding males are immigrants (Cooke *et al.* 1975, Rockwell and Cooke 1977). The growing body of information documenting the extent of non-random mating in nature (chapter 9) underscores the need to examine mating patterns of immigrants rather than tacitly assuming that they are random.

In addition to its dependence on the effective immigration rate, the effect of gene flow is dependent on the level of genetic difference between the recipient population and the immigrants. As is clear from the above equations that if there is no genetic difference, there is no effect of gene flow. For a constant rate of effective immigration, increasing the genetic difference between populations increases the effect of gene flow. Of course, this continues only up to a point because eventually the recipient and donor populations become sufficiently divergent that either mating fails to occur (e.g. immigrants are not recognized as conspecifics) or "hybrid" offspring fail to survive because of genetic incompatibility (Endler 1977, Merrell 1981). The point at which genetic divergence between recipient and donor populations becomes sufficient that gene flow "within species" becomes gene flow "between species" presents a problem (e.g. Spiess 1977, Corbin 1983). In this chapter we have restricted ourselves to general issues of gene flow and its measurement and to the examination of gene flow among populations that are not so genetically distinct that species recognition and genic incompatibility are potential problems.

There is one final issue involving genetic differences that is crucial to gene flow. We have assumed that the immigrants are a random sample of the gene pool of the donor population. If they are not, then it is obvious that genetic characteristics of the donor population are inappropriate for the evaluation of gene flow. Leptokurtic dispersal from a population that does not display random genetic distribution over its range could lead to non-random genetic representation among "immigrants". It is also possible that certain genotypes may be more likely to emigrate than others (Fisher 1958, chapter VI). Although there are numerous examples of sexual differences in dispersal (Greenwood and Harvey 1982), we are unaware of any avian examples in which a particular genotype is more likely to emigrate. Genotype-specific emigration has been suggested for small mammals (Krebs *et al.* 1973; but see McGovern and Tracy 1981, Parsons 1983).

In summary, even the simplest model of gene flow can become complex when one considers the possibilities that immigrants' genes are not randomly incorporated into the recipient gene pool or that they do not reflect the total gene pool of the donor population. Although these factors complicate the examination and even the conceptualization of gene flow, they do not preclude its study. Consideration of them here is meant as both a warning and a challenge—their potential impact is real, the extent of their existence requires further examination.

3   EVOLUTIONARY IMPORTANCE

There is little doubt that gene flow can have a profound effect on the evolutionary process. This notion was evident in the early work of Fisher (1958) and Wright (1931) and is supported by a substantial body of subsequent theoretical research. That literature has considered gene flow operating alone under a variety of geographical structures (e.g. Moran 1962, Kimura and Weiss 1964, Wright 1969, Crow and Kimura 1970) and operating in consort with genetic drift (e.g. Maynard Smith 1970, Spieth 1974), with selection (e.g. Felsenstein 1976, Karlin 1976, Karlin and Richter-Dyn 1976, Endler 1977) and with both (e.g. Malecot 1969, Wright 1977). Much of the emphasis of this work has centred on clarifying the conditions under which gene flow will have major or minor effects. Although many of the models are not presently applicable to natural populations, Barrowclough (1980 a) has shown that some of the simpler models can be used to begin an empirical investigation of the relative roles of gene flow and selection, particularly along clines involving hybrid zones. In the following we review some of the major effects that gene flow can have as an evolutionary determinant.

3.1 Genetic continuity

Many species do not occur continuously over their entire ranges. Rather, they occupy patches of more or less suitable habitat that may be distributed in a uniform or clumped fashion. The ecologies of the various patches and the sizes of the local populations will no doubt differ. Under the combined effects of mutation, genetic drift and selection for adaptation to local conditions, these more or less isolated populations are expected to diverge genetically. Gene flow among the populations will reduce this divergence. At one level, therefore, gene flow can be viewed as evolutionary "glue", genetically binding together fragments of the species. At another level, gene flow can be seen as a force retarding or even precluding local adaptation through the constant input of foreign alleles (e.g. Rockwell and Cooke 1977). From either perspective, gene flow is integral to the substructuring of species and operates such that some level of genetic continuity is maintained.

   In theory, the same effects of gene flow are seen in species that occur continuously over extensive regions (e.g. Wright 1943, 1951, 1977). This is because mating (and resulting gene flow) is more likely to occur between individuals that come from local neighbourhoods than randomly from the total area occupied by the species. Consequently, genetic differentiation will exist across the range of the species owing to a balance between finite gene flow and the random drift of allelic frequencies. The greater the extent of gene flow, the less the degree of this random differentiation. More precisely, the extent of differentiation will be determined by both the level of gene flow and the density of breeding birds.

   Thus, the principal effect of gene flow is to maintain a genetic continuity throughout the range of a species. The degree of such coherence is known as the *genetic population structure*. This notion, or its converse, the extent of genetic differentiation among conspecific populations, is of such intrinsic interest to those interested in the genetics and evolution of populations that it is a major field of empirical research *per se* (e.g. Wright 1976, Barrowclough 1983, Selander and Whittam 1983). Estimates of variables associated with it enter many of the equations of population genetics and an empirical understanding of the subject is essential.

The genetic structure of populations is most frequently described by a measure known as the among-population component of genetic variance, F_{ST}. F_{ST} can be developed in many different ways (see, for example, Spiess 1977, chapter 12; for a more complete development, see Wright 1969, chapter 12, or Crow and Kimura 1970, section 3.12). One way to think of F_{ST} is as the correlation of genes within a single population relative to the universe of populations. Values of F_{ST} can vary from zero to one. If a species is organized into many strongly differentiated demes, i.e. if gene flow is not maintaining alleles at roughly the same frequency throughout a species' range, then the correlation of alleles sampled from within the same population will be high relative to two alleles drawn from two arbitrary populations. If different alleles are fixed in the various demes, then F_{ST} will equal 1·0. Alternatively, if gene flow is large, allelic frequencies will be similar across the range of a species; hence there will not be local neighbourhoods of correlated genomes, and F_{ST} will be small. Identical allelic frequencies in all populations will yield an F_{ST} of 0·0. In an alternative, but equivalent, statistical derivation, F_{ST} can be shown to be the ratio of observed genetic variance among populations to its maximum possible value.

3.2 Clines

When examined over some broad portion of their range, many species display continuous patterns of variation for conspicuous polymorphisms, morphological characters or allozymic frequencies. If that variation can be related in a monotonic fashion to a convenient geographical feature (e.g. elevation, latitude, longitude), the distribution is described as clinal. Historically, clines have been assumed to reflect adaptive responses to gradients in often unknown environmental variables. Although this may afford a partial explanation of some clines, it is more reasonable to assume that clines reflect the interaction of selection with gene flow (Merrell 1981); not selection alone. The interplay between these two factors has been examined extensively at the theoretical level (e.g. Jacquard 1974, May *et al.* 1975, Felsenstein 1976, Karlin 1982). By combining various patterns or intensities of selection with different levels of gene flow, clines of varying shapes, slopes and stabilities can be generated. Unfortunately, any given cline can be the result of several such combinations. Endler's (1977, page 95) point that, "It is impossible to interpret a natural cline without knowing the geography of absolute survival values (the shape of the fitness curves) or the extent of gene flow", remains critical in the application of theory to field studies. Although there has been progress on this front in plants (e.g. Antonovics and Bradshaw 1970), avian studies that address these issues in any detail are scarce (Barrowclough 1980 a, Wunderle 1981, O'Donald 1983).

3.3   Inbreeding and allelic frequencies

Gene flow can retard the rate and effect of inbreeding in local populations. The extent of this effect depends in part on the geographic relationships of the populations and on their genetic divergence. It also depends on whether the recipient population is sufficiently inbred to display or be susceptible to inbreeding depression. If so, then selection favouring more outbred progeny, possessing at least some immigrant alleles, would increase the effect of gene flow. In contrast, selection operating either to enhance or in consort with "optimal inbreeding" would tend to reduce the level and effect of gene flow (Shields 1982).

Endler (1977) points out that "the comparative rarity of introduced genes means that once established they may be lost by chance in the first few generations". Clearly, this effect would be countered by selection favouring an allele or those at closely linked loci. Further, Endler's point must be viewed in the light of the effective size of the recipient population. The chance of loss decreases as the recipient population's effective size declines. The chance fixation (or rapid increase in frequency) of rare alleles, introduced in small populations by gene flow (or mutation), is central to Wright's models of evolution. In those models, such chance events followed by gene flow to other populations are seen as one mechanism for rapidly altering the genetic composition of a subdivided species or population. Discussions of this and other aspects of the shifting-balance theory are found in Wright (1977, 1980).

3.4   Theoretical versus empirical importance

The theoretical evolutionary impact of gene flow is still well summarized by Mayr's (1963, page 178) view that, "Gene flow and its consequences are essentially a retarding element as far as evolution is concerned. Gene flow thus has far-reaching effects on geographic variation, ecotypic adaptation, speciation and long-time evolution." Unfortunately, evidence that gene flow has had or does have these effects in nature is not abundant. As a consequence, opinions on the *actual importance* of gene flow, particularly in relation to selection, vary considerably (see Spiess 1977, Merrell 1981). Absence of relevant evidence stems in part from the difficulty of estimating gene flow in nature. This, in turn, is related to the restrictive definition of gene flow that requires estimates to reflect not only movement of alleles between populations but also their incorporation.

Referring to the joint effects of gene flow and genetic drift, Spieth (1974) states, "In terms of gene flow, the distinction between absolutely none and almost none is enormous." Although this is true, there is also a great distinction between a little gene flow and a little more. The precise quantification of such differences will allow us to assess gene flow in nature and to understand its historical and actual role rather than just its potential as an evolutionary determinant. In the following sections, several approaches and methods for such quantification are presented.

4 ESTIMATION OF GENE FLOW AND GENETIC POPULATION STRUCTURES

For the various reasons outlined in the earlier sections of this chapter, gene flow and genetic structure are important parameters of natural populations that may affect the way we think about avian ecology and evolution, and the way in which we model and even manage populations of, for example, game, non-game and endangered species of birds. Any such application, however, will require quantitative, at least order of magnitude, estimates of these variables. In spite of all the cautions outlined above, the potential complexities and the necessity to quantify abstract aspects of population biology, there has been some empirical work on estimating aspects of the genetic structure of avian populations.

4.1 Gene flow

4.1.1 Direct measurement

At least in theory, it is possible to measure gene flow among avian populations or demes directly through labour-intensive banding and field observations. In practice this is usually done by banding nestlings. In a subsequent breeding season, adjacent and more distant demes or colonies can be checked for the presence of banded birds. If these individuals are successful in breeding in a non-natal area with a local resident, then gene flow is indicated. If the birds are colonial, then the fraction of the total number of recruits into the breeding population that are from other colonies represents the estimate of gene flow. If the birds are distributed in more or less continuous habitat, then more complicated calculations are required. For such cases, gene flow is quantified by a measure of the variance of distances moved by individuals from their natal site to their breeding site: the root-mean-square dispersal distance, σ_n (Endler 1977). This is estimated as

$$\sigma_n = \sqrt{\left(\frac{1}{2N} \sum_{i=1}^{N} x_i^2\right)}$$

where x_i is the distance moved by individual i from its natal site to its breeding site (Wright 1946, Crumpacker and Williams 1973). If adults shift their breeding site from year to year, then overall gene flow, σ_T, can be calculated as

$$\sigma_T = \sqrt{[\sigma_n^2 + \lambda\sigma_a^2]}$$

where σ_a is the annual root-mean-square distance moved by adults from nest site to nest site, and λ is the expected number of years that adults live (Barrowclough 1980 b). (The σ_T computed here is technically the component of dispersal along a single axis of a two-dimensional Cartesian coordinate system. If dispersal were strictly limited to one dimension, or if an r–θ coordinate system were used, then the proper estimate of dispersal would be $\sqrt{2}$ times the value computed here; e.g. Crumpacker and Williams 1973.)

Example 1

Verner (1971) studied Marsh Wrens (*Cistothorus palustris*) nesting in eastern Washington. These birds are confined to the marshes surrounding the numerous small lakes in the area, and they can be modelled as having a colonial population structure. Verner found that although most surviving adults nested in consecutive years in the same marsh, nine out of ten yearlings had immigrated to non-natal marshes. Thus, assuming that a random sample of yearlings had been banded, the gene flow fraction in these birds was 0·9.

Example 2

Nice (1937) studied Song Sparrows (*Melospiza melodia*) in the area surrounding her home near Columbus, Ohio. These birds are widespread and their habitat can be treated as continuous. Nice banded many nestlings and adults and then searched for nests in subsequent breeding seasons. She found 34 banded nestlings and 117 adults that survived and bred. These data are summarized in Fig. 2. For example, eight yearlings had moved between 0 and

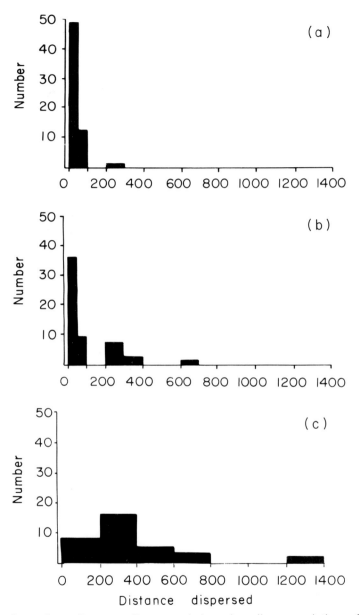

Fig. 2. Gene flow distances (in metres) in a breeding population of Song Sparrows (*Melospiza melodia*) in Ohio based on the study of Nice (1937). (*a*) Distances moved by adult males between years. (*b*) Distances moved by adult females between years. (*c*) Distances moved by yearlings from their natal sites to their first breeding site.

200 metres from their natal site to their breeding sites, 16 had moved 200 to 400 metres, etc. Thus,

$$\sigma_n = \sqrt{[(8 \times 100^2 + 16 \times 300^2 + \cdots)/2 \times (8 + 16 + \cdots)]} = 334 \cdot 8 \text{ m}$$

Adult survival was estimated as 50% per year. If life expectancy is exponentially distributed in birds (Deevey 1947), then 50% annual survival is equivalent to an expected 1·50 years of adult survival. The small amount of adult movement between seasons yields a $\sigma_{\male}$ of 27·3 metres and a $\sigma_{\female}$ of 101·2 metres. σ_a is computed as $\sqrt{[(\sigma_{\male}^2 + \sigma_{\female}^2)/2]}$ or 74·2 metres. Thus, overall gene flow was estimated as

$$\sigma_T = \sqrt{[334 \cdot 8^2 + 1 \cdot 50 \times (74 \cdot 2)^2]} = 346 \cdot 9 \text{ m}$$

Status

Obtaining estimates of gene flow in this manner requires a great deal of field work. In practice, each such estimate is normally the result of a minimum of 3 to 4 years of work in an intensive study of a single species' breeding biology. Thus, only a few such estimates are available for birds (mainly for temperate-zone species). Results from such studies have been summarized by Barrowclough (1980 b). For continuously distributed passerine birds, σ_T was of the order of 10^2 to 10^3 metres per year. For several species of owls (Barrowclough and Coats 1985), σ_T was of the order of 10 to 10^2 kilometres per year. For colonial species, gene flow to adjacent colonies varied widely, from 0·0001 in Manx Shearwaters (*P. puffinus*) in the eastern Atlantic to 0·9 in Verner's Marsh Wrens. No generalizations seem to be warranted for the colonial birds based on species studied to date.

Caveats

In practice, the actual fact of gene flow is often not established. Usually the existence of a mated pair is used to infer successful breeding and, hence, the incorporation of immigrant alleles. This obviously represents an assumption that may not always be justified.

This direct approach to the estimation of gene flow avoids some of the assumptions of less direct methods. However, many such studies involve inherent bias towards underestimation of actual gene flow. In reality, intensive field studies of the breeding biology of a species involve a study site of finite size. Consequently, dispersers outside this area are less likely to be observed and there is, thus, a systematic underestimation of longer distance dispersal. Barrowclough (1978) has discussed this problem and offers a partial remedy.

An additional problem with the direct approach is that gene flow is estimated only for the period during which the study takes place. If gene flow varies stochastically, or even in concert with an environmental variable, such as a food resource, then the short-term estimate may not be of the same magnitude as the actual long-term value that is relevant on an evolutionary time-scale.

4.1.2   Indirect measurement

Slatkin (1981, 1985) has shown that it is possible to get indirect estimates of gene flow rates in natural populations using data from electrophoretic surveys of protein polymorphisms. The underlying idea is that if gene flow is extensive, then there will be a tendency for all alleles that segregate in a species to be found in all populations. Thus, the frequency of alleles found only in single populations ("private polymorphisms") can be high only if there is little gene flow. There is not a solid theoretical basis for the estimates obtained using this approach, rather the quantitative estimates of gene flow obtained are based on Slatkin's (1985) observation (from computer simulations) of a linear regression of the log of the average frequency of alleles found only in single populations, p_1, on the logarithm of the product of m, the gene flow rate, and N_e, the population size. In particular, Slatkin found that

$$\ln(p_1) = -0\cdot505 \ln(N_e m) - 2\cdot44$$

Thus, $N_e m$ can be estimated as

$$(N_e m) = \exp\left[(\ln(p_1) + 2\cdot44)/(-0\cdot505)\right]$$

The product $N_e m$ is the number of individuals exchanged between adjacent demes per generation.

Example

In a study of geographic variation in Yellow-rumped Warbler (*Dendroica coronata*) across North America, Barrowclough (1980 a) found six alleles at four loci that were present in single-population samples. These had frequencies of 0·019, 0·024, 0·019, 0·024, 0·039 and 0·044. Thus, the average frequency of private alleles was 0·028. Consequently, $N_e m$ is estimated to be

$$\exp\left[(\ln(0\cdot028) + 2\cdot44)/(-0\cdot505)\right] = 9\cdot475$$

That is, the frequencies of these alleles are equivalent to those expected if demes exchanged about ten immigrants per generation.

Status

Avian electrophoretic data have not previously been analysed using this method. However, we analysed the data reported by Corbin *et al.* (1979) for Northern Oriole (*Icterus galbula*) of North America and by Handford and Nottebohm (1976) for Rufous-crowned Sparrow (*Zonotrichia capensis*) of Argentina. Our results based on their data yielded estimates of the numbers of individuals exchanged between demes per generation as about eight and two, respectively. In his initial survey using the method, Slatkin (1984) found values in a wide range of animal species varying from 0·86 (in relatively sedentary pocket gophers) to 42·0 (in pelagically dispersed marine mussels).

Caveats

A general problem with electrophoretic surveys is that it is difficult to get sufficient data to show that the "alleles" behave as Mendelian genes (see chapters 1 and 4). However, for the cases that have been studied in detail, at least in birds, consistency with Mendelian ratios has usually been the case (Matson 1984).

In practice, the numbers of demes sampled, the size of the samples, the spatial geometry of colonies or demes, and the actual magnitude of gene flow can all affect the accuracy of the estimate obtained using this method. Slatkin (1985) provides guidelines and correction factors to counter, partially, some of these problems. If, however, gene flow is too great, or sample sizes are too small, then no private polymorphisms will be observed, and so no estimate of gene flow will be obtained. On the other hand, if the populations sampled have been completely isolated, physically or behaviourally, for an evolutionarily short period of time, then they will still share many alleles but also have some new private alleles. For such a case, the estimate of gene flow obtained would be an overestimate as a result of the taxa's shared past history (e.g. Larson *et al.* 1984).

An assumption of this method is that selection does not act to maintain an allele in one population and eliminate it from all others. Also, because the estimate depends on the existence of a stochastic balance between mutation and gene flow, the estimates will accurately reflect current levels of gene flow only if population dynamics have been unchanged for a sufficiently long period of time that an equilibrium obtains. This may take 10^5 years or more (approximately the reciprocal of the mutation rate). If population sizes and connectedness have fluctuated substantially, then estimates obtained using this method may be more reflective of past levels of gene flow than of present ones.

Finally, the estimate itself is something of a problem; it is the product of *m* and N_e that is estimated, not m alone. This is a major difficulty if an estimate of m is needed for purposes of modelling using the standard equations of population genetics. Two additional methods for obtaining estimates of gene flow using the results of electrophoretic surveys (Larson *et al.* 1984) suffer from this limitation.

4.2 Genetic structure of populations

Although estimates of gene flow are useful in some genetic applications, estimates of the genetic structure of avian populations will be of at least equal concern to investigators interested in the population, evolutionary and ecological genetics of birds.

4.2.1 Direct approach

By the "genetic structure of populations", we refer to the correlation of genotypes and allelic frequencies both among and within populations. Thus, estimates of the genetic structure of populations tell us how effective the genetic "glue"—gene flow—is in a particular situation. The results of electrophoretic studies yield information on the frequencies of genotypes within and among populations and so can be used to estimate F-statistics directly. F_{ST} is the particular statistic relevant to studies of the extent of differentiation of populations; it is a measure of the standardized among-population component of genetic variance (see section 3.1). There are several slightly different methods of estimating F_{ST} from data obtained using electrophoresis; we prefer the method of Wright (1978) because it includes a correction for sampling error due to the finite numbers of individuals. Let q_{ijk} be the frequency of allele k at locus i in population j, and let $q_{i.k}$ be the average frequency of this allele over all populations sampled. That is, $q_{i.k} = (1/J)\sum q_{ijk}$, where J is the total number of populations samples. Wright estimates F_{ST} as

$$\sum_i \sum_k \sigma_{ik}^2 \Big/ \left(\sum_i \sum_k [q_{i.k}(1 - q_{i.k})] \right)$$

Here the numerator is the actual variance in allelic frequencies among populations; the denominator the limiting variance. Its effect is to standardize the actual variance. σ_{ik}^2 is estimated as

$$(1/J)\left[\sum_j q_{ijk}^2 - Jq_{i.k}^2 \right] - (1/J)\left[\sum_j [q_{ijk}(1 - q_{ijk})/n_{ij}] \right]$$

where n_{ij} is twice the number of individuals sampled for locus i in population

j (i.e. the total number of genomes sampled in diploids). The first term is the observed variance due to both differentiation among populations and sampling variance; the second term is that sampling variance. Note that here we use the mean sampling variance across populations. Wright (1978, page 86) suggested using an harmonic mean, but later advocated (personal communication), and in practice used, the arithmetic mean sampling variance. The computations are normally performed using a computer.

Example

Ferguson (1971) studied electrophoretic variation at the transferrin locus in Woodpigeons (*Columba palumbus*) in Ireland. Two alleles were found segregating in each of two populations. At Antrim, 30 birds were sampled; the *S* allele had a frequency of 0·717; the *F* allele, 0·283. From Fermanagh, 50 birds were analysed. The allelic frequencies were 0·470 and 0·530, respectively. Therefore,

$$q_{1.1} = (1/2)[0·717 + 0·470] = 0·594$$

and

$$q_{1.2} = 1 - 0·594 = 0·406$$

The limiting variance can be computed:

$$[0·594(1 - 0·594) + 0·406(1 - 0·406)] = 0·4824$$

Finally,

$$\sigma^2_{11} = (1/2)[(0·717^2 + 0·470^2) - 2 \times 0·594^2]$$
$$- (1/2)[0·717(0·283)/60) + (0·470(0·530)/100)]$$
$$= 0·0118$$

and

$$\sigma^2_{12} = (1/2)[(0·283^2 + 0·530^2) - 2 \times 0·406^2]$$
$$- (1/2)[(0·283(0·717)/60) + (0·530(0·470)/100)]$$
$$= 0·0128$$

Thus,

$$F_{ST} = [0·0118 + 0·0128]/(0·4824) = 0·0510$$

About 5% of the total genic variance can be explained by the population the pigeon came from; 95% of the variance is common to all populations.

Status

A review of direct estimates of F_{ST} values from avian populations, along with some comparative results from other vertebrates, can be found in

Barrowclough (1983). These results indicate that most avian species have values of F_{ST} of the order of 0·1 or less. For other taxa, however, estimates vary more widely: estimates as high as 0·9 have been obtained in salamanders. For birds, the results suggest that less than 10% of the total genic variation can be attributed to locality. This implies substantial gene flow.

Caveats

Although this approach avoids many of the assumptions inherent in less direct estimates of F_{ST} (see the following), it does involve the assumption that selection does not substantially affect geographic patterns of allelic frequencies. Recent work by Barrowclough *et al.* (1984) does suggest that the variation uncovered by avian electrophoretic surveys is, if not precisely neutral, nearly so. In fact, the great difficulty encountered in the last twenty years (Lewontin 1974) in discriminating between selective and neutral maintenance of electrophoretic variation suggests that the neutral theory is a reasonably accurate approximation for describing patterns of genic variation.

As with Slatkin's method of estimating gene flow, this approach to measuring genetic population structure relies on the existence of a balance between mutation and gene flow. Thus, if the population structure has recently changed, the estimates may not accurately reflect current conditions.

4.2.2   Indirect approaches

Demographic data can be used to estimate aspects of the genetic structure of populations. Three variants of this approach are relevant to avian populations (Fig. 3). Which of the three demographic models should be used depends on the geographical connectedness of the populations. Continuously distributed populations are analysed using Wright's "isolation-by-distance" model; colonial populations are analysed using either a "stepping-stone" model or an "island" model. The former applies to situations in which most gene flow is to adjacent colonies; the latter is relevant if gene flow, when it occurs, is approximately equally probable to all non-natal colonies regardless of their geographical location. In practice, of course, the use of any particular model will require a more or less procrustean solution to the dilemma of forcing a complex biological and geographical situation into the exigencies of simple mathematical models. Nevertheless, in many situations even knowing the order of magnitude of a parameter such as F_{ST} will represent a major advance. Some knowledge, after all, is better than complete ignorance. In addition, the results may suggest further projects to be investigated

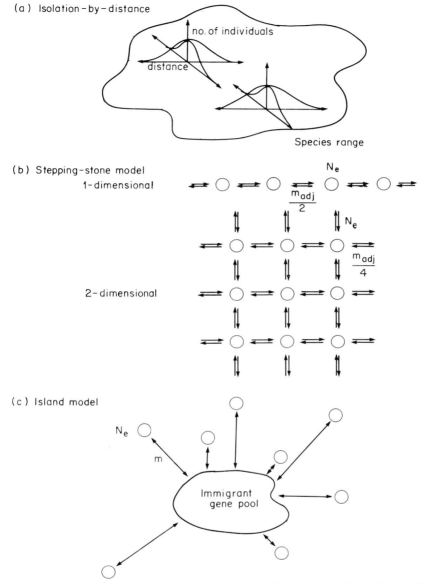

(a) Isolation – by – distance

no. of individuals

distance

Species range

(b) Stepping-stone model
1-dimensional

N_e

$\dfrac{m_{adj}}{2}$

N_e

$\dfrac{m_{adj}}{4}$

2-dimensional

(c) Island model

N_e

m

Immigrant
gene pool

Fig. 3. Isolation-by-distance, stepping-stone and island models of genetic population structure. (*a*) In the isolation-by-distance model, populations are assumed to be continuously distributed throughout their range, and gene flow from any point is assumed to have some continuous probability distribution function. (*b*) In the one- and two-dimensional stepping-stone models of population structure, populations are assumed to be colonial, of equal sizes, and gene flow is predominantly to adjacent colonies. (*c*) In the island model of population structure, gene flow among the equal-sized colonies is independent of distance between the colonies. Thus, it is equivalent to drawing immigrant individuals from a common gene pool consisting of a mixture of all genotypes.

empirically, and may also encourage theoreticians to develop more specialized and realistic models.

(i) Isolation-by-distance

Birds that are not colonial must be more or less continuously distributed, at least to the extent that their habitat is uniform. Even though such populations may be continuous over large expanses, geographical differentiation can develop owing to the finite distances moved by birds during dispersal. It may take many generations for genes to move across the range of the species owing to the restricted distance genes move in any one generation. Thus, populations are isolated by distance if not by actual barriers or gaps in the habitat. Wright (1943, 1946, 1951) suggested that such situations could be modelled by dividing up the continuous distribution of breeding organisms into a set of "neighbourhoods" or demes, each with an effective population size, N_e. The quantity N_e is determined by gene flow, population density, mean life expectancy and fecundity schedules (including the effect of overlapping generations), variances of these schedules and sex ratio. The effective size of these demes and the number of such demes in the total range are sufficient to compute F_{ST}, the expected degree of genetic differentiation in the taxon. In particular, Wright showed that neighbourhood or deme size could be computed as

$$N_e = 4\pi\rho\sigma_T^2$$

where ρ is the density of breeding birds. Then F_{ST} can be calculated as

$$(1 - Kt_k)/(1 + Kt_k)$$

where Kt_k is defined as the infinite series:

$$\exp - [(1/N_e) \times [\ln{(K - 0\cdot5)} + 0\cdot5772]$$
$$+ (1/(2N_e^2)) \times [1\cdot6449 - 2/(2K - 1)]$$
$$+ (1/(3N_e^3)) \times [1\cdot202 - 2/(2K - 1)^2]$$
$$+ (1/(4N_e^4)) \times [1\cdot082 - 2/(2K - 1)^3] + \cdots]$$

In practice, the series converges sufficiently rapidly that only the first two or three terms are necessary. Here K is the total number of demes in the species' range.

Example

Kluijver (1951) studied a population of Great Tit (*Parus major*) in The Netherlands. He gave distances dispersed between breeding sites in consecutive years by adults and between natal site and first breeding site by yearlings. We can calculate the root-mean-square dispersal distance from these data using the method described previously. (A slight correction is necessary here because the study site was finite in area; Barrowclough 1978.) Adult survival was approximately 50% per year. σ_T is estimated to be 811·4 metres. Because average territory size was 2·15 hectares, density, ρ, equals $9·3 \times 10^{-5}\,\text{m}^{-2}$. Thus,

$$N_e = 4\pi(9·3 \times 10^{-5}) \times 811·4^2 = 769·6$$

Note that in this simple example several potentially important effects have been ignored. These include variance among individuals in offspring number and kurtosis of the dispersal distribution. For examples in which these complications are analysed, see Barrowclough and Coats (1985). In practice they may have a substantial effect on estimates of N_e.

Finally, if we assume there are of the order of 10^6 demes of Great Tits in their range, then

$$Kt_k = \exp - [(1/769·6) \times [\ln(10^6 - 0·5) + 0·5772] \\ + (1/(2 \times 769·6^2))[1·6449 - 2/(2 \times 10^6 - 1))]$$

Thus, $Kt_k = 0·981$ and $F_{ST} = 0·009$. This result is actually fairly robust to the estimate of the number of demes; for estimates between 10^5 and 10^8, F_{ST} varies only between 0·008 and 0·012.

Status

Barrowclough (1980 b) reviewed estimates of neighbourhood size and F_{ST} for continuously distributed species of birds that had been the subject of long-term studies. Only eight such studies were found at that time; estimates of N_e varied from 176 to 7700. Estimates of F_{ST} were all small, on the order of 0·04 and less. Since that paper appeared, Baker (1981) has computed an N_e of about 36 for White-crowned Sparrows (*Zonotrichia leucophrys*) using a slightly different method. Barrowclough and Coats (1985) have considered such complications as non-normal dispersal distributions, overlapping generations and non-Poisson distributions of the number of offspring in their analysis of the population genetics of six species of owls. For these birds, estimates of N_e varied over three orders of magnitude, but estimates of F_{ST} remained small for all cases.

Caveats

Problems with all three demographic approaches (isolation-by-distance, stepping-stone and island models) include the theoretical necessity to correct estimates of N_e for the effects of the variables listed above (sex-ratio, non-normal dispersal, and life table schedule means and variances). Unfortunately, these parameters are rarely known, and so default assumptions must be made in the absence of specific estimates. Also, the demographic estimates, and especially the estimate of gene flow, may be subject to large sampling errors. In general, estimates of N_e are best considered accurate only to an "order of magnitude", i.e. to about a factor of ten.

The general problem of time and equilibrium arises again. Estimates of the genetic structure of populations based on studies of breeding biology done today give us information on what the structure should be in the future (or would be today, if patterns have been constant over the last tens of thousands of years). If any parameters have varied with past environments, or if for any reason the study was not representative of the "typical" pattern, then the estimates may not be evolutionarily useful.

Finally, the isolation-by-distance model has a serious problem all of its own (Felsenstein 1975): the computation of F_{ST} given N_e is not well defined mathematically. The precise magnitude of the problem is unknown; however, simulations by Rohlf and Schnell (1971) suggest the estimates obtained are probably of the correct order of magnitude.

(ii) Stepping-stone models

In the vast majority of colonial species of birds, those individuals effecting gene flow by moving to other colonies will settle with greater probability in adjacent or nearby colonies rather than in more distant ones. The genetic structure of such species is investigated using stepping-stone models (Crow and Kimura 1970). Both one- and two-dimensional versions of the models exist; which is the more appropriate to a particular case depends on the geography of the colonies. Colonies distributed along a river or coastline are effectively one-dimensional. Those on arrays of freshwater lakes, mountain tops and oceanic islands are more reasonably considered using two-dimensional models.

Although the mathematical treatment of this model is quite different from the isolation-by-distance one, the underlying ideas are closely allied. Here each colony is treated as a deme, with an effective population size determined by census size and modified, as in the isolation-by-distance case, to reflect patterns of mean and variance of life expectancy and fecundity, sex-ratio, etc. The effective size of colonies, the gene flow fraction to adjacent colonies and the long-distance gene flow fraction are sufficient information in the computation of the expected amount of differentiation among colonies. The particular model we will discuss here, that of Kimura and Weiss (1964), treats a lattice of colonies, each of size N_e. In practice, not all colonies will be identical in size; because smaller colonies are subject to greater divergence due to drift than are larger ones, they require more weight in computing an average colony size. This can be accomplished by substituting the harmonic mean of colony sizes in the computations (Wright 1969). For simplicity, it is assumed that gene flow, m_{adj}, is equally probable to each of the adjacent colonies. Long-distance gene flow, m_∞, formally equivalent to mutation, is the rate at which genes are uniformly spread over the entire species' range. This must be a very small number and, in the absence of data to the contrary, should be treated as of the order of magnitude of mutation, e.g. 10^{-6}.

Following Kimura and Weiss (1964), we can estimate the expected component of genetic variance distributed among colonies as

$$F_{ST} = 1/[1 + 2N_e C_0]$$

where C_0 is a function of N_e, m_{adj} and m_∞. For a one-dimensional situation,

$$C_0 = 2[2m_{adj}m_\infty]^{1/2}$$

For the two-dimensional case, C_0 is a complex function involving elliptical integrals, and is given on page 567 of Kimura and Weiss (1964). Also provided in that paper is a correction factor used to estimate F_{ST} for a reduced portion of a species range. In practice, the expression for the two-dimensional case must be evaluated with a computer and numerical algorithms.

Example

Murray and Carrick (1964) and Wheeler and Watson (1963) studied Silver Gulls (*Larus novaehollandiae*) along the coast of Australia. Of 88 birds banded as nestlings and subsequently observed breeding, Murray and Carrick report that 16 emigrated from their natal colony. Thus, m_{adj} is approximately 0·181. The 47 colonies surveyed by Wheeler and Watson varied greatly in size. The harmonic mean of these sizes was 194. Again, m_∞ is taken to be 10^{-6}. Consequently, C_0 can be computed as

$$2[2(0·181) \times 10^{-6}]^{1/2} = 1·20 \times 10^{-3}$$

Thus, F_{ST} ought to be approximately

$$1/[1 + 2(194)1·20 \times 10^{-3}] = 0·682$$

In practice, two further complications need to be considered. First, these gulls are long-lived and have overlapping generations. A method for correcting for this effect is given in Emigh and Pollak (1979); for this case it results in a reduction of effective colony size from 194 to about 174, and an increase in F_{ST} to 0·705. This is for an infinite number of colonies. In fact, however, in Australia there are about 50 colonies. A method for correcting for this latter factor, given in Kimura and Weiss (1964), reduces the expected F_{ST} to 0·04 for the Australian region of the species' distribution.

Status

Barrowclough (1980 b) computed estimates of F_{ST} for studies of birds whose geographical distributions were compatible with stepping-stone models. In the two-dimensional cases, F_{ST} varied from 0·0001 to 0·06 for seven species of birds. The sole one-dimensional case, Silver Gull, is discussed above. Fleischer (1983) studied House Sparrow (*Passer domesticus*) colonies in barns in north-eastern Kansas. He estimated an F_{ST} for the birds of 0·014; the actual value, based on his independent electrophoretic study, was of the same order of magnitude. Thus, all stepping-stone analyses to date suggest F_{ST}, at least for finite numbers of colonies, should be small.

Caveats

The general problems of unknown or large standard errors on the demographic parameters, especially gene flow, apply, as do the questions of whether the populations are in long-term demographic and geographic equilibrium. The use of the harmonic mean when colonies differ in effective size by an order of magnitude or more represents a partial solution; more complex models are needed.

(iii) Island model

For a few species of birds, including some waterfowl, gene flow does not occur in a stepwise fashion from colony to colony across the species' range. Rather, in birds such as Lesser Snow Goose, pair-formation takes place on wintering grounds that are common to all breeding colonies. Following pairing, females return to their natal colony; males go to the colony of their mate. Thus, if this pair-formation is random among individuals of the various colonies, then genes from any one colony will be dispersed, via the males, throughout the species' range each generation. This wide-ranging type of gene flow restricts the potential extent of genetic differentiation of populations.

The general development of this model of population structure originated with Wright (1943) and the theory has been subsequently elaborated upon by Nei *et al.* (1977). If m is the gene flow fraction from one colony to the others and N_e is the size of each colony, then the expected genetic differentiation among colonies is

$$F_{ST} = (1 - m)^2/[2N_e - (2N_e - 1)(1 - m)^2]$$

In practice, all colonies will not have a common effective population size. If the colonies differ substantially in size, then an harmonic mean ought to be used. Also, if data are available, these colony sizes ought to be corrected for the effects of overlapping generations, unequal sex ratios and variance in offspring numbers (Crow and Kimura 1970).

Example

Cooke and his associates (Cooke et al. 1975, Rockwell and Cooke 1977) have been investigating the demographics and genetics of Lesser Snow Geese since 1968. As pointed out above, pair formation in this species occurs on the Gulf Coast of the United States in early spring; the male then follows the female to her natal colony in the Hudson's Bay region of the central Canadian arctic. Thus, gene flow, mediated through males, is massive. Quantitatively, it is 0·50 times one minus the fraction of males returning to their own colonies due to chance mating with females from their own colony.

The locations and sizes (in number of breeding pairs) of the colonies are shown in Fig. 4. The harmonic mean of these colony sizes is 8657·26 pairs, or 17 314·51 individuals. These geese are long-lived; consequently it is appropriate to correct for the existence of overlapping generations. A correction for this effect, based on the life table shown in Table 1, was computed using the method of Emigh and Pollak (1979). In practice this factor is found by computer, as the algebra is quite involved. The results indicate that for a species with these demographic schedules, the ratio of effective population size to breeding size is 0·982. Hence, the effective size of the colonies is taken as 17 002·8.

There are, in fact, a finite number of colonies, each of finite size. Therefore, actual gene flow among colonies must be less than 0·5 as some males will, by chance, pair with females from their natal colony, and hence return with them to that natal colony. For example, La Perouse Bay represents 0·0069 of the total population. Assuming random mixing on the wintering grounds, gene flow through males into this colony must be approximately 0·5(1 − 0·0069) or 0·4966. A large colony, such as the Baffin Island colony, represents 0·393 of the total population. Consequently, gene flow into that population is only 0·5(1 − 0·393) or 0·304. For the seven colonies in the central Canadian arctic, the average fraction of males returning to their natal colony is 0·143. Thus, overall gene flow is estimated as 0·5(1 − 0·143) or 0·429.

The biological scheme shown in Fig. 4 is modelled, in this simplified

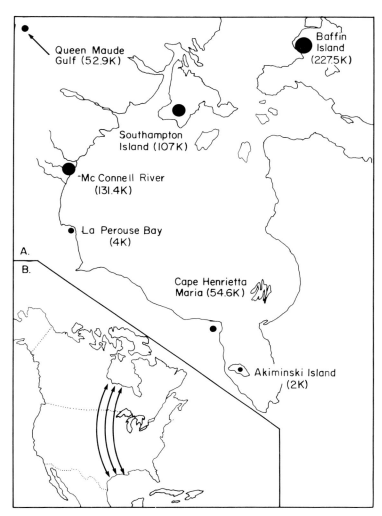

Fig. 4. Breeding, migration and wintering areas of Lesser Snow Goose. A. Locations of breeding colonies in the Hudson Bay region of the central Canadian arctic. Colony sizes (in thousands of pairs) are indicated, based on data provided by Cooch (personal communication). B. Location of migration and wintering areas. Mate selection takes place on the wintering grounds, not at the breeding colonies.

Table 1. Approximate life history schedule for female Lesser Snow Geese at La Perouse Bay

Age	0	1	2	3	4	5	$\cdots$	15
$m(X)$	0	0	1·25	1·45	1·45	1·45	$\cdots$	1·45
$s(X)$	0·45	0·74	0·74	0·74	0·81	0·81	$\cdots$	0·81

Notes

(1) $m(X)$, the age-specific fecundity, is the average number of female goslings brought to the stage immediately prior to fledging by successful females of age X. Successful females are those which brought at least one gosling to this stage. The estimates are averaged over six years and those for $X > 4$ are averaged over age (Rockwell *et al.* 1983).

(2) $s(X)$, the age-specific survival probability, is the probability that a female of age X at time t reaches age $X + 1$ at time $t + 1$. The estimates are based on both cohort and census analyses of females recaptured at La Perouse Bay and have been averaged over several years and cohorts. The estimates for $X = 0, 1, 2, 3$ were obtained by apportioning the overall mortality of the first four years among these age classes (Tanner 1978). The differential weights for $X = 0$ versus $X = 1, 2, 3$ were empirically determined from band recovery analyses. For $X > 3$, a standard Type II survivorship curve was assumed and the average survival probability was estimated with regression (Tanner 1978).

(3) This life history schedule is a first approximation for this species and its accuracy is predicated on the validity of a number of assumptions required by the sampling and estimation procedures. In addition, the schedule does not allow for the variable age of first breeding in this species nor for the irregularity of subsequent breeding attempts. It also does not account for those females which lose their entire clutch or brood before the prefledging stage.

treatment, as an infinite number of colonies, each of effective size 17 002·8, and each of which exchanges a fraction, 0·429, of its members randomly with the other colonies each generation (Fig. 5). Hence, F_{ST} can be estimated as

$$(1 - 0·429)^2 / [2(17\,002·8) - [2(17\,002·8) - 1](1 - 0·429)^2]$$

The estimate of the among-colony component of genetic variance is then 0·000 014 2. The combination of relatively large colony sizes, and extensive gene flow results in the prediction that, at equilibrium, allelic frequencies will be very nearly equal among colonies. The approach to equilibrium will be tempered by such factors as selection and non-random mating and the effects of these factors will, no doubt, vary from locus to locus. The positive assortative mating practised by this dichromatic species is a good case in point. Given the present conditions and distributions, it will take considerable time for the colour phase ratios of the Hudson Bay–Foxe Basin colonies to equilibrate.

Status

The preliminary analysis of Lesser Snow Geese, described above, is the only use this model has received by avian geneticists. It may be applicable to some

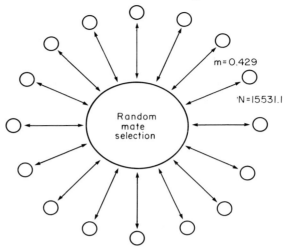

Fig. 5. Simplified model used to analyse the genetic structure of Lesser Snow Goose populations. An infinite number of equal-sized (15 531·1 individuals) colonies are each assumed to exchange randomly a fraction, 0·429, of their members with a common gene pool each generation.

other ducks in which pair formation does not occur on the breeding grounds, e.g. Canvasback (*Aythya valisineria*).

Caveats

The general cautions discussed for the isolation-by-distance and stepping-stone models apply. These include the problems of the effects of unknown variation of the demographic parameters in the computation of N_e and the assumption of a long-term equilibrium of the demographic and geographic structure.

Additionally, the model implicitly involves the assumption of an infinite number of colonies. In a theoretical investigation of a model with a finite colony number, F_{ST} eventually declined to zero (Nei *et al.* 1977). This was because there was no mutation in the model; thus the joint action of gene flow and drift eventually resulted in the global fixation of a single allele. Consequently, the actual effect of the assumption of a very large number of colonies must await the development of island models simultaneously treating mutation, as well as finite colony number, and drift of allelic frequencies.

5 SUMMARY

Gene flow is the movement and incorporation of alleles among local populations. Empirical demonstration of gene flow requires the existence of an individual only one of whose parents is endemic to the local population. Although the *potential importance* of gene flow as an evolutionary determinant is firmly established, the *actual role* of gene flow in the evolution of specific lineages remains a problem. This reflects a paucity of evidence from natural populations. There is no doubt that gene flow occurs in nature. The important question here is: How much gene flow is there? This question is central to a more basic issue in evolutionary biology, namely, the elucidation of the genetic structure of natural populations.

The assessment of gene flow involves more than simply measuring movement of individuals among populations. Consideration must be given to such factors as randomness of movement from point of origin, distribution of immigrants in the range of the recipient population, and, of course, mating propensities and opportunities of immigrants relative to endemics.

There are several approaches for the estimation of gene flow that depend, in part, on basic mathematical models of *theoretical* genetic population structure. In our discussions of methods for obtaining quantitative estimates of gene flow and the genetic structure of populations, we have distinguished between direct, observational methods and indirect, inferential approaches. All involve many assumptions and abstractions, some of which are more realistic than others. Direct measurements of gene flow involve field observations, at their breeding site, of birds originally banded as nestlings. For colonial species, the small number of studies to date include estimates of gene flow among colonies ranging over four orders of magnitude. Consequently, no generalizations seem warranted. For more or less continuously distributed passerines, gene flow, measured as the root-mean-square dispersal distance, is of the order of 10^2 to 10^3 metres per year for the seven species studied to date. For some owls the estimates are two orders of magnitude larger. The results of indirect methods of estimating gene flow, based on biochemical observations of the frequencies of rare alleles in populations, are consistent with the exchange of approximately ten individuals per year among adjacent populations.

The genetic cohesiveness of conspecific populations is reflected in a measure termed the "genetic population structure". Direct methods of analysing aspects of the genetic structure of populations involve electrophoretic estimates of the variance of allelic frequencies among populations. Results to date suggest the among-population component of genetic variance (F_{ST}) is small; less than 0·10, in most cases. Indirect methods of estimating genetic population structure involve inferences based on demographic parameters, such as life tables, and gene flow. Isolation-by-distance, stepping-stone and island models have been used for analysing avian species. Which particular model is appropriate depends on the geographic nature of the population and habitat. The results of the limited analyses to date, using all three models, are in agreement with the generalizations based on the direct approach; they suggest avian populations, when in equilibrium, should have a relatively small component of genetic variance distributed among populations. That is, different avian populations are not very different in their genetic composition.

Results such as those summarized above are only first approximations and involve many assumptions; nevertheless, they increase our understanding of the actual genetic population structure. This understanding ought to lead to the construction of more realistic models that will, in turn, allow for more accurate estimates in the future. Ultimately, our level of knowledge may surpass our level of ignorance.

For the present, field workers are urged to estimate quantitatively the level of gene flow in their study species, paying heed to its precise definition. They should also try to assess the extent of confounding effects such as non-random mating. More data are critically needed if our understanding of these important topics is to increase; every additional study will be helpful. Finally, it is hoped that theoreticians will develop models that will both account for and aid in the detection of such complexities.

ACKNOWLEDGMENTS

We thank Graham Cooch, Fred Cooke, Peter Evans, James L. Patton, John Reynolds and Robert M. Zink for information, helpful comments and discussions concerning the manuscript.

REFERENCES

Antonovics, J. and Bradshaw, A. D. (1970). Evolution in closely adjacent plant populations. VIII. Clinal patterns at a mine boundary. *Heredity* **25**, 349–362.

Baker, M. C. (1981). Effective population size in a songbird: some possible implications. *Heredity* **46**, 209–218.

Barrowclough, G. F. (1978). Sampling bias in dispersal studies based on finite area. *Bird-Banding* **49**, 333–341.

Barrowclough, G. F. (1980a). Genetic and phenotypic differentiation in a wood warbler (genus *Dendroica*) hybrid zone. *Auk* **97**, 655–668.

Barrowclough, G. F. (1980b). Gene flow, effective population sizes, and genetic variance components in birds. *Evolution* **34**, 789–798.

Barrowclough, G. F. (1983). Biochemical studies of microevolutionary processes. *In*

"Perspectives in Ornithology" (eds A. H. Brush and G. A. Clark Jr), pp. 223–261. Cambridge University Press, New York.

Barrowclough, G. F. and Coats, S. L. (1985). The demography and population genetics of owls, with special reference to the conservation of the spotted owl (*Strix occidentalis*). *In* "Ecology and Management of the Spotted Owl in the Pacific Northwest" (eds R. J. Gutiérrez and A. B. Carey), pp. 74–85. U.S. Forest Service, Portland, Oregon.

Barrowclough, G. F., Johnson, N. K. and Zink, R. M. (1984). On the nature of genic variation in birds. *Current Ornithol.* **2**, 135–154.

Bateman, A. J. (1951). Is gene dispersal normal? *Heredity* **4**, 353–363.

Bateson, P. (1983). Optimal outbreeding. *In* "Mate Choice" (ed. P. Bateson), pp. 257–277. Cambridge University Press.

Cooke, F., MacInnes, C. D. and Prevett, J. P. (1975). Gene flow between breeding populations of Lesser Snow Geese. *Auk* **92**, 493–510.

Corbin, K. W. (1983). Genetic structure and avian systematics. *Current Ornithol.* **1**, 211–244.

Corbin, K. W., Sibley, C. G. and Ferguson, A. (1979). Genic changes associated with the establishment of sympatry in orioles of the genus *Icterus*. *Evolution* **33**, 624–633.

Crow, J. F. and Kimura, M. (1970). "An Introduction to Population Genetics Theory". Harper & Row, New York.

Crumpacker, D. W. and Williams, J. S. (1973). Density, dispersion, and population structure in *Drosophila pseudoobscura*. *Ecol. Monogr.* **43**, 499–538.

Deevey, E. S. Jr (1947). Life tables for natural populations of animals. *Q. Rev. Biol.* **22**, 283–314.

Ehrlich, P. R. and Raven, P. H. (1969). Differentiation of populations. *Science* **165**, 1228–1232.

Ehrman, L. (1972). Genetics and sexual selection. *In* "Sexual Selection and the Descent of Man" (ed. B. Campbell), pp. 105–135. Aldine, Chicago.

Emigh, T. H. and Pollak, E. (1979). Fixation probabilities and effective population numbers in diploid populations with overlapping generations. *Theor. Pop. Biol.* **15**, 86–107.

Endler, J. A. (1977). "Geographic Variation, Speciation, and Clines". Princeton University Press.

Felsenstein, J. (1975). A pain in the torus: some difficulties with models of isolation by distance. *Am. Natur.* **109**, 359–368.

Felsenstein, J. (1976). The theoretical population genetics of variable selection and migration. *Ann. Rev. Genet.* **10**, 253–280.

Ferguson, A. (1971). Geographic and species variation in transferrin and ovotransferrin polymorphism in the Columbidae. *Comp. Biochem. Physiol.* **38B**, 477–486.

Fisher, R. A. (1958). "The Genetical Theory of Natural Selection" (Second Revised Edition). Dover Publications, New York.

Fleischer, R. C. (1983). A comparison of theoretical and electrophoretic assessments of genetic structure in populations of the house sparrow (*Passer domesticus*). *Evolution* **37**, 1001–1009.

Greenwood, P. J. and Harvey, P. H. (1982). The natal and breeding dispersal of birds. *Ann. Rev. Ecol. Syst.* **13**, 1–21.

Greenwood, P. J., Harvey, P. H. and Perrins, C. M. (1978). Inbreeding and dispersal in the great tit. *Nature* **271**, 52–54.

Handford, P. and Nottebohm, F. (1976). Allozymic and morphological variation in population samples of rufous-collared sparrow, *Zonotrichia capensis*, in relation to vocal dialects. *Evolution* **30**, 802–817.

Howard, W. E. (1960). Innate and environmental dispersal of individual vertebrates. *Am. Midl. Natur.* **63**, 152–161.

Jacquard, A. (1974). "The Genetic Structure of Populations". Springer-Verlag, New York.

Jain, S. K. (1976). Patterns of survival and microevolution in plant populations. *In* "Population Genetics and Ecology" (eds S. Karlin and E. Nevo), pp. 49–89. Academic Press, New York.

Johnson, C. G. (1969). "Migration and Dispersal of Insects by Flight". Methuen, London.

Karlin, S. (1976). Population subdivision and selection migration interaction. *In* "Population Genetics and Ecology" (eds S. Karlin and E. Nevo), pp. 617–657. Academic Press, New York.

Karlin, S. (1982). Classifications of selection–migration structures and conditions for a protected polymorphism. *Evol. Biol.* **14**, 61–204.

Karlin, S. and Richter-Dyn, N. (1976). Some theoretical analyses of migration selection interaction in a cline: a generalized two-range environment. *In* "Population Genetics and Ecology" (eds S. Karlin and E. Nevo), pp. 659–706. Academic Press, New York.

Kimura, M. and Ohta, T. (1971). "Theoretical Aspects of Population Genetics". Princeton University Press.

Kimura, M. and Weiss, G. H. (1964). The stepping stone model of population structure and the decrease of genetic correlation with distance. *Genetics* **49**, 561–576.

Kluijver, H. N. (1951). The population ecology of the Great Tit, *Parus m. major* L. *Ardea* **39**, 1–135.

Krebs, C. J., Gaines, M. S., Keller, B. L., Myers, J. H. and Tamarin, R. H. (1973). Population cycles in small rodents. *Science* **179**, 35–41.

Larson, A., Wake, D. B. and Yanev, K. P. (1984). Measuring gene flow among populations having a high level of genetic fragmentation. *Genetics* **106**, 293–308.

Levin, D. A. and Kerster, H. W. (1974). Gene flow in seed plants. *Evol. Biol.* **7**, 139–220.

Lewontin, R. C. (1974). "The Genetic Basis of Evolutionary Change". Columbia University Press, New York.

Malecot, G. (1969). "The Mathematics of Heredity". Freeman, San Francisco.

Matson, R. H. (1984). Applications of electrophoretic data in avian systematics. *Auk* **101**, 717–729.

May, R. M., Endler, J. A. and McMurtrie, R. E. (1975). Gene frequency clines in the presence of selection opposed by gene flow. *Am. Natur.* **109**, 659–676.

Maynard Smith, J. (1970). Population size, polymorphism, and the rate of non-Darwinian evolution. *Am. Natur.* **104**, 231–237.

Mayr, E. (1963). "Animal Species and Evolution". Harvard University Press, Cambridge, Massachusetts.

McGovern, M. and Tracy, C. R. (1981). Phenotypic variation in electromorphs previously considered to be genetic markers in *Microtus ochrogaster*. *Oecologia* **51**, 276–280.

Merrell, D. J. (1981). "Ecological Genetics". Minnesota University Press, Minneapolis.

Moran, P. A. P. (1962). "The Statistical Processes of Evolutionary Theory". Clarendon Press, Oxford.

Murray, M. D. and Carrick, R. (1964). Seasonal movements and habitats of the Silver Gull, *Larus novaehollandiae* Stephens, in South-Eastern Australia. *CSIRO Wildl. Res.* **9**, 160–188.

Nei, M., Chakravarti, A. and Tateno, Y. (1977). Mean and variance of F_{st} in a finite number of incompletely isolated populations. *Theor. Pop. Biol.* **11**, 291–306.

Nice, M. M. (1937). Studies in the Life History of the Song Sparrow, Vol. 1. *Trans. Linn. Soc. N.Y.* **4**, 1–247.

O'Donald, P. (1983). "The Arctic Skua". Cambridge University Press.

Parsons, P. (1983). "The Evolutionary Biology of Colonizing Species". Cambridge University Press.

Rockwell, R. F. and Cooke, F. (1977). Gene flow and local adaptation in a colonially nesting dimorphic bird: the lesser snow goose (*Anser caerulescens caerulescens*). *Am. Natur.* **111**, 91–97.

Rockwell, R. F., Findlay, C. S. and Cooke, F. (1983). Life history studies of the lesser snow goose (*Anser caerulescens caerulescens*). I. The influence of age and time on fecundity. *Oerologia* **56**, 318–322.

Rockwell, R. F. and Levine, L. (1987). Chromosomal polymorphism in natural populations of *Drosophila pseudoobscura*. *In* "Evolutionary Genetics of Invertebrate Behavior" (ed. M. Huettel), pp. 19–32. Plenum, New York.

Rohlf, F. J. and Schnell, G. D. (1971). An investigation of the isolation-by-distance model. *Am. Natur.* **105**, 297–324.

Selander, R. K. and Whittam, T. S. (1983). Protein polymorphisms and the genetic structure of populations. *In* "Evolution of Genes and Proteins" (eds M. Nei and R. K. Koehn), pp. 89–114. Sinauer Associates, Inc., Sunderland, Massachusetts.

Shields, W. M. (1982). "Philopatry, Inbreeding, and the Evolution of Sex". State University of New York Press, Albany, New York.

Slatkin, M. (1981). Estimating levels of gene flow in natural populations. *Genetics* **99**, 323–335.

Slatkin, M. (1985). Rare alleles as indicators of gene flow. *Evolution* **39**, 53–65.

Spiess, E. (1977). "Genes in Populations". John Wiley, New York.

Spieth, P. T. (1974). Gene flow and genetic differentiation. *Genetics* **78**, 961–965.

Tanner, J. T. (1978). "Guide to the Study of Animal Populations". University of Tennessee Press, Knoxville, Tennessee.

Verner, J. (1971). Survival and dispersal of male Long-billed Marsh Wrens. *Bird-Banding* **42**, 92–98.

Wheeler, W. R. and Watson, I. (1963). The Silver Gull *Larus novaehollandiae* Stephens. *Emu* **63**, 99–173.

Wright, S. (1931). Evolution in Mendelian populations. *Genetics* **16**, 97–159.

Wright, S. (1943). Isolation by distance. *Genetics* **28**, 114–138.

Wright, S. (1946). Isolation by distance under diverse systems of mating. *Genetics* **31**, 39–59.

Wright, S. (1951). The genetical structure of populations. *Ann. Eugenics* **15**, 323–354.

Wright, S. (1969). "Evolution and the Genetics of Populations", Vol. 2. University of Chicago Press.

Wright, S. (1977). "Evolution and the Genetics of Populations", Vol. 3. University of Chicago Press.

Wright, S. (1978). "Evolution and the Genetics of Populations", Vol. 4. University of Chicago Press.

Wright, S. (1980). Genic and organismic selection. *Evolution* **34**, 825–843.

Wunderle, J. M. Jr (1981). An analysis of a morph ratio cline in the bananaquit (*Coereba flaveola*) on Grenada, West Indies. *Evolution* **35**, 333–344.

8

Selection in Natural Populations of Birds

Trevor D. Price

Department of Biology, C-016, University of California, San Diego, La Jolla,
California 92093, USA

and Peter T. Boag

Department of Biology, Queen's University, Kingston, Ontario, Canada K7L 3N6

1 INTRODUCTION

Birds are proving to be one of the best groups for the study of selection in natural vertebrate populations. This is because the fates of uniquely banded

AVIAN GENETICS
ISBN 0-12-187570-9

individuals can be followed over extended periods, and because phenotypic characters of interest can often be accurately measured. Morphological characters in particular show rapid and determinate growth. In this chapter we shall discuss the measurement of selection and illustrate the methods with an example from our own studies on a population of Darwin's finches. The reader is urged to consult recent books by Manly (1985) and Endler (1986) for fully detailed accounts of methods for measuring selection.

Selection on a character arises when that character correlates with a component of fitness. For example, large body size (a character) may correlate with probability of survival (a component of fitness); in this case, size can be said to be under selection to increase over a period of mortality. Commonly studied components of fitness in birds include variance in fertility (e.g. clutch size, number of surviving offspring, etc.), age at reproduction, survival and mating success. Sexual selection on a character arises as a correlation of that character with mating success while natural selection arises from correlations with other components of fitness.

Selection has commonly been studied in the investigation of poly-morphisms and clines (e.g. O'Donald 1983), and less often in the investigation of levels of population variation in continuously varying traits (Grant and Price 1981). However, studies of selection have a number of other applications.

Measurements of selection are useful in interpreting the adaptive significance of characters. They in effect provide a measure of adaptation (Arnold 1983, Lande and Arnold 1983). For example, hypotheses about the adaptive significance of body size can be directly tested by observing selection on size, and such tests may be particularly useful when combined with functional, behavioural or physiological studies.

Selection occurs on phenotypic characters regardless of their genetic basis (Haldane 1954, Lande and Arnold 1983). Studies on the inheritance of characters can be combined with measurements of selection to ask questions about the evolution of these characters, and there has been some success with this approach in bird populations (van Noordwijk *et al.* 1981b, Boag and Grant 1981, Boag 1983, O'Donald 1983, Price *et al.* 1984a). For example, processes of speciation can be inferred from studies of selection on those characters that differentiate closely related species (Price *et al.* 1984a).

Life history evolution

There is usually variation in components of fitness in natural populations: for example, not all individuals have the same mating success or number of fledglings. Understanding how the mean and variance of fitness components are maintained at their expressed levels is important for many behavioural, ecological and evolutionary studies. A first step in this understanding comes from asking how much of the variance in a component of fitness can be attributed to chance events, and how much to phenotypic differences among individuals. The question can be answered by measuring selection. If a phenotypic character is found to be under selection then variation in that character or other correlated characters can be causally related to variation in the component of fitness under investigation.

As we see later, natural selection tends to act on suites of correlated characters, and this introduces several theoretical and methodological complications. These complications have stimulated much recent research into new models of natural selection based on quantitative genetics. Nowhere is this interest more obvious than in the study of life history traits (Dingle and Hegmann 1982). Thus, an important theory of life history evolution is termed "antagonistic pleiotropy" (Rose 1983). Under this theory there may be little genetic variation in overall fitness but substantial amounts of additive genetic variation for specific traits correlated with different fitness components, because components of fitness genetically covary negatively (Lande 1982). This is equivalent to saying that selection on heritable characters may change in magnitude or even sign at different stages of a bird's life cycle within generations; such patterns can be tested for by combining measurements of selection with studies on patterns of inheritance (see chapter 2).

2 DETECTING SELECTION

If the "antagonistic pleiotropy" theory of life history evolution is correct, selection should be common in natural populations. However, selection has rarely been properly documented. This is partly attributable to the difficulties involved in measuring individual fitnesses (evolutionarily significant selection coefficients may be small, and hard to measure in a short-term study), but it also reflects the failure of many field workers to examine the causes and consequences of intraspecific phenotypic variation (Grant and Price 1981).

However, there have been careful studies that have failed to detect selection (e.g. Ross and McLaren 1981, Cooke *et al.* 1985, Rockwell *et al.* 1985). Furthermore such negative results are almost certainly under-represented in the literature, both because they have been considered "uninteresting", hence not worth publishing, and because it is difficult to assess the statistical power lying behind the acceptance of a null hypothesis of no selection. Inability to detect selection may be because selection is indeed weak or absent on the characters being measured. Selection may also not be detected because components of fitness are combined. For example, the net selection over a whole generation on a combination of many heritable traits is theoretically expected to be small, but there may be large opposing selection pressures at different life history stages. In the past, no avian study has measured selection at all or even most of the stages in a single species' life cycle. But long-term population studies, such as those of Lesser Snow Goose (*Anser c. caerulescens*) and Song Sparrow (*Melospiza melodia*) (Smith 1987, Schluter and Smith 1986), are now nearing that goal (e.g. see Fig. 2 in Cooke *et al.* 1985).

A major difficulty arises in accurately measuring the phenotype. Coefficients of variation for morphological measurements in birds are often low, in the region of 4%, and half this variation may be due to errors of measurement (e.g. Smith and Zach 1979). Other characters, such as clutch size, are known to have a large between-year environment component to their variation (van Noordwijk *et al.* 1981 a). In such cases, selection on the phenotype may become obscured. Studies of selection in hybrid zones, or in populations subject to occasional hybridization, have the advantage that characters are often very variable and highly heritable. One example of this is the Galápagos Medium Ground Finch (*Geospiza fortis*) on Daphne Major Island, which we discuss presently (see also chapter 2).

The choice of organisms, characters and components of fitness for a study of selection will be a compromise between the question being asked, and the ease with which it can be investigated. Thus, studies on mating success are becoming more common both because of current interest in sexual selection, and because variation in mating success among individuals can be rather easily measured (Price 1984).

3 OBSERVING SELECTION

Table 1 lists some examples of selection observed in natural bird populations. The list is designed to illustrate methods and the types of characters and selection that have been observed. More extensive lists from a variety of taxa are given by Johnson (1976) and Endler (1986). Three distinct methods have been used to infer or detect selection (see Table 1).

3.1 Longitudinal analysis

The method requiring the least number of assumptions is longitudinal analysis, when a single group of individuals is followed over a life stage or stages, and a fitness value can be assigned to each individual (e.g. whether the individual survived or died, or the number of eggs it laid).

Table 1. Some observations of selection in natural populations

Species	Character	Component of fitness	Analysis	Reference
Passer domesticus	Morphology	Survival	Longitudinal	Johnston et al. (1972), O'Donald (1973)
Geospiza scandens	Morphology	Survival	Longitudinal	Boag and Grant (1984)
Geospiza conirostris	Morphology	Survival	Longitudinal	Grant (1985)
Passer domesticus	Morphology	Survival	Cross-sectional	Johnston and Fleischer (1981), Fleischer and Johnston (1982), Rising (1970)
Parus major	Laying date	Reproductive success	Longitudinal	van Noordwijk et al. (1981 b)
	Clutch size	Reproductive success	Longitudinal	van Noordwijk et al. (1981 a)
	Morphology	?	Microevolution	Dhondt et al. (1979)
Stercorarius parasiticus	Plumage colour	Mating success	Longitudinal	O'Donald (1983)
	Plumage colour	Age at first breeding	Longitudinal	O'Donald (1983)
Geospiza fortis	Morphology	Survival	Longitudinal	Boag and Grant (1981)
	Territory size	Mating success	Longitudinal	Price (1984)
	Morphology	Survival	Longitudinal	Price and Grant (1984)
Anser caerulescens	Hatch date	Reproductive success	Longitudinal	Cooke and Findlay (1982)
Sturnus vulgaris	Clutch size	Reproductive success	Longitudinal[1]	Flux and Flux (1982)
Dendragapus obscurus	Ng locus	Survival	Cross-sectional	Redfield (1973)
Quiscalus quiscula	Morphology	Survival	Microevolution	Baker and Fox (1978 b)
Melospiza melodia	Morphology	Survival	Longitudinal	Schluter and Smith (1986)
Ficedula hypoleuca	Morphology	Survival	Cross-sectional	Alatalo and Lundberg (1986)
Molothrus ater	Morphology	Survival	Longitudinal	Johnson et al. (1980)
Agelaius phoeniceus	Morphology	Survival	Longitudinal	Weatherhead et al. (1984)
	Morphology	Survival	Longitudinal	Searcy (1979 b)
Blackbird spp.	Morphology	Survival	Microevolution	Searcy and Yasukawa (1981)
Xanthocephalus xanthocephalus	Morphology	Survival	Longitudinal	Searcy (1979 a)

[1] Artificial selection.

3.2   Cross-sectional analysis

Cross-sectional analysis involves a comparison of two or more samples drawn from the population at the same or at different times. The essential difference between this and longitudinal analysis is that individuals cannot be assigned a fitness value; groups are compared instead. For instance, Lowther (1977) compared the morphology of groups of House Sparrows (*Passer domesticus*) biased towards younger birds with groups of older birds. In these cases it is necessary to carefully exclude the possibility of age-correlated changes in the character (e.g. growth and wear, differential migration of young birds, etc.).

3.3   Microevolution

Observations of across-generation change in the mean value of characters (microevolution) have been used to infer selection. As in some examples of cross-sectional analysis, independent samples of the same population are taken at two or more points in time, but in this case samples extend across generations. Assumptions such as no migration and no direct effect of the environment on the phenotype, have to be made. These may be reasonable in cases where the study organism is known to have a low rate of dispersal (e.g. the butterfly *Maniola* examined by O'Donald (1970)). But the high mobility of birds makes it difficult to unambiguously interpret differences between two independent samples as being the result of selection and not immigration. Observations on selection within a generation are needed to establish its cause.

4   DESCRIBING AND COMPARING SELECTION

4.1   Single loci

Selection is a change in phenotypic frequencies caused by the environment, mediated through one or more fitness components. Selection regimes are described in terms of the shape of the function relating fitness to phenotypic value. The three main types of selection traditionally recognized by evolutionary biologists are *directional, stabilizing* and *disruptive*, as shown in Fig. 1. These models are most obviously applicable to continuous approximately normally distributed phenotypic characters such as beak or body size. However, these three types of selection do bear some similarity to situations found in Mendelian genetics. With a single locus and two alleles, selection favouring one or the other homozygote is clearly directional, with the rate of approach to fixation depending on the strength of selection,

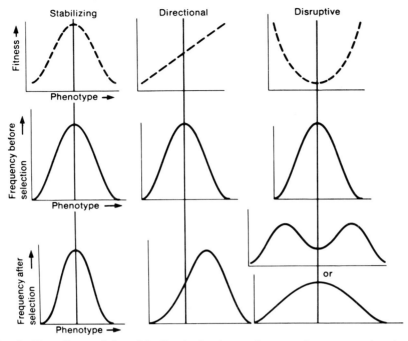

Fig. 1. The effects of three idealized selection regimes on the mean and variance of a continuous character. Solid lines show frequency distributions of a phenotypic character, while broken lines show fitness as a function of that character. Most real examples of natural selection probably involve selection functions displaying more than one of these models. From "The Genetics of Human Populations" by L. L. Cavalli-Sforza and W. F. Bodmer (W. H. Freeman & Co., Copyright, 1971).

dominance relationships and initial gene frequencies. Heterozygote superiority looks like stabilizing selection, although the genetic outcomes are reversed—in the Mendelian case, variation is maintained by a stable polymorphism, whereas in the continuous case, variation is depleted. Likewise, disruptive selection resembles heterozygote disadvantage. In this case, in the absence of frequency dependence or morph-dependent habitat selection, both types may lead to a depletion of genetic variation, although disruptive selection may increase variation in non-equilibrium situations, which may persist for a long time (Felsenstein 1979).

The measurement of selection at a single locus is relatively straightforward, at least in principle. Complications arise if changes in phenotype frequency are measured across generations and it is not understood how the trait in question is inherited, i.e. the number of alleles involved and whether or not sex linkage or dominance exists and the extent of variable penetrance (O'Donald 1983). The nature of the fitness component involved also

Table 2. An example of the calculation of selection intensity at a single locus. The data are for the "bridled" plumage polymorphism in Common Murre, taken from Järvinen and Vepsäläinen (1973) and Brun (1971)

	Phenotypes		Totals	Frequency of $A(p)$
	Normal (AA or Aa)	Bridled (aa)		
1948 frequencies	397 (0·461)	465 (0·539)	862	0·266
1970 frequencies	3 869 (0·506)	3 772 (0·494)	7 641	0·297
Totals	4 266	4 237	8 503	
Relative fitness	1·00	0·832 $= (3\,772 \times 397)/(3\,869 \times 465)$		
Mean fitness $(\bar{w})$[1]		0·909 $= [(397 \times 1·0) + (465 \times 0·832)]/862$		
Variance in fitness (V_w)[1]		0·007 7 $= [\{(397 \times (1·0)^2) + (465 \times (0·832)^2)\} - \{862 \times (0·909)^2\}]/861$		
Increase in mean fitness $(\Delta\bar{w}/\bar{w})$[1]		0·009 3 $= 0·007\,7/(0·909)^2$		

[1] See O'Donald (1970).

determines how easy it is to measure selection. Thus it is relatively easy to measure the survival rate of one morph compared to another between generations one and two of a semelparous insect. It can be much more difficult to measure the relative fitnesses of two morphs over the entire life cycle of an iteroparous bird with overlapping generations. O'Donald (1983) provides an excellent example of the relatively involved demographic model one must build to assess selection acting on morphs of a complex organism such as Arctic Skua (*Stercorarius parasiticus*).

If we take the simplest example of selection acting against a recessive homozygote, the analysis is set up as shown in Table 2. The data here are from Järvinen and Vepsäläinen's (1973) study of selection acting on the "bridling" plumage polymorphism in Common Murre (*Uria aalge*). (See chapter 1 for additional discussion of this character.) Until Jeffries and Parslow (1976) later evaluated the necessary crosses using hand-reared chicks, it was not known for certain that bridling was caused by an autosomal recessive gene. Thus Järvinen and Vepsäläinen (1973) had to carry out four different selection analyses based on different assumptions (see p. 24 in Johnson (1976) for classification of Mendelian selection models). In this case the data consist of independent samples of morph frequencies estimated in 1948 and again in 1970 by Brun (1971). To estimate selection intensities based on independent sample data, relative fitnesses must be calculated; the most fit phenotype(s) are assigned a fitness of $1\cdot0$, while the fitness(es) of the selected phenotype(s) are calculated using cross-product ratio techniques (Manly *et al.* 1972, Johnson 1976).

Having established the fitness differences between the morphs in Table 2, it remains to scale the data that were gathered 22 years apart to something resembling a contemporary annual selection pressure. There is often disagreement as to whether the proper scale to use is years or generations. Järvinen and Vepsäläinen (1973) used years and eqn. (5.3.14) from Crow and Kimura (1970) for selection with overlapping generations:

$$t = [\ln \{ p_t(1 - p_0)/p_0(1 - p_t)\} + 1/(1 - p_t) - 1/(1 - p_0)]/s$$

Here t is the number of years, p_0 is the frequency of allele N in year zero, p_t the frequency of N after t years, and s is the selection intensity (one minus the relative fitness). Based on this model of selection, an annual selection pressure of only 1% against the homozygote recessive genotype (bridled phenotype) would explain the observed decline in the frequency of bridled birds on Bear Island. The authors speculate that the polymorphism could be maintained by selection for bridling in the northern part of the cline, balanced by selection for the "normal" phenotype in the warmer south. Unfortunately little hard evidence exists that could be used to evaluate this possibility, and the more parsimonious explanation is that small changes in gene flow or sampling regime are responsible for temporal shifts in the pattern of this polymorphism. In a similar vein, Cooch (1961) has speculated that selection is responsible for changes in morph frequency of Lesser Snow Goose, an observation which Rockwell *et al.* (1985) have since shown to be better explained by gene flow (see also Geramita *et al.* 1982). It cannot be overemphasized that it is difficult to measure selection pressures unambiguously using data collected by means other than a carefully designed longitudinal study. Furthermore, in cases involving clinal variation, the analysis of selection is especially complex and reference should be made to selection models developed specifically for these situations (Endler 1973, Johnson 1976).

There are in fact few avian examples in which selection has been conclusively shown to act on either a conspicuous (plumage) polymorphism or on electromorphs (see Table 1 and chapters 1, 4 and 15 for additional discussion). O'Donald's (1983) study of the Arctic Skua remains the best example of selection for an avian plumage polymorphism, while the most often cited example of selection acting on an avian biochemical polymorphism is Redfield's (1973) study of variation at the Ng locus in Blue Grouse (*Dendragapus obscurus*). However, selection intensities were not actually calculated for the grouse, and no plausible mechanism for the postulated heterozygote advantage was found. One possibility is the explanation suggested by Lucotte and Kaminski (1978) for the maintenance of a high frequency of heterozygotes at a lysozyme locus in Japanese Quail (*Coturnix japonicus*). They suggested that heterozygotes were favoured because two alleles were codominant, and each had distinct temperature/pH optima. Thus a measure of biochemical homeostasis or flexibility was conferred on heterozygotes that neither homozygote alone possessed. Without such experimental data to suggest the adaptive basis of Blue Grouse polymorphism, coupled with the fact that Redfield's (1973) data do not strictly conform to the longitudinal analysis technique outlined earlier, we cannot dismiss the possibility that some non-adaptive sampling bias or non-random dispersal process may be responsible for the changes observed in Blue Grouse electromorph frequencies. In a more recent study of Willow Grouse (*Lagopus lagopus*) in Scandinavia, Gyllensten (1985) also found significant spatial and temporal variation in electromorph frequencies; in this case he stated explicitly that this probably resulted from stochastic processes, such as drift and non-random sampling of family groups.

4.2 Continuously varying characters

There have been many different suggestions for the best way to measure selection on metric characters—too many to review in detail here (see

Johnson 1976, Manly 1985, Endler 1986). We shall however review enough of the literature to give the reader an intuitive grasp of the problems involved, and then quickly move to a detailed discussion of one of the most recent techniques, based on the work of Lande and Arnold (1983).

The traditional way animal breeders have measured selection is by changes in the mean value of a character, with the difference (i.e. before and after selection) being referred to as the selection *differential*. To compensate for changes in scale, selection differentials are usually divided by the standard deviation of the character before selection, resulting in the standardized selection *intensity* (i). This relatively simple approach to the measurement of selection is intertwined with the methods and models used in applied quantitative genetics. It is used primarily for describing directional artificial selection on a single character. However, as long as a character has a normal distribution before selection, i is closely related to some of the more elaborate indices of selection discussed below (O'Donald 1970), and may in simple cases be adequate as a measure of directional natural selection. Lande and Arnold (1983) do in fact use this index as the starting point for their recently developed model of multivariate natural selection.

In the single-locus example, selection intensity was evaluated as the change in phenotypic frequencies relative to some optimum phenotype. The properties of the normal distribution make it possible to define selection on a continuous character in an analogous fashion (Van Valen 1965). Figure 2 shows that by raising the post-selection distribution until it intersects the pre-selection curve, one can determine the optimum phenotypic value. As in the Mendelian case, selection intensity can be thought of as the proportion of the population that disappeared because it lacked the optimum phenotype. In Fig. 2, this quantity (I) is the shaded area lying between the before-selection curve and the raised after-selection curve; O'Donald (1970) has called this the "phenotypic load". Van Valen (1965) goes on to give several formulae based on integral calculus from which these areas can be calculated, given assumptions about normality before selection, and the shape of the fitness function involved.

Van Valen's (1965) approach has a number of shortcomings, principally it assumes that selection occurs by truncation, i.e. his fitness curves were step functions. Though this may be adequate for standard artificial-selection procedures, natural selection is unlikely to operate on a metric trait in this manner. Moreover, the method does not allow for a reasonable definition of an optimal phenotype in the case of true disruptive selection, where two optima exist, and where the fitness function has more than one inflection point. O'Donald (1970, 1973) developed a series of extensions to Van Valen's (1965) work, which took into account the shapes of the distributions before and after selection, and introduced a second measure of selection intensity,

Selection Intensity — Continuous Case

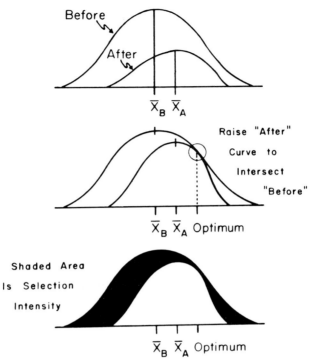

Fig. 2. Van Valen's (1965) definition of selection intensity for a metric trait. Here $\bar{x}_B$ is the mean of the population before selection and $\bar{x}_A$ the mean after. The optimum phenotype is that value experiencing the highest survival rate, found by raising the post-selection curve until it intersects the pre-selection curve. The shaded area between the curves measures the selection intensity, I. This is the phenotypic load, or that portion of the population which died because it lacked the optimum phenotype.

$\Delta\bar{w}/\bar{w}$, giving the increase in the mean fitness of a population as a result of the selection event (see also Table 2). This was needed for the case in which pure directional selection was due to a linear fitness function, meaning that no optimum phenotype currently existed in the population (e.g. Fig. 1). One can intuitively picture this index as measuring the percentage by which survival (or any other fitness component) would be increased if a scaled-up version of the surviving population could be rerun through a given selective event in the place of the entire original population, assuming mortality to be density-independent. O'Donald (1973) used this approach to analyse selection in

Bumpus's (1898) famous House Sparrow (*Passer domesticus*) winter-kill data set, and several other recent tests of selection on passerine morphology (Lowther 1977, Boag and Grant 1981, Fleischer and Johnston 1982) have also used his methodology.

O'Donald took predetermined models of fitness functions about as far as is practicable. Yet disruptive selection was still not explicitly addressed; indeed the method has no real way of determining the actual *shape* of the fitness function a population is exposed to, which may be of as much interest as the selection intensity itself. Moreover, while in artificial selection the experimenter knows which character is under selection, natural selection by definition acts on the entire phenotype. In the usual *a posteriori* analyses of selection we would like to know which of several (usually correlated) characters has experienced the most intense selection. Manly (1976) used a variety of multiple-regression techniques to explain variation in fitness, based on a class of double exponential fitness functions. Although some trial and error was involved, analysis of the Bumpus (1898) sparrow data, amongst others, suggested that the approach was on the right track towards beginning to assess which characters were most closely associated with fitness.

4.3 A multivariate model of selection on quantitative characters

A breakthrough in measuring selection came when Lande and Arnold (1983) adapted Lande's (1979) theory for the evolution of continuous characters to the specific problem of measuring selection on correlated characters. The approach is in principle simple, consisting of the calculation of partial-regression coefficients between relative fitness and one or more characters thought to be correlated with fitness. Thus an empirical model of the fitness function is constructed, and the weights of each character in that model indicate their contribution to fitness. Significance tests of higher-order coefficients can be used to assess curvilinearity in the function, with the signs of these terms indicating whether the curvilinearity reflects disruptive or stabilizing selection. Most importantly, all the coefficients can be shown to have meaning in a multivariate quantitative genetic model for the evolution of metric traits previous developed by Lande (1979, 1980). This means that, given knowledge of heritabilities and genetic correlations between characters, the evolutionary trajectory of a character in response to past and future selective episodes can be predicted.

If the character(s) being examined are single-gene polymorphism(s) where the heterozygote can be identified (i.e. most cases of electrophoretic polymorphism), changes in gene frequencies (hence evolution) can of course still be recorded directly. However, the Lande–Arnold method can be applied

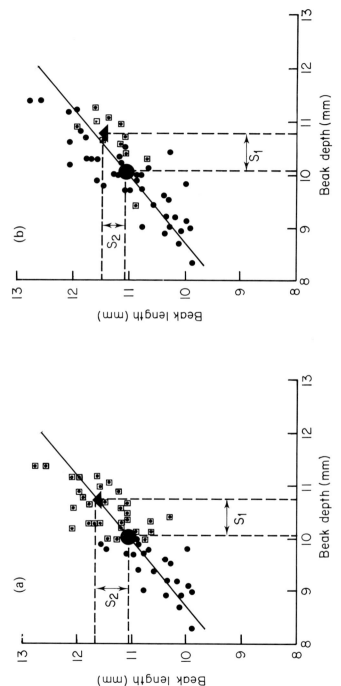

Fig. 3. Scatterplots illustrating selection differentials and targets of selection. The line is the regression of beak length on beak depth from a sample of *G. fortis*. The two characters are significantly correlated ($r = 0.82$). Boxed points representing surviving individuals after hypothetical mortality. ● is the population mean before selection; ▲ the mean after selection. (*a*) An example of truncation selection, where all individuals with a depth <10 mm die, and all those with a beak depth ⩾10 mm survive. (*b*) A possible example of natural selection, where the joint mean for the selected individuals lies below the regression line.

in these situations also, and may have to be if one wants to include continuous characters in the selection analysis simultaneously (e.g. Baker and Fox 1978 a,b). In the remainder of this chapter we review this new methodology in some detail.

4.4 Directional selection

The difference in the mean value of a character in a sample before and after a period of selection (the *selection differential*; Falconer 1981) includes a component due to selection acting directly on that character, and a component due to selection on other phenotypically correlated characters. This important distinction is illustrated in Fig. 3, which is a scatterplot of beak length against beak depth from measurements of Darwin's Medium Ground Finches.

In Fig. 3 (*a*) the results of an imaginary truncation selection experiment are depicted: all individuals with a beak depth $\geqslant 10$ mm survive, while those with a beak depth < 10 mm do not. In this case, selection has clearly been based only on the criterion of beak depth, and there is a positive selection differential, s_1, on that character. Note that beak length is under no selection, yet there is a positive selection differential, s_2, for this character by virtue of its positive phenotypic correlation with beak depth. Apart from sampling error, the joint mean of beak length and beak depth is expected to lie on the regression line of beak length on beak depth (Fig. 3) (any pattern of mortality, not just truncation selection, which resulted in the joint mean lying on this regression line, would indicate that mortality was essentially random with respect to beak length, and had acted directly on beak depth). The selection differentials can be placed in a vector, **S**, (which can be extended to include as many characters as are in the analysis):

$$\mathbf{S} = (s_1, s_2, \ldots, s_n)^\mathrm{T}$$

Lande and Arnold (1983) show that pre-multiplication of this vector by the inverse of the phenotypic variance–covariance matrix of characters ($\mathbf{P}^{-1}$), gives a vector whose entries measure the forces of selection acting directly on each character, apart from phenotypic responses due to selection on other characters included in the analysis. This new vector, $\boldsymbol{\beta}$, is termed the *directional selection gradient*

$$\boldsymbol{\beta} = \mathbf{P}^{-1}\mathbf{s}$$

In the example illustrated in Fig. 3, the selection gradient would have entries,

$$\boldsymbol{\beta} = (s_1/P_1, 0)^\mathrm{T}$$

where P_1 is the phenotypic variance for the character beak depth. These entries indicate positive selection on beak depth, and none on beak length. In this case, the reader can derive the β vector by substituting $s_2 = bs_1$ in the vector of selection differentials, where b is the regression coefficient of beak length on beak depth, which is written as the ratio of the covariance between beak length and beak depth to the variance of beak depth. The selection differential vector can then be pre-multiplied by the inverse of the phenotypic variance–covariance matrix, to yield the selection gradient shown above.

In Fig. 3 (*b*) we illustrate a hypothetical example of natural selection. Here the joint mean value of the two characters after selection lies below the regression line of beak length on beak depth: the selection differential for beak length, although positive is actually less than it would have been had beak length been subject to no selection. Beak length has in fact been under direct selection to decrease. The selection gradient in this instance would contain a *positive* value for beak depth, but a *negative* value for beak length. Alternatively, if the joint mean lay above the regression line, there would have been some direct selection to increase beak length, and the amount and direction of selection on beak depth would depend on the relation of this joint mean to the regression line of beak depth on beak length.

When longitudinal data are available, the selection gradient can be estimated by a simple regression technique, which is described below. The selection gradient (β) is valuable in that it provides the measure of phenotypic selection included in equations for the evolution of the mean phenotype:

$$\Delta \bar{z} = \mathbf{G}\beta$$

where $\mathbf{G}$ is the genetic variance–covariance matrix, and $\Delta\bar{z}$ is the vector of predicted responses in the mean values of the characters across a generation (Lande 1979).

4.5   Stabilizing selection

Just as changes in the mean of a character can be attributed to selection on that character and also to selection on other correlated characters, changes in the variance include components due to direct selection on the character, to selection on other correlated characters, and selection on the correlation itself. The fact that directional selection alone leads to changes in the variance is not made clear in some examples of selection. The Lande–Arnold technique measures forces of stabilizing selection on a character, except for any changes due to selection on other correlated characters and any changes due to directional selection (Fig. 4). The actual estimation involves pre- and post-multiplication of the change in variance (after subtracting the change

Before   After

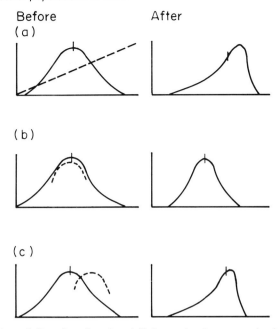

Fig. 4. Examples of directional and stabilizing selection on a single character. In each example the variance is reduced by selection. The solid lines give the phenotypic distribution before and after selection, while the dotted line gives the relative fitness of individuals during the selection period. (*a*) Pure directional selection. The coefficient of directional selection, β, is positive, and the coefficient of stabilizing selection, γ, is zero. (*b*) Pure stabilizing selection, $\beta = 0$, and γ is negative. (*c*) Mixed directional and stabilizing selection, β is positive, and as the mean positions of distributions (*a*) and (*c*) are the same before and after selection, the βs for (*a*) and (*c*) are numerically equal. γ is negative and numerically equal to the γ in (*b*) because the fitness curves are identical, although one is displaced in mean position with respect to the other.

due to directional selection) by $\mathbf{P}^{-1}$, the inverse of the phenotypic variance covariance matrix. This gives a matrix (the *stabilizing selection gradient*) whose diagonal entries measure the force of stabilizing selection acting directly on each character, and whose off-diagonal entries measure the force of selection to strengthen or weaken the correlation between pairs of characters. Lande and Arnold (1983) also provide a simple regression technique to estimate the coefficients of stabilizing selection when longitudinal data are available. The stabilizing selection gradient also appears in equations for the evolution of the variances and covariances of characters (Lande 1980).

When cross-sectional data are available, the directional selection gradients are calculated by pre-multiplication of the vector of inferred selection differentials by the inverse of the phenotypic variance–covariance matrix in the population before selection. The stabilizing selection coefficients can be estimated in a similar manner (Lande and Arnold 1983), but their estimation requires the more tentative assumption that the characters in question follow a multivariate normal distribution, which will often be violated.

We will here outline the regression technique used to obtain coefficients of directional and stabilizing selection when longitudinal data are available. The mathematical justification is given by Lande and Arnold (1983). It is assumed that several. phenotypic characters (e.g. morphological characters, territory size, etc.; for examples, see Table 1) have been measured on each individual.

(1) Ascribe a fitness value to each individual in the sample. "Fitness" as used here and in following sections actually refers not to total fitness, but to some major *component of fitness*. For example, this may be the number of mates an individual acquires, or the number of eggs an individual laid, or 1 or 0 depending on the survival or death of an individual over a period of mortality.

(2) Calculate the average fitness, by summing the fitness of each individual in the sample, and dividing by the total number of individuals in the sample.

(3) Divide each individual's fitness value by the average fitness. The purpose of steps (2) and (3) is to scale each individual's relative fitness value such that average relative fitness in the sample is $1\cdot0$. The covariance of relative fitness with each character is then equal to the selection differential (Price 1970); this is the simplest way to estimate the selection differential when there are more than two fitness classes. (Note that the measure of relative fitness used here is different from that used on p. 264. When discussing evolution at single loci, it is more informative to scale relative fitness such that the *maximum* relative fitness is $1\cdot0$; this contrasts with the *average* fitness scaled to $1\cdot0$, as used here).

(4) Regress the relative fitness values obtained on the measured characters as the independent variables. Partial-regression coefficients for each character are the change in relative fitness that would occur per unit change in the character, statistically holding the effects of all other characters fixed. The vector of partial-regression coefficients is equal to the directional selection gradient.

(5) To measure the forces of stabilizing or disruptive selection the squared value of each character is included in the regression together with all paired cross-products. For two characters only (x and y) in the analysis we have the regression,

$$w = c + \beta_1 x + \beta_2 y \tag{1}$$

to estimate coefficients of directional selection, and the regression,

$$w = c + \beta'_1 x + \beta'_2 y + \tfrac{1}{2}\gamma_{11}x^2 + \tfrac{1}{2}\gamma_{22}y^2 + \gamma_{12}xy \tag{2}$$

to estimate coefficients of stabilizing selection. In these equations w is the relative fitness, c is a constant term, the βs are coefficients of directional selection, and the γs are coefficients of stabilizing selection. If the distribution of the characters in the regression (apart from the dependent variable, fitness) is not multivariate normal (i.e. there is some skewness in the data, as will often be the case), the directional selection coefficients (β'_1) and (β'_2) in equation (2) will not be equivalent to the directional selection coefficients in the selection gradient, as estimated from equation (1), and should be ignored unless steps have been taken to correct for deviations from multivariate normality (see Appendix in Lande and Arnold (1983)).

When the sign(s) of the stabilizing selection coefficient(s) $(\gamma_{11}, \gamma_{22})$ is (are) negative, there is stabilizing selection; otherwise there is disruptive selection influencing the character. Consider, for example, the distribution of a character centred at zero by the subtraction of the sample mean. Squared character values will then be large and positive for individuals in either tail of the distribution. Stabilizing selection (low fitness in the tails of the distribution) would therefore be measured as a negative correlation of fitness with these squared values, and disruptive selection (high fitness in the tails) as a positive correlation. Regression coefficients for x^2 and y^2 have to be doubled to give estimates as they appear in equations for the evolution of variances and covariances. The "correlating selection" coefficient (γ_{12}) is a measure of the extent to which there is selection to increase or decrease the correlation between two characters.

The coefficients of the stabilizing selection gradient are a measure of the fitness surface (for example, the selection curves in Fig. 4). If the characters follow a multivariate normal distribution, the tangent to this surface pointing in the steepest upward direction at the joint mean value for all characters is the directional selection gradient. Thus the coefficients of directional and stabilizing selection describe an adaptive surface in the vicinity of the population's multivariate mean. We illustrate this below with an example.

Techniques of regression can be used to estimate coefficients of directional and stabilizing selection, but there are several difficulties with the assessment of statistical significance and interpretation.

4.6   Statistical testing

Measurements of fitness may be almost continuous (e.g. survival of fledglings from hatching in weeks) or highly discontinuous, as in the case of selection associated with mortality when there are just two fitness classes: those surviving and those not. Assumptions for testing the significance of regression coefficients require an expected normal distribution of errors from the regression line, with constant variance for all values of the independent variables. When there are few fitness classes, this is clearly violated. One way to avoid the problem is to assess significance using probit analysis (Finney 1971), which uses maximum likelihood to best separate groups (this analysis may be used only for statistical testing, and not to obtain coefficients).

When fitness falls into several classes, significance of selection differentials may be assessed by correlations between fitness and each character. (The correlation analysis should be non-parametric if the assumption of normality for the distribution of either variable is violated. However, transformation of data may allow parametric analysis.) When fitness falls into two or a few classes, *t*-tests, or ANOVAs (or their non-parametric equivalents) should be used in comparisons among the classes, to assess significance of selection differentials.

A classic problem with the interpretation of partial-regression coefficients arises when the independent variables are highly correlated (multi-collinearity) (Snedecor and Cochran 1980, Sokal and Rohlf 1981). Few statisticians agree on what "highly correlated" means in this context, but caution is probably warranted if more than 25% of the entries in a correlation matrix lie within ± 0.8–0.99. In such cases, a significant difference between partial regression coefficients can be so interpreted, but it is difficult to compare strengths of selection among coefficients that do not significantly differ, because the magnitudes of the coefficients are highly susceptible to small changes in the data. Multicollinearity among the independent variables can be reduced through use of principal components or the omission of one or more variables (Lande and Arnold 1983).

Another statistical problem comes from the assumption that the regressions of the independent variables are approximately linear and homoscedastic on each other. For example, suppose that the regression of beak length on beak depth in Fig. 3 was actually curvilinear. The selection restricted to beak depth (Fig. 3 (*a*)) would be accompanied by a correlated response in beak length to a mean position that would lie off the linear-regression line, and there would be a non-zero partial-regression coefficient of fitness on beak length. The assumption of linearity is best tested by regressing one independent variable on the others and plotting the residuals from the regression against the predicted values of the dependent variable. Often simple transformations of the data can result in near-bivariate linearity. Thus it is traditional to take the logarithm ($\log_e$) of morphological measurements prior to analysis, after first reducing the characters to a common dimensionality, for instance by taking the cube root of weights or volume measurements.

4.7 Missing characters

This technique can only disentangle the effects of direct and correlated responses to selection among the characters included in the analysis. Further inclusion of an important variable may completely alter the relationships among all the characters. It is necessary to appeal to both biological and statistical reasoning to interpret partial-regression coefficients in any analysis.

Finally, a problem can arise when too many characters are included in the analysis, in that the power of the statistical tests rapidly decreases. Two positively correlated characters may both be under selection to increase, but the detection of any significant selection at all may depend on the exclusion of one of the characters. Furthermore, large numbers of characters may require large sample sizes; this is particularly true for the calculation of stabilizing selection coefficients, where the number of coefficients is greatly increased by the square and product terms (Lande and Arnold 1983). Thus in a full analysis, the expected number of coefficients is $\frac{1}{2}(p^2 + 3p)$, where p is the number of correlated characters measured; the sample size (N) should greatly exceed the total number of coefficients being estimated.

4.8 Comparing selection intensities

The partial-regression coefficients, as measures of the intensity of selection, are best compared by transforming all the independent variables to standard-deviation units. This is because, under truncation selection, and with a normal distribution for each character, a given selection differential in standard-deviation units results from a given proportion of the population being culled (Falconer 1981); thus it gives a direct measure of the selective mortality. Standardization can be accomplished by transforming the data such that they have unit variance before analysis, or by multiplying the regression coefficient by the standard deviation of the character (see Lande and Arnold 1983).

Measurement error inflates phenotypic variances but will not affect covariances if randomized over phenotypes. Therefore it will lower the partial-regression coefficients, which are ratios of covariances to variances. If measurement error varies among traits it may be difficult to compare directly the partial-regression coefficients. An estimate of the measurement error variance can be obtained by making multiple measurements on the same individual and calculating repeatabilities (see chapter 2; Falconer 1981), and the magnitude of the partial-regression coefficients can be adjusted accordingly. However, statistical testing becomes more difficult, and it is also important to ensure that the measurement "error" is not also included in the

Table 3. The correlation matrix for the morphological measurements (log-transformed data; $N = 640$). A correlation of $r = 0.08$ is significant ($P < 0.05$). Principal components were extracted from the covariance matrix of the log-transformed variables (the cube root of weight was first taken). The phenotypic variance for each character is given on the diagonal, after being multiplied by 100. PC1 accounted for 67·9% of the total variance, and PC2 for a further 19·8%

		1	2	3	4	5	6	7	8	9
Weight (g^{-3})	1	0·11								
Wing (mm)	2	0·67	0·13							
Tarsus (mm)	3	0·58	0·52	0·16						
Beak length (mm)	4	0·69	0·55	0·55	0·16					
Beak depth (mm)	5	0·72	0·60	0·52	0·86	0·77				
Beak width (mm)	6	0·75	0·63	0·55	0·80	0·89	0·48			
LA4 (mm)*	7	−0·31	−0·30	−0·15	−0·19	−0·47	−0·46	0·68		
PC1	8	0·78	0·67	0·58	0·87	0·97	0·94	−0·57	1·91	
PC2	9	0·16	0·09	0·25	0·40	0·09	0·08	0·82	0·00	0·56

* LA4 is beak length at a depth of 4 mm, a measure of beak pointedness (Boag 1983).

variation as perceived by a selective agent. Unless repeatabilities differ greatly among traits it may be best not to correct for measurement error.

4.9 Comparing selection episodes

Draper and Smith (1981) give a method for comparing two multiple regressions statistically, and a similar method can be applied using probit analysis. The procedure has low power, and significant differences require striking differences in the partial-regression coefficients and/or very large samples.

5 SELECTION ON WILD POPULATIONS OF DARWIN'S FINCHES

Between 1975 and 1977 one of us (P.T.B., in collaboration with P. R. Grant) banded and measured a large number of Medium Ground Finches on Isla Daphne Major in the Galápagos. In a drought in 1977, many of these finches died, and the mortality was accompanied by directional selection for large size. Boag and Grant (1981) describe the ecological circumstances, and the evidence that the selection was a result of mortality due to starvation. The correlation matrix for the seven measured variables is given in Table 3 together with phenotypic variances. The population is variable, with some morphological measurements having coefficients of variation of up to 9% (Grant and Price 1981). An analysis of the selection is presented in Table 4. Survivors were significantly larger than those dying, for all characters except beak length at a depth of 4 mm, which is negatively correlated with measures of body size (Table 3). The selection gradient shows that the direct targets of selection for increased size were body weight and beak depth. There was some selection for a stubbier beak, and most surprisingly beak width was selected to *decrease*—in the opposite direction to the selection differential.

The results of omitting characters from the analysis are shown in columns 3–6 of Table 4. The exclusion of characters under weak or no selection (wing, tarsus and beak length) has little effect on the partial-regression coefficients, and may aid interpretation. If weight and beak width only are included in the analysis, a negative partial-regression coefficient for beak width is not observed; selection favouring a relatively narrower beak appears to be largely with respect to beak depth. This shows how significant countervailing selection on beak width would not have been observed if beak depth had not been measured.

Are there characters that were not measured which could affect the results? The seven characters appear to summarize much of the size and shape

Table 4. Standardized directional selection differentials (*s*) and standardized directional selection gradients (*β*) for *G. fortis* associated with mortality over the drought of 1977 on Daphne Major, Galápagos. Original measurements were in g for weight, mm for the other characters. The measurements were log-transformed, and separately standardized to have zero mean and unit variance. Columns 3 to 6 give the selection gradients when only a subset of the characters are included in the analysis. The sample size was $N = 640$. 97 individuals survived the drought. The dependent variable (relative fitness) thus has values of zero (for individuals dying) or $640/97 = 6.6$ for individuals surviving. Significance of the selection differentials was assessed by *t*-tests comparing survivors with dead, and of the selection gradients by probit analysis.

	s	β	β	β	β	β
Weight	0·62**	0·46**	0·51**	0·58**	—	0·49**
Wing	0·50**	0·13	—	—	—	—
Tarsus	0·36**	−0·01	—	—	—	—
Beak length	0·49**	−0·03	—	—	—	—
Beak depth	0·61**	0·57*	0·60**	—	0·82**	0·69**
Beak width	0·49**	−0·57**	−0·54**	0·05	−0·24	−0·49*
LA4 (mm)	−0·42**	−0·22	−0·22*	—	—	—

* $P < 0.05$.
** $P < 0.01$.

variation within populations (Boag 1984) and between species (Grant *et al.* 1985). Thus, much of the selection on morphology may be summarized by our measurements. There may also have been selection on other correlated characters, for example behavioural and physiological variables (e.g. territory size or blackness of male plumage; see Price 1984), and this selection may directly account for some of the observed selection on morphology and would alter the partial-regression coefficients if included. Nevertheless, the resolution of the pattern of selection pressures within the morphological data allows us to interpret these pressures functionally.

The selection favouring relatively narrower beaks is surprising, and it is important to investigate the assumptions of the regression further. A scatterplot of beak width against beak depth did not suggest any non-linearity in the regression of one character on the other. More convincingly, a scatter of the residuals from a regression of beak width on the other six characters shows no pattern (Fig. 5). Thus the selection to decrease beak width appears to be a real phenomenon.

Selection to increase beak depth and body weight cannot be distinguished from selection to increase either beak depth or body weight or both, or a character with which these characters are both correlated. The identification of beak depth as a probable selection target supports the hypothesis that seed-cracking ability was an important selective force in an environment

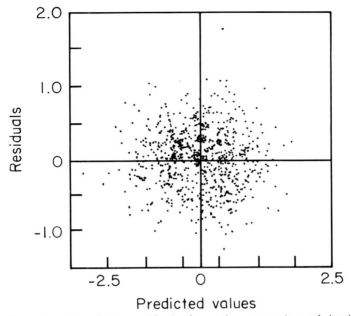

Fig. 5. A scatterplot of the residuals from the regression of beak width (dependent variable) on body weight, wing, tarsus, beak length, beak depth and beak length at a depth of 4 mm (independent variables), all in standard-deviation units. The samples are as in Table 2.

where large seeds remained disproportionately common (Boag and Grant 1981). The partial-regression coefficient for beak width, which is significantly different from those for beak depth and weight, may also be associated with fruit- and seed-cracking ability (Price *et al.* 1984 b). The discovery of these targets of selection suggests further experiments to investigate the function of the beak in feeding.

An analysis of stabilizing selection is very difficult to interpret with a large number of characters. The first two principal components (PC1 and PC2) from the covariance matrix of log-transformed variables (Table 3) were used. PC1 provides a summary measure of overall size, while PC2 measures beak pointedness and length (Table 3). PC1 and PC2 were first separately standardized to have zero mean and unit variance. The regression equations were then,

$$w = 1 \cdot 00 + 0 \cdot 61 \, \text{PC1}** - 0 \cdot 08 \, \text{PC2} \tag{3}$$

and

$$w = 0 \cdot 83 + 0 \cdot 64 \, \text{PC1}** - 0 \cdot 06 \, \text{PC2} + 0 \cdot 22 \, (\text{PC1})^{2}** \\ - 0 \cdot 05 \, (\text{PC2})^{2} + 0 \cdot 04 \, \text{PC1} \times \text{PC2} \tag{4}$$

where w is relative fitness, and "**" indicates the regression coefficient is significant at $P < 0.01$. The positive coefficients for PC1 and (PC1)^2 ($\gamma_{11} = 0.44$) indicates strong directional and disruptive selection on PC1 only.

These results can be rather completely pictured in the form of a three-dimensional fitness surface (Fig. 6). The surface is exactly given by equation (4). The joint mean of the population lies to one side of a valley. The directional selection gradient is approximately equal to the tangent to the

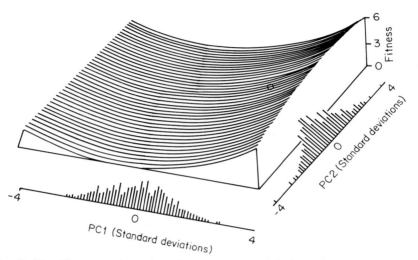

Fig. 6. The fitness surface, based on equation (4) for PC1 and PC2. The frequency distributions of the two characters are shown approximately, and the joint mean position (O) on the fitness surface.

fitness surface, pointing in the steepest upward direction at this mean position (if it were exactly given by the tangent, the coefficients for PC1 and PC2 in equations (3) (4) would be the same). This demonstrates strong selection to increase PC1, arising because the population is on the side of an adaptive peak. There was no significant selection on PC2, or to correlate PC1 and PC2. The surface very gently slopes in the plane of PC2, indicating that there is little variance in fitness among individuals that vary in this character.

The results for PC1 show how the variance can change as a result of both directional and disruptive selection. The variance of PC1 before selection was 1.0 and after selection 0.94, and the difference in variance between survivors and dead was not significant by Levene's test (Van Valen 1978). The significant disruptive selection to increase the variance was effectively countered by directional selection which decreased the variance.

6 SUMMARY AND CONCLUSIONS

Our example illustrates some of the diverse applications of selection studies. The adaptive significance of beak depth/body size and beak width over a drought has been clearly demonstrated and suggests how behavioural and physiological experiments might profitably be organized. The observation of disruptive selection provides part of the explanation for the high levels of morphological variation found in this population (Grant and Price 1981), and the relatively small mean size of *G. fortis* on Daphne (Schluter *et al.* 1985). This selection can be related to the feeding ability of different-sized individuals, and changes in the quantity and quality of food available in the environment. Body size of *G. fortis* is heritable (Boag 1983). Thus, much of the genetic variance in probability of adult mortality can be attributed to body size, and covariance with other life history traits can be determined by measuring selection on body size at other life stages (Price and Grant 1984). Finally the role of selection in the adaptive radiation of Darwin's Finches is better substantiated (Price *et al.* 1984 a).

This is not to say that the Lande–Arnold (1983) approach is the last word in selection analysis. Earlier we suggested that it had the advantage of linking selection analysis to a model for the evolution of continuous traits. Yet several assumptions underlying their model for the evolution of quantitative genetics traits, such as the ability of mutation to maintain polygenic variation (Turelli 1984), the stability of genetic variance–covariance matrices over evolutionary time (Lande 1979), and the assumption that genetic values, in particular, follow the multivariate normal distribution, remain controversial. There are practical problems as well. Evolutionary applications of the approach depend on one's being able to estimate heritabilities and the genetic correlation structure of characters in natural populations; the correlations in particular are notoriously difficult to estimate accurately under even the most ideal laboratory conditions (Falconer 1981, Dingle and Hegmann 1982). Coupled with this are other problems which we described earlier in this chapter, such as the need to choose the right type and number of characters for analysis, to be able to acquire very large sample sizes for all but the simplest situations, and to be able to place the selection process under study in its proper perspective within the entire life cycle of the species in question. In this regard, Arnold and Wade (1984 a,b) have recently described methods for partitioning selection taking place at more than one stage of an organism's life cycle. Other extensions of the methodology might include alternative curve-fitting algorithms given that the linear or parabolic fitness functions assumed here may not always match observed fitness functions precisely (e.g. Fig. 10 in Boag and Grant 1984).

Ornithologists are becoming increasingly aware of the need to mark, measure and follow the fates of individuals. If the problems of accurately measuring traits of potentially high repeatability and controlling for emigration can be satisfactorily resolved, studies of selection are likely to be increasingly applied to problems such as those outlined above. Careful measurement of selection in natural populations, coupled with functional analyses of the relationship between character variation and performance (Bock 1980, Arnold 1983) will help add rigour to the study of adaptation in avian evolutionary biology (Lewontin 1979, Wake 1982).

ACKNOWLEDGMENTS

We thank S. J. Arnold, B. R. Grant, P. R. Grant and R. Lande for much discussion. A. J. van Noordwijk, L. M. Ratcliffe, D. Schluter and C. S. Findlay provided constructive criticism of the manuscript. Our studies on Darwin's Finches were supported by a grant from the National Science and Engineering Research Council of Canada (NSERC) to P.R.G., and a grant from the Chapman Fund to P.T.B. P.T.B. is currently funded by NSERC operating grant U-0315.

REFERENCES

Alatalo, R. V. and Lundberg, A. (1986). Heritability and selection on tarsus length in the Pied Flycatcher (*Fidecula hypoleuca*). *Evolution* **40**, 574–583.

Arnold, S. J. (1983). Morphology, performance and fitness. *Am. Zool.* **23**, 347–361.

Arnold, S. J. and Wade, M. J. (1984 a). On the measurement of natural and sexual selection: Theory. *Evolution* **38**, 709–719.

Arnold, S. J. and Wade, M. J. (1984 b). On the measurement of natural and sexual selection: Applications. *Evolution* **38**, 720–734.

Baker, M. C. and Fox, S. F. (1978 a). Dominance, survival, and enzyme polymorphism in dark-eyed juncos, *Junco hyemalis*. *Evolution* **32**, 697–711.

Baker, M. C. and Fox, S. F. (1978 b). Differential survival in common grackles sprayed with Turgitol. *Am. Natur.* **112**, 675–682.

Boag, P. T. (1983). The heritability of external morphology in Darwin's Ground Finches (*Geospiza*) on Isla Daphne Major, Galápagos. *Evolution* **37**, 877–894.

Boag, P. T. (1984). Growth and allometry of external morphology in Darwin's finches (*Geospiza*) on Isla Daphne Major, Galápagos. *J. Zool.* **204**, 413–441.

Boag, P. T. and Grant, P. R. (1981). Intense natural selection in a population of Darwin's finches (Geospizinae) in the Galápagos. *Science* **214**, 82–85.

Boag, P. T. and Grant, P. R. (1984). The classical case of character release: Darwin's finches (*Geospiza*) on Isla Daphne Major, Galápagos. *Biol. J. Linn. Soc.* **22**, 243–287.

Bock, W. J. (1980). The definition and recognition of biological adaptation. *Am. Zool.* **20**, 217–227.

Brun, E. (1971). Change in dimorph-ratio of bridled guillemots (*Uria aalge*) on Bear Island. *Astarte* **4**, 1–6.

Bumpus, H. C. (1898). The elimination of the unfit as illustrated by the introduced sparrow *Passer domesticus*. Biological Lectures No. 11, The Marine Biological Laboratory, Woods Hole.

Cavalli-Sforza, L. L. and Bodmer, W. F. (1971). "The Genetics of Human Populations". W. H. Freeman & Co., San Francisco.

Cooch, F. G. (1961). Ecological aspects of the blue-snow goose complex. *Auk* **78**, 72–89.

Cooke, F. and Findlay, C. S. (1982). Polygenic variation and stabilizing selection in a wild population of Lesser Snow Geese (*Anser caerulescens caerulescens*). *Am. Natur.* **120**, 543–547.

Cooke, F., Findlay, C. S., Rockwell, R. F. and Smith, J. A. (1985). Life history studies of the lesser snow goose (*Answer caerulescens caerulescens*). III. The selective value of plumage polymorphism: Net Fecundity. *Evolution* **39**, 165–177.

Crow, J. F. and Kimura, M. (1970). "An Introduction to Population Genetics Theory". Harper & Row, New York.

Dhondt, A. A., Eyckeman, R. and Hublé, J. (1979). Will great tits become little tits? *Biol. J. Linn. Soc.* **11**, 289–294.

Dingle, H. and Hegmann, J. P. (1982). "Evolution and Genetics of Life Histories". Springer-Verlag, New York.

Draper, N. R. and Smith, H. (1981). "Applied Regression Analysis". 2nd edn. Wiley, New York.

Endler, J. A. (1973). Gene flow and population differentiation. *Science* **179**, 243–250.

Endler, J. A. (1986). "Natural Selection in the Wild". Princeton University Press.

Falconer, D. S. (1981). "Introduction to Quantitative Genetics". 2nd edition. Longman, London.

Felsentein, J. (1979). Excursions along the interface between disruptive and stabilizing selection. *Genetics* **93**, 773–795.

Finney, D. J. (1971). "Probit Analysis". 3rd edn. Cambridge University Press.

Fleischer, R. C. and Johnston, R. F. (1982). Natural selection on body size and proportions in house sparrows. *Nature* **298**, 747–749.

Flux, J. E. C. and Flux, M. M. (1982). Artificial selection and gene flow in wild starlings, *Sturnus vulgaris*. *Naturwissenschaften* **69**, 96–97.

Geramita, J. M., Cooke, F. and Rockwell, R. F. (1982). Assortative mating and gene flow in the lesser snow goose: a modelling approach. *Theoret. Pop. Biol.* **22**, 177–203.

Grant, B. R. (1985). Selection on bill characters in a population of Darwin's finches: *Geospiza conirostris* on Isla Genovesa, Galápagos. *Evolution* **39**, 523–532.

Grant, P. R., Abbott, I., Schluter, D., Curry, R. L. and Abbott, L. K. (1985). Variation in the size and shape of Darwin's finches. *Biol. J. Linn. Soc.* **23**, 1–39.

Grant, P. R. and Price, T. D. (1981). Population variation in continuously varying traits as an ecological genetics question. *Am. Zool.* **21**, 795–811.

Gyllensten, U. (1985). Temporal allozyme frequency changes in density fluctuating populations of Willow grouse (*Lagopus lagopus* L.) *Evolution* **39**, 115–121.

Haldane, J. B. S. (1954). The measurement of natural selection. *Proc. IX Intl Cong. Genet.* **1**, 480–487.

Järvinen, O. and Vepsäläinen, K. (1973). Intensity of selection in bridled guillemots (*Uria aalge*) on Bear Island. *Astarte* **6**, 35–41.

Jeffries, D. J. and Parslow, L. J. F. (1976). The genetics of bridling in guillemots from a study of hand-reared birds. *J. Zool.* **179**, 411–420.

Johnson, C. (1976). "Introduction to Natural Selection". University Park Press, Baltimore.

Johnson, D. M., Stewart, G. L., Corley, M., Ghrist, R., Hagner, J., Ketterer, A., McDonnell, B., Newsom, W., Owen, E. and Samuels, P. (1980). Brown-headed Cowbird (*Molothrus ater*) mortality in an urban winter roost. *Auk* **97**, 299–320.

Johnston, R. F. and Fleischer, R. C. (1981). Overwinter mortality and sexual size dimorphism in the house sparrow. *Auk* **98**, 503–511.

Johnston, R. F., Niles, D. M. and Rohwer, S. A. (1972). Herman Bumpus and natural selection in the house sparrow *Passer domesticus*. *Evolution* **26**, 20–31.

Lande, R. (1979). Quantitative genetic analysis of multivariate evolution, applied to brain:body size allometry. *Evolution* **33**, 402–416.

Lande, R. (1980). The genetic covariance between characters maintained by pleiotropic mutations. *Genetics* **94**, 203–215.

Lande, R. (1982). A quantitative genetic theory of life history evolution. *Ecology* **63**, 607–615.

Lande, R. and Arnold, S. J. (1983). The measurement of selection on correlated characters. *Evolution* **37**, 1210–1226.

Lewontin, R. C. (1979). Sociobiology as an adaptationist program. *Behav. Sci.* **24**, 1–10.

Lowther, P. E. (1977). Selection intensity in North American house sparrows (*Passer domesticus*). *Evolution* **32**, 649–656.

Lucotte, G. and Kaminski, M. (1978). Biochemical homeostasis of the heterozygote at the lysozyme locus in Japanese quail. *Biochem. Syst. Ecol.* **6**, 145–147.

Manly, B. F. J. (1976). Some examples of double exponential fitness functions. *Heredity* **36**, 228–234.

Manly, B. F. J. (1985). "The Statistics of Natural Selection". Chapman & Hall, London.

Manly, B. F. J., Miller, P. and Cook, L. M. (1972). Analysis of a selective predation experiment. *Am. Natur.* **106**, 719–736.

O'Donald, P. (1970). Change of fitness by selection for a quantitative character. *Theor. Pop. Biol.* **1**, 219–232.

O'Donald, P. (1973). A further analysis of Bumpus' data: the intensity of natural selection. *Evolution* **27**, 398–404.

O'Donald, P. (1983). "The Arctic Skua". Cambridge University Press.

Price, G. R. (1970). Selection and covariance. *Nature* **227**, 520–521.

Price, T. D. (1984). Sexual selection on body size, territory and plumage variables in a population of Darwin's finches. *Evolution* **38**, 327–341.

Price, T. D. and Grant, P. R. (1984). Life history traits and natural selection for small body size in a population of Darwin's finches. *Evolution* **38**, 483–494.

Price, T. D., Grant, P. R. and Boag, P. T. (1984a). Genetic changes in the morphological differentiation of Darwin's Ground finches. *In* "Population Biology and Evolution" (Eds K. Wöhrmann and V. Löschke), pp. 49–66. Springer-Verlag, Berlin.

Price, T. D., Grant, P. R., Gibbs, H. L. and Boag, P. T. (1984b). Recurrent patterns of natural selection in a population of Darwin's finches. *Nature* **309**, 787–789.

Redfield, J. A. (1973). Demography and genetics in colonizing populations of Blue grouse (*Dendragapus obscurus*). *Evolution* **27**, 576–592.

Rising, J. D. (1970). Age and seasonal variation in dimensions of the house sparrow,

Passer domesticus (L.) from a single population in Kansas. *In* "Productivity, Population Dynamics and Systematics of Granivorous Birds". (Eds S. C. Kendeigh and J. Pinowsky), Institute of Ecology, Dziekanow, Poland.

Rockwell, R. F., Findlay, C. S., Cooke, F. and Smith, J. A. (1985). Life history studies of the lesser show goose (*Anser caerulescens caerulescens*). IV. The selective value of plumage polymorphism: Net viability, the timing of maturation, and breeding propensity. *Evolution* **39**, 178–189.

Rose, M. R. (1983). Theories of life history evolution. *Am. Zool.* **23**, 15–23.

Ross, H. A. and McLaren, I. A. (1981). Lack of differential survival among young Ipswich Sparrows. *Auk* **98**, 495–502.

Schluter, D., Price, T. D. and Grant, P. R. (1985). Ecological character displacement in Darwin's finches. *Science* **227**, 1056–1059.

Schluter, D. and Smith, J. N. M. (1986). Natural selection on beak and body size in the Song Sparrow. *Evolution* **40**, 221–231.

Searcy, W. A. (1979a). Size and mortality in male yellow-headed blackbirds. *Condor* **81**, 304–305.

Searcy, W. A. (1979 b). Sexual selection and body size in male red-winged blackbirds. *Evolution* **33**, 649–661.

Searcy, W. A. and Yasukawa, K. (1981). Sexual size dimorphism and survival of male and female blackbirds (Icteridae). *Auk* **98**, 457–465.

Smith, J. N. M. (1987). Determinants of lifetime reproductive success in the song sparrow. *In* "Lifetime Reproductive Success" (ed. T. H. Clutton-Brock). University of Chicago Press.

Smith, J. N. M. and Zach, R. (1979). Heritability of some morphological characters in a Song sparrow population. *Evolution* **33**, 460–467.

Snedecor, G. W. and Cochran, W. G. (1980). "Statistical Methods". 8th edn. Iowa State Press, Ames.

Sokal, R. R. and Rohlf, F. J. (1981). "Biometry". 2nd edn. Freeman, San Francisco.

Turelli, M. (1984). Heritable genetic variation via mutation–selection balance: Lerch's zeta meets the abdominal bristle. *Theor. Pop. Biol.* **25**, 138–193.

van Noordwijk, A. J., van Balen, J. H. and Scharloo, W. (1981a). Genetic and environmental variation in clutch size of the Great tit *Parus major*. *Neth. J. Zool.* **31**, 342–372.

van Noordwijk, A. J., van Balen, J. H. and Scharloo, W. (1981 b). Genetic variation in the timing of reproduction in the Great tit. *Oecologia* **49**, 158–166.

Van Valen, L. (1965). Selection in natural populations. III. Measurement and estimation. *Evolution* **19**, 514–528.

Van Valen, L. (1978). The statistics of variation. *Evol. Theory* **4**, 33–43.

Wake, D. B. (1982). Functional and evolutionary morphology. *Persp. Biol. Med.* **25**, 603–620.

Weatherhead, P. J., Greenwood, H. and Clark, R. G. (1984). On the use of avian mortality patterns to test sexual selection theory. *Auk* **101**, 134–139.

9

Non-random Mating: A Theoretical and Empirical Overview with Special Reference to Birds

C. Scott Findlay†

Department of Biology, Queen's University, Kingston, Ontario, Canada K7L 3N6

†Present address: Departments of Zoology and Medicine, University of Toronto, Toronto, Ontario, Canada M5S 1A1.

AVIAN GENETICS
ISBN 0-12-187570-9

1   INTRODUCTION

Random models are invariably used as first approximations to the behaviour of many natural systems. The concept figures prominently in two phenomena of particular interest to population geneticists: genetic drift ("random walk") and random mating. Genetic drift is discussed in Chapters 4 and 7. What follows is an introduction to the general topic of mating paradigms that violate the randomness ideal, namely, systems of non-random mating.

In this chapter, I present an operational definition of the phenomenon, and a simple analytical classification of systems of non-random mating. Secondly, I outline the expected influence of these systems on the genetic composition of populations. Here, I draw heavily on previous general treatments of the subject, notably the excellent volumes by Karlin (1969), Crow and Kimura (1970), Cavalli-Sforza and Bodmer (1971), Jacquard (1974) and Bulmer (1980). Thirdly, I provide some empirical examples of non-random mating in natural populations, paying particular (although not exclusive) attention to avian studies. Finally, I include a representative bibliography concerned with both theoretical and empirical aspects of non-random mating.

2   NON-RANDOM MATING

2.1   Definition

While the observation that individuals do not mate randomly with respect to particular traits is not new, to my knowledge there is no clear definition of what exactly constitutes non-random mating. This may, of course, reflect the general belief that the definition is implicit to the term itself, and so defined, the concept is sufficiently nebulous as to be of negligible empirical utility. In view of the latter, there is an overwhelming tendency for investigators to define (or more precisely, to redefine) the term in the context of their own studies.

At the empirical level, the question appears to be not "What is non-random mating?", but rather "How do I know when it is present?" The term is applied to those situations in which the observed frequencies of various mating combinations cannot be predicted solely from the joint distribution of male and female phenotypes or genotypes. Suppose, for example, we observe a population comprising two distinct phenotypes (A, B) at relative frequencies (f_A, f_B) in both sexes. If mating is random with respect to the trait determining A and B, we predict that

$$\text{Freq}(A \times A) = f_A^2$$
$$\text{Freq}(A \times B) = 2f_A f_B \quad \text{(since we may have } A\female \times B\male \text{ or } B\female \times A\male \text{)}$$
$$\text{Freq}(B \times B) = f_B^2$$

that is, mating combinations occur in standard binomial proportions. If observed frequencies deviate from these proportions, we can legitimately conclude that there exists some element of non-random mating in the system. (I must here add the caveat that failure to demonstrate significant deviations from binomial proportions is, unfortunately, *not* sufficient proof of random mating.)

Several points should be made concerning the above definition. First, non-random mating is trait- (or trait complex)-specific. That is, we speak of individuals mating non-randomly *with respect to* one or more characters. Clearly, all individuals in natural populations labour under various constraints that preclude their mating randomly with respect to all phenotypic attributes. When examining populations, therefore, it is reasonable to begin with the premise that mating may well occur randomly with respect to some traits and non-randomly with respect to others. This does not, of course, preclude the possibility that non-random mating can occur simultaneously for two or more traits which may or may not show some phenotypic correlation.

Secondly, the term represents nothing more than a *description* of an empirically observable pattern. Unfortunately, one often encounters situations in which, having demonstrated non-random mating for some trait, researchers (myself included) are tempted to conclude that they have demonstrated, say, female choice. Such conclusions usually exceed the available data; generally, one cannot infer the underlying mechanism solely from population patterns.

Finally, the proposed definition clearly relegates non-random mating to the status of a *population* phenomenon. Populations (except in monoclonal organisms) invariably comprise individuals of diverse genetic and cultural ancestries often exploiting heterogeneous environments. Under such conditions, it is unlikely that all individuals will manifest the same behaviours. Suppose, for example, that we examined a population and found that for some trait there were considerably more matings between phenotypically similar individuals than we would expect by chance alone. Suppose further that we managed to capture some of these creatures, culture them in the laboratory and conduct an experiment which indicated that females prefer to mate with males phenotypically similar to themselves. While this helps to explain the observed population pattern, it cannot be the whole story, in as much as if *all* females always selected mates like themselves, we would never find mated pairs of *dissimilar* phenotypes. Perhaps in the wild some females cannot obtain the males they desire because such males are in short supply. Or maybe some small proportion of females (who remain uncaptured in our original sample) actually prefer males phenotypically *dissimilar* to themselves! In either case, statistical inferences at the population level do not tell the whole story.

2.2   Preference or prevalence?

The detection of non-random mating for a particular trait involves fitting a random model to observed mating frequencies. If the model provides an ill fit, we conclude that there is some element of non-random mating in the system. This procedure appears simple enough, but the onus is on the researcher to provide the *appropriate* null model. Suppose, for example, we have a population comprising N_T individuals of each sex distributed between two niches i and j, with population sizes N_i and N_j, respectively, such that $N_T = N_i + N_j$. The population comprises two phenotypes (A, B) at relative proportions (A_i, B_i) in niche i and (A_j, B_j) in niche j, with phenotype frequencies assumed equal for each sex. Individuals mate randomly within each niche, so that the observed frequencies of the three mating types (A × A, A × B, B × B) are as given in Table 1. The frequencies of A and B individuals in the *total* population are

$$\text{Freq}(A) = (A_iN_i + A_jN_j)/N_T,$$
$$\text{Freq}(B) = (B_iN_i + B_jN_j)/N_T, \tag{1}$$

Suppose we failed to realize the population was structured and blithely calculated expected mating frequencies based on the overall (total) frequency of the two phenotypes, i.e.

$$\text{Freq}(A \times A)_E = A^2 = [(A_iN_i + A_jN_j)/N_T]^2,$$
$$\text{Freq}(A \times B)_E = 2AB = 2[(A_iN_i + A_jN_j)/N_T][(B_iN_i + B_jN_j)/N_T], \tag{2}$$
$$\text{Freq}(B \times B)_E = B^2 = [(B_iN_i + B_jN_j)/N_T]^2$$

From Table 1, our observed mating-type frequencies are

$$\text{Freq}(A \times A)_0 = (A_i^2 N_i + A_j^2 N_j)/N_T,$$
$$\text{Freq}(A \times B)_0 = 2(A_iB_iN_i + A_jB_jN_j)/N_T, \tag{3}$$
$$\text{Freq}(B \times B)_0 = (B_i^2 N_i + B_j^2 N_j)/N_T.$$

Under what circumstances are the observed and expected mating frequencies equal? Setting, say, $\text{Freq}(A \times A)_0 = \text{Freq}(A \times A)_E$ we have

$$\frac{(A_iN_i + A_jN_j)^2}{N_T} = \frac{(A_i^2N_i + A_j^2N_j)}{N_T},$$

which eventually reduces to

$$A_i^2 + A_j^2 = 2A_iA_j,$$

or more simply

$$A_i = A_j = A \qquad B_i = B_j = B.$$

Hence, unless phenotype frequencies are constant from niche to niche, it is inappropriate to use global phenotype frequencies in order to generate the

Table 1. Observed frequencies and numbers of each mating type for a dimorphic population occupying two niches (i, j)

Mating type	Niche i		Niche j	
	Frequency	Number of matings	Frequency	Number of matings
A × A	A_i^2	$A_i^2 N_i$	A_j^2	$A_j^2 N_j$
A × B	$2A_i B_i$	$2A_i B_i N_i$	$2A_j B_j$	$2A_j B_j N_j$
B × B	B_i^2	$B_i^2 N_i$	B_j^2	$B_j^2 N_j$

expected proportions of each mating type under random mating. Clearly, homogeneity across niches is a rather restrictive condition. As such, it is possible to observe significant deviations from binomial proportions which arise not from mating *preferences* but rather from spatiotemporal variation in the distribution of various phenotypes.

Traditionally, avian researchers have underplayed the "prevalence" (Cooke *et al.* 1976) hypothesis in deference to the "preference" hypothesis. There are, however, several exceptions. Coulson and Thomas (1983), for example, concluded that the observed non-random mating for age in Black-legged Kittiwake (*Rissa tridactyla*) was most readily explained by differential availability rather than true mating preferences. Similarly, patterns of non-random mating for plumage coloration in Lesser Snow Geese (*Anser caerulescens caerulescens*) are at least partially attributable to clinal variation in phenotype frequencies during the period of pair formation (Cooke 1978). It cannot be overemphasized that mating preferences can be inferred from population data only when the distribution of phenotypes (or genotypes) among mated pairs is a non-random sample of the distribution of available mates *when and where mating occurs*. Even then our troubles are not over, because it is entirely possible that the preferences are based on some correlated character rather than the character we are concerned with. Given these ambiguities (which are inherent to virtually any population-level analysis), a concrete demonstration of true mating preferences for particular characters invariably entails careful laboratory or experimental field work.

3 AN ANALYTICAL CLASSIFICATION OF NON-RANDOM MATING SYSTEMS

Consider a polymorphic trait controlled by a single diallelic autosomal locus. In this simplified model, any system of non-random mating is classified on the basis of a set of assorting parameters which give the proportion of all

Table 2. A generalized one-locus two-allele mating paradigm (after Karlin 1978, p. 285)

Female (♀♀) genotype	Male (♂♂) genotype			
	AA	Aa	aa	R
AA	α_1	α_2	α_3	$1 - \sum_{i=1}^{3} \alpha_i$
Aa	β_1	β_2	β_3	$1 - \sum_{i=1}^{3} \beta_i$
aa	γ_1	γ_2	γ_3	$1 - \sum_{i=1}^{3} \gamma_i$

individuals of a particular genotype (AA, Aa or aa) who prefer mates genotypically AA, Aa or aa (Table 2). For example, from Table 2 we see that the proportion of all individuals genotypically AA who prefer mates genotypically aa is α_3. For each genotype, we must also include a parameter R which specifies the proportion of all individuals of that genotype who have no preference, i.e. mate at random with respect to the locus in question.

Systems of non-random mating (Table 3) can be distinguished by reference to the preference array, as follows.

3.1 Sexual selection/assortative mating

Sexual selection occurs when the probability of an individual selecting a particular type of mate is *independent* of its own phenotype (or genotype) (or, at least, of its *perception* of its own phenotype). Conversely, assortative

Table 3. An analytical classification of systems of non-random mating for a single-locus trait

Level	Classification	Analytic formulation
I	Sexual selection	$\alpha_i = \beta_i = \gamma_i$ for all $i = 1, \ldots, 3$
	Assortative mating	$\alpha_i \neq \beta_i \neq \gamma_i$ for some i
II	Genotypic	E.g. $\alpha_1 = \alpha_2 = \alpha_3$, etc.
	Phenotypic	E.g. $\alpha_1 = \alpha_2 \neq \alpha_3$, etc.
III	Complete	$R_i = 0$ for all $i = $ AA, Aa, aa
	Partial	Some $R_i > 0$
IV	Negative assortative	E.g. $\alpha_1 = 0$, (α_2 and/or α_3) > 0, etc.
	Mixed mating	E.g. α_1, α_2 and/or $\alpha_3 > 0$, etc.
	Positive only	E.g. $\alpha_1 = \alpha$, (α_2, α_3) $= 0$, etc.

mating occurs when individuals assess prospective mates on the basis of some real or perceived similarlity or dissimilarity to their own phenotype or genotype.

3.2   Genotypic/phenotypic

Under a genotypic system of non-random mating, individual *genotypes* are perceived as being different and preferences are genotype-specific. This might, for example, be expected when there are no dominance relations among the various allelic forms such that each genotype produces an individually identifiable phenotype. Phenotypic non-random mating, on the other hand, occurs when individuals are unable (or unwilling) to distinguish between two or more different genotypes because of their similar phenotypes (as would be expected, say, in situations of complete dominance, or when environmental variation tends to obscure genotypic differences).

3.3   Complete/partial

Systems of non-random mating can be classified according to whether they are partial or complete. In the former, all individuals express a preference for a particular genotype or phenotype; that is, there are *no* individuals in the population who mate at random. Alternatively, under partial non-random mating, some individuals do mate randomly with respect to the trait in question.

3.4   Assortative mating: positive, negative, mixed

Finally, any assortative mating system can be classified according to whether there is a tendency of individuals to select mates genotypically (phenotypically) similar to themselves (positive assortment), dissimilar to themselves (negative assortment) or some amalgam thereof (mixed assortment).

The scheme presented in Table 3 is intended to serve only as a general paradigm for distinguishing *analytically* among various systems of non-random mating. Obviously, it is difficult (often impossible) to pigeonhole an empirical system into one or another category. Suppose, for example, we observe a population which, though dominated by homogamous (i.e. AA × AA, aa × aa, etc.) matings, also comprised a number of heterogamous (e.g. AA × aa) matings. While the system is probably not one of complete positive assortment, it is not clear whether we are dealing with partial positive assortment, partial mixed assortment, complete mixed assortment, etc. Only by examining the preferences of the individuals themselves can we ascertain the true nature of the system.

4 NON-RANDOM MATING AND THE GENETIC STRUCTURE OF POPULATIONS: THE SINGLE-LOCUS MODELLING APPROACH

Since the days of Jennings (1916) and Fisher (1918), geneticists have been concerned with the influence of non-random mating on the genetic composition of populations. Originally, theoretical treatments were relatively simple and easily followed (Fisher's 1918 paper being a notable exception). The humble beginnings have, however, spawned a plethora of derivatives examining not only the effects of non-random mating *per se* but also non-random mating in concert with selection, drift, inbreeding depression and related phenomena. Certainly the modelling approach has aided our understanding of how non-random mating can affect genotype frequencies. Yet rarely does a model provide a completely accurate representation of reality. To ensure mathematical tractability, various simplifying assumptions must be made—some are biologically reasonable, others less so. Consequently, models are generally useful in describing only the *qualitative* behaviour of the system. The strength of the analytic approach thus lies not in its *quantitative* predictive power but rather in its heuristic value. While some researchers (e.g. O'Donald and co-workers) have successfully fitted analytic models to observed frequencies of mating combinations in natural populations, we should realize that the procedure involves estimating preference parameters assuming that the underlying model is reasonably correct. Since different mechanisms may generate similar observed mating frequencies, this technique does not allow for an independent assessment of the models' validity. Though a model may adequately *describe* the system in question, it may not provide the correct causal *explanation*. Nevertheless, it is worthwhile to briefly review some analytic investigations of the influence of non-random mating on the genetical structure of populations.

4.1 Models of sexual selection

4.1.1 Under polygamous mating systems with female choice

Suppose (Table 3) we designate α_1, α_2 and α_3 as the proportion of all females in the population who prefer and mate with males genotypically AA, Aa and aa, respectively. Assume further a polygamous mating system, a balanced sex-ratio, complete fertilization of all females and a large (effectively infinite) population with discrete generations. Under these conditions, Karlin (1978) has shown that if all preference parameters are greater than zero, there exists a unique stable equilibrium state in which genotype frequencies conform to standard Hardy–Weinberg proportions. (A stable equilibrium means that if genotype frequencies are perturbed from the equilibrium, they will eventually return to it.) Fixation of the population in the homozygous AA or aa state occurs only if no females prefer aa males in the former, or AA and Aa males in the latter.

Karlin (1978) has also investigated a set of relatively simple models of phenotypic sexual selection combined with viability natural selection, which are particularly relevant to sexual selection in birds. One can, for example, readily imagine a situation in which some male trait (e.g. bright plumage coloration) is attractive to females but nevertheless confers a selective disadvantage, perhaps through enhanced visibility to predators. In this instance, the system evolves towards a unique globally stable polymorphism, *independent* of the natural selection differentials, provided that all preference parameters are greater than zero. When only one phenotype is preferred, natural selection can, under certain conditions, lead to fixation of the *non-preferred* phenotype. Finally, if sexual selection and natural selection operate only within the male sex, the system exhibits a unique polymorphic equilibrium in Hardy–Weinberg proportions. However, if selection acts on both sexes, the equilibrium deviates from Hardy–Weinberg proportions immediately following natural selection but before sexual selection.

4.1.2   Under monogamous mating systems

Polygamy implies that the frequency of males available for mating is unaffected by the frequencies of those who have already mated. In general, this does not hold for monogamous systems, where pair bonds last at least the length of the breeding season. Here, males already paired are removed from the pool of available mates, thereby affecting subsequent mating frequencies.

It is unnecessary here to provide the details of various treatments examining the influence of sexual selection under a monogamous mating system. Those readers interested in the mathematical details should consult O'Donald (1963 a,b, 1967, 1973, 1974, 1977 b, 1978 a,b, 1980 a), Karlin (1978) and Karlin and O'Donald (1979). From these works, the following general conclusions have emerged: irrespective of whether sexual selection is genotypic or phenotypic and whether preferential matings occur first (followed by random matings), or vice versa, the system evolves towards a unique polymorphic equilibrium in Hardy–Weinberg proportions, provided that all preference parameters are greater than zero. In the case where those females with preferences mate before those who are indifferent or ambivalent (i.e. have no preference), the rate of convergence mimics that of the polygamous case. When mating order is reversed (i.e. random mating precedes preferential mating), the convergence rate is reduced relative to the polygamous case.

4.1.3 Evolutionary dynamics of sexual selection

The models described above represent only a portion of a substantial literature examining the evolutionary dynamics of sexual selection on single-locus traits. They were selected because they represent serious attempts to construct analytical models which incorporate parameters of particular interest to avian ecologists, e.g. the type of mating system, the timing of preferential and random matings, etc. Despite these laudable efforts, however, mathematical tractability is (inevitably) ensured only through various simplifying (but ecologically suspect) assumptions (see, for example, Taylor and Williams 1981). Recall, for example, that in Karlin's (1978) model of sexual selection under a polygamous mating system (section IV.*a.a.*) he implicitly assumes that the probability of a particular type of female mating with a particular type of male (i.e. her "preference") is independent of the number of females with which the male has already mated. Yet we know, for example, that in some polygynous systems harem size *does* influence subsequent mating probabilities. Note also that in this model there are no allowances made for the possibility (probability?) that a female possessing an intrinsic preference for, say, a genotypically aa male may abandon her search after some interval and mate with the next encountered male irrespective of his phenotype. One can easily imagine a situation in which some females prefer a male phenotype which is present at low frequencies in the population. If there is a reproductive cost of delayed breeding (e.g. O'Donald 1972 a,b) it is perhaps not in a female's best interest to search indefinitely for a mate of the preferred phenotype. Under these circumstances, we might expect the expression of individual preferences to be, at least to some extent, frequency-dependent.

An attempt to incorporate some element of frequency dependence has been made by O'Donald (1977 b, 1978 b, 1980 a) and Karlin and Raper (1979) (see also Raper *et al.* 1979) through a generalized "encounter" model of mating behaviour. Here, different response thresholds to the courtship of particular male phenotypes determine female mating preferences. Females have a lower threshold to males they prefer. The stimulation to mate is derived through encounters with the opposite sex. Females who prefer a particular type of male require fewer encounters before mating with these males, and more encounters before mating with a "non-preferred" male. Females express their preference only if they encounter a preferred male before being stimulated to the higher threshold. Once the higher threshold is exceeded, even females with an intrinsic preference mate at random. A somewhat different model of frequency-dependent sexual selection has been investigated by Eshel (1979).

4.2   Models of assortative mating

As with sexual selection, there is a formidable literature detailing the evolutionary dynamics of systems subject to, e.g., negative assortment (Moree 1953, Workman 1964, Falk and Li 1969, Karlin and Feldman 1968 a,b, Karlin 1969), positive assortment (O'Donald 1960, Scudo and Karlin 1969, Karlin and Scudo 1969, Ghai 1974, Matessi and Scudo 1975, Karlin and Farkash 1978 a,b, Karlin 1978, Campbell 1980), mixed assortment (Otto 1978), and the combined effects of assortative mating and sexual selection (Karlin and O'Donald 1978). Assortative mating for metric and continuously varying traits has also been a source of considerable concern among quantitative geneticists (Fisher 1918, Wright 1921, Wilson 1973, Feldman and Cavalli-Sforza 1979, Bulmer 1980, Felsenstein 1981). In the following sections, I briefly review some pertinent conclusions that have arisen from this analytical investigation of systems of assortative mating, concentrating primarily on the simplest case of single-locus traits.

4.2.1   Positive

For a model of positive assortative mating under a polygamous mating system, we assume a proportion α, β and γ of each female genotype (AA, Aa and aa, respectively) prefer to mate with their own kind (see Table 3). The dynamics of the system depend primarily on the magnitudes of the preference parameters (Karlin and Scudo 1969, Karlin 1978), insofar as only with specific values of α, β and γ does there exist a unique stable polymorphic equilibrium (Karlin 1969). Otherwise, the system evolves towards fixation of one or the other homozygous states. Where all females exercise positive genotypic assortment (i.e. complete positive assortment), the system rapidly evolves towards homozygosity with the deviation from equilibrium being halved every generation (Jacquard 1974, p. 249).

The situation becomes somewhat more complex under a monogamous breeding system. Here, several models can be formulated in which assorting individuals pair first, followed by random-mating individuals, and vice versa. It appears, however, that the mating order makes little difference: in both instances, we find the system generally converging to the corresponding homozygous structure (AA or aa) depending on the initial genotype frequencies (Karlin 1969). (Under certain restrictive conditions, however, there may exist a unique stable polymorphic equilibrium; for details, see Karlin and Scudo 1969, Scudo and Karlin 1969 and Karlin 1969, pp. 39–45). Models of positive phenotypic assortment under polygamous mating yield similar results. Once again, the monogamous situation generally mimics the polygamous system, except that rates of convergence to the homozygous state are reduced (again, however, there are several conditions under which a unique polymorphic equilibrium results (Karlin 1969, pp. 30–37)). Jacquard (1974, p. 253) notes that under complete positive phenotypic assortative mating, the rate of elimination of heterozygotes is relatively low, particularly if the initial frequency of the dominant allele is high. In general, any system of positive assortment tends to degenerate to a pure homozygous state, with heterozygotes being eliminated in each successive generation. The major difference between genotypic and phenotypic assortment relates not to the ultimate equilibrium state but rather to the rate of convergence. The same conclusion applies for the mating system of the population, with convergence proceeding faster under polygamy than monogamy.

4.2.2   Negative

The dynamics of negative assortment have been investigated in considerable detail by Moree (1953), Workman (1964), Karlin and Feldman (1968 a,b) and Karlin (1968, 1969). The models are generally of two types. In one case, a proportion of each female genotype or phenotype is assumed to mate only with males genotypically (phenotypically) dissimilar to themselves. Alternatively, certain matings between individuals of the same genotype may be prohibited. Karlin (1969) has coined the term "incompatibility models" to describe the latter.

In the case of total negative genotypic assortment, the population usually evolves towards a stable equilibrium in which half of all individuals are heterozygous, the other half homozygous. An unstable equilibrium with all three genotypes present occurs only if the initial frequencies of the two homozygotes are equal. Whichever homozygote is present in lowest frequencies initially is eventually eliminated from the population.

Results from models examining the influence of phenotypic negative assortment are similar to those for genotypic assortment. With partial negative assortment by phenotype, we again find a stable polymorphic equilibrium, with convergence occurring at a much slower rate, and with the equilibrium gene frequencies being functions only of the proportion of female phenotypes practising negative assortment. Furthermore, they are relatively insensitive to variation in the preference parameters (Jacquard 1974).

4.2.3   Mixed

Karlin (1969, pp. 58–60) and Otto (1978) have both investigated systems subject to both positive and negative assortment. As we might expect, the tendency for positive assortment to eliminate heterozygotes is balanced by the tendency of negative assortment to promote heterozygosity, generally leading to a unique globally stable polymorphic equilibrium.

4.3   Comparing sexual selection and assortative mating models

Karlin (1978) has provided a lucid comparison of single-locus sexual selection and assortative mating models. The major conclusions of his and other investigations can be summarized as follows.

(1) Sexual selection occurs when the tendency of a female to prefer mating with a particular male genotype (phenotype) is independent of her own (real or perceived) genotype (phenotype). In assortative mating, preferences depend on the genotype (phenotype) of the individual doing the choosing. So construed, sexual selection can be considered a special case of generalized assortative mating (Karlin 1978). Both sexual selection and pure assortment may result in observable deviations from random mating at the population level.

(2) Positive assortative mating generally results in a deficiency of heterozygotes. In some cases, e.g. total positive assortment by genotype (Jacquard 1974) and positive assortment by phenotype (Scudo and Karlin 1969), heterozygotes are eliminated very rapidly and the population state tends towards fixation. In other cases, the system may admit stable polymorphisms, but equilibrium genotype frequencies are almost never in Hardy–Weinberg proportions. In some cases, negative assortment leads to polymorphic equilibria in which one homozygote is eliminated (Jacquard 1974); in other instances, fixation of one allele occurs, albeit rather slowly (Workman 1964, Karlin and Feldman 1968 a,b). Like systems of positive assortment, polymorphic equilibria generally do not conform to Hardy–Weinberg proportions. By contrast, systems subject to sexual selection consistently evolve towards a unique globally stable equilibrium with genotype frequencies in Hardy–Weinberg proportions. Karlin (1978, pp. 305–308) has provided an explanation of why sexual selection equilibria invariably manifest Hardy–Weinberg proportions.

(3) For both assortment and sexual selection, equilibrium outcomes are similar under monogamy or polygamy. In general, convergence rates are reduced under monogamous mating systems relative to polygamous systems (Karlin 1978).

(4) Finally, the timing of preferential versus random mating influences the equilibrium outcomes under assortment (Karlin 1969), whereas equilibria under sexual selection are unaffected.

5 NON-RANDOM MATING AND THE EXISTENCE OF MATING PREFERENCES

5.1 Evolution of mating preferences

If patterns of non-random mating reflect—at least to some degree—the expression of mating preferences, the question arises as to why such preferences exist, particularly when preferences are often for extreme characters (e.g. extravagant plumage) which would appear to be of negative survival value. Fisher (1930) proposed an ingenious solution to the puzzle by suggesting that the joint evolution of mating preferences and the preferred trait (or trait complex) arises from a genetic correlation between the sexes. The correlation implies that those segregating factors affecting female mating preferences would to some extent be transmitted to the male offspring *in addition* to the preferred trait itself. The greater the preference, the greater the advantage of the sons possessing the trait. Hence, Fisher concluded that the preferred trait and the mating preferences for it would evolve simultaneously in a "runaway" fashion, slowing only when the trait had evolved to the point where its possessor now suffered *reduced* reproduction fitness. Lande (1981) points out that, at the outset, there need not have existed a genetic correlation between the preferred trait and its preference, since such a correlation could arise through assortative mating (e.g. by more discriminating females selecting more extreme males). Furthermore, there is no need to postulate an initial advantage to females choosing mates with the trait(s) in question, since mating preferences can evolve purely as a correlated response to selection in males. However, the scheme does rest on the implicit assumption that there exists sufficient additive genetic variance for both mating preferences and the preferred trait in the original population.

Fisher's theory regarding the evolution of mating preferences was well received by behaviourists and population geneticists alike (e.g. O'Donald 1963 b, 1967, 1980 a, Lande 1981). Yet, clearly the theory is couched in terms of sexual selection, *not* assortative mating. In the Fisherian scheme, the fitness of a male is independent of the genotype of the female who is doing the assessing. As such, the theory does not touch upon the evolution of mating preferences that are based on an individual's perception of her (or his) own genotype.

Several mechanisms have been advanced to explain the evolution of assortative mating preferences. Suppose, for example, that in a polymorphic population there are some individuals who have a genetic predisposition to select a mate genotypically similar to themselves and, in so doing, enjoy a selective advantage relative to their non-assorting counterparts. Then, assuming the tendency to mate by positive assortment is heritable, we expect an increase in the frequency of positively assorting genotypes in subsequent generations.

This scenario contrasts with the Fisherian scheme for sexual selection in several important ways. First, there is no need to postulate that different male or female genotypes have different intrinsic fitnesses. Indeed, the fitness of a male is, in part, determined by the genotype of the female with which he mates (and vice versa). (This does not, of course, preclude the possibility that there exists variation in male or female fitness, but this condition is not necessary as it is in Fisher's model.) Suppose, for example, that matings between two individuals homozygous for the same allele (i.e. AA × AA, aa × aa) produce, on average, four offspring, whereas matings between individuals homozygous for *different* alleles (i.e. AA × aa) produce only three offspring. Clearly, individuals involved in the first type of mating enjoy a selective advantage, but only because some mating *combinations* are more fertile than others, not because some *individuals* are more fertile than others.

Secondly, there need not be any "runaway" co-evolutionary process between mating preferences and the preferred trait (or traits). In fact, such a situation occurs only if the probability of an individual mating assortatively depends on his or her own genotype. Suppose, for example, that all homogametic matings (i.e. AA × AA, Aa × Aa and aa × aa) confer equal fitnesses on the individuals so involved, as do all heterogametic matings (i.e. AA × aa, Aa × AA, Aa × aa), but that the mean fitness of individuals in the first class exceeds that of the second. Suppose further that a constant proportion of each genotype is involved in each class of matings. If the tendency to mate by positive assortment is heritable, we expect an increase in the proportion of assorting genotypes in the next generation. Note, however, that since there is no selective advantage *per se* to being genotypically AA, Aa or aa, allele frequencies will remain unchanged. If, however, the probability of mating by positive assortment is genotype specific, then a greater proportion of, say, AA individuals will be involved in homogametic matings. As such, there is a net advantage gained by the A allele over its recessive counterpart, and subsequent generations will see a change in allele frequencies.

The hypothesis that assortative mating preferences have evolved through the selective advantage accrued to individuals obtaining a mate genotypically similar (or dissimilar) to themselves is based on two fundamental assumptions, namely, that there exists additive genetic variation for mating preferences (or at least for traits genetically correlated with mating preferences) in the population, and that the effects of the male and female genotypes on the reproductive fitness of the "pair" are non-additive. Potential evidence of the former was obtained by Thoday and Gibson (1962) in their selection for high and low numbers of bristles in a laboratory population of *Drosophila melanogaster*. Despite ample opportunity for mixed matings, complete reproductive isolation between the high and low lines was achieved very rapidly, though it was not clear whether the decline in the frequency of "hybrids" (i.e. low × high) reflected strong mating preferences or a reduced competitive ability of hybrid larvae. More direct evidence of genetic variation for mating preferences comes from a recent study by Majerus *et al.* (1982) of positive assortative mating in Ladybirds. By selecting those females actually observed mating with melanic males, they obtained a significant increase in the frequency of individuals mating with such males over five generations.

The second premise is even more problematical. Suppose, for example, we are dealing with a system of negative assortment. Why should, say, an AA individual who mates with an aa individual be accrued a selective advantage over one who chooses a genotypically AA mate? One possible explanation involves the avoidance of inbreeding. Like positive assortment, consanguinity (matings between related individuals, e.g. first cousins) increases population homozygosity as a function of the coefficient of kinship between mated individuals and the frequency of the trait in question. The results of consanguinity are manifest. For example, while many diseases are caused by recessive genes, the disease is manifested only in homozygotes. As such, incidence rates among the offspring of consanguineous matings may suffer because of their generally reduced levels of heterozygosity, particularly if various loci are subject to heterosis (Jacquard 1974).

As Karlin (1978) has pointed out, systems of positive assortment are similar to (in some cases, indistinguishable from) systems of partial selfing (see also Karlin and McGregor 1974, pp. 90–94). If there are deleterious effects associated with the increased homozygosity among the offspring of positively assorting (or inbred) parents, then there may be some selective advantage to choosing a mate of *dissimilar* phenotype (genotype) to oneself. Under such conditions, we might expect an increase in the proportion of negatively assorting genotypes in the population.

Empirical evidence for enhanced fitness among negatively assorting genotypes is very sparse. The most recent (and convincing) data can be found in Serradilla and Ayala's (1983) investigation of the influence of mating type of fecundity in *Drosophila melanogaster*. For two of three loci investigated, they found enhanced fecundity associated with mated pairs *homozygous* for *different* alleles, and reduced fecundity among pairs homozygous for the *same* allele. Similar results (albeit at a somewhat cruder level) were obtained in the study by Findlay *et al.* (1985) of assortative mating on reproductive fitness in

A. c. caerulescens. While pair type has no influence on most components of fitness (see chapter 13), pairs comprising individuals of different genotypes consistently enjoyed greater nesting success than did their positively assorting counterparts. Furthermore, for two of seven cohorts examined, offspring from heterochromatic pairs showed significantly higher recruitment rates into the breeding segment of the population. These results suggest that there may in fact be some selective advantage(s) to negative assortment, though the magnitude and importance of these pressures remain unknown. Along somewhat similar lines, Murton *et al.* (1973) reported reduced hatching success among homochromatic pairs of *Columbia livia* in comparison to their heterochromatic counterparts.

But what of positive assortment? Again, we return to the theory of inbreeding, but this time we adopt the premise that a small level of inbreeding may in fact be advantageous. While inbreeding tends to increase homozygosity, it nevertheless reduces the recombinational load associated with the disruption of co-adapted gene complexes under outbreeding (Williams 1975, Maynard-Smith 1978). In other words, outbreeding may entail a certain "outbreeding depression". Several authors (e.g. Bateson 1978, Price and Waser 1979, Shields 1983) have argued that fitness is maximized through a genetically optimal balance between negative and positive assortment. If indeed this is the case, there may well be a selective advantage to positive assortment. Bateson (1979) has argued that, when genetic relatedness is manifested in phenotypic similarity, optimal outbreeding implies a balance between negative and positive assortment. While there is some evidence of outbreeding depression in natural populations (see Shields (1983) for a review), direct evidence of enhanced fitness accruing to positively assorting genotypes in avian populations is very scarce. To my knowledge, the only tentative evidence of increased reproductive success associated with positive assortment in birds comes from Boag and Grant's (1978) investigation of assortative mating for external morphology in Darwin's Finches.

5.2   Imprinting and mating preferences

In many species, offspring imprint on various aspects of parental (or sibling) phenotypes (for a comprehensive review, see Colgan (1983), pp. 123–140). Such early experiences often determine mating preferences once an individual attains reproductive maturity. Assortative mating may then persist because of mating preferences based on early experience. As such, imprinting may have considerable effect on the genetic structure of populations (Kalmus and Maynard-Smith 1966, Seiger 1967, Matessi and Scudo 1975).

It is all very well to accept the premise that some patterns of non-random mating reflect sexual preferences based on imprinting. This hypothesis has certainly been borne out by studies of natural populations. But, in so doing, we have simply transformed the question "Why do patterns of non-random mating exist (and persist)?" into "Why do sexual preferences (which give rise to assortment and are based on early experience) exist (and persist)?". If there is no selective advantage to selecting a mate phenotypically similar (or dissimilar) to onself, why then do individuals show preferences for particular types of mates? Surely these preferences must entail some selective cost, insofar as the time and energy required to locate a "preferred" mate (particularly if that phenotype is rare) might perhaps be better spent, say, increasing one's stored food reserves or producing more eggs.

One potential explanation involves the evolution of species-recognition mechanisms in polymorphic species. Lorenz (1935) first pointed out that imprinting on various characteristics of the parental (or sibling) phenotypes provides offspring with a species image, allowing them to recognize conspecifics as such. In monomorphic species, this image is representative of each and every member of the population. But in polymorphic species, the species image may well include cues which are morph-specific, in addition to species-specific. As a result, an individually phenotypically P may simply not recognize an individual phenotypically p as a conspecific. In a polymorphic population, the imprinting process would lead to assortative mating for those phenotypic cues that are morph-specific.

This explanation for the existence of assortative mating preferences is fundamentally different from the preceding explanation insofar as there is no need to postulate any selective advantage to assortment *per se*. As long as the species-recognition mechanism persists, so too will mating preferences leading to assortative mating. Thus, Cooke *et al.* (1976) have argued that current mating preferences for plumage colour in Lesser Snow Geese simply represent extensions of an ancestral species-recognition mechanism (see also Findlay *et al.* 1985).

6 ASSORTATIVE MATING AND POLYGENIC VARIATION

Fisher (1918) first investigated the influence of assortative mating on the correlation among relatives in what Bulmer (1980) has legitimately described as a "notoriously difficult paper". Subsequent treatments include Crow and Felsenstein (1968), Crow and Kimura (1970, pp. 158–161), Cavalli-Sforza and Feldman (1979), Bulmer (1980, pp. 126–131) and Felsenstein (1981). Generally, if we assume that assortative mating acts through the phenotypic values (i.e. depends on genotypic values only indirectly through the influence of the genotype on the phenotype), then positive assortment will tend to inflate the estimated additive variance of the trait, V_a. The recursion equation relating additive variance at generation $g + 1$ and g is relatively simple:

$$V_a(g + 1) = 0·5V_a(g)(1 + rh^2(g)) + 0·5V_a \quad \text{(Bulmer 1980)}$$

where $V_a(g)$ is the additive variance at generation g, $h^2(g)$ the heritability of the trait at generation g, V_a the additive variance under random mating, and r the correlation between the maternal and paternal phenotypic values. From the above equation, it is clear that, under positive assortment (where $r > 0$), $V_a(g + 1) > V_a(g)$, i.e. the estimated additive genetic variance of the trait is enhanced. Under negative assortment, V_a decreases. Apart from the inflated (or deflated) additive variance, assortative mating can modify the correlation between relatives insofar as the phenotypic correlation between parents will, say, enhance the correlation of offspring with a single parent because of influences operating through the other parent.

The situation is complicated further if assortative mating occurs not for the trait in question but rather for some correlated character. Suppose, for example, we are attempting to estimate the heritability of trait *a*, which is phenotypically correlated with trait *b*. Suppose further that mating proceeds randomly with respect to *a* but non-randomly with respect to *b*. Here, there are two possible outcomes. If the phenotypic covariance between *a* and *b* is entirely of environmental origin, then the estimated heritability of *a* will be unaffected, since environmental deviations are not influenced by non-random mating (Bulmer 1980, pp. 121–143). Alternatively, the phenotypic covariance between *a* and *b* may arise from pleiotropy. Here, there will be a correlation between the maternal and paternal phenotypes in the additive component of *a*, and a corresponding increase (or decrease) in the estimated heritability of the trait.

7 EXAMPLES OF NON-RANDOM MATING IN WILD BIRDS

7.1 Assortative mating

Several avian studies have indicated assortative mating for a variety of traits. Coulson (1966) and Newton *et al.* (1979) both reported a tendency of mated pairs to comprise individuals of similar age. Positive assortment for plumage coloration has been documented in several species, including Domestic Fowl (*Gallus gallus*; Lill 1968 a,b), Swainson's Hawk (*Buteo swainsoni*; Dunkle 1977), Western Grebe (*Aechmophorus* cf. *occidentalis*; Nuechterlein 1981 a,b), feral Rock Doves (*Columba livia*; Goodwin 1958), Lesser Snow Geese (Cooch and Beardmore 1959, Cooke *et al.* 1976), Brant (*Branta bernicla*; Abraham *et al.* 1983) and Arctic Skuas (*Stercorarius parasiticus*; Davis and O'Donald 1976, O'Donald 1959, 1960, 1974). Baker and Mewaldt (1978) report an interesting example of how positive assortment for song dialects restricts interdemic gene flow and permits local adaptation of two populations of White-crowned Sparrows (*Zonotrichia leucophrys*). Weak positive assortment for various morphological characters has also been documented in Darwin's Finches (Boag and Grant 1978).

Negative assortment in birds has been less well documented. Lowther (1961) provided strong evidence of negative assortment for plumage coloration in White-throated Sparrows (*Zonotrichia albicollis*). Of 110 mated pairs, 106 comprised individuals of dissimilar phenotype (white-striped × tan-striped, and vice versa). Moreover, there appeared to be considerable consistency in mate selection. Of 15 individuals recaptured with two different mates, in all but one instance the second mate was phenotypically similar to the first. Negative assortment for plumage variation has also been documented in Rock Doves (Murton *et al.* 1973). Weak negative assortment for beak width has apparently been observed by Smith and Zach (1979) in an island population of Song Sparrows (*Melospiza melodia*).

7.2   Sexual selection

Although sexual selection has been investigated in a wide variety of organisms, birds have historically been a favourite target. The literature on sexual selection in birds is vast and varied, reaching as far back as Darwin's (1871) original formulation of the theory. Many earlier works, particularly those pertaining to the evolution of sexual dimorphism, have been summarized by Selander (1972). Excellent recent reviews concerning various aspects of sexual selection (in birds and non-birds alike) include Halliday (1978), Blum and Blum (1979), Andersson (1982 b), Searcy (1982), Arnold (1983) and Partridge (1983).

In light of these extensive reviews, the present section will focus only on one aspect of the theory of sexual selection, namely female choice. Recall that, in section 4, systems of non-random mating were classified on the basis of their preference configurations. In particular, the Darwin–Fisher theory of sexual selection holds that females select their mates on the basis of some (real or perceived) quality (e.g. Ryan 1980, Petrie 1983). Unfortunately, it is notoriously difficult to document if—and for what character(s)—female choice is occurring, principally because it is often impossible to distinguish between the effects of intersexual selection and intrasexual competition. Invariably, data purporting to demonstrate the former can be accommodated by the latter and vice versa, so that which hypothesis is advanced generally depends on the author's state of mind.

Much evidence of female choice is indirect. A good example is the study by O'Donald and co-workers (O'Donald 1972 a,b, 1974, 1976, 1977 a, 1980 b,

O'Donald and Davis 1977) on sexual selection in Arctic Skuas. Here, evidence of female choice is based on the fact that analytical models of female preference generally provide a good fit to—and presumably a good explanation of—field data. But as Halliday (1978) points out, the conclusions are *not* based on direct observation of male and female mating behaviour.

There are, however, several ways in which the potential effects of intrasexual competition are minimized (Searcy 1982). One design involves restraining males so that they cannot interact, with females then being allowed to choose among prospective mates (e.g. Burley 1977, 1981). An alternative approach is to isolate a particular male character that appears to confer a selective advantage, and then present females with the character abstracted from its natural context. In Brown-headed Cowbirds (*Molothrus ater*), females apparently mate preferentially with dominant males whose songs are distinct from subordinate males. Isolated females showed an increased frequency of a copulatory response to the recorded song of dominant males relative to the song of subordinate males (West *et al.* 1981), indicating that preferences were indeed being exercised by females on the basis of the male song phenotype.

Perhaps the most convincing data on intersexual selection comes from Andersson's (1982 a) unique investigation of female preferences in the Long-tailed Widowbird (*Euplectes progne*). In his experiment, one treatment group of males had their tails cut; others received new feathers that elongated their tails. Males with "supernormal" tails showed higher breeding success than both normal and "curtailed" (pun intended) males. Moreover, the alternate hypothesis that intrasexual competition maintains tail length was inconsistent with the observation that shortening the tail did *not* influence the ability of a male to retain his territory. Since long tails are presumably of little or no value in intrasexual competition, tail length must have evolved through female mating preferences.

The studies cited above indicate that there are indeed some clear examples of female preference leading to sexual selection for various male traits. This does not, however, imply that male choice does not exist (see, for example, Burley 1981, Gwynne 1981, Colgan 1983). For example, in long-lived permanently monogamous species, male investment may well equal that of the female. Here, we might expect the sexes to be equally discriminating in their choice of mates, such that sex-specific traits evolve in response to mating preferences expressed by the opposite sex.

8 NON-RANDOM MATING AND SYMPATRIC SPECIATION

Although the pervasiveness of sympatric speciation in natural populations is a source of endless debate (e.g. Maynard-Smith 1966, Bush 1975, White 1978), this has not discouraged researchers from postulating non-random mating as ancillary mechanism. Fisher (1930) suggested that the "runaway" process of sexual selection could rapidly lead to species formation through the establishment of sexual reproductive isolation. Though it seems unlikely that sexual selection *per se* can induce population subdivision on its own accord, there is some evidence that it may be responsible for the rapid divergence of two (or more) allopatric populations. Carson (1978) suggests that genetic drift arising from inbreeding or small initial population sizes may have resulted in intensified sexual selection for complex behavioural "mate recognition" systems within geographically isolated populations of Hawaiian *Drosophila*. Population differentiation with respect to these syndromes then provides the foundations for sexual isolation and subsequent speciation.

Clearly, *once* reproductive isolation has been achieved, non-random mating may ensure that the evolutionary dynamics of two sympatric (or allopatric, for that matter) populations are independent. Of greater interest is whether non-random mating can bring about reproductive isolation in the first place. Theoretically, a system of complete positive assortment could produce two monomorphic isolates from an ancestral polymorphic population. Problems arise, however, when we consider the level of preferential mating required to reduce inter-morph gene flow to the level of effective reproductive isolation. This is particularly true if preferences arise from imprinting on parental or sibling phenotype. Seiger (1967) showed that subdivision of an ancestral population into two reproductively isolated monomorphic populations requires *absolute* imprinting (see also Kalmus and Maynard-Smith 1966). Fixation of the population in a purely homozygous state is a general characteristic of most isophenogamous mating systems in which all females imprinted on a particular male phenotype *always* mate with such males (Matessi and Scudo 1975). Since during pure sympatric speciation, selection pressures are not expected to be a factor (at least initially), population subdivision and the establishment of complete reproductive isolation through non-random mating will generally occur only via an efficient, well-canalized imprinting mechanism inducing very high levels of preferential mating.

Empirically, then, the question is whether or not such strong sexual preferences exist in polymorphic populations. Though the jury is not yet in, there is good evidence that imprinting mechanisms are less than absolute. Immelmann (1975) cites several studies which indicate considerable inter-individual variation in "imprintability", notably those by Schutz (1965) with cross-fostered mallard ducklings and Goodwin (1971) with cross-fostered female Blue-headed Waxbills (*Uraeginthus cyanocephalus*). Individual differences in the duration of the sensitive period and in the level of social experience required for sexual imprinting also occur in populations of Zebra Finch. Baptista (1974) suggested that observed differences in song-learning dispositions among White-crowned Sparrows may have some genetic component. Certainly, there is no evidence that sexual preferences based on imprinting on the familial environment are absolute in Lesser Snow Geese (Cooke 1978) or Japanese Quail (*Coturnix japonicus*; Bateson 1978).

Despite the documented environmental lability of most imprinting mechanisms, some authors maintain that imprinting has indeed led to sympatric speciation. One example is Payne's (1973) study of speciation in the parasitic African indigo birds (genus *Hypochera*). Non-interbreeding sympatric forms are ethologically isolated by fixations to different hosts, which have ostensibly arisen from host imprinting and vocal mimicry. Reproductive isolation has in turn allowed morphological differentiation among adjacent sympatric groups, and allowed further speciation to proceed.

In summary, non-random mating can, under certain circumstances, promote sub-population differentiation. However, the establishment of complete reproductive isolation *solely* through non-random mating requires levels of preferential mating which are unrealistic for many traits. In concert with other factors (particularly genetic drift and selection), however, non-random mating may well contribute to incipient sympatric speciation.

9 MIXED ASSORTMENT IN SNOW GEESE: PREFERENCE AND PREVALENCE

As outlined in the introductory section of this chapter, non-random mating is a population phenomenon. But, despite clear patterns of non-random mating at the population level, researchers are often unable to uncover the underlying mechanism(s). There are, however, several exceptions. A good example is the study by Cooke and co-workers of assortative mating in Lesser Snow Geese, a dimorphic anatid breeding in geographically isolated colonies throughout the Canadian arctic. The plumage dimorphism is controlled by a single diallelic locus, such that all phenotypically blue individuals are homozygous dominant or heterozygous, whereas all white individuals are homozygous recessive (Cooke and Cooch 1968). Non-random mating for plumage colour was first documented by Cooch and Beardmore (1959) at the extensive Boas River colony on Baffin Island, and subsequently by Cooke *et al.* (1976) at the smaller La Perouse Bay colony near Churchill, Manitoba. In both instances, more homochromatic (B × B, W × W) matings were observed than would otherwise be expected by chance. In a series of experiments, Cooke and McNally (1975) were able to show that the observed pattern of positive assortment in part reflected the tendency of offspring to select mates of the same colour as their parents. Later, Cooke (1978) demonstrated that sibling colour was another important cue in the imprinting process. The current wisdom can be summarized as follows: offspring of monomorphic families (i.e. parents and sibs all the same colour) generally select mates of that colour, whereas we expect the offspring of mixed families to show no imprinting preference (at the population level, then, offspring from mixed families effectively mate at random; see Geramita *et al.* 1982).

Clearly, the imprinting process results in most individuals selecting mates who are phenotypically similar to themselves (i.e. mating by positive assortment). However, some individuals are apparently indifferent to the phenotype of their mate (i.e. mate at random). Still others mate by negative assortment. In matings between heterozygotes, one-quarter of the offspring will be phenotypically white, the other three-quarters blue. As such, we expect a proportion of families to comprise a lone white gosling in an otherwise blue environment. Since this individual imprints on parental or sib colour, it perceives itself as being phenotypically blue, and will tend to select a mate accordingly.

The observed pattern of assortment is not, however, completely explained by individual mating preferences. Cooke (1978; chapter 13) and Findlay *et al.* (1985) have shown significant asymmetry in the frequency of mixed matings at the La Perouse colony; that is, $B\male \times W\female$ pairs significantly outnumber $W\male \times B\female$ pairs. Cooke (1978) has suggested that the asymmetry reflects the non-random distribution of the phenotypes on the wintering grounds where pair formation occurs. Cooke *et al.* (1975) documented a preponderance of blue-phase individuals in the eastern section of the wintering range, while white-phase individuals dominated the western regions. Furthermore, the La Perouse colony is about 30% blue, whereas the global population is approximately 40% blue. Clinal variation in phenotype frequencies on the wintering grounds, combined with the discrepancy between the global and local phase ratios, implies that a random-mating white female from La Perouse Bay is more likely to obtain a blue male than if she were selecting her spouse entirely from within the La Perouse segment of the global population. As such, we expect to find an excess of $B\male \times W\female$ relative to $W\male \times B\female$ pairs on the breeding colony. (In Snow Geese, only the females are philopatric, with the male accompanying the female back to her natal colony to breed.)

Two lines of evidence support the prevalence hypothesis. If the observed asymmetry in mixed matings reflects differential availability of mates as a function of discrepancies between global and local phenotype frequencies, we would expect that in colonies where the proportion of blue individuals exceeds the global phase ratio, the asymmetry should be reversed; that is, $W\male \times B\female$ matings should outnumber $B\male \times W\female$ matings. And indeed, this is the case. Using data from four colonies, Cooke and Davies (1983) showed a linear relationship between local phenotype distributions and the asymmetry in mixed matings.

Secondly, the prevalence hypothesis predicts that with temporal changes in the phase ratio of a given local population we should observe a change in the asymmetry of mixed matings, provided of course that global changes over the same period are negligible. In particular, as the global and local phase ratios equilibrate, we expect a concomitant reduction in the asymmetry of mixed matings within local populations. Again, this prediction holds for the La Perouse population. While Cooke *et al.* (1985) showed a significant increase in the proportion of blue individuals between 1969 and 1977, Findlay *et al.* (1985) have documented, over the same time interval, a significant decrease in the asymmetry of mixed matings.

10 SUMMARY AND CONCLUSIONS

Non-random mating can have substantial effects on the structure of populations. Though simple single-locus models of various systems of non-random mating are of considerable heuristic value, their applicability in the "real" world remains suspect. Many traits for which preferential matings occur exist not as discrete phenotypic classes but rather as continuous distributions on some appropriate scale. Such variation may be more realistically modelled as a polygenic system, a likelihood which had been largely ignored until quite recently (e.g. Lande 1981). Even more probable is that mating preferences are not for individual traits but for trait complexes whose elements may (or may not) be highly correlated. In the case of low correlations, it is not legitimate to model the system in a univariate space; rather, we require a multivariate formulation in which factors responsible for changes in a vector of phenotypic attributes are considered. This approach is proving to be a powerful tool in the analysis of natural selection and despite its inherently more complex nature, nonetheless imparts an element of general applicability to current models of preferential mating.

Non-random mating is a population phenomenon. It is not legitimate to conclude that population patterns of non-random mating reflect true mating preferences, since such patterns can arise purely from the differential availability of various phenotypic classes when and where mating occurs. Mate choice can only be demonstrated at the individual level by means of experimental manipulation. Even here, however, the researcher must proceed cautiously. Often, experimental outcomes are such that it is impossible to attribute unambiguously the results to intersexual selection versus intrasexual selection. Moreover, there is considerable difficulty involved in determining exactly what traits determine sexual preferences. This is particularly true in birds where many life-history traits are highly correlated (e.g. male size and/or dominance and territory size). Randomizing environmental variation over phenotypes may be possible in the field but, for highly correlated morphological or behavioural characters, one usually must rely on laboratory protocols designed to determine the mechanism(s) of mating preferences by considering each trait in isolation and in various combinations. At the risk of advancing an undeniably biased opinion, it is this combination of laboratory and field work which has made the Snow Goose study a model for the investigation of non-random mating in natural populations. Moreover, this study provides a clear illustration of a situation in which several different ecological constraints and modes of assortment combine to generate the observed population patterns.

ACKNOWLEDGMENTS

I thank Genevieve Menard, Rocky Rockwell, Lou Levine, Ethan Akin, Sievert Rohwer, George Williams and Fred Cooke for advice and discussion.

REFERENCES

Abraham, K. F., Ankney, C. D. and Boyd, H. (1983). Assortative mating by Brant. *Auk* **100**, 201–202.
Andersson, M. (1982 a). Female choice selects for extreme tail length in a widowbird. *Nature* **299**, 818–820.
Andersson, M. (1982 b). Sexual selection, natural selection and quality advertisement. *Biol. J. Linn. Soc.* **17**, 375–393.
Arnold, S. (1983). Sexual selection: the interface of theory and empiricism. *In* "Mate Choice" (ed. P. P. G. Bateson). Cambridge University Press.
Baker, M. C. and Mewaldt, L. R. (1978). Song dialects as barriers to dispersal in white-crowned sparrows, *Zonotrichia leucophrys nuttalli*. *Evolution* **32**, 712–722.
Baptista, L. F. (1974). The effects of songs of wintering white-crowned sparrows on song development in sedentary populations of the species. *Z. Tierpsych.* **34**, 147–171.
Bateson, P. P. G. (1978). Sexual imprinting and optimal outbreeding. *Nature* **273**, 659–660.
Bateson, P. P. G. (1979). How do sensitive periods arise and what are they for? *Anim. Behav.* **27**, 470–486.
Blum, M. S. and Blum, N. A. (eds) (1979). "Sexual Selection and Reproductive Competition in Insects". Academic Press, New York.
Boag, P. T. and Grant, P. R. (1978). Heritability of external morphology in Darwin's finches. *Nature* **274**, 793–794.
Bulmer, M. G. (1980). "The Mathematical Theory of Quantitative Genetics". Oxford University Press.
Burley, N. (1977). Parental investment, mate choice and mate quality. *Proc. Natl Acad. Sci. USA* **74**, 3476–3479.
Burley, N. (1981). Mate choice by multiple criteria in a monogamous species. *Am. Natur.* **117**, 515–528.

Bush, G. L. (1975). Modes of animal speciation. *Ann. Rev. Ecol. Syst.* **6**, 339–364.

Campbell, R. B. (1980). Polymorphic equilibria with assortative mating and selection in sub-divided populations. *Theor. Pop. Biol.* **18**, 94–111.

Carson, H. L. (1978). Speciation and sexual selection in Hawaiian *Drosophila*. In "Ecological Genetics: The Interface" (ed. P. F. Brussard). Springer-Verlag, New York.

Cavalli-Sforza, L. L. and Bodmer, W. F. (1971). "The Genetics of Human Populations". Freeman, San Francisco.

Colgan, P. (1983). "Comparative Social Recognition". John Wiley & Sons, New York.

Cooch, F. G. and Beardmore, J. A. (1959). Assortative mating and reciprocal difference in the blue-snow goose complex. *Nature* **183**, 1833–1834.

Cooke, F. (1978). Early learning and its effect on population structure. Studies of a wild population of Snow Geese. *Z. Tierpsych.* **46**, 344–358.

Cooke, F. and Cooch, F. G. (1968). The genetics of polymorphism in the goose *Anser caerulescens. Evolution* **22**, 289–300.

Cooke, F. and Davies, J. C. (1983). Assortative mating, mate choice and reproductive fitness in Snow Geese. *In* "Mate Choice" (ed. P. P. G. Bateson). Cambridge University Press.

Cooke, F., Findlay, C. S., Rockwell, R. F. and Smith, J. A. (1985). Life history studies of the Lesser Snow Goose. III. The selective value of plumage polymorphism: net fecundity. *Evolution* **39**, 165–177.

Cooke, F., Finney, G. H. and Rockwell, R. F. (1976). Assortative mating in Lesser Snow Geese. *Behav. Genet.* **6**, 127–140.

Cooke, F., MacInnes, C. D. and Prevett, J. P. (1975). Gene flow between breeding populations of Lesser Snow Geese. *Auk* **93**, 493–510.

Cooke, F. and McNally, C. M. (1975). Mate selection and colour preferences in Lesser Snow Geese. *Behaviour* **53**, 151–170.

Coulson, J. C. (1966). The influence of the pair-bond and age on the breeding biology of the Kittiwake gull *Rissa tridactyla. J. Anim. Ecol.* **35**, 269–279.

Coulson, J. C. and Thomas, C. (1983). Mate choice in the Kittiwake Gull. *In* "Mate Choice" (ed. P. P. G. Bateson). Cambridge University Press.

Crow, J. F. and Felsenstein, J. (1968). The effect of assortative mating on the genetic composition of a population. *Eugenics Quart.* **15**, 85–97.

Crow, J. F. and Kimura, M. (1970). "An Introduction to Population Genetics Theory". Harper & Row, New York.

Darwin, C. (1871). "The Descent of Man, and Selection in Relation to Sex". Murray, London.

Davis, J. W. F. and O'Donald, P. (1976). Estimation of assortative mating preferences in the Arctic Skua. *Heredity* **36**, 235–244.

Dunkle, S. W. (1977). Swainson's Hawks on the Laramie plains, Wyoming. *Auk* **94**, 65–71.

Eshel, I. (1979). Sexual selection, population-density and availability of mates. *Theor. Pop. Biol.* **16**, 301–314.

Falk, C. and Li, C. C. (1969). Negative assortative mating: exact solution to a simple model. *Genetics* **62**, 215–223.

Feldman, M. W. and Cavalli-Sforza, L. L. (1979). Aspects of variance and covariance analysis with cultural inheritance. *Theor. Pop. Biol.* **15**, 276–309.

Felsenstein, J. (1981). Continuous-genotype models and assortative mating. *Theor. Pop. Biol.* **19**, 341–357.

Findlay, C. S., Rockwell, R. F., Smith, J. A. and Cooke, F. (1985). Life history studies of the Lesser Snow Goose. VI. Plumage polymorphism, positive assortative mating and fitness. *Evolution* **39**, 904–914.

Fisher, R. A. (1918). The correlation between relatives on the supposition of Mendelian inheritance. *Trans. Roy. Soc. Edinb.* **52**, 399–433.

Fisher, R. A. (1930). "The Genetical Theory of Natural Selection". Clarendon Press, Oxford.

Geramita, J., Cooke, F. and Rockwell, R. F. (1982). Assortative mating and gene flow in the Lesser Snow Goose: A modelling approach. *Theor. Pop. Biol.* **22**, 177–203.

Ghai, G. L. (1974). Analysis of some non-random mating models. *Theor. Pop. Biol.* **6**, 76–91.

Goodwin, D. (1958). The existence and causation of colour-preferences in the pairing of feral and domestic pigeons. *Bull. Br. Ornithol. Club* **78**, 136–139.

Goodwin, D. (1971). Imprinting, or otherwise, in some cross-fostered Red-cheeked and Blue-headed Cordon-bleus. *Avic. Mag.* **77**, 26–31.

Gwynne, D. T. (1981). Sexual difference theory: Mormon crickets show role reversal in mate choice. *Science* **213**, 779–780.

Halliday, T. R. (1978). Sexual selection and mate choice. *In* "Behavioural Ecology" (eds J. R. Krebs and N. B. Davies). Sinauer, Sunderland, Massachusetts.

Immelman, K. (1975). Ecological significance of imprinting and early learning. *Ann. Rev. Ecol. Syst.* **6**, 15–37.

Jacquard, A. (1974). "The Genetic Structure of Populations". Springer-Verlag, Berlin.

Jennings, H. S. (1916). The numerical results of diverse systems of breeding. *Genetics* **1**, 53–89.

Kalmus, M. and Maynard-Smith, S. (1966). Some evolutionary consequences of pegmatypic mating systems (imprinting). *Am. Natur.* **100**, 619–635.

Karlin, S. (1968). Equilibrium behaviour of population genetic models with non-random mating. Part I: Preliminaries and special mating systems. *J. Appl. Prob.* **5**, 231–313.

Karlin, S. (1969). "Equilibrium Behavior of Population Genetic Models with Non Random Mating". Gordon & Breach, New York.

Karlin, S. (1978). Comparisons of positive assortative mating and sexual selection models. *Theor. Pop. Biol.* **14**, 281–312.

Karlin, S. and Farkash, S. (1978 a). Analysis of partial assortative mating and sexual selection models for a polygamous species involving a trait based on levels of heterozygosity. *Theor. Pop. Biol.* **14**, 430–445.

Karlin, S. and Farkash, S. (1978 b). Some multiallele partial assortative mating systems for a polygamous species. *Theor. Pop. Biol.* **14**, 446–470.

Karlin, S. and Feldman, M. W. (1968 a). Analysis of models with homozygote × hetero-zygote matings. *Genetics* **59**, 105–116.

Karlin, S. and Feldman, M. W. (1968 b). Further analysis of negative assortative mating. *Genetics* **59**, 117–136.

Karlin, S. and McGregor, J. (1974). Towards a theory of the evolution of modifier genes. *Theor. Pop. Biol.* **5**, 59–103.

Karlin, S. and O'Donald, P. (1978). Some population genetic models combining sexual selection with assortative mating. *Heredity* **41**, 165–174.

Karlin, S. and Raper, J. K. (1979). Sexual selection encounter models. *Theor. Pop. Biol.* **15**, 246–256.

Karlin, S. and Scudo, F. M. (1969). Assortative mating based on phenotype: II. Two autosomal alleles without dominance. *Genetics* **63**, 499–510.

Lande, R. (1981). Models of speciation by sexual selection on polygenic traits. *Proc. Natl Acad. Sci. USA* **78**, 3721–3725.

Lill, A. (1968 a). An analysis of sexual isolation in the domestic fowl: I. The basis of homogamy in males. *Behaviour* **30**, 107–126.

Lill, A. (1968 b). An analysis of sexual isolation in the domestic fowl: II. The basis of homogamy in females. *Behaviour* **30**, 127–145.

Lorenz, K. (1935). Der Kumpan in der Umwelt des Vogels. *J. f. Ornithologie* **83**, 137–213, 289–413.

Lowther, J. K. (1961). Polymorphism in the white-throated sparrow, *Zonotrichia albicollis* (Gmelin). *Can. J. Zool.* **39**, 281–292.

Majerus, M. E. N., O'Donald, P. and War, J. (1982). Female mating preference is genetic. *Nature* **300**, 521–523.

Matessi, C. and Scudo, F. M. (1975). The population genetics of assortative mating based on imprinting. *Theor. Pop. Biol.* **7**, 306–337.

Maynard-Smith, J. (1966). Sympatric speciation. *Am. Natur.* **100**, 637–650.

Maynard-Smith, J. (1978). "The Evolution of Sex". Cambridge University Press.

Moree, R. (1953). An effect of negative assortative mating on gene frequency. *Science* **118**, 600–601.

Murton, R. K., Westwood, N. J. and Thearle, R. J. P. (1973). Polymorphism and the evolution of continuous breeding season in the pigeon *Columba livia. J. Reprod. Fert. Suppl.* **19**, 563–577.

Newton, I., Marquiss, M. and Moss, D. (1979). Habitat, female age, organo-chlorine compounds and breeding of European Sparrowhawks. *J. Appl. Ecol.* **16**, 777–793.

Nuechterlein, G. L. (1981 a). Variations and multiple functions of the advertising display of Western Grebes. *Behaviour* **76**, 289–317.

Nuechterlein, G. L. (1981 b). Courtship behaviour and reproductive isolation between Western Grebe color morphs. *Auk* **98**, 335–349.

O'Donald, P. (1959). Possibility of assortative mating in the Arctic Skua. *Nature* **183**, 1210–1211.

O'Donald, P. (1960). Assortative mating in a population in which two alleles are segregating. *Heredity* **15**, 389–391.

O'Donald, P. (1963 a). The theory of sexual selection. *Heredity* **17**, 541–552.

O'Donald, P. (1963 b). Sexual selection for dominant and recessive genes. *Heredity* **18**, 451–457.

O'Donald, P. (1967). A general model of sexual and natural selection. *Heredity* **22**, 499–518.

O'Donald, P. (1972 a). Natural selection of reproductive rates and breeding times and its effect on sexual selection. *Am. Natur.* **106**, 368–379.

O'Donald, P. (1972 b). Sexual selection by variations in fitness at breeding time. *Nature* **237**, 349–351.

O'Donald, P. (1973). Models of sexual and natural selection in polygamous species. *Heredity* **31**, 145–156.

O'Donald, P. (1974). Polymorphisms maintained by sexual selection in a monogamous species of bird. *Heredity* **32**, 1–10.

O'Donald, P. (1976). Mating preferences and their genetic effects in models of sexual selection. *In* "Population Genetics and Ecology" (eds S. Karlin and E. Nevo). Academic Press, New York.

O'Donald, P. (1977 a). Mating preferences and sexual selection in the Arctic Skua. II. Behavioural mechanisms of the mating preferences. *Heredity* **39**, 111–119.

O'Donald, P. (1977 b). Theoretical aspects of sexual selection. *Theor. Pop. Biol.* **12**, 298–334.

O'Donald, P. (1978 a). A general model of mating behaviour with natural selection and female preference. *Heredity* **40**, 427–438.

O'Donald, P. (1978 b). Theoretical aspects of sexual selection: A generalized model of mating behaviour. *Theor. Pop. Biol.* **13**, 226–243.

O'Donald, P. (1980 a). "Genetic Models of Sexual Selection". Cambridge University Press.

O'Donald, P. (1980 b). Sexual selection by female choice in a monogamous bird: Darwin's theory corroborated. *Heredity* **45**, 201–217.

O'Donald, P. and Davis, J. W. F. (1977). Mating preferences and sexual selection in the Arctic Skua. III. Estimation of parameters and tests of heterogeneity. *Heredity* **39**, 121–132.

Otto, P. A. (1978). Studies on assortative mating. II. Effects of admixture of positive and negative systems. *J. Hered.* **69**, 207–209.

Partridge, L. (1983). Non-random mating and offspring fitness. *In* "Mate Choice" (ed. P. P. G. Bateson). Cambridge University Press.

Payne, R. B. (1973). Behavior, mimetic songs and song dialects, and relationships of the parasitic Indigo birds (*Vidua*) of Africa. *Ornithol. Monogr.* **11**, 1–333.

Petrie, M. (1983). Female moorhens (*Gallinula chloropus*) compete for small fat males. *Science* **220**, 413–415.

Price, M. V. and Waser, N. M. (1979). Pollen dispersal and optimal outcrossing in *Delphinium nelsoni*. *Nature* **277**, 294–297.

Raper, J. K., Karlin, S. and O'Donald, P. (1979). An assortative mating encounter model. *Heredity* **43**, 27–34.

Ryan, M. J. (1980). Female mate choice in neotropical frog. *Science* **209**, 523–525.

Schutz, F. (1965). Sexuelle Prägung bei Anatiden. *Z. Tierpsych.* **22**, 50–103.

Scudo, F. M. and Karlin, S. (1969). Assortative mating based on phenotype: I. Two alleles with dominance. *Genetics* **63**, 479–498.

Searcy, W. A. (1982). The evolutionary effects of mate selection. *Ann. Rev. Ecol. Syst.* **13**, 57–85.

Seiger, M. B. (1967). A computer simulation study of the influence of imprinting on population structure. *Am. Natur.* **101**, 47–57.

Selander, R. K. (1972). Sexual selection and dimorphism in birds. *In* "Sexual Selection and the Descent of Man" (ed. B. Campbell). Heinemann, London.

Serradilla, J. M. and Ayala, F. J. (1983). Alloprocoptic selection: A mode of natural selection promoting polymorphism. *Proc. Natl Acad. Sci. USA* **80**, 2022–2025.

Shields, W. (1983). *In* "The Ecology of Animal Movement" (eds I. R. Swingland and P. J. Greenwood). Oxford University Press.

Smith, J. N. M. and Zach, R. (1979). Heritability of some morphological characters in a song sparrow population. *Evolution* **33**, 460–467.

Taylor, P. D. and Williams, G. C. (1981). On the modelling of sexual selection. *Quart. Rev. Biol.* **56**, 305–313.

Thoday, J. M. and Gibson, J. B. (1962). Isolation by disruptive selection. *Nature* **193**, 1164–1166.

West, M. J., King, A. P. and Eastzer, D. H. (1981). Validating the female bioassay of cowbird song: Relating differences in song potency to mating success. *Anim. Behav.* **29**, 490–501.

White, M. J. D. (1978). "Modes of Speciation". W. H. Freeman, San Francisco.

Williams, G. C. (1975). "Sex and Evolution". Princeton University Press.

Wilson, S. R. (1973). The correlation between relatives under the multifactorial model with assortative mating. *Ann. Hum. Genet.* **37**, 189–204.

Workman, P. L. (1964). The maintenance of heterozygosity by partial negative assortative mating. *Genetics* **50**, 1369–1382.

Wright, S. (1921). Systems of mating. III. Assortative mating based on somatic resemblance. *Genetics* **6**, 144–161.

10
Geographic Variation and Speciation

Kendall W. Corbin

Department of Ecology and Behavioral Biology, 318 Church Street South East, University of Minnesota, Minneapolis, Minnesota 55455, USA

1 INTRODUCTION

As a result of the pioneering documentation of variation of allelic frequencies in natural populations (Hubby and Lewontin 1966, Lewontin and Hubby 1966) and in human populations (Harris 1966), a new and exciting approach developed for the characterization of geographic variation within species and the quantification of genetic differences among taxa. The method of analysis providing this kind of information is the electrophoresis of allozymes. The data obtained are the genotypes of structural gene loci; the electrophoresis of proteins yields quantifiable information about the frequencies of alleles in natural populations. The data on genetic variation in natural populations accumulated rapidly, and we now have a great deal of information about the allelic frequencies of taxa at all levels of classification. This body of data makes possible the study of geographic variation of proteins and, by inference, of the genes that encode them. The genetic structure of local populations, demes,

AVIAN GENETICS
ISBN 0-12-187570-9

subspecies and species, can now be analysed in great detail, with intra- and interspecific comparisons being made with a precision that was impossible twenty years ago.

The variation associated with gross morphological structures (i.e. organelles, cells or higher levels of integration) is controlled by unknown numbers of genes acting alone and epistaticly. By contrast, there is essentially a one-to-one relationship between structural genes and their protein products. The use of genetic information, gained through the analysis of variation in protein structure, therefore, provides a more precise means for discriminating between genetically differentiated taxa. This potential for quantifying genetic differences between even the most closely related taxa, i.e. local neighbour-hoods, is now being realized, and many studies of the genetic differences among taxa at higher levels of classification have been carried out on a wide diversity of organisms.

The first such studies of birds were those of Bush (1967) on the House Sparrow (*Passer domesticus*). Since that time, not only have the techniques for the electrophoretic analysis of protein variants improved markedly, but also the methods for analysing the information from such studies have matured. It was once sufficient to detail the distribution of genotypes at polymorphic loci, estimate their deviation from expected equilibrium frequencies, provide rough estimates of the per cent heterozygosity within populations and calculate the percentage of loci that were polymorphic within the taxon. Now however, more sophisticated methods for the analysis of allelic frequency data are available. While this chapter will focus on these techniques and their application to the analysis of geographic variation, it will emphasize the methods of statistical analysis of allelic frequency data rather than the methods of biochemical analysis.

The early sections of the chapter will deal with the relationship between heterozygosity and polymorphism in natural populations, the various methods used to estimate heterozygosity, estimates of genetic distance and similarity, and the examination of genetic structure in avian populations (see also chapter 7 for a thorough discussion of genetic structure). The final sections of this chapter will deal with (1) clinal variation in natural avian populations, (2) heterozygosity as an index to boundaries between subspecies, (3) the disruption of clines in allelic frequencies resulting from secondary introgression between subspecies or species, and (4) genetic distances between species and the reorganization of genomes and gene pools during speciation.

2   ESTIMATION OF GENETIC VARIATION IN NATURAL POPULATIONS

The electrophoresis of even a moderate number of polymorphic proteins obtained from 20 or so individuals from each of a dozen populations, can provide an amazing amount of genetic information. Such data may be obtained in any of several ways depending upon the size of the organism, the expertise of the investigator and the resolving power of the electrophoretic technique employed. In avian studies one can easily assay the protein products of up to 40 gene loci from each individual (e.g., see Corbin 1981, Zink 1983), but fewer gene loci are often examined (see chapter 4). The size of the tissue samples one obtains from birds is normally more than adequate to carry out many electrophoretic comparisons. However, in those cases in which there is a limited amount of tissue from each individual, such as when tissue biopsies are made, each sample may provide genetic information on only a few gene loci. In such cases, an adequate sample can be obtained by repeatedly sampling the population.

In any event, the initial data set will consist of the distribution of observed genotypes, arranged by locus and population. Usually, and lamentably, such distributions are not published. Instead they are converted to allelic frequency distributions, which are the initial input for commonly used computer programs, that use the formulae of Nei (1972, 1978) for the estimation of genetic distance between taxa, of Farris (1972, 1973) for the reconstruction of evolutionary relationships, and of Wright (1978) for the estimation of the effects and extent of genetic exchange between populations. This section will deal with those statistics that one normally calculates in order to analyse geographic variation in the genetic structure of taxa.

2.1 Per cent polymorphism

The simple ratio of the number of polymorphic loci to the total number of loci examined electrophoretically is known as the per cent polymorphism of a taxon. What constitutes a polymorphic locus is not universally agreed upon, however. Conservative authors consider a locus to be polymorphic only if the frequency of the most abundant allele is 0·95 or less. Others, including myself and Evans (chapter 4) would set this limit at 0·99. Nevertheless, in comparison to some of the other statistics discussed below, per cent polymorphism may be a descriptive statistic of minimal interest in the context of a discussion of geographic variation.

In general, there is a positive correlation between per cent polymorphism and the overall level of genetic variability within a taxon. This is illustrated in Figs 1 and 2, in which the per cent polymorphism of the taxon is plotted as a function of genetic variability, expressed in terms of average heterozygosity (see below for more discussion about measures of heterozygosity). Within a species, per cent polymorphism may vary geographically, as seen in the variation among populations of White-crowned Sparrow (*Zonotrichia leucophrys*) (Table 1, based on the unpublished data of Corbin and Wilkie).

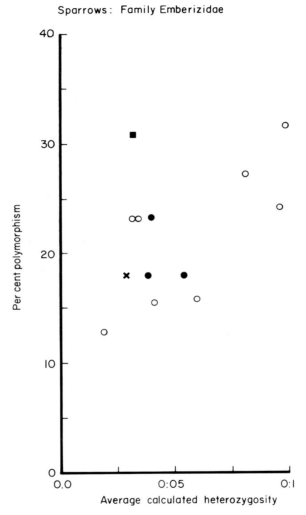

Fig. 1. The relationship between average calculated heterozygosity and per cent polymorphism for the avian subfamily Emberizinae, family Emberizidae: ○ comparisons for species and subspecies of the genus *Zonotrichia*; ● species of the genus *Melospiza*; ■ the genus *Passerella*; x the genus *Junco*. This analysis is based on the data of Baker (1975), Corbin (1981), Zink (1982), and Corbin and Wilkie (in preparation).

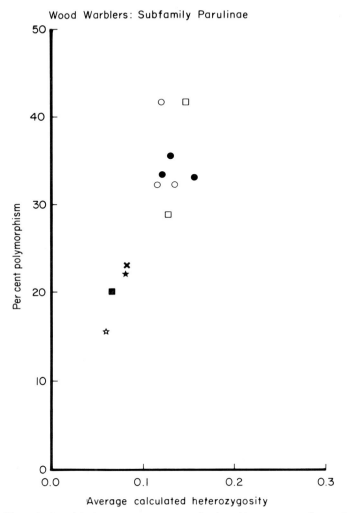

Fig. 2. The relationship between average calculated heterozygosity and per cent polymorphism for the avian subfamily Parulinae, family Emberizidae: ○ comparisons for species of the genus *Dendroica*; ● the genus *Vermivora*; □ the genus *Seiurus*; ■ the genus *Setophaga*; x the genus *Geothlypis*; ☆ the genus *Mniotilta*; ★ the genus *Oporornis*. This analysis is based on the data of Barrowclough and Corbin (1978).

Table 1. Per cent polymorphism, average observed heterozygosity, H_o, and average calculated heterozygosity, H_c, for populations of the White-crowned Sparrow, *Zonotrichia leucophrys*

Population	Number of genomes	Number of loci	Per cent polymorphism	$H_o \pm$ SD	$H_c \pm$ SD
California					
Jalama	36	45	0·244	0·044 ± 0·030	0·090 ± 0·192
Pt. Piedras Blancas	30	46	0·217	0·043 ± 0·028	0·065 ± 0·165
Marina	20	46	0·217	0·047 ± 0·035	0·071 ± 0·168
Pt. Reyes	42	46	0·304	0·057 ± 0·030	0·098 ± 0·175
Manchester	40	45	0·244	0·078 ± 0·034	0·096 ± 0·190
Rockport	20	46	0·174	0·056 ± 0·019	0·068 ± 0·163
Ferndale	30	45	0·244	0·062 ± 0·019	0·091 ± 0·193
Oregon					
Yachats	32	46	0·239	0·059 ± 0·040	0·099 ± 0·210

This variation in per cent polymorphism appears to be a result of the exchange of different alleles between subspecies of White-crowned Sparrow. In some cases, unique aspects of life history parameters of the species, such as high levels of inbreeding, may affect the per cent polymorphism, as in Lesser Prairie Chicken (*Tympanuchus pallidicinctus*), which has a per cent polymorphism of 0·0 (Gutiérrez *et al.* 1983). This is probably the result of having a small effective breeding population perpetuated by only one or a few breeding males.

Among all avian species examined, per cent polymorphism varies from a high value of 0·714 for the steamer duck, *Tachyeres patachonicus* (Corbin 1983), to the lower limit of 0·0 mentioned above for Lesser Prairie Chicken (Gutiérrez *et al.* 1983). The average value for birds, based on the taxa and studies listed in Table 2, is 0·222 ± 0·128. This is slightly below the range of per cent polymorphisms found for other groups of organisms (Selander 1978, Nevo 1978), but among the best studied groups of birds, such as the wood warblers of the subfamily Parulinae (Barrowclough and Corbin 1978) and the sparrows of the genus *Zonotrichia* (Baker 1975, Corbin 1981, Avise *et al.* 1980 b, Zink 1982), per cent polymorphisms are well within the range of polymorphism for all other groups (Figs 1 and 2).

2.2 Genic heterozygosity

Heterozygosity is a parameter whose value will vary with the particular method of calculation. Unfortunately, a distinction between methods used to estimate heterozygosity usually has not been made in the literature, and some confusion exists, therefore, concerning both the interpretation and usefulness of this statistic. Obviously, any attempt to compare values of heterozygosity calculated by means of different methods will lead to confusion. It is less obvious that levels of variance differ greatly among the different kinds of estimate of heterozygosity. This may lead to some difficulty, if not the impossibility, of demonstrating the existence of significant patterns of geographic variation in heterozygosity.

Heterozygosity is an estimate of the average number of loci within an individual that are in a heterozygous state. In its simplest method of calculation, the observed heterozygosity of individuals is the ratio of the number of heterozygous loci to the total number of loci examined in an individual. By averaging the observed individual heterozygosity over individuals, one obtains what I call the "average observed heterozygosity", $\bar{H}_0$, for a taxon (Corbin 1981). The variance associated with this estimate can be reduced both by increasing the number of loci examined electrophoretically and by increasing the number of individuals sampled from the population. A second method is to calculate the observed frequency of heterozygotes per

Table 2. Per cent polymorphism and average calculated heterozygosity, H_c, for avian species. The classification is according to the Thirty-fourth Supplement to the A.O.U. Check-list of North American Birds. Species are included if at least five individuals have been examined by means of electrophoresis. Updated from "Current Ornithology", Vol. 1, pp. 211–244 (Plenum Press, Copyright 1983).

Family and species	Number of genomes	Number of loci	Per cent polymorphism	$H_c \pm$ SD	Reference
Procellariidae					
Thalassoica antarctica	16	16	25·0	0·114 ± 0·240	Barrowclough *et al.* (1981), Corbin (1983)
Daption capense	16	16	31·3	0·143 ± 0·239	
Pagodroma nivea	22	16	43·8	0·175 ± 0·231	
Pachyptila desolata	16	16	31·3	0·134 ± 0·225	
Hydrobatidae					
Oceanites oceanicus	24	16	25·0	0·096 ± 0·180	Barrowclough *et al.* (1981), Corbin (1983)
Anatidae					
Tachyeres patachonicus	68	14	71·4[a]	0·307 ± 0·017	Corbin, Humphrey and Livezey (unpublished work)
T. leucocephalus	12	14	64·3	0·164 ± 0·154	
Phasianidae					
Tetraoninae					
Tympanuchus pallidicinctus	26	27	0·0	0·0	Gutiérrez *et al.* (1983)
Phasianinae					
Phasianus colchicus	26	27	11·1	0·031 ± 0·100	
Coturnix coturnix	60	27	19·7	0·075 ± 0·031	
Alectoris chukar	24	27	14·8	0·052 ± 0·138	
Lophortyx californicus	72	27	18·5[a]	0·025 ± 0·008	
L. gambelii	44	27	18·5	0·031 ± 0·098	
Callipepla squamata	58	27	13·0[a]	0·037 ± 0·023	
Colinus virginianus	30	27	14·8[a]	0·034 ± 0·004	
Oreortyx pictus	32	27	11·1	0·024 ± 0·092	
Cyrtonyx montuzumae	62	27	20·4[a]	0·039 ± 0·009	

Taxon					Reference
Picidae					
Sphyrapicus r. ruber	26	39	15.4	0.046 ± 0.021[b]	Johnson and Zink (1983)
S. ruber daggetti	30	39	15.4	0.044 ± 0.019	
S. nuchalis	68	39	17.1[a]	0.048 ± 0.020	
S. v. varius	14	39	12.8	0.032 ± 0.015	
S. thyroideus	36	39	7.7	0.015 ± 0.013	
Tyrannidae					
Empidonax flaviventris	38	38	28.2	0.084 ± 0.024[b]	Zink and Johnson (to be published)
E. virescens	20	38	30.8	0.091 ± 0.027	
E. alnorum	34	38	28.2	0.079 ± 0.026	
E. traillii	40	38	28.2	0.088 ± 0.025	
E. euleri	44	38	20.5	0.065 ± 0.022	
E. minimus	36	38	15.4	0.054 ± 0.019	
E. hammondii	26	38	15.4	0.060 ± 0.025	
E. wrightii	36	38	17.9	0.047 ± 0.019	
E. oberholseri	34	38	23.1	0.073 ± 0.025	
E. difficilis	32	38	15.4	0.054 ± 0.022	
E. flavescens	12	38	7.7	0.021 ± 0.014	
E. atriceps	36	38	12.8	0.043 ± 0.020	
Contopus borealis	16	38	28.2	0.079 ± 0.022	
C. sordidulus	10	38	23.1	0.079 ± 0.026	
C. virens	14	38	30.8	0.096 ± 0.026	
Mimidae					
Dumetella carolinensis	16	24	20.8	0.028 ± 0.059	Avise et al. (1980a)
Muscicapidae					
Turdinae					
Catharus ustulatus	34	27	29.6	0.065 ± 0.140	Avise et al. (1980a)
C. guttatus	26	27	25.9	0.045 ± 0.089	
C. fuscescens	10	27	18.5	0.048 ± 0.107	
Hylocichla mustelina	10	27	14.8	0.060 ± 0.150	
Turdus migratorius	10	26	7.7	0.031 ± 0.108	
Sialia sialis	14	27	14.8	0.045 ± 0.121	

Table 2–*continued*

Family and species	Number of genomes	Number of loci	Per cent polymorphism	$H_c \pm$ SD	Reference
Sylviinae					
Regulus calendula	20	23	17·4	0·037 ± 0·097	Corbin *et al.* (1974)
Sturnidae					
Aplonis m. metallica	372	18	11·8[a]	0·054 ± 0·157	
A. m. nitida	278	18	11·1[a]	0·046 ± 0·136	
A. m. purpuriceps	58	18	11·1	0·027 ± 0·100	
A. cantaroides	188	18	12·5[a]	0·016 ± 0·061	
Emberizidae					
Parulinae					
Vermivora peregrina	26	30	33·3	0·158 ± 0·243	Barrowclough and Corbin (1978)
V. celata	16	31	35·5	0·130 ± 0·203	
V. ruficapilla	44	31	33·5	0·123 ± 0·186	
Mniotilta varia	16	26	15·4	0·064 ± 0·157	
Dendroica magnolia	28	31	32·3	0·117 ± 0·208	
D. coronata	70	31	41·9	0·121 ± 0·175	
D. palmarum	24	31	32·3	0·134 ± 0·214	
D. striata	12	31	3·2	0·016 ± 0·090	
Seiurus auricapillus	20	31	29·0	0·126 ± 0·209	
S. noveboracensis	48	31	41·9	0·147 ± 0·219	
Oporornis philadelphia	16	27	22·2	0·081 ± 0·163	
Geothlypis trichas	32	30	23·3	0·084 ± 0·169	
Setophaga ruticilla	24	30	20·0	0·069 ± 0·159	
Dendroica c. coronata	96	32	15·6[a]	0·031 ± 0·003	Barrowclough (1980 a)
D. c. auduboni	114	32	16·7[a]	0·034 ± 0·003	
Icterinae					
Icterus g. galbula	246	19	10·5	0·071 ± 0·005	Corbin *et al.* (1978)
I. g. bullockii	132	19	10·5	0·073 ± 0·001	

Emberizinae					
Zonotrichia leucophrus nuttalli	298	19	31·6	0·098 ± 0·158	Baker (1975)
Z. l. oriantha	156	19	15·8	0·065 ± 0·100	
Z. l. nuttalli	128	46	24·6[a]	0·085 ± 0·013	Corbin (1981, 1983)
Z. l. pugetensis	82	46	21·9[a]	0·096 ± 0·005	
Z. capensis hypoleuca	390	14	42·8	0·099 ± 0·009	Handford and Nottebohm (1976)
Z. c. carabayae	126	45	48·9[a]	0·096 ± 0·159	Corbin (1983)
Z. albicollis	20	21	33·3	0·062 ± 0·109	Avise et al. (1980 b)
Z. leucophrys	38	39	23·1	0·032 ± 0·081	Zink (1982)
Z. albicollis	24	39	23·1	0·034 ± 0·075	
Z. atricapilla	30	39	15·4	0·041 ± 0·117	
Z. querula	36	39	12·8	0·019 ± 0·058	
Ammodramus sandwichensis	20	20	25·0	0·042 ± 0·089	Avise et al. (1980 b)
A. savannorum	20	20	20·0	0·051 ± 0·132	
Spizella passerina	22	21	14·3	0·030 ± 0·083	
S. pusilla	21	21	14·3	0·054 ± 0·150	
Amphispiza bilineata	14	21	9·5	0·028 ± 0·101	
Pipilo fuscus	10	21	4·8	0·009 ± 0·039	
Junco hyemalis	20	21	14·3	0·045 ± 0·138	
J. hyemalis	96	39	17·9	0·029 ± 0·095	Zink (1982)
Melospiza melodia	14	20	5·0	0·007 ± 0·029	Avise et al. (1980 b)
M. melodia	28	39	17·9	0·038 ± 0·097	Zink (1982)
M. lincolnii	16	39	17·9	0·054 ± 0·128	
M. georgiana	20	21	19·0	0·031 ± 0·071	Avise et al. (1980 b)
M. georgiana	32	39	23·1	0·040 ± 0·087	Zink (1982)
Passerella iliaca	114	39	30·8	0·032 ± 0·069	

[a] These values of per cent polymorphism are the averages of two or more populations.

[b] Values for the Picidae and Tyrannidae are $H_c \pm$ SE.

locus, and then average these values over loci (Corbin *et al.* 1974, 1979, Barrowclough and Corbin 1978). Given a data set identical to that used in the first method, the average observed heterozygosity estimated by the two methods will be identical, but the variance associated with the second method will be significantly larger, owing to the inclusion of a large interlocus component; that is, much of the variance of the second kind of estimate is a consequence of the high diversity in the number of alleles per locus, some loci being monomorphic, whereas others are highly polymorphic.

The third and fourth methods for estimating heterozygosity both assume that the distribution of genotypes within a population conforms to an expected Hardy–Weinberg equilibrium. The third method is to use the equilibrium frequencies of heterozygotes to approximate the heterozygosity per locus. These estimates are then averaged to obtain the average heterozygosity for the taxon (e.g., see Avise *et al.* 1980 a). As in the second method, the variance associated with this estimate will be large owing to the inclusion of a large interlocus component. The fourth method is perhaps the most commonly used, although the variances associated with this measure are also large. With this method, proposed by Nei (1975), one uses the allelic frequencies at each locus to calculate the heterozygosity per locus, which equals $1 - \sum x_i^2$, where x_i is the frequency of the ith allele at locus x. As in the two previous methods, the values are averaged over loci to obtain the average heterozygosity for the taxon. Table 1 gives a comparison, based on the same data set, of the variances associated with average heterozygosities estimated by the first and fourth methods. For a more detailed description of these four methods, see Corbin (1981) and chapter 4.

By the early 1970s it was obvious that a significant positive correlation existed between the per cent polymorphism and heterozygosity. In general, vertebrate populations exhibit relatively low heterozygosities and low per cent polymorphisms whereas invertebrates, and especially insects, are highly polymorphic and have high levels of heterozygosity within most taxa (Nevo 1978, Selander 1978). There are many exceptions to this general pattern, however. For example, within birds, there are representative taxa that span almost the entire range found in all other phyla. This is illustrated in Fig. 3, in which the values, with a few exceptions, are the averages for several species within each genus.

Correlations between heterozygosity and biological or environmental factors have been sought almost since the earliest studies of allelic frequencies in natural populations. Few hard and fast relationships have been found. Basically, the hypotheses proposed invoke either a selectionist or neutralist explanation. Only a few of these hypotheses are relevant to a discussion of geographic variation in birds.

Calculated heterozygosity will be maximized at a locus when the alleles at

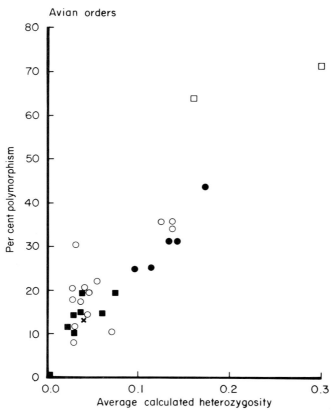

Fig. 3. The relationship between per cent polymorphism and average calculated heterozygosity for genera of birds representing 11 families and 5 orders of birds: ○ comparisons for the order Passeriformes; ● the order Procellariiformes; □ the order Anseriformes; ■ the order Galliformes; x the order Piciformes. This analysis is based on the data of Barrowclough and Corbin (1978), Corbin *et al.* (1979), Avise *et al.* (1980 a,b), Barrowclough *et al.* (1981), Zink (1982), Gutiérrez *et al.* (1983), Johnson and Zink (1983), and Corbin, Livezey and Humphrey (unpublished work).

that locus are equal in frequency (Corbin 1981). For observed heterozygosity, the same will be true if the alleles are selectively equivalent and the population is in Hardy–Weinberg equilibrium. If two populations or subspecies are genetically differentiated, and if they exchange alleles via juvenile or adult dispersal, the level of genetic variability should be highest at some point within the zone of contact between the two differentiated populations. In nature, however, gene flow between populations may be greater in one direction than the other, and thus, the peak of heterozygosity will not fall exactly mid-way

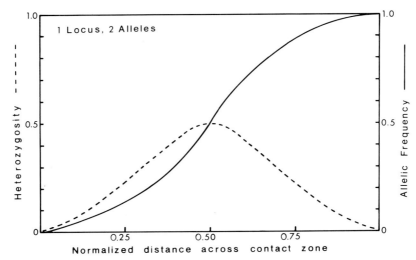

Fig. 4. A theoretical model showing how heterozygosity at a single gene locus might vary as a function of clinal variation in allelic frequencies within a zone of intergradation between two genically differentiated populations, subspecies or species in secondary contact. In this model, heterozygosity, shown by the dashed line, is calculated as $1 - \sum x_i^2$, where the x_is are the frequencies of only two alleles, each of which is fixed in one or the other of the two, intergrading populations. The solid line shows the variation at one of these two alleles. Heterozygosity is maximized when the frequencies of the two alleles are identical. In general, this relationship is true for any number of alleles, greater than one.

between the two taxa. This relationship between allelic frequencies and heterozygosity within a zone of contact between genetically differentiated populations is shown in Fig. 4. In this model the values of calculated heterozygosity $\bar{H}_c$ at only one locus are calculated from the allelic frequencies at each point according to the equation $\bar{H} = 1 - \sum x_i^2$. It is assumed here that the genetically differentiated populations are fixed for alternative alleles.

Within populations, heterozygosity will be maximized when allelic frequencies at all polymorphic loci are equalized or when all polymorphic loci are heterozygous within individuals. The latter is unlikely to occur except under conditions of selective neutrality or selective equality. The data from natural populations suggest that the second of these limits is not reached, but under certain conditions allelic frequencies may approach equality. Such conditions potentially exist whenever one population having allelic frequencies above 0·5 introgresses with another having frequencies below 0·5. This is particularly likely to occur in zones of intergradation between subspecies in secondary contact. At least one example of this kind of geographic variation in heterozygosity has been found, and is described in greater detail under section 3.

2.3 Genetic similarity and distance

In 1972, Rogers and Nei independently derived measures of genetic similarity and distance between taxa (Rogers 1972, Nei 1972). Although both utilized allelic frequencies to estimate genetic similarity and difference, their distance parameters have very different properties. Rogers' method calculates an index of genetic distance, D, which is the mean geometric distance between taxa, but it is unclear what this means in biological terms (see chapter 4 for a detailed presentation of the equations used). The limiting values taken by D are 0·0, in the case of taxa that share all of their alleles at identical frequencies, and 1·0 for taxa that do not share any alleles. Rogers' genetic similarity is equal to $1 - D$. The principal value of the distance measure D is that it is a metric and, therefore, satisfies the triangle inequality (Barrowclough and Corbin 1978, Farris 1981). That is, in the comparison of three taxa, A, B and C, the sum of the genetic distances between any two pairs, e.g., A–B and B–C, will be equal to or greater than the genetic distance between the third pair, A–C. This is convenient when reconstructing evolutionary trees because branch lengths in a cladogram will always have positive values.

The method of Nei (1972), which estimates the normalized genetic identity, I, of allelic frequencies for alleles shared by a pair of taxa at a locus, is not a metric. However, I does have a clear biological meaning; the probability that alleles drawn at random from two populations or taxa are identical. Nei's standard genetic distance, D, is a non-linear function of I, and is estimated as the negative natural logarithm of I (Nei 1972, 1978).

Values of Nei's normalized genetic identity range between 1·0 for pairs of populations or taxa that have identical allelic frequencies at all loci, to 0·0 for pairs of taxa that do not share any alleles. Standard genetic distance, on the other hand, ranges between 0·0 for pairs of taxa that have identical allelic frequencies, to infinity for those that do not share any alleles. Among avian taxa, however, it is rare to find pairs of species having values of D greater than 0·9. Interestingly, D is thought to be an estimate of the number of nucleotide base-pair substitutions per gene locus that have accumulated during evolutionary time since the divergence of taxa from their common ancestor (Nei 1972). This, however, assumes that evolutionary rates are identical along lineages and among loci. Viewed in this way, in the comparison of two taxa, a D-value of 0·01 would indicate that one allelic substitution had occurred per 100 gene loci since the divergence of these taxa from their common ancestor. A value of 0·5 would indicate that 50 allelic substitutions had occurred per 100 gene loci, and so on.

2.4   Genetic structure and geographic variation

In chapter 7 of this volume, Rockwell and Barrowclough define the "genetic structure of populations" as the degree of genetic continuity or correlation maintained throughout the range of a species. They consider in detail the calculation and use of the parameter F_{ST} for the description of genetic structure in taxa at or below the level of species. In this chapter I describe the application of this statistic to the analysis of geographic variation in natural populations, and describe its relationship to Nei's indices of genetic distance and similarity.

As discussed in detail by Wright (1921, 1951, 1965, 1978) there are various components of genetic variance associated with allelic frequency estimates of populations, natural or artificial. The measure F_{ST} deals specifically with the among-population component of the total variance (Wright 1951). It is the correlation between the alleles of randomly sampled individuals, obtained from two or more subdivisions of a taxon, to the allelic distribution of the entire taxon. The taxa usually considered are subdivisions of the species, i.e. local populations, demes and subspecies. In practice, one should consider F_{ST} as the probability that allelic frequency distributions, drawn at random for one or more loci from two or more populations, are unique. If the allelic frequency distributions are identical, then F_{ST} will equal 0·0. If no alleles are shared in common, i.e. if alternative alleles are fixed in the different subdivisions of the taxon, then the value of F_{ST} will be 1·0. As such, F_{ST} is very similar to and highly correlated with Nei's standard genetic distance (Corbin 1983), and it is inversely related to Nei's normalized genetic identity. Further, it shows little or no correlation with Rogers' indices.

Although Nei's indices provide one with a rigorous measure of the degree of similarity between taxa, they are not related to any of the usual test statistics with their associated levels of confidence. On the other hand, if only two alleles exist at each polymorphic locus (or if there are more than two alleles, they are treated as though there were only two alleles having frequencies p and $1 - p = q$), and if the sample size, n, of each subdivision is identical, then F_{ST} is readily transformed to chi-squared:

$$\chi^2 = 2NF_{ST}$$

where N equals $\sum n$. However, when there are more than two alleles at polymorphic loci, which is often the case, then a particularly powerful test of whether or not F_{ST} is significantly different from zero is the log-likelihood chi-squared test (or G test) of homogeneity of the allele distributions themselves. Here one is essentially asking whether the distributions of alleles among subdivisions of a taxon are homogeneous. As such, a G-statistic is calculated for the distribution of alleles, not allelic frequencies, at each locus, with each subdivision being a replicate to yield a replicated goodness of fit test for the locus. Values for individual polymorphic loci are then pooled to estimate the total G-statistic or log-likelihood chi-squared value. The equation and associated degrees of freedom for the ith locus involving the comparison of two or more subdivisions, as based on Sokal and Rohlf (1969, pp. 575–581), is as follows:

$$G_i = 2\left[\sum_j \sum_k (x_{jk} \ln x_{jk}) - \sum_k (b \ln b) - \sum_j (n \ln n) + (N \ln N)\right]$$

with $(k-1)(j-1)$ degrees of freedom, where j is the number of subdivisions, k is the number of alleles at locus i, x_{jk} is the number of kth alleles in the jth subdivision, b equals $\sum_j x_{jk}$ and is the total number of kth alleles summed over all subdivisions, n equals $\sum_k x_{jk}$ and is the total number of copies of all k alleles at the ith locus of the jth subdivision, and N equals $\sum_j \sum_k x_{jk}$, which is the total number of copies of all alleles within all subdivisions. The G-statistic for all loci taken simultaneously, which is the best measure of whether F_{ST} deviates significantly from zero, is the sum of the G_is for individual loci, with $\sum[(k-1)(j-1)]$ degrees of freedom.

3 CLINAL VARIATION IN NATURAL POPULATIONS

With the background provided above, we shall now look at a few examples of geographic variation involving (1) variation in allelic frequencies, (2) variation in heterozygosity, and (3) subdivision within a species based on the F_{ST} statistic. Before beginning this discussion, however, it may be helpful to define a few of the terms that will be used here. Through time a population may divide into two or more geographically isolated populations. During the period of geographic isolation, the frequencies of alleles shared by the different populations may diverge and new mutations, i.e., new alleles, may arise and increase in frequency in one population and not in the others. This process of divergence with respect to allele types and frequencies is called "genetic differentiation". If at some time following geographic isolation, two populations have re-established a zone of contact, this is known as a "secondary zone of intergradation". Finally, if those populations in secondary contact have become genetically differentiated during the period of isolation and then subsequently exchange genes via the dispersal of reproductively active individuals, the movement of genes is known as "gene flow" and the introduction of new alleles from one population into another is called "introgression".

3.1   Clines in allelic frequencies

Several electrophoretic studies of avian species have involved the analysis of geographic variation in allelic frequencies. These include the studies of Corbin *et al.* (1974), Baker (1975), Corbin *et al.* (1979), Barrowclough (1980), Corbin (1981), Johnson and Zink (1983) and Zink (1983). In several of these, little or no significant geographic variation of allelic frequencies was found, even when there was obvious geographic variation in plumage pattern and coloration or skeletal morphology. Among those cases in which allelic frequencies vary geographically, the patterns of variation appear to fall into one of two categories; one of which might have been predicted, the other unexpected, and not yet explained.

The first pattern is that zones of intergradation and introgression based on variation in allelic frequencies span broader geographic regions than do those based on clines for other morphological characters of the same organism. There may or may not be a generalized concordance among clines in allelic frequencies. For example, clines based on plumage pattern and coloration resulting from hybridization in the orioles of the genus *Icterus* are most evident over a distance of about 80 km across the Great Plains of North America (Sibley and Short 1964, Rising 1970, 1973, Corbin and Sibley 1977). By contrast, the zone of intergradation based on allelic frequency variation at two esterase loci extends from the Rocky Mountains to the central-midwestern states (Corbin *et al.* 1979), a distance of 750 km or more. Likewise, in the case of White-crowned Sparrow, Banks' (1964) morphological study of the contact zone between the subspecies *nuttalli* and *pugetensis* defined a zone of intergradation of about 160 km along the California coast, whereas Corbin's (1981) study of allelic variation at 46 loci showed that the zone of intergradation was about 300 km in length (see Fig. 5; based on data of Corbin and Wilkie (in preparation)).

The second pattern emerges from studies involving introgression between genetically differentiated taxa in secondary contact. Within zones of intergradation between such taxa, there may be abrupt, and unpredictable changes in allelic frequencies, as illustrated by the data for the two subspecies of White-crowned Sparrow, *Z. l. nuttalli* and *Z. l. pugetensis* (Fig. 5). Contrary to expectation, the clinal patterns observed outside of the zone of intergradation completely disintegrate within the zone; these patterns are unlike any pattern predicted by cline theory (Endler 1977). Three plausible explanations for this observation are (1) that populations within the zone of intergradation are both small and isolated from one another, thus resulting in significant effects of drift, (2) that gene complexes co-adapted outside the zone of contact are disrupted by even low levels of gene flow into the zone, with the new arrangements responding differentially to novel selective regimes, or (3)

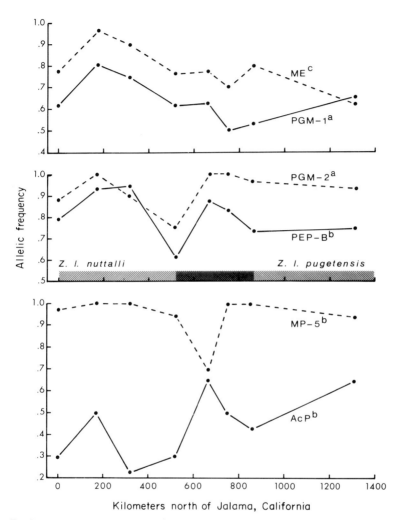

Fig. 5. Geographic variation in the allelic frequencies of selected polymorphic loci of the White-crowned Sparrow subspecies *Zonotrichia leucophrys nuttalli* and *Z. l. pugetensis,* which intergrade in northern California (Corbin and Wilkie, in preparation). Localities, left to right, are as given in Table 1 and shown in Fig. 7. Not only is there significant geographic variation in allelic frequencies among the different populations, but also frequencies within the zone of contact between the two subspecies (indicated by the overlapped hatching) do not conform to theoretical expectations for *Pgm-2, Pep-B, MP-5,* and *Acp.*

that local populations within the zone of intergradation possess gene complexes that are well adapted to local conditions in the transition zone and natural selection offsets the effects of gene flow.

Where the subspecies are poorly differentiated or completely isolated, such as on separate islands, then such erratic shifts in allelic frequency may or may not be found. For example, the allelic variation at the lactate dehydrogenase locus of Metallic Starling (*Aplonis metallica*) involves three subspecies inhabiting both mainland New Guinea and the islands of the Bismarck Archipelago. Changes in allelic frequencies among these populations and subspecies follow a predictable pattern (Corbin *et al.* 1974). At Talasea, on New Britain in the southern part of the archipelago, the frequency of $Ldh\text{-}H^b$ is 0·58. Moving northward along the archipelago, the frequency of this allele increases to 0·63 at Rabaul, New Britain, to 0·74 at Kavieng on New Ireland, and to 0·96 at Lorengau on Manus Island. Simultaneously, the frequency of $Ldh\text{-}H^a$ decreases from 0·42 to 0·04.

In the comparison of five populations of Yellow-rumped Warbler (*Dendroica coronata*), Barrowclough (1980) found polymorphisms at 8 out of 32 gene loci, with five of these eight loci having three or four alleles. In spite of this amount of variation and although the subspecies *D. c. coronata* and *D. c. auduboni* are readily distinguished on the basis of plumage differences, only one of the eight polymorphic loci showed significant levels of heterogeneity among the five localities, and none of the allelic frequencies at these eight loci varied clinally. Therefore, populations of the parental subspecies were not significantly different from one another, nor were there abrupt changes in allelic frequency within the zone of intergradation between them.

In an exhaustive analysis of the genic variation of eight subspecies of Fox Sparrow (*Passerella iliaca*), Zink (1983) could not detect significant geographic variation either among local populations or among subspecies. This is particularly interesting given that variation in other morphological traits is extensive among subspecies of Fox Sparrows.

With regard to variation in allelic frequencies as a function of environmental parameters, an analysis of genic variation at 55 loci of Rufous-collared Sparrow (*Zonotrichia capensis*; (Corbin, in preparation)) revealed that only one locus, out of 21 that were polymorphic, varied significantly as a function of elevation above sea level. This is to be expected by chance alone, however. In addition, there was no significant variation among the major vegetational communities, including humid montane forest, montane cloud forest, montane chaparral and alpine grassland.

The above results, taken together with those of Evans (chapter 4), point to a single general pattern of geographic variation in allelic frequencies among bird populations. Namely, it appears that gene flow among populations offsets local variation due to drift and selective differences. This supposition is

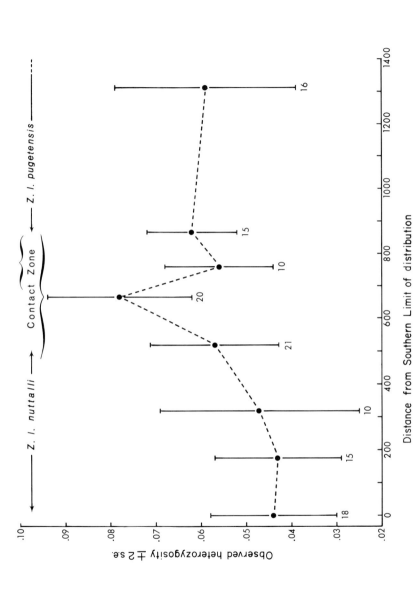

Fig. 6. Geographic variation in observed heterozygosity, based on the allelic variation at 46 gene loci, in White-crowned Sparrow (*Zonotrichia leucophrys*). The vertical lines indicate ±2 standard errors of the mean heterozygosity values, and the number of individuals sampled from a locality is given at the bottom of each line. Localities from left to right are as given in Table 1. The zone of intergradation based on morphological studies is indicated by the upper bracket, and constitutes only the northern half of the zone of intergradation based on the variation in heterozygosity, as indicated by the lower bracket. Based on Corbin (1981).

supported by the findings of Barrowclough (1980) who was unable to detect differences in selection coefficients among the alleles of polymorphic loci of the Yellow-rumped Warbler.

3.2   Clinal variation in heterozygosity

As discussed in section 2.2 above, there are theoretical reasons to believe that heterozygosity should vary within zones of secondary contact between either hybridizing species or between genetically differentiated subspecies. Only one study of avian species has dealt specifically with this phenomenon. That analysis (Corbin 1981) examined the contact zone between the coastal subspecies of White-crowned Sparrow, *Z. l. nuttalli* and *Z. L. pugetensis*. The results are shown in Fig. 6, in which the average observed heterozygosity, estimated by means of the first method described in section 2.2 above, peaks at or near the mid-point within the zone of intergradation between these two subspecies. It is of interest to note that the zone of intergradation defined on the basis of variation in external morphology constitutes only the northern half of this zone of contact defined by the variation in heterozygosity.

It seems plausible that heterozygosity might also vary geographically as a function of any of several environmental parameters. However, such relationships could not be demonstrated for different populations of Rufous-collared Sparrow (*Zonotrichia capensis carabayae*) that were sampled from five different biomes or ecotones over an elevational gradient extending from 2040 to 3900 metres in the Cordillera Oriental of the Bolivian Andes (Corbin, in preparation).

4   GENETIC STRUCTURE AS A MEASURE OF GEOGRAPHIC VARIATION

Wright's *F*-statistic, F_{ST}, has now been used in a number of avian studies to measure the degree of genetic divergence among subdivisions of a species. Much of this work has been reviewed by Barrowclough (1983). Here I call attention to the potential use of this statistic as an aid in partitioning homogeneous subdivisions of a species. Since the log-likelihood χ^2 statistic is composed of nested sets of additive values, these values can be examined for homogeneous subsets, which correspond to local populations, demes and subspecies. Obviously, if one looks at enough combinations of these subsets, non-homogeneous groupings of populations may be found by chance alone. Thus, the level of confidence must be sufficiently rigorous to guarantee the reliability of this method. The data for White-crowned Sparrows (Corbin

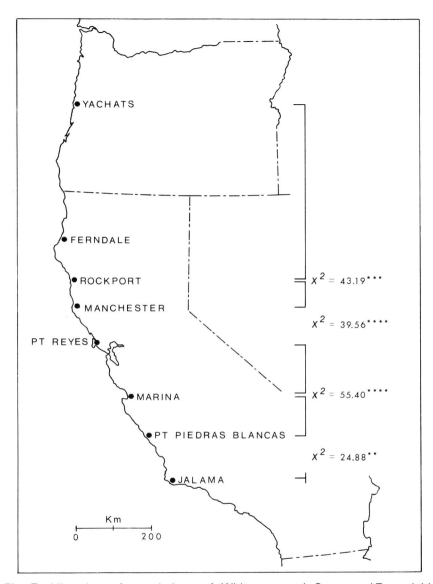

Fig. 7. Allocation of populations of White-crowned Sparrow (*Zonotrichia leucophrys*) to genically homogeneous subsets, as based on chi-squared values associated with F_{ST} values calculated for various combinations of local populations. Any combination of populations not included within a bracket yields values of F_{ST} that are significantly different from zero. The χ^2 values shown are for cases where the next adjacent population outside of a bracket is included in the calculation of F_{ST}. The corresponding levels of significance are indicated by the stars, where ** is for $P \leq 0.025$, *** is for $P \leq 0.01$, and **** is for $P \leq 0.005$.

1981, Corbin and Wilkie, in preparation) again may be used to illustrate this approach to the recognition of genetic structure, and thereby geographic variation, within the taxon.

When the coastal populations of White-crowned Sparrows in California and Oregon were examined by means of an F_{ST} analysis, several groups of populations formed homogeneous subsets. Since the natural distribution of these subspecies of White-crowned Sparrow consists of a narrow north–south linear sequence of populations along the coast of California and Oregon, sampled populations were compared pairwise north to south and then blocked into larger and larger sets of populations based on whether or not the F_{ST} values were significantly different from zero. The results of this type of analysis are shown in Fig. 7, in which homogeneous subsets of populations are delimited by brackets. Comparisons of populations within brackets have values of F_{ST} that are not significantly different from zero, whereas the inclusion of one or more populations from different sets of brackets yields values that are significantly different from zero. The result of the analysis is that the southernmost population sampled from Jalama, California apparently is part of a deme that is distinct from one that includes the three populations at Point Piedras Blancas, Marina and Point Reyes, California. These, in turn, are distinct from a third deme that includes the four populations to the north. Taken together, the two southern demes constitute the subspecies *Zonotrichia l. nuttalli*, and the northern deme is part of the subspecies *Z. l. pugetensis*. It remains to be determined whether these genetically differentiated demes coincide with physiographic or ecological discontinuities that might restrict gene flow. It is clear, however, that the major differentiation between the subspecies occurs between populations that are migratory (*Z. l. pugetensis*) and those that are non-migratory (*Z. l. nuttalli*).

5 SPECIATION

Speciation has been defined as the acquisition of reproductive isolation by a population or group of populations (Mayr 1963). Among other definitions, the taxon species has been defined as "groups of actually or potentially interbreeding natural populations which are reproductively isolated from other such groups" (Mayr 1940). In his definition of species, Dobzhansky (1961) stressed the homogeneity of the gene pool shared by different subdivisions of a population. Namely, "a species is the most inclusive Mendelian population" (Dobzhansky 1961). In the absence of information concerning the breeding biology of interacting populations, these definitions do not, however, greatly aid us in distinguishing species. For populations that cannot come into contact because of geographic isolation, these definitions are almost meaningless. Aside from a biological definition of the species, what we should like to know is how different must such populations be genetically to be considered as distinct species. How different are the genotypic and allelic frequency distributions of populations before and after speciation? An answer to the latter question provides us with some guidelines relative to the first.

Over the last decade and a half, the study of allelic variation in natural populations by means of electrophoresis has led to the accumulation of remarkable information about the genetic differences between species (see reviews in Powell (1975), Ayala (1976), Corbin (1978, 1983), Barrowclough (1983)). Nevertheless, with the exception of fruit flies in the genus *Drosophila* (Ayala *et al.* 1974 a,b,c, Carson 1978, 1982), and in the genus *Rhagoletis* (Berlocher and Bush 1982), we do not yet have good estimates of genetic distances between species at the time of and shortly following speciation. (In this context, even a speciation event as long ago as the Pleistocene might be considered recent.) Instead, what we do know rather well is the extent of genetic differentiation between and among species that have had separate evolutionary histories for extremely long periods of time. In all likelihood, there is no single degree of genetic differentiation that characterizes species level differences among congeners. Rather, it is probable that the number of genetic differences (i.e. accumulated mutations) that distinguish one species from another varies among organisms and taxonomic groups. That is to say, there is probably no single threshold number of nucleotide base-pair substitutions that results in the cladogenesis of one species into two. Nevertheless, it is of interest to determine the range and magnitude of the genetic distances that separate species.

For most pairs of avian species, with the exception of sibling species, it is rather easy to distinguish the different species within a genus by means of classical methods. With some exceptions, even closely related species are remarkably different from one another in terms of their morphology, physiology and behaviour. The differences themselves may be either the result of the slow accumulation and fixation of new alleles both prior to and following speciation or they have developed rapidly during speciation. In either case, abrupt increases in genetic distance should be associated with speciation events.

In 1954, Mayr hypothesized that emerging species may undergo genetic revolutions during speciation following the reproductive isolation of a small peripheral, founder population. Although this mode of speciation is merely one form of allopatric speciation, Mayr later (1982) coined the term "peripatric speciation" to distinguish it from those situations in which a population is divided into two or more large, but reproductively isolated, populations that subsequently undergo speciation. Mayr's hypothesis was later criticized by Carson and Templeton (1984), and shown to be an unlikely means by which significant differences might evolve between species. Carson and Templeton (1984) have demonstrated, however, that under a limited set of conditions, a small founder population may undergo a genetic revolution during speciation. Clearly, when speciation of this type occurs, genetic distances should then increase rapidly. In such cases, if it were possible to measure a progression of genetic distances between taxa at various taxonomic levels, beginning with intrademic comparisons and ending with interspecific comparisons, then the smallest interspecific genetic distances should be significantly larger than the largest intraspecific distances. On the other hand, if speciation occurred as a result of reaching some threshold level of genetic differentiation, then there should be a continuum in intertaxa genetic distances, without gaps or abrupt changes in the distribution of distance values. The smallest distances would be between local neighbourhoods, the next greater being amongst local populations, and so on through the largest values, i.e. those amongst species.

The detection and quantification of genetic differentiation requires more than the simple analysis of the distribution of genetic distance measurements that was the approach of earlier studies such as those of Ayala (1975), Avise (1976) and Barrowclough and Corbin (1978). This is a non-trivial problem for two reasons. First, the soluble proteins examined in electrophoretic studies are assumed to be representative of their genomes with respect to variation and extent of genetic differentiation between species, i.e. there is the implicit assumption that the evolution of genes that code for these proteins does not differ from that of regulatory genes. If this is not true, then an examination of genetic distances between and among taxa that represent various stages in the speciation process cannot offer significant information about the extent of genetic reorganization that occurs within genomes and gene pools during speciation. Second, the basic data of such analyses, i.e. the distributions of alleles possessed by individuals, that are used to estimate allelic frequencies within the lowest taxonomic level, such as a local population, must also be used to estimate the allelic frequencies of all higher taxa that include these data. This is because the alleles possessed by a given individual are simultaneously a part of the allele distributions of a local population, the deme containing this local population, a subspecies that contains the deme, and so on. The individual is the basic unit of each of these taxonomic levels. Therefore, the allelic frequency data sets of the different taxonomic levels are not independent, and statistical procedures such as the t-test cannot be used to determine whether or not the mean genetic distances among taxa are significantly different. In order to circumvent this statistical problem, I have begun to explore an alternative method in which two measures of genetic differentiation are regressed against one another to yield patterns of evolutionary rate and divergence that seem to be associated with speciation events (Fig. 8; Corbin 1983).

The analyses were performed by regressing F_{ST} against Nei's standard genetic distance. Although these two parameters are highly correlated (Corbin 1983), they manipulate the allelic frequency data in different ways. The *F*-statistic is the product of an analysis of variance, whereas Nei's indices are basically correlation coefficients. By presenting the results in two dimensions there is an enhancement of the differences between the methods, as in a discriminant-function analysis, but to a lesser degree. In the analysis illustrated in Fig. 8, intraspecific comparisons define one line of points having a gentle slope near the origin, interspecific comparisons define a second line having a greater slope at some distance from the origin, and the brackets mark off a region that lacks potential intermediate values between the smallest interspecific and the largest intraspecific values. Corbin (1983) examined these relationships for several genera of birds, and subsequently for a variety of other taxonomic groups (work to be published), including mammals, fish, reptiles and insects. Figure 9, in which the brackets of Fig. 8 have been replaced by a solid line, summarizes the results for each of these major groups.

In each taxonomic group, significant gaps in genetic distances exist between one set of comparisons that result from intraspecific comparisons and a second set comprising interspecific comparisons, with an obvious absence of potential values in between the two sets. This has been true for each of the genera examined thus far, and the phenomenon can be taken as evidence that a major reorganization of genomes occurs either during or following speciation. Because the species involved in these particular comparisons have had independent evolutionary histories for extremely long periods of time the presence of these gaps between intra- and interspecific comparisons is not sufficient evidence that genetic revolution has occurred during speciation *per se*. However, from the perspective of this chapter it is of interest to emphasize that the range of intraspecific values is significantly different among organisms; intrageneric genetic distances between species of birds are substantially smaller than such comparisons among species in all other groups examined. Indeed, the intraspecific genetic distances in the lizard genus *Anolis* and the fish genus *Catostomus* are usually greater than the interspecific distances within genera of birds.

We now have a preliminary answer to the first of the questions posed above; namely, within a genus it is possible to recognize the limits of genetic distance that define intraspecific versus interspecific differences. Once the genetic variation within a genus has been determined, it appears possible to judge whether or not two taxa of unknown relationship should be placed within the same species. Furthermore, these limits that define the genetic distances expected among the various subdivisions of a species vary considerably

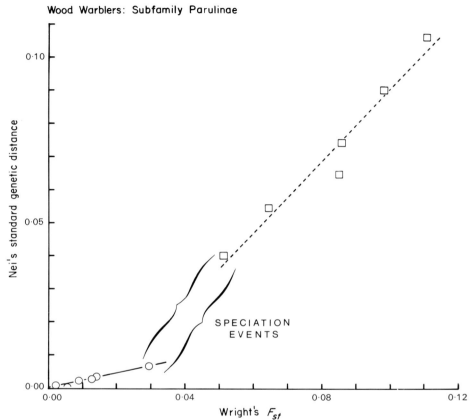

Fig. 8. The hypothesis that allopatric speciation is accompanied by significant genetic differentiation is examined here for wood warblers of the subfamily Parulinae. For each pair of taxa, values of F_{ST} are regressed against Nei's standard genetic distance. These two parameters are highly correlated with one another, and therefore the data points tend to fall along one or the other of the two lines. The solid line at the lower left involves only intraspecific comparisons (○), which are based on the data of Barrowclough (1980). The dashed line at the upper right involves only comparisons between species of the same genus (□). The latter comparisons are based on the data of Barrowclough and Corbin (1978). The brackets serve to emphasize the absence of potential values between the largest intraspecific values and the smallest interspecific values; the distance between these points is an index to the extent of genetic reorganization that occurs during or following speciation. (After Corbin 1983.)

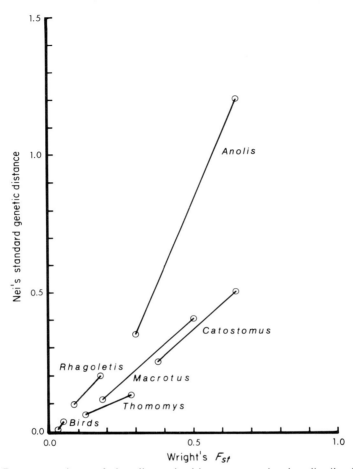

Fig. 9. Representations of the discontinuities or gaps in the distributions of genetic differences that are the result of genetic differentiation during or following speciation. The lower left point on each line is the largest observed intraspecific genetic distance, expressed as a function of both Nei's standard genetic distance and Wright's F_{ST}, whereas the upper right point on each line is the smallest interspecific genetic distance observed. The length of each line is an index to the extent of genetic differentiation that occurred within any given taxon during or following speciation events. The analysis for birds is based on the data of Barrowclough and Corbin (1978), Barrowclough (1980), Corbin (1981) and Zink (1982). The analysis for the pocket gophers of the genus *Thomomys* is based on the data of Patton *et al.* (1972). That for American Leaf-nosed Bats (*Macrotus*) is based on the data of Greenbaum and Baker (1976). That for the New World Lizards (*Anolis*) is based on the data of Webster *et al.* (1972). The analysis for Fruit Flies of the genus *Rhagoletis* is based on the data of Berlocher and Bush (1982), and that for the suckers of the genus *Catostomus* is based on the data of Ferris *et al.* (1982).

among the major groups of organisms, with the genetic distances among species of birds being substantially smaller than those found in other classes and phyla.

6 SUMMARY AND CONCLUSIONS

Electrophoretic studies of allozyme variation yield information about the distribution of genotypes and alleles in natural populations, and thereby provide a powerful means of studying geographic variation. The observed distributions of alleles and genotypes themselves vary geographically and they also can be used to calculate and estimate population statistics of three general types. These are (1) per cent polymorphism, which is the ratio of the number of loci that exhibit two or more alleles within a taxon, to the total number of loci sampled from that taxon, (2) the heterozygosity of a taxon, which is an estimate of the ratio of the number of loci that are heterozygous within individuals to the total number of loci sampled from individuals, and (3) various indices of genetic similarity or difference, which approximate either the number of gene substitutions that distinguish one taxon from another or the amount of genetic exchange between taxa. Each of the parameters may vary geographically.

Per cent polymorphism and heterozygosity are positively correlated with one another. Thus, taxa that are highly polymorphic tend to exhibit relatively high levels of heterozygosity, and vice versa. How these parameters relate to life-history phenomena is much less certain, however. Among avian examples there is at least one case in which extremely low values of heterozygosity and per cent polymorphism can be attributed to the breeding structure of the population, i.e. a small effective breeding population having only one or very few active males. Toward the opposite end of the scale, it has been shown that higher levels of heterozygosity may be found within the contact zones between subspecies.

Within species, allelic frequencies may vary clinally, but within zones of secondary contact and intergradation between subspecies or species there may be abrupt changes in allelic frequencies. Three plausible explanations for these abrupt shifts are (1) that populations within zones of intergradation are small and geographically isolated from one another, which results in significant effects of genetic drift, (2) that gene complexes within the zone of contact are continually being disrupted by gene flow into the zone of contact, with the new gene arrangements responding differentially to novel selective regimes within the zone of contact, or (3) that local populations within zones of intergradation have gene complexes which are well adapted to local conditions in the transition zone and natural selection offsets the effects of gene flow.

ACKNOWLEDGMENTS

I am especially grateful to Patricia J. Wilkie for her critical comments on the manuscript, and to Robert M. Zink for the use of unpublished information in his doctoral thesis. Portions of this study were supported by grants from the National Geographic Society, Grant 8599 from the Penrose Fund of the American Philosophical Society, Grant DEB 82-05371 from the National Science Foundation, and a subcontract to NSF Grant DEB 80-12403.

REFERENCES

Avise, J. C. (1976). Genetic differentiation during speciation. *In* "Molecular Evolution" (ed. F. J. Ayala), pp. 106–122. Sinauer Publishers, Sunderland, Massachusetts.

Avise, J. C., Patton, J. C. and Aquandro, C. F. (1980a). Evolutionary genetics of birds. I. Relationships among North American thrushes and allies. *Auk* **97**, 135–147.

Avise, J. C., Patton, J. C. and Aquadro, C. F. (1980 b). Evolutionary genetics of birds. II. Conservative protein evolution in North American sparrows and relatives. *Syst. Zool.* **29**, 323–334.

Ayala, F. J. (1975). Genetic differentiation during the speciation process. *In* "Evolutionary Biology" (eds T. Dobzhansky, M. K. Hecht and W. C. Steere), Vol. 8, pp. 1–78. Plenum Press, New York.

Ayala, F. J. (1976). "Molecular Evolution". Sinauer Publishers, Sunderland, Massachusetts.

Ayala, F. J., Tracey, M. L., Barr, L. G. and Ehrenfeld, J. G. (1974 a). Genetic and reproductive differentiation of the subspecies *Drosophila equinoxialis caribbensis. Evolution* **28**, 24–41.

Ayala, F. J., Tracey, M. L., Barr, L. G., McDonald, J. F. and Perez-Salas, S. (1974 b). Genetic variation in natural populations of five *Drosophila* species and the hypothesis of the selective neutrality of protein polymorphisms. *Genetics* **77**, 343–384.

Ayala, F. J., Tracey, M. L., Hedgecock, D., and Richmond, R. C. (1974 c). Genetic differentiation during the speciation process in *Drosophila. Evolution* **28**, 576–592.

Baker, M. C. (1975). Song dialects and genetic differences in white-crowned sparrows (*Zonotrichia leucophrys*). *Evolution* **29**, 226–241.

Banks, R. C. (1964). Geographic variation in the White-crowned Sparrow, *Zonotrichia leucophrys. Univ. Calif. Publ. Zool.* **70**, 1–123.

Barrowclough, G. F. (1980). Genetic and phenotypic differentiation in a wood warbler (Genus *Dendroica*) hybrid zone. *Auk* **97**, 655–668.

Barrowclough, G. F. (1983). Biochemical studies of microevolutionary processes. *In* "Perspectives in Ornithology" (eds A. H. Brush and G. A. Clark, Jr), pp. 223–261. Cambridge University Press, New York.

Barrowclough, G. F. and Corbin, K. W. (1978). Genetic variation and differentiation in the Parulidae. *Auk* **95**, 691–702.

Barrowclough, G. F., Corbin, K. W. and Zink, R. M. (1981). Genetic differentiation in the Procellariiformes. *Comp. Biochem. Physiol.* **69B**, 629–632.

Berlocher, S. H. and Bush, G. L. (1982). An electrophoretic analysis of *Rhagoletis* (Diptera: Tephritidae) phylogeny. *Syst. Zool.* **31**, 136–155.

Bush, F. M. (1967). Developmental and populational variation in electrophoretic properties of dehydrogenases, hydrolases and other blood proteins of the House Sparrow, *Passer domesticus. Comp. Biochem. Physiol.* **22**, 273–287.

Carson, H. L. (1978). Speciation and sexual selection in Hawaiian *Drosophila. In* "Ecological Genetics" (ed. P. F. Brussard), pp. 93–107. Springer-Verlag, New York.

Carson, H. L. (1982). Evolution of *Drosophila* on the newer Hawaiian volcanoes. *Heredity* **48**, 3–25.

Carson, H. L. and Templeton, A. R. (1984). Genetic revolutions in relation to speciation phenomena: The founding of new populations. *Ann. Rev. Ecol. Syst.* **15**, 97–131.

Corbin, K. W. (1978). Genetic diversity in avian populations. *In* "Endangered Birds: Management Techniques for Preserving Threatened Species" (ed. S. A. Temple), pp. 291–302. University of Wisconsin Press, Madison.

Corbin, K. W. (1981). Genic heterozygosity in the White-crowned Sparrow: A potential index to boundaries between subspecies. *Auk* **98**, 669–680.

Corbin, K. W. (1983). Genetic structure and avian systematics. *In* "Current Ornithology" (ed. R. F. Johnston), Vol. 1, pp. 211–244. Plenum Press, New York, London.

Corbin, K. W. and Sibley, C. G. (1977). Rapid evolution in orioles in the genus *Icterus. Condor* **79**, 335–342.

Corbin, K. W., Sibley, C. G. and Ferguson, A. (1979). Genic changes associated with the establishment of sympatry in orioles of the genus *Icterus. Evolution* **33**, 624–633.

Corbin, K. W., Sibley, C. G., Ferguson, A., Wilson, A. C., Brush, A. H. and Ahlquist, J. E. (1974). Genetic polymorphism in New Guinea starlings of the genus *Aplonis. Condor* **76**, 307–318.

Dobzhansky, Th. (1961). "Genetics and the Origin of Species". Columbia University Press, New York.

Endler, J. A. (1977). "Geographic Variation, Speciation, and Clines". Princeton University Press.

Farris, J. S. (1972). Estimating phylogenetic trees from distance matrices. *Am. Natur.* **106**, 645–668.

Farris, J. S. (1973). A probability model for inferring evolutionary trees. *Syst. Zool.* **22**, 250–256.

Farris, J. S. (1981). Distance data in phylogenetic analysis. *In* "Advances in Cladistics" (eds V. A. Funk and D. R. Brooks), pp. 3–23. New York Botanical Garden, Bronx, New York.

Ferris, S. D., Buth, D. G. and Whitt, G. S. (1982). Substantial genetic differentiation among populations of *Catostomus plebeius. Copeia* 444–449.

Greenbaum, I. F. and Baker, R. J. (1976). Evolutionary relationships in *Macrotus* (Mammalia: Chiroptera): Biochemical variation and karyology. *Syst. Zool.* **5**, 15–25.

Gutiérrez, R. J., Zink, R. M. and Yang, S. Y. (1983). Genic variation, systematic, and biogeographic relationships of some galliform birds. *Auk* **100**, 33–47.

Handford, P. and Nottebohm, F. (1976). Allozymic and morphological variation in population samples of rufous-collared sparrow, *Zonotrichia capensis*, in relation to vocal dialects. *Evolution* **30**, 802–817.

Harris, H. (1966). Enzyme polymorphisms in man. *Proc. Roy. Soc., Lond. B* **174**, 298–310.

Hubby, J. L. and Lewontin, R. C. (1966). A molecular approach to the study of genic heterozygosity in natural populations. I. The number of alleles at different loci in *Drosophila pseudoobscura. Genetics* **54**, 577–594.

Johnson, N. K. and Zink, R. M. (1983). Speciation in sapsuckers (*Sphyrapicus*): I. Genetic differentiation. *Auk* **100**, 871–884.

Lewontin, R. C. and Hubby, J. L. (1966). A molecular approach to the study of genic heterozygosity in natural populations. II. Amount of variation and degree of heterozygosity in natural populations of *Drosophila pseudoobscura*. *Genetics* **54**, 595–609.

Mayr, E. (1940). Speciation phenomena in birds. *Am. Natur.* **74**, 249–278.

Mayr, E. (1954). Change of genetic environment and evolution. *In* "Evolution as a Process" (eds J. Huxley, A. C. Hardy and E. B. Ford), pp. 157–180. Allen & Unwin, London.

Mayr, E. (1963). "Animal Species and Evolution". Belknap Press, Harvard University, Cambridge, Massachusetts.

Mayr, E. (1982). Processes of speciation in animals. *In* "Mechanisms of Speciation" (ed. C. Barigozzi), pp. 1–19. Alan R. Liss, Inc., New York.

Nei, M. (1972). Genetic distance between populations. *Am. Natur.* **106**, 283–292.

Nei, M. (1975). "Molecular Population Genetics and Evolution". North-Holland, Amsterdam.

Nei, M. (1978). Estimation of average heterozygosity and genetic distance from a small number of individuals. *Genetics* **89**, 583–590.

Nevo, E. (1978). Genetic variation in natural populations: Patterns and theory. *Theoret. Pop. Biol.* **13**, 121–177.

Patton, J. L., Selander, R. K. and Smith, M. H. (1972). Genic variation in hybridizing populations of gophers (genus *Thomomys*). *Syst. Zool.* **21**, 263–270.

Powell, J. R. (1975). Protein variation in natural populations of animals. *Evol. Biol.* **8**, 79–119.

Rising, J. D. (1970). Morphological variation and evolution in some North American orioles. *Syst. Zool.* **19**, 315–351.

Rising, J. D. (1973). Morphological variation and status of the orioles, *Icterus galbula*, *I. bullockii*, and *I. abeillei*, in the northern Great Plains and in Durango, Mexico, *Can. J. Zool.* **51**, 1267–1273.

Rogers, J. S. (1972). Measures of genetic similarity and genetic distance. *University of Texas Publication No. 7213*, pp. 145–153.

Selander, R. K. (1978). Genic variation in natural populations. *In* "Molecular Evolution" (ed. F. J. Ayala), pp. 21–45. Sinauer Associates, Sunderland, Massachusetts.

Sibley, C. G. and Short, L. L. Jr (1964). Hybridization in the orioles of the Great Plains. *Condor* **66**, 130–150.

Sokal, R. R. and Rohlf, F. J. (1969). "Biometry". W. H. Freeman & Co., San Francisco.

Webster, T. P., Selander, R. K. and Yang, S. Y. (1972). Genetic variability and similarity in the *Anolis* lizards of Bimini. *Evolution* **26**, 523–535.

Wright, S. (1921). Systems of mating. *Genetics* **6**, 111–178.

Wright, S. (1951). The genetical structure of populations. *Ann. Eugenics* **15**, 323–354.

Wright, S. (1965). The interpretation of population structure by *F*-statistics with special regard to systems of mating. *Evolution* **19**, 395–420.

Wright, S. (1978). "Evolution and the Genetics of Populations", Vol. 4, "Variability within and among Natural Populations". University of Chicago Press.

Zink, R. M. (1982). Patterns of genic and morphologic variation among sparrows in the genera *Zonotrichia*, *Melospiza*, *Junco* and *Passerella*. *Auk* **99**, 632–649.

Zink, R. M. (1983). Patterns and evolutionary significance of geographic variation in the Schistacea Group of the Fox Sparrow (*Passerella iliaca*). Ph.D. Dissertation. University of California, Berkeley.

Synthesis II—Moulding Genetic Variation

F. Cooke

In the second five chapters we have seen the various ways in which the genetic variation present in all bird populations may be modified or maintained as a result of natural processes. Ecological and ethological influences can modify the genetic structure of a population and lead to evolutionary change. Since it is seldom, if ever, possible to observe the genetical structure of populations over several generations in birds, we must independently analyse various factors, such as gene flow, selection, drift, non-random mating and inbreeding, in order to understand what it is that moulds the genetic structure of avian populations.

In many ways birds are the ideal group of vertebrates to use for such an investigation, and it is surprising that so few reviews have focused on avian genetics. The value of birds lies mainly in the fact that they have been well studied both ecologically and ethologically. We have more detailed knowledge of the different stages in the life cycle of birds than of most other animals and this allows, as Price and Boag point out in chapter 8, a detailed analysis of selection for life-history traits. There have been relatively few attempts to partition the life histories of birds into their components and to measure the ways in which diverse segments of the population (e.g. large versus small individuals within a population) respond differently to selection during the various stages of the life history. Yet, the theoretical framework pioneered by Lande, Arnold and co-workers allows this to be done, and many ornithologists possess data that would allow this sort of analysis to be carried out. Avian ecologists are becoming increasingly familiar with the techniques of population genetics and are advancing our understanding of evolutionary processes. Even so, much more is possible, and one can still find ecological studies where unwarranted assumptions about the genetic structure of the population are made. For example, if a sample of birds in an area is examined in two successive years and is found to differ in some way in the two years, it is usually assumed that the differences are due to some environmental variable. It is possible, though admittedly less likely, that the samples differed genetically from one another in the two years. Unless the same individuals comprised both samples, a genetical explanation for the differences could not be ruled out. The example of the changes in the bill measurements in a sample of Darwin's Finches in successive years is an important one. In this case, and not surprisingly since we are dealing with a morphological trait, the differences in mean bill shape in the two years were ascribed to differences in the genetic composition of the population, and not to some environmental factor acting directly on the phenotype of the birds. In similar fashion, differences in mean clutch size in two different seasons could be due to differences in the genetic composition of the population sample rather than to environmental differences, the usually preferred explanation.

Ethologists, too, have studied birds in considerable detail, and the interface between ethology and genetics is evident in the previous five chapters. Birds can clearly recognize one another at various levels (from species to the individual), as Colgan (1983) has documented. This recognition is important in terms of mate choice and, in turn, influences the genetic structure of the population. The avoidance of inbreeding or outbreeding affects the frequency of heterozygosity and the rate at which genetic drift may occur, as pointed out by Greenwood in chapter 6. Other types of non-random mating may be due to sexual selection where certain types of individuals are preferred by members of the opposite sex, or assortative mating (positive or negative) where mates are chosen in relation to the chooser's own phenotype. This is discussed by Findlay in chapter 9. Birds offer wide opportunities to investigate the ways in which mates are selected, as important studies by Andersson (1982) and Petrie (1983) have shown. Few studies have documented the population consequences of such choices, although two examples, Lesser Snow Geese and Arctic Skua, are documented later in this volume (chapters 13 and 14).

The wealth of ecological and ethological knowledge of bird populations in the field contrasts markedly with the poor understanding of the field habits of most species of *Drosophila*. In the case of those species like *D. melanogaster* and *D. pseudoobscura*, an understanding of the genetics in experimental conditions has vastly outstripped our knowledge of the species in the wild. With birds, the reverse is true, and this book may help to redress the balance by encouraging field ornithologists to consider the genetic implications of their studies.

What generalizations about avian genetics emerge from the preceding chapters? Perhaps the one with the most far-reaching consequences is that birds are in general highly mobile and that gene flow among most populations is considerable. The interchange of individuals among populations, as pointed out by several authors (e.g. Rockwell and Cooke 1977), is high enough to restrict local differentiation and to reduce the effects of local adaptation. As such, it is difficult to find isolated populations of birds where the effects of gene flow can be ignored. Only by having a well-marked population or one where immigration and emigration are highly restricted is it possible to investigate selection with confidence. Several authors in this volume (Greenwood,

Rockwell and Barrowclough, and Corbin) have made use of Wright's *F*-statistics (e.g. F_{IT} or F_{ST}), which define the genetic structure of populations. Most local bird populations have low F_{ST} values, implying considerable genetic similarity among populations of the same taxon. This strengthens the view expressed by Rockwell and Barrowclough that gene flow is the evolutionary "glue" binding together segments of the species and thus retarding the process of speciation.

Chapters 6 (Inbreeding) and 7 (Gene Flow) discuss topics which are to some extent mirror images of one another. Greenwood asks whether genetic differentiation is a consequence of philopatry, or does philopatry arise, as Shields (1982) believes, in order that birds can choose a mate with an appropriate genetic constitution? Whatever the explanation, the tendency of birds to return to breed close to where they were hatched increases the possibility of inbreeding and the possibility of local differentiation, but in most cases this differentiation is not strong. Data are currently available on the coefficient of inbreeding for only two species, Yellow-eyed Penguin (*Megadyptes antipodes*) and Great Tit (*Parus major*). In both cases the values are low, and the deleterious effects of such inbreeding are of little consequence.

Greenwood points out a number of questions regarding inbreeding which need to be pursued further. For example, if one is to examine the fitness consequences of philopatry, an attempt should be made to investigate the effects of dispersal on components of fitness. What are the costs of dispersal? Secondly, inbreeding is low in most populations, but is it actively avoided by birds in the wild? There is now strong evidence of such avoidance in laboratory situations but there may be little need for it in the field, and there may even be advantages in choosing a mate with a similar genetic composition.

Rockwell and Barrowclough (chapter 7) point out the complexities of measuring gene flow and then suggest a number of practical ways in which it has been or might be carried out. When investigating gene frequency changes for possible evidence of selection, it is crucial to be aware of the effects of gene flow. It would be wise to consider how gene flow might be measured before embarking on a detailed population study if the aim of the study is an evolutionary one.

One question underlying several of the methods of investigating gene flow and the genetic structure of populations is the question of neutrality. Are the alleles used to estimate the degree of relatedness of the similarity of populations selectively neutral? Chapters in the first two sections of this text do little to contribute to the neutrality-selectionist debate (but see chapters 4 and 15), although Price and Boag (chapter 8) have documented some of the few cases where selection in birds has been effectively demonstrated; other examples are mentioned in chapter 4. What becomes obvious is that selection, whether directional, normalizing or disruptive, has rarely been convincingly shown and there are several examples which suggest that, on the contrary, gene frequencies tend to remain constant over time. This does not of course imply neutrality, but does suggest that the large amount of genetic variability which occurs in bird populations is likely to persist.

Price and Boag stress the importance of investigating traits that vary quantitatively since these are likely to be the ones which respond readily to selection. Life-history traits, in addition to morphometric differences, fit into this category. Selection on a character arises when that character correlates with a component of fitness. The authors emphasize the problems of covariance and suggest ways in which it may be assessed. Selection acting on one trait can produce a correlated response on another trait if the traits covary in some way. This may sometimes lead to results which are counter-intuitive, as has been pointed out by Arnold and Wade (1984 a,b). Chapter 8 effectively summarizes the ways in which selection in natural populations may be most effectively examined. Selection at the phenotypic level can occur in the absence of genetic variation but, if the traits examined show heritable variation, then field studies can give an effective *demonstration* of adaptation in action. This is a considerable scientific advance over studies which *invoke* adaptation to explain biological phenomena, but without evidence.

One aspect of non-random mating, inbreeding, was considered in chapter 6 by Greenwood, but Findlay, in chapter 9, examines other facets of the phenomenon. Ecological and ethological factors which space birds out non-randomly lead to non-random mating even if choices are random within the non-random spacing. Non-random mating may be further enhanced if certain individuals within the population are preferred as mates, either absolutely or relative to the chooser's phenotype. Non-random mating as a population phenomenon modifies gene or genotype frequencies and, as such, it can enhance or retard the effects of gene flow and local differentiation.

It is this local differentiation which is examined in detail by Corbin in chapter 10. He probes geographic variation at the intra- and interspecific levels. In general, the relatedness of taxa as deduced by morphology and as determined by allozyme studies show a similar pattern. The degree of morphological similarity corresponds to the degree of allozymic similarity, but there are some surprising anomalies that require further investigation. When morphological evidence suggests introgression of two taxa, the evidence from allozymes indicates much wider gene flow than one would deduce from morphology. In other cases, morphology suggests considerable local differentiation while allozyme patterns indicate otherwise. These discrepancies present a fruitful way of investigating genetic variation further, and make us realize that our understanding of speciation is still far from complete.

In the next section of the book we examine four case histories that illustrate some of the ways in which bird populations can be studied, with an emphasis on genetics. Each example has its own special approach and no population of birds has been examined using all the methods described in this book. The chapter on Arctic Skua by Peter O'Donald differs from the others in that he has recently completed a fine monograph on this species (O'Donald 1983). His chapter, rather than repeating the main points of that book, concentrates on some of the recent ideas which have emerged since the book's publication. Those readers wishing a more complete picture should read the original book as well.

REFERENCES

Andersson, M. (1982). Female choice selects for extreme tail length in a widowbird. *Nature* **299**, 818–820.

Arnold, S. J. and Wade, M. J. (1984 a). On the measurement of natural and sexual selection: Theory. *Evolution* **38**, 709–719.

Arnold, S. J. and Wade, M. J. (1984 b). On the measurement of natural and sexual selection: Applications. *Evolution* **38**, 720–734.

Colgan, P. (1983). "Comparative Social Recognition", J. Wiley & Sons, New York.

O'Donald, P. (1983). "The Arctic Skua". Cambridge University Press.

Petrie, M. (1983). Female moorhens (*Gallinula chloropus*) compete for small fat males. *Science* **220**, 413–415.

Rockwell, R. F. and Cooke, F. (1977). Gene flow and local adaptation in a colonially nesting dimorphic bird: The Lesser Snow Goose. *Am. Natur.* **111**, 91–97.

Shields, W. M. (1982). "Philopatry, Inbreeding and the Evolution of Sex". State University of New York Press, Albany, New York.

Part III

Genetic Case Histories

11

Quantitative Ecological Genetics of Great Tits

Arie J. van Noordwijk†

*Department of Population and Evolutionary Biology, University of Utrecht,
PO Box 80.055, 3508 TB Utrecht, The Netherlands*

1 INTRODUCTION

The population ecology of Great Tit (*Parus major*) has probably been studied
more extensively than that of any other bird species. In the past decades there
have been major population studies in several European countries. Many of
the results obtained in these studies are summarized and reviewed by Perrins
(1979). In this chapter I refer only to those populations where genetic analyses
have been made. These are the Wytham population near Oxford in England,
the population near Oulu in Northern Finland, and the Dutch populations in
Hoge Veluwe, on the island of Vlieland, and in Liesbos and Oosterhout.

†Present address: Zoologisches Institut der Universität Basel, Rheinsprung 9, CH-4051 Basel,
Switzerland.

AVIAN GENETICS
ISBN 0-12-187570-9

There are two main reasons why Great Tit has been the object of many studies. It is a good choice from many practical points of view and, because it has already been well studied, there is a good frame of reference to compare one's results with. When Kluyver first started his seminal population study, he was looking for a common insectivorous passerine in woodlands. His aim was to investigate the contribution of birds in controlling insect pests in woodlands. The methods developed by Kluyver (1950, 1951, 1952) became standard tools. Lack copied them and gave them wide publicity (see Lack 1951). The outstanding feature is that the population level is linked to the individual level by studying populations in which all birds are individually marked. All nestlings are ringed, and both parents are identified while feeding their nestlings.

This not only makes it possible to trace the survival of the nestlings in relation to properties of the parents—which was the original intention—but also allows the construction of family trees for the locally born breeding birds. These genealogical data are the basis for the investigation of the heritable nature of the observed variation in many traits.

Kluyver (1951) analysed the constancy of clutch size and of clutch initiation date in individual females. From the data in his Table 31 a repeatability for clutch size of 0·29 for 104 females can be calculated. After recognizing the potential effect of laying subsequent clutches in the same territory, his conclusion is "... that in the Great Tit any individual (hereditary) disposition to lay a clutch of fixed size is not predominating, and adaptation to environmental factors is evidently of great importance" (Kluyver 1951). In contrast, his conclusion for date of first egg laying is that "individual disposition probably plays a more important part. This is corroborated by the fact that there is often a very early brood at a particular place for several years in succession and then not again. This can be explained by supposing that the clutches in question were all laid by the same female, which then died." Data are given for 10 females, for which there is a Spearman rank correlation of 0·948 between the initiation dates in 1938 and in 1939 (calculated from data in Table 14 in Kluyver (1951)). Lack (1954) interpreted the clutch size estimate as suggesting "that different individuals differ somewhat in the hereditary factors influencing clutch size", but he also stated that there was no proof yet. Kluyver (1963) expressed the view, without any data or reference, that genetic variation in clutch size does not play any role in Great Tit.

In recent years more extensive genetic analyses have led to the conclusion that the repeatability and the heritability for clutch size are a little higher than Kluyver's original repeatability estimate. However, the question is mainly whether or not a heritability of 0·3 is high. There are two ways to answer this question: by reference to heritability estimates in agricultural practice, and by referring to the consequences for potential speed of evolutionary change. The latter will be discussed in the section on clutch size, the former leads (also) to a positive answer, many traits with heritabilities of around 0·1 can still be successfully selected for, and this way of improving traits is of commercial importance.

There are several problems in the application of the methods of quantitative genetics to data from natural populations. These are extensively discussed in chapter 2 on quantitative genetics. In the trait-by-trait discussion of heritability estimates below, attention will be given only to the special problems that are important in each case. It will be assumed that the reader is familiar with the general problems, and the ways to solve them.

In the following sections the heritabilities of several traits will be described, together with a short summary of their ecology. As a general background it must be borne in mind that Great Tits are rather small birds, which means that they have little capacity for accumulating food reserves. Their daily food intake is about half their own body weight, and in winter the overnight weight loss may be as high as 10% (van Balen 1967). The food consumption of nestlings depends on age and brood size; on average a brood above the age of seven days consumes over 50 g of insects (mainly caterpillars) per day (van Balen 1973). This is about three times the weight of the female or the male. The female lays a clutch that is equal to her own body weight.

Thus, the physiology of breeding is entirely different from that of a larger bird such as Snow Goose (*Anser caerulescens*) where much of the energy needed for egg-laying, and even incubation, can be stored in the weeks prior to the breeding season. One may expect that environmental effects act on a much shorter time-scale in the Great Tit.

2 SUCCESSFUL DEMONSTRATION OF GENETIC VARIATION

2.1 Clutch size

The size of first clutches usually varies between 7 and 12 eggs, on occasion being as small as 5 or as large as 15 eggs. There is a tendency for late first clutches to be smaller than early ones, but this explains only some 10% of the variation in clutch size (van Noordwijk *et al.* 1981 a). The evidence for an effect of age on clutch size is equivocal. Jones (1973) reported that one-year-old females lay smaller clutches than older birds in Wytham, confirming earlier analyses (see Perrins 1979). In both the principal Dutch populations there is no evidence for an effect of age on mean clutch size (van Balen 1973, van Noordwijk *et al.* 1981 a). There are considerable differences in mean clutch size between years within a population, e.g. varying from a low 8·0 to a high 11·2 in a quarter-century in the Hoge Veluwe population. One aspect of these

Table 1. Heritability and repeatability estimates for reproductive traits in Great Tit. The estimates are in percentages of the total phenotypic variance. The number of observed clutches and the number of individuals in the repeatability, and the number of daughters in the heritability, estimated are given in brackets.

Population	Repeatability	Heritability	Reference
Clutch size			
Wytham	51 (696/267)	48 ± 10 (256/–)	1
Hoge Veluwe	36 (1277/480)	34 ± 13 (1242/336)	2
Vlieland	54 (509/189)	46 ± 14 (1327/362)	2
Liesbos	30 (422/178)	25 ± 21 (–/139)	2
Oosterhout	46 (165/62)	50 ± 30 (–/57)	2
Clutch initiation date			
Wytham	35 (767/267)	14 ± 10 (359/232)	1
Hoge Veluwe	38 (1277/480)	18 ± 9 (1270/371)	3
Vlieland	44 (504/189)	45 ± 15 (1350/371)	3
Liesbos	33 (422/178)	-8 ± 27 (–/129)	3
Oosterhout	19 (165/62)	14 ± 36 (–/56)	3
Egg volume			
Wytham	72 (–/84)	72 ± 22 (–/81)	1
Oulu	58 (421/–)	86 ± 29 (–/45)	4
Hoge Veluwe	70 (118/59)	66 ± 24 (93/60)	5
Vlieland	61 (84/42)	72 ± 30 (110/54)	5

References: 1—Jones 1973; 2—van Noordwijk *et al.* 1981 a; 3—van Noordwijk *et al.* 1981 b; 4—Ojanen *et al.* 1979; 5—van Noordwijk *et al.* 1981 c.

differences in mean clutch size is that, together with the fact that the mean clutch sizes in subsequent years are positively correlated, they will increase the resemblance between parents and offspring (see chapter 2).

The repeatability and heritability estimates reported by Jones (1973) are not fully comparable with the estimates by van Noordwijk *et al.* (1981 a). Different approaches were taken to eliminate the effects of differences in clutch size due to age, and due to local and temporal environmental conditions. Jones used corrected clutch sizes (equal to the observed clutch size plus three constants for age, year of breeding and area, respectively). In one of his analyses van Noordwijk used a correction for year effects similar to that of Jones, but he mainly relied on calculating "control" resemblances between unrelated individuals that share environmental conditions, of which year-to-year differences seem to be the most important, judging from that part of the variation in mean clutch sizes that could be explained. The estimates for both repeatability and heritability are given in Table 1. All estimates are reasonably close and suggest that about 40% of the observed variation is inherited. Both Jones and van Noordwijk found that males have no effect on the clutch size of their female partner. This was concluded from the absence of a correlation between the clutch sizes of the subsequent female partners of the same male. If either the male had a substantial effect on its partner's clutch size, or consistent differences in territory quality had existed, a positive correlation between different female partners of the same male would have been expected. In their study of Eurasian Sparrowhawks (*Accipiter nisus*) Newton and Marquiss (1984) found high repeatabilities for males with different partners. There are two aspects that may explain this contrast between species. The range of territory qualities included in the study is much wider in the sparrowhawk (see Newton *et al.* 1981) and courtship feeding is much more important in the sparrowhawk as well, giving the male a direct effect on the caloric intake of the female during the egg formation period.

This heritability of some 40%, together with the rather high coefficient of variation (the within-year standard deviation is on average 1·7 and the mean is 9·6 eggs, giving a coefficient of variation of 18%), suggests that rapid response to directional selection is possible. A rate of change in the mean clutch size by almost two eggs per decade (about five generations) is quite possible. The similar results for the British and the Dutch Great Tit populations are different from those for Eurasian Starlings (*Sturnus vulgaris*) in New Zealand (Flux and Flux 1982). The heritability was virtually the same (0·37), but the coefficient of variation was much lower for the starlings. Therefore the time (cumulative selection differential) needed to obtain a comparable change in clutch size is far greater in the starling (Flux and Flux 1982).

The evidence that the resemblance in clutch size between relatives is genetic, and is not caused by sharing environments, is better than that for other traits. In the two large Dutch populations there were sufficient data to calculate the regression of granddaughters on the maternal and on the paternal grandmothers separately. Although the standard errors of the resulting heritability estimates are high, there is no indication of a difference in resemblance of granddaughters to the two types of grandmothers. So the conclusion must be that the genes with an effect on clutch size are transmitted through the male in a normal way, but are not expressed since the male has no effect on the clutch size of its female partner.

2.2   Egg size

In continental Europe, a female Great Tit weighs about 17–19 g, a little more in Great Britain. Eggs are laid at a rate of one per day and eggs weigh between 1·5 and 1·8 g. It is thus not uncommon for a female to lay more than her body weight in eggs within a fortnight. There is no correlation between egg weight and clutch size (A. J. van Noordwijk, unpublished work). For practical purposes, egg volume is more convenient than egg weight, owing to the weight loss before and during incubation. The variation in the specific weight of freshly laid eggs is much less than the weight loss even before incubation (van Noordwijk *et al.* 1981 c).

The repeatability of egg dimensions can be studied at two levels: the variation in egg dimension within clutches compared with the variation between clutches, or at the level of comparing the variation in clutch means within and between females. The second way of estimating repeatabilities is best comparable with heritability estimates obtained from mother–daughter regression. Estimates from several studies are given in Table 1. It is evident that heritabilities are high. There is no evidence for an effect of the male on the egg size of its partner. It is worth mentioning that egg-size heritabilities in poultry are in general also high in comparison with other traits.

2.3   Date of laying

The date on which the first egg of a clutch is laid is used as a measure of the timing of the breeding season in many studies. An alternative parameter would be the date of hatching, which in Great Tit is equal to the date of first egg laying plus the clutch size plus the incubation period, which is about 13 days. In first clutches, incubation usually starts on the day that the last egg was laid, but depending on the weather it may start from one day earlier to two days later. In repeat and second clutches, incubation usually starts one or two days before the last egg has been laid.

The date of first egg laying is difficult to analyse. The median date may vary by as much as three weeks between years. Most of the distributions of dates within a single year are distinctly non-normal. There is, however, no single pattern, which might suggest transformations. Positive as well as negative skewness regularly occurs, while platykurtosis as well as leptokurtosis is observed. One of the reasons for the oddly shaped distributions is that dates on a human calendar form an artificial scale. There are three factors involved in determining the initiation of clutches: day-length, temperature, and the abundance of food. These are correlated, which makes it difficult to distinguish the importance of each individually. Availability of (insect) food causes particular problems, since the development of the insects is strongly temperature-dependent and, furthermore, the fact that caterpillars are more active on warm days probably makes them more conspicuous to the tits. Attempts to calculate repeatabilities on initiation dates transformed to temperature sums have so far been unsuccessful (A. J. van Noordwijk, unpublished work).

A typical example of the problems encountered is shown in Fig. 1 (four

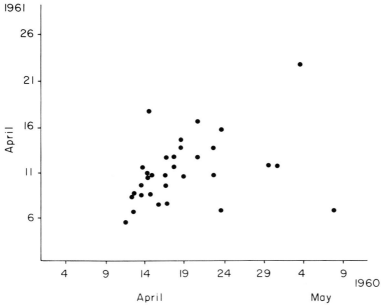

Fig. 1. An example of the constancy of individual females in laying date. For all females that were recorded breeding on the Hoge Veluwe in both 1960 and 1961, the date on which the first egg was laid in 1961 is plotted against the first egg date of the same female in 1960. It is possible that the latest four dates in 1960 were preceded by an undiscovered earlier breeding attempt. The correlation for the points as given is $r = 0.33$ ($n = 32$).

similar figures can be found in van Noordwijk *et al.* 1981 b). It shows that for the majority of the females there is a positive correlation between the dates of first egg-laying in the two subsequent years, but also a few outlying points that have a large effect on the calculated correlations. These outliers represent a biologically meaningful part of the variation, but the strong effect of few points results in lack of robustness in the estimates. Nevertheless, four of the five repeatability estimates in Table 1 are grouped around 0·37. In the heritability estimates, a few similarly deviating points have a much stronger effect. The estimates are very sensitive to the inclusion or exclusion of a few observations. Only the heritability estimates for the Vlieland and the Hoge Veluwe populations are significantly different from zero, and only the Vlieland estimate is closely similar to the repeatability estimate. There are reasons to believe that this is largely a data problem (van Noordwijk *et al.* 1981 c). Only on Vlieland is it possible to relate the large majority of failing early first clutches to the subsequent repeat clutches of the same female, thus avoiding the observation that an early repeat clutch is interpreted as a late first clutch.

The only good way to accommodate the effect of outliers is to collect many more data until the effect of every individual outlying point becomes very small. For the time being, the heritability estimates should be regarded as less reliable than those given for the other traits.

2.4   Body size

There are several parameters that are often used as an index for overall body size, such as weight, tarsus length and wing length. These three parameters are positively correlated, with phenotypic correlations typically close to $r = 0.5$. From the point of view of a genetic analysis, the most interesting difference between the three parameters lies in the period from which the environmental conditions are reflected in the measurement. Tarsus length does not change following completion of growth at an age of 13 days after hatching at the latest (van Noordwijk *et al.* 1988). It may therefore be seen as an indication of conditions during the nestling stage that is still measurable on adults. Wing length is equal to the length of the longest primaries and may thus be seen as a reflection of the nutritional conditions during the last moult period (van Balen 1967). Weight changes continuously, and the non-genetic part of the variation may be seen as the condition at the time of measurement. These different types of environmental variance are reflected in the differences between the repeatability and the heritability estimates (see Table 2).

Repeatability estimates for tarsus lengths are always high. The non-genetic variance is almost exclusively measurement error. Heritability estimates are rather variable: they are high (around 0.6) if the birds involved grew up under favourable conditions (e.g. Hoge Veluwe in 1978), but if feeding conditions were poor in the breeding season, no genetic variation can be demonstrated (e.g. Vlieland in 1979). Similar observations can be made for the heritability estimates for weight. The only difference is that the repeatability estimates are much lower than for tarsus length. They not only contain measurement error, but also variation that can be correlated with feeding conditions, temperature on the day of capture, and time of day (see, for example, van Balen 1967).

It is quite possible that offspring resemble their parents in body size through non-genetic causes. Big individuals are better able to secure the better territories, and therefore their offspring grow up under better conditions and become in turn relatively big. This can be investigated by cross-fostering experiments. Eggs or hatchlings are swapped between nests and are thus brought up by other individuals. It is then possible to compare the body sizes with those of the foster-parents and those of the biological parents. Smith and Dhondt (1980) found no effect of the foster-parents in Song Sparrow (*Melospiza melodia*) and similar results were obtained for Blue Tit (*Parus*

Table 2. Heritability and repeatability estimates for body size traits in Great Tit. The numbers in brackets following the repeatability estimates are the number of measurements and the number of individuals, respectively. The numbers following the heritability estimates are the number of offspring individuals and the number of broods, respectively. If only the latter number is given the heritability estimate is based on regression of brood means on mid-parent.

Population		Repeatability	Heritability	Reference
Adult weight				
Hoge Veluwe	F	55 (6666/1372)	57 ± 9 (156/–)	1
	M	56 (10453/1882)	46 ± 7 (244/–)	1
	T	70 (18945/4058)		1
Fledging weight				
Hoge Veluwe 1975			38 ± 28 (347/34)	1
1976			47 ± 28 (734/68)	1
1977			26 ± 40 (892/89)	1
1978			29 ± 22 (531/53)	1
Tarsus length				
Wytham		96 (298/96)	76 ± 16 (460/61)	2
Hoge Veluwe 1978		85 (2355/821)	52 ± 13 (568/59)	1
Vlieland 1979		93 (82/41)	-7 ± 9 (–/63)	3
1980			47 ± 18 (–/70)	4
1981			38 ± 12 (–/75)	4
1982			13 ± 11 (–/98)	4

Bill measurements from Vlieland 1979

Trait	Repeatability	Heritability	Reference
Length	25 (58/29)	49 ± 20 (56/–)	3
Width	33 (58/29)	68 ± 18 (56/–)	3
Depth	76 (58/29)	71 ± 16 (54/–)	3

References: 1—van Noordwijk *et al.* 1988; 2—Garnett 1981; 3—van Noordwijk and Klerks 1983; 4—Koelewijn, unpublished work.

caeruleus) by Dhondt (1982). In contrast, Ricklefs and Peters (1981), working with Eurasian Starlings and using a different design, in that they compared unrelated nestlings brought up in a single brood with full sibs brought up in different broods, found little evidence for a genetic component and an overriding effect of the brood. I have argued that the latter result is to be expected under poor feeding conditions and the former under good feeding conditions, and there is some circumstantial evidence that this has been the case in these studies (van Noordwijk *et al.* 1988). It must be noted that the resemblance to relatives seems to be dependent upon environmental conditions, but there is no evidence for a resemblance with forest-parents.

The interactions between environmental conditions during the nestling growth and heritability estimates are currently being investigated experimentally. This is done through manipulation of brood size simultaneously with cross-fostering. The first results (J. Schoemaker, unpublished work; van Noordwijk 1984 b) indicate that the heritabilities are lower in the larger broods and higher in the smaller broods for both tarsus length and body weight. This line of research is still at a preliminary stage, but I believe that such experiments will not only enhance our knowledge of the importance of genetic variation, but will also lead to new insights into the breeding ecology.

2.5   Bill size

Bill size can, of course, be seen as a part of the variation in body size, but since it is closely associated with the feeding niche, it is, at least between species, much more variable than overall body size. In titmice there is a difference in bill size and shape between species from broadleaved and species from coniferous habitats. The former have relatively short and stout bills, while the latter have long and slender bills (Snow 1954, Lack 1968). These differences are less spectacular than those in Darwin's Finches, because tits are smaller, but on the other hand the same differences are found in both Europe and North America. Moreover, between populations of Coal Tit (*Parus ater*) inhabiting the two habitats the same difference is found as between species. Of all the European tits, Great Tit is the species that lives in both habitats most often. It is therefore interesting to know to what extent genetic variation in bill dimensions can be demonstrated.

Measuring bills is not without problems. Bills continuously grow and wear and there are no standardized ways of taking measurements. The heritability estimates in Table 2 are results from a pilot study. The heritability estimates seem to be very high, especially considering the absence of genetic variation for tarsus length in the same group of birds. It is unexpected (and inexplicable) that the heritability estimates for two of the traits are much higher than the corresponding repeatability estimates. The measurements were made from photographs of the bills, so measurement error cannot be a source of variation. More data will have to be collected.

2.6   Other traits

There is one aspect in which quantitative genetics is an art rather than a science: in answering the question of what is a *suitable* trait. In principle, every characteristic that is countable or measurable can be used as a trait. However, many of such traits will lead to disappointing results, by which I mean lack of reproducibility rather than demonstration of the absence of genetic variation. This is because, although often unspoken, it is assumed that there are physiological mechanisms involved in the observed variation, as an underlying cause of the genetic variation. It is not necessary to know, or even to guess, what physiological mechanisms are involved. To give an outlandish example of a mechanism underlying variation in clutch size: it is possible that a difference in eye pigments leads to differences in foraging efficiency and hence to differences in clutch size. If the difference in eye pigments is genetic and if it is an important factor in determining clutch size, it would be sufficient to let us observe genetic variation in clutch size. This consideration of physiological mechanisms provides a link between quantitative genetics and Mendelian genetics. We assume that the DNA codes the structure of enzymes and is involved in the regulation of the amounts of active enzymes present. There are numerous examples of mutants in single genes where effects on quantitative traits are observable. There are few, if any, examples where the variation in quantitative traits has been broken down into the individual genes involved, although especially in *Drosophila* it is a standard technique to localize the chromosomes, or even chromosome segments that contribute to the genetic variation.

It is unlikely that mapping of quantitative genetic variation to chromosomes will be feasible in birds, if only because the number of chromosomes is generally high (cf. chapter 3). However, it is useful to keep potential mechanisms in mind when selecting traits for quantitative genetic analysis. The following two traits are examples where the effects of environmental conditions are overwhelming and where quantitative genetic analysis has failed to show the presence of genetic variation: the tendency to lay second clutches and the natal dispersal distance.

3 UNSUCCESSFUL DEMONSTRATION OF GENETIC VARIATION

3.1 Second clutches

Great Tits may lay more than one clutch per year. A distinction is usually made between repeat clutches following a first clutch that failed, and second clutches that are produced after a first clutch that produced fledglings. The production of repeat clutches is, of course, mainly determined by the cause and manner of failure of the first clutch. These failures are too infrequent to be able to determine whether or not there is variation between individuals in the way they react to a similar situation.

The ecology of true second clutches is also complicated. The proportion of second clutches is usually low in broadleaved woods and much higher in mixed and coniferous habitats. It varies strongly from year to year within populations. Many second clutches are produced in years when laying starts early and when the population density is low (Kluyver *et al.* 1977, J. den Boer Hazewinkel, in preparation). It is, of course, possible that innate differences exist between individuals in the tendency to produce second clutches. A first step towards demonstrating such a tendency is to analyse two-by-two tables for pairs of subsequent years scoring whether or not each female had a second clutch in either year. Such tables do not show a significant tendency (A. J. van Noordwijk, unpublished work). This means either that there is no variation between individuals in their tendency to produce second clutches or that such variation is overshadowed by variation in the ecological situations of the individuals. The fact that more second clutches are produced if the relative success (defined as number of fledglings divided by clutch size) of the first clutch is lower points in the latter direction. In any case the statement is correct that no innate variation, whether genetic or not, in the tendency to produce second clutches has been demonstrated.

3.2   Natal dispersal distance

Great Tits breed in nestboxes in the study area. The positions of these boxes are known. It is thus possible to calculate the distance moved from the place of birth to that of first breeding for all individuals born in one of the boxes. Moreover, if the parents were also born locally, it is possible to compare the distances moved by parents and offspring. Greenwood *et al.* (1979) made such an analysis on data from Wytham and they found a resemblance in the distance moved from the birth site to site of first breeding, which they called "natal dispersal". There is insufficient evidence for a genetic cause of such a resemblance, however, because it can be demonstrated with simple simulations that similar resemblances arise while assuming that all individuals behave according to the same rules (van Noordwijk 1984 a). The observed resemblance is a property of the position of the nestbox in which the parents bred and the offspring were hatched.

There may be aspects of the behaviour involved in the natal dispersal for which genetical variation exists. The only point I want to make here is that the available data on movements from the nestbox of birth to the nestbox of breeding for half the population (about 50% of the breeding birds are immigrants) are too crude to demonstrate a genetic component. Furthermore, there is evidence for cultural transmission of geographical knowledge from parents to offspring (Drent 1983).

4 DETECTION OF INBREEDING

Whether inbreeding can be detected is highly dependent upon the completeness of the pedigrees of the breeding birds. Only if the family trees of both the male and the female are known can it be decided whether or not they have ancestors in common. In this respect the data from the Great Tit population on the island of Vlieland are unique. About 85% of the breeding birds in this population were ringed as nestlings and have known ancestors. In the larger mainland population such as that in the Hoge Veluwe and Wytham half the breeding birds are immigrants, which means that breeding pairs for which all eight grandparents are known are very rare. In the Vlieland population data from 1965 until 1978, 200 pairs out of 611 have the pedigrees of both male and female complete to the grandparents of the breeding birds. In 102 of these pairs a family relation between the male and the female is known. In the 411 pairs with less complete pedigrees, a further 62 cases are known to be related (van Noordwijk and Scharloo 1981). There is no simple answer to the question as to whether or not there is more or less inbreeding than expected. The detected amount of inbreeding is higher than the amount of inbreeding expected for a closed random-mating population of the same size in which the number of offspring per parent is binomially distributed. However, the population is not closed, which makes inbreeding less likely; mating is not entirely random because of subdivision of the population which makes inbreeding more likely; but by far the most important factor is that the variance in offspring number is much higher than in the ideal population from theoretical population genetics. Some families produce a great number of breeding birds, and the members of these families have a high chance of mating with a relative, simply because a high proportion of the potential mates are relatives. That this is an important factor is demonstrated by the fact that individuals that are inbred (its parents being relatives) are much more likely to be related to their partners than outbred individuals. Further, it has been shown that for those individuals that had two or more partners, the chance of being related to the second partner is much higher for individuals related to their first partner. Thus some individuals have a much higher chance of becoming involved in inbreeding (van Noordwijk and Scharloo 1981).

Some recent results (from the largest wooded area on Vlieland "bos bij dorp", containing some 70% of all breeding pairs on Vlieland) support the above conclusions. As a control for the occurrence of inbreeding, the degrees of relatedness with the neighbours were calculated (van Noordwijk et al. 1985). If the males are taken as focal birds and the mean degree of relatedness with the nearest female neighbour is calculated (or the other way round), the values are the same as the value for the average degree of relatedness of partners. Moreover, if one substitutes a randomly chosen individual for the nearest neighbour, the values are still very similar. In contrast, if one calculates the relatedness between male neighbours one obtains a higher value, and for female neighbours the average degree of relatedness is substantially lower. Again, there is no difference between the degree of relatedness with the nearest neighbour and with a randomly chosen bird (P. H. van Tienderen, in preparation; van Noordwijk *et al.* 1985).

The data from Vlieland allow a quantitative analysis of the effect of inbreeding. It is expected that the effects of inbreeding are dependent on the degree of relatedness of the parents. This is usually expressed in Wright's coefficient of inbreeding F, which is equal to the average proportion of the genes in the inbred individual that consist of two identical copies of the genes in the common ancestor (see chapter 6). Thus regressing, for example, the number of eggs failing to hatch on the degree of inbreeding, will indicate whether there is an effect of inbreeding.

Inbreeding results in increased homozygosity. Many deleterious genes are recessive, which implies that they are more frequently expressed in inbred genomes. Many properties of eggs are due to the genotype of the laying female. It is therefore possible that if the laying female is inbred, the hatchability of its eggs is lower, because, for example, the shell is more permeable and the embryo dries out. Hatchability may also be reduced as a consequence of the embryo being inbred. In this case, development may be stopped, for example, owing to a lack of some enzyme.

Both effects of inbreeding on the hatching of eggs are, in fact, detectable. There is a difference in the patterns that are observed. In both cases the chance that the clutch contains one or more eggs failing to hatch is significantly related to the degree of inbreeding, but only if the embryo is inbred is the mean number of eggs failing to hatch related to the degree of inbreeding. This is expected, because if the laying female being inbred is the cause of failure, then this female will either produce good eggs or bad eggs, but she will not change

Table 3. The effects of inbreeding on reproductive output at several ages of the offspring (data from van Noordwijk and Scharloo 1981)

---

(1) *The parents are related, the offspring inbred*
    Hatching failure $0.77 F + 0.15$
    Brood reduction $0.59 F + 0.29$
    Recruitment/fledgling $(2.0 F + 0.9)$ (average recruitment)

(2) (a) *F inbred*   (b) *M inbred*
       Hatching failure $0.16 F + 0.10$ No effect
    Recruitment for offspring from 2(a) and 2(b) combined is 1.7 times average recruitment

The net effect over two generations is that related pairs have twice as many grandchildren at breeding age as unrelated pairs.

---

her own genes while in the process of egg-laying. If the hatching failure is due to the embryo, then one expects Mendelian ratios for the deleterious genes in the clutch, and thus on average a quantitative relationship between the mean number of eggs failing and the degree of inbreeding.

In Table 3 a summary of the effects of inbreeding on the reproductive output is given. To take both effects of inbreeding (the egg being inbred and the laying female being inbred) into account, one can look at the number of grandchildren that reach breeding age produced by related and by unrelated pairs. The result is surprising in that related pairs produce twice as many grandchildren. The negative effects of inbreeding at egg hatching are more than compensated for by higher survival after fledging in both generations.

5 PROSPECTS FOR FUTURE RESEARCH

So far genetic variation has been demonstrated for many traits in several species of birds. At present, examples indicating the absence of genetic variation will probably be more interesting than further results that show the presence of heritable variation in these same traits in other species. These negative examples will, of course, have to be comparable in depth of analysis and in the definition of traits. In this respect the reports by Ricklefs and Peters (1981) and Smith (1981) are difficult to interpret because of differences in methods, and differences in the analysed trait, respectively. If there are comparable estimates indicating the absence of genetic variation, this will help towards an understanding of when genetic variation can be expected. In this sense the estimates of nestling body size in Great Tit are interesting, because of the differences between years.

Several lines of further research suggest themselves. It is quite possible to combine many of the classical experiments of evolutionary ecology with genetic analysis. Our current investigations into the ontogeny of body size variation combining cross-fostering with manipulation of brood size will help us to understand the interactions with environmental conditions; in this case, the amount of available food per nestling. In quantitative genetics the concept of "reaction norm" (i.e. the set of phenotypes produced by a single genotype in different environments) is very important (see, for example, Falconer 1960, Gupta and Lewontin 1982, Robertson 1960). The experiment described above is well suited to the calculation of reaction norms over the range of naturally occurring environments. It is not too difficult to extend it to other traits as well. The great advantage of undertaking such experiments with birds in a natural environment, rather than typical laboratory species, is that much more is known and understood of wild birds' natural ecology, and thus about the relevant range of environmental conditions. The interest in reaction norms for ecologically important traits (life-history traits), will certainly re-emerge in the next few years.

6   CONCLUSIONS

The results reviewed in this chapter show that there is ample genetic variation in ecologically important traits for evolutionary change to occur rapidly, if there is selection in a constant direction. Thus, the absence of systematic changes in many populations that have been studied over a long time is due to an absence of directional selection, rather than to an absence of genetic variation. This implies that there is a potential for adjusting to changes in the environmental circumstances. Apart from this broad statement, the main conclusion must be that the interactions between the processes traditionally studied in either ecology or genetics are manifold. This is true of the genetic process of inbreeding being responsible for a large number of the eggs failing to hatch (at least in the island population of Vlieland), as well as the heritability of nestling body size being high in years with abundant food, and being zero in poor breeding seasons. It is still too early to predict what new insights further integrated studies will give us.

REFERENCES

Dhondt, A. A. (1982). Heritability of blue tit tarsus length from normal and cross-fostered broods. *Evolution* **36**, 418–419.

Drent, P. J. (1983). The functional ethology of territoriality in the Great Tit *Parus major* L.). D.Sc. Thesis, Gröningen.

Falconer, D. S. (1960). Selection of mice for growth on low and high planes of nutrition. *Genet. Res.* **1**, 91–113.

Flux, J. E. C. and Flux, M. M. (1982). Artificial selection and gene flow in Wild Starlings, *Sturnus vulgaris. Naturwissensch.* **69**, 96–97.

Garnett, M. C. (1981). Body size, its heritability and influence on juvenile survival among Great Tits, *Parus major. Ibis* **123**, 31–41.

Greenwood, P. J., Harvey, P. H. and Perrins, C. M. (1979). The role of dispersal in the Great Tit (*Parus major*): The causes, consequences and heritability of natal dispersal. *J. Anim. Ecol.* **48**, 123–142.

Gupta, A. P. and Lewontin, R. C. (1982). A study of reaction norms in natural populations of *Drosophila pseudobscura. Evolution* **36**, 934–938.

Jones, P. J. (1973). Some aspects of the feeding ecology of the Great Tit, *Parus major.* D.Phil. Thesis, Oxford.

Kluyver, H. N. (1950). Daily routines of the Great Tit (*Parus m. major*). *Ardea* **38**, 99–135.

Kluyver, H. N. (1951). The population ecology of the Great Tit, *Parus major* L. *Ardea* **39**, 1–135.

Kluyver, H. N. (1952). Notes on body weight and time of breeding in the Great Tit, *Parus major* L. *Ardea* **40**, 123–141.

Kluyver, H. N. (1963). The determination of reproductive rates in paridae. *Proc. XIII Int. Ornith. Congress*, pp. 706–716.

Kluyver, H. N., van Balen, J. H. and Cavé, A. J. (1977). The occurrence of time-saving mechanisms in the breeding biology of the Great Tit, *Parus major. In* "Evolutionary Ecology" (eds B. Stonehouse and C. M. Perrins), pp. 153–169. Macmillan Press, London.

Lack, D. (1951). Reproductive rate and population density in the Great Tit: Kluijver's study. *Ibis* **94**, 167–173.

Lack, D. (1954). The evolution of clutch size. *In* "Evolution as a Process" (eds J. Huxley, A. C. Hardy and E. B. Ford). Allen & Unwin, London.

Lack, D. (1968). "Ecological Adaptations for Breeding in Birds". Methuen, London.

Newton, I., Marquiss, M. and Moss, D. (1981). Age and breeding in Sparrowhawks. *J. Anim. Ecol.* **50**, 839–853.

Newton, I. and Marquiss, M. (1984). Seasonal trends in the breeding performance of Sparrowhawks. *J. Anim. Ecol.* **53**, 809–829.

Ojanen, M., Orell, M. and Väisänen, R. A. (1979). The role of heredity in egg size variation in the Great Tit, *Parus major*, and the Pied Flycatcher, *Ficedula hypoleuca. Ornis Scand.* **10**, 22–28.

Perrins, C. M. (1979). "British Tits". Collins, London.

Robertson, F. W. (1960). The ecological genetics of growth in *Drosophila*. 2. Selection of large body size on different diets. *Genet. Res.* **1**, 305–318.

Ricklefs, R. E. and Peters, S. (1981). Parental components of variance in growth rate and body size of nestling European Starlings (*Sturnus vulgaris*) in eastern Pennsylvania. *Auk* **98**, 39–48.

Smith, J. N. M. (1981). Does high fecundity reduce survival in Song Sparrows? *Evolution* **35**, 1142–1148.

Smith, J. N. M. and Dhondt, A. A. (1980). Experimental confirmation of heritable morphological variation in a natural population of song sparrows. *Evolution* **34**, 1155–1158.

Snow, D. W. (1954). Trends in geographical variation in palearctic members of the genus *Parus. Evolution* **8**, 19–28.

van Balen, J. H. (1967). The significance of variations in body weight and wing length in the Great Tit, *Parus major. Ardea* **55**, 1–59.

van Balen, J. H. (1973). A comparative study of the breeding ecology of the Great Tit, *Parus major*, in different habitats. *Ardea* **61**, 1–93.

van Noordwijk, A. J. (1984 a). Problems in the analysis of dispersal and a critique on its heritability in the Great Tit. *J. Anim. Ecol.* **53**, 533–544.

van Noordwijk, A. J. (1984 b). Quantitative genetics in natural populations of birds, illustrated with examples from the Great Tit, *Parus major. In* "Population Biology and Evolution" (eds K. Wöhrman and V. Löschke), pp. 67–79. Springer-Verlag, Berlin, Heidelberg.

van Noordwijk, A. J., van Balen, J. H. and Scharloo, W. (1981a). Genetic and environmental variation in clutch size of the Great Tit. *Neth. J. Zool.* **31**, 342–372.

van Noordwijk, A. J., van Balen, J. H. and Scharloo, W. (1981 b). Genetic variation in the timing of reproduction in the Great Tit. *Oecologia* **49**, 158–166.

van Noordwijk, A. J., Keizer, L. C. P., van Balen, J. H. and Scharloo, W. (1981 c). Genetic variation in egg dimensions in natural populations of the Great Tit. *Genetica* **55**, 221–232.

van Noordwijk, A. J. and Klerks, P. L. M. (1983). Heritability of bill dimensions in the Great Tit. *Verh. Kon. Ned. Akad. Wetensch., Afd. Natuurk. 2e reeks 81 Prog. Rep. I.O.O.*, pp. 7–12.

van Noordwijk, A. J. and Scharloo, W. (1981). Inbreeding in an island population of the Great Tit. *Evolution* **35**, 674–688.

van Noordwijk, A. J., van Tienderen, P. H., de Jong, G. and van Balen, J. H. (1985). Genealogical evidence for random mating in a natural population of the Great Tit (*Parus major* L.). *Naturwissensch.* **72**, 104–106.

van Noordwijk, A. J., van Balen, J. H. and Scharloo, W. (1988). Heritability of body size in a natural population of the Great Tit and its relation to age and environmental conditions during growth. *Gen. Res. (Camb.)* (in press).

12

Evolutionary Genetics of House Sparrows

David T. Parkin

Department of Genetics, Medical School, Queen's Medical Centre, Nottingham NG7 2UH

1 INTRODUCTION

The palaearctic House Sparrow (*Passer domesticus*) is probably one of the most familiar birds in the world. It is found endemically across most of Europe, north Africa, central Asia and the Indian subcontinent, and following deliberate introductions by man and its subsequent dispersal, it now occurs in north and south America, southern Africa, Australia and New Zealand, in addition to a series of smaller island groups. Taxonomically, it is a member of the genus *Passer* alongside 17 other species, one of which (*P. predomesticus*) is an extinct form known only by fossil remains from Palestine (Tchernov 1962, Markus 1964). The genus *Passer* has traditionally been placed in the family Ploceidae together with the weavers and estrildine finches, and separate from the new world sparrows that belong to the Emberizidae. More recently, however, it has been suggested that *Passer* belongs in a separate family, the Passeridae, on the basis of anatomical, behavioural and serological data (see Summers-Smith (1985) for a review and references).

The detailed taxonomy of the genus *Passer* is still a matter for debate. *P. domesticus* is by far the most widespread, although it interbreeds with at least two other members of the genus in endemic populations (Meise 1936). For example, it hybridizes "very freely" with Spanish or Willow Sparrow (*P.*

AVIAN GENETICS
ISBN 0-12-187570-9

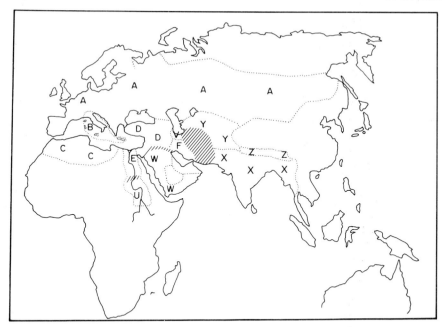

Fig. 1. The distribution of endemic populations of House Sparrow (*Passer domesticus*) showing subspecies and subspecies groups. *Domesticus* group: (A) *domesticus*; (B) *italiae*; (C) *tingitanus*; (D) *biblicus*; (E) *niloticus*; (F) *persicus*. *Indicus* group: (U) *rufidorsalis*; (V) *hyrcanus*; (W) *hufufae*; (X) *indicus*; (Y) *bactrianus*; (Z) *parkini*. (After Vaurie 1956.)

hispaniolensis) over wide areas of their range in north-west Africa, some Mediterranean islands and Italy (Vaurie 1956). In Spain, the Balkans and parts of Asia, the two forms co-exist with less (if any) interbreeding.

 P. domesticus itself shows a considerable amount of morphological variation, and has been divided into a series of subspecies, of which Vaurie (1956) recognizes 12 (Fig. 1). These fall into two groups on the basis of their morphology and, to a lesser extent, distribution. The western forms tend to have longer bill and wings, while the cheeks are greyish and do not become paler with wear. They are grouped together in the *domesticus* subspecies group, separate from the *indicus* group that also has a darker, richer chestnut colour in the mantle. Within these two groups, the subspecific differentiation is relatively slight, being largely morphometric. Vaurie (1956) considers that the size and colour variations manifest within and between subspecies may be explained in terms of adaptations following the so-called ecogeographic rules of Bergmann, Allen and Gloger (Mayr 1963). Thus, the more southerly populations tend to be smaller, and to have increased amounts of reddish pigment.

Because of its general abundance and familiarity, House Sparrow has been the subject of extensive research through the years. Its close association with man and its frequent superabundance have combined to facilitate field and laboratory study and experimentation. For example, its general population ecology and dynamics have been studied in North America by Anderson (1978), Lowther (1979 a,c), McGillivray (1980, 1983) and Murphy (1978 a,b). In western Europe it has been studied by Seel (1960, 1966, 1968 a,b) and Schifferli (1978), and in Poland by Pinowski and his colleagues (see, for example, Pinowski and Myrcha 1977). Endemic populations in India have been studied by Naik and Mistry (1970). Its movement and dispersal have been examined by Cheke (1972) and Lowther (1979 b), and its migratory behaviour by Broun (1972). The spread of sparrows into new areas either naturally or, more usually, following human introduction has been reported many times. A recent review by Long (1981) draws many of these together, and gives documentary information on dates and numbers. The subsequent increase to pest status in many areas has attracted much attention, notably from Kalmbach (1940), Dawson (1970), and Dawson and Bull (1970), while its possible role in the spread of parasitic and fungal diseases has been reported by Cornelius (1969), Gustafson and Moses (1953) and Hubalek (1977), amongst others. Finally, its karyotype has been examined by Castrowiejo *et al.* (1969) and Bulatova *et al.* (1972), who have also compared this with related passerine species.

The ease with which samples of live birds can be obtained, and their experimental convenience, has resulted in a considerable amount of physiological research, especially into aspects of metabolic adaptation and bioenergetics by Kendeigh and his colleagues (e.g. Kendeigh 1944, Kendeigh and Blem 1974, Blem 1973). The species has not escaped the attention of behaviourists, with studies of flock structure (Barnard 1980 a,b), time-budgets (Barnard 1980 c) and feeding behaviour (Barnard and Sibly 1981).

While this is inevitably a somewhat brief and subjective list, it does nevertheless make the point that a great deal of very diverse information is available concerning this species, which forms a sound basis for studies of evolutionary and population genetics. Over most of its range, House Sparrow is more or less an obligate commensal of man. Indeed, in the more extreme habitats such as semi-desert, sub-arctic farms and jungle settlements of South America, it only occurs in towns and on agricultural land where cereals are grown or are available for domestic livestock. It is generally a colonial species, breeding in natural holes and cavities when these are available, or when necessary constructing large and untidy nests of twigs, grasses and straw. It can be fairly easily induced to breed in nestboxes, which facilitates the study of its reproductive biology. Pairs are formed, and the species is territorial around the nest site, but this behaviour is relaxed away from the nest, and there is now an accumulation of data indicating that successful extra-pair copulation may be widespread (e.g. Yom Tov 1980, Manwell and Baker 1975, Burke 1984).

This wealth of background information has led a series of scientists to choose (either consciously or unconsciously) to study the evolutionary biology of House Sparrows. It is possible to use the data to assist in the interpretation of patterns of size and allele variation, and thereby learn a great deal about the evolution of bird populations in general, and sparrows in particular. This chapter will review some aspects of this research, and examine the various studies in the light of current understanding of evolutionary genetics.

2   SELECTION BY EXTREMES OF CLIMATE

One of the first examples of natural selection was provided by a study of House Sparrow at the end of the last century. In a, now classic, analysis, Hermon Bumpus (1899) observed the effects of a severe winter snowstorm upon the birds around the campus of Brown University at Providence, Rhode Island. This storm lasted for several hours and, towards its end, samples of moribund House Sparrows were brought into the laboratory. About half of these animals died from the effects of the blizzard conditions, and Bumpus made specimens of all of the birds noting their age, sex, weight and survival, and subsequently recording a series of body dimensions from every individual. From the analysis of these data, Bumpus postulated the existence of the phenomenon that is now known as "stabilizing" or "centripetal" selection. He suggested that the surviving birds were closer to the population mean, and that more extreme individuals had a reduced viability.

The data were published in full and have been re-assessed on several occasions as statistical methodology became more rigorous (e.g. Harris 1911, Calhoun 1947), and as its techniques became more sophisticated (e.g. Grant 1972, Johnston *et al.* 1972, O'Donald 1973). The three more recent re-analyses took rather different approaches. Grant (1972) examined the data character by character, whereas Johnston *et al.* (1972) applied principal-components analysis to assess the effects of overall size upon survival. In the most imaginative approach, O'Donald (1973) attempted to estimate the intensity of selection imposed upon the birds by the fierce winter conditions.

In the first of these, Grant (1972) showed that there were differences in the pattern of survival between the sexes, and also between the age classes among the males. He found that the female sparrows did indeed confirm Bumpus' suggestion of stabilizing selection, for the survivors have a lower variance for weight, and humeral, sternal and tibiotarsal lengths. He also found differences in the length and weight of surviving and non-surviving males, and concluded that the result was probably real, although the former is difficult to measure consistently, while the latter fluctuates diurnally and with the physiological condition of the bird. Johnston *et al.* (1972) applied principal-components analysis to the skeletal data alone, and confirmed Grant's findings for both sexes.

Grant (1972) commented that the females seemed to have survived less well than the males, and suggested that this might be because they had been denied access to food before the storm by the socially dominant males. There is, however, evidence that females are more aggressive and displace males from feeding sites (Johnston 1969 b), so Grant's idea may be wrong, although his suggestion that the enhanced mortality among the younger and smaller males may have been due to this social hierarchy is probably correct. Grant also suggested that the smallest females perished because they used up their energy reserves, whereas the largest birds could not mobilize these fast enough, and so suffered the same fate. While this is an attractive proposition that would account for the enhanced survival of the intermediate females, there does not seem to be much evidence to support it.

O'Donald (1973) approached the data set in a completely different way. He applied a series of models of selection to the measurements, both by taking them one at a time and also collectively through principal-components analysis. By comparing the means and variances of survivors and non-survivors, he was able to estimate the intensity of selection for most characters. He calculated that some 20% of deaths in the storm had been selective, and commented that this value was higher than had previously been recorded (although see Boag and Grant 1981). His results are open to some question, however, since he was obliged to pool the data over age and sex because the sample sizes were rather small. A higher mortality among the centripetally selected females combined with a lower mortality among directionally selected males could in fact give a lower overall intensity of selection than the values for the two sexes taken separately.

The general problem of selection upon multivariate characters has recently been examined in some detail by Lande and Arnold (1983). They point out that many traits are intercorrelated, which complicates their individual analysis. They have developed a statistical model that allows the dissection of a series of such intercorrelated characters and the estimation of selection differentials upon each of them. In an attempt to assess the value of their model to field biology, they have applied it to the sparrow data collected by Bumpus. They found (Lande and Arnold 1983) that "the winter storm apparently favoured small birds", which contrasts markedly with Johnston *et al.* (1972), who concluded that "large males have a selective advantage over small ones". Since these conclusions are apparently based upon precisely the same data set, they warrant further comment.

In fact, the cause of the discrepancy is not hard to find. Lande and Arnold (1983) utilized the entire set of nine measurements taken from each bird by Bumpus. One of these is body weight, which fluctuates considerably during a normal day, and is generally regarded as needing cautious interpretation. Johnston *et al.* reported that surviving birds weighed less than non-survivors, but considered that this result was produced artefactually. They pointed out that the "survivors" in the study were taken into the laboratory and held there for some time before their despatch and preparation. During this period, they were presumably not fed, but continued to lose weight by respiration and defaecation. Consequently, the apparently lower weight of these individuals compared with those found dead in the storm outside could have been produced by differential handling, and may thus be artefactual.

The other two metrics included by Lande and Arnold (1983), and excluded by most other analysts, were wing span and total body length. These are notoriously difficult measurements to take in a standard fashion, depending upon the attitude of the bird and the pressure exerted upon its body. They are thus not normally used by avian anatomists and taxonomists, and were accordingly excluded by Johnston *et al.* Thus, the different result obtained by Lande and Arnold could be due to the difference in the character set included in their analysis. It is unfortunate that they have approached the problem in this way, for it would be interesting to see the effects of character interaction analysed separately.

Returning to the study in general, Johnston *et al.* (1972) pointed out that the concept of stabilizing selection was generated from the results of this study. It is thus developed *a posteriori*, and so the data are responsible for the hypothesis and cannot be regarded as testing it. Consequently, there have been several attempts to repeat the study, with varying success. Two of these are worth discussing since they illustrate the problems inherent in this kind of research. Both were undertaken in the area around Lawrence, Kansas, and involved the comparison of an autumn sample with one taken in the spring. In the first, Rising (1970) took 57 birds in the autumn and a further 45 in the spring, of which 15 came from a site four miles from that of the rest. He found no difference in survival among the females, but the males in the spring were significantly bigger for a variety of skeletal characters. Some of these differences might have been due to the continued growth of the birds during the winter, but other changes seem to have been due to the disappearance of smaller individuals. Whether this arose from differential mortality or unrecognized patterns of movement could not be resolved. However, the result agreed with that from the earlier study, and could have been due to difficulties with thermoregulation or food acquisition. The second study, by Fleischer and Johnston (1982), utilized the same experimental design but is more conclusive. Their analysis followed O'Donald (1973) in the statistical comparison of biometrics and principal components, followed by the estimation of selection intensities from the means and variances of autumn and spring birds. Fleischer and Johnston examined many more birds than Rising (240 in autumn and 196 in spring), and, since a considerable number had been ringed in the course of an alternative study, it was possible to separate some of the spring birds into first year and older. Despite this, they too had problems over sample size, for only 15 males and 10 females were known to be first years in the spring sample. They were compelled to pool the spring birds, irrespective of age, and justified this by suggesting that all of them had undergone at least one winter of selection. They proceeded to demonstrate striking differences between the juveniles in the autumn, and these spring birds. Males were considerably bigger in body core in the spring, with a parallel but lesser increase in limb length. Females showed a different pattern, having a slight reduction in body core with a dramatic decrease in limb length. Combining these results indicates that the appendicular/core ratio is reduced over the winter. Such a result is similar to Bumpus' findings, and is predictable from Allen's ecogeographic rule.

The problem with this kind of field research is the awful heterogeneity and unpredictability of nature, particularly in cool temperate environments. Thus, both experiments were essentially opportunistic in that they were set up in the hope that suitable winter conditions would occur for selective mortality to be detectable. In this, Fleischer and Johnston were more fortunate than Rising, but even they were obstructed by the need to obtain sufficient individuals of each age class to be able to compare like with like in the subsequent analysis. The pre- and post-selection samples should be as nearly similar in number as possible, and of course the samples should be of the same age and sex, and come from the same population. It is almost impossible to age sparrows after the midwinter of their first year, so ageing in the spring is only possible if the bird was ringed as a youngster. The limited size of sparrow populations (Fleischer 1983, Parkin and Cole 1984), combined with a low first-year survival rate (Summers-Smith 1963), make it almost impossible to accumulate sufficient first-year birds in spring to compare with an autumn sample from the same population. This is perhaps the most critical period in a sparrow's life, and yet the data have to be pooled, and the analysis becomes very complex. The results obtained by Rising (1970) and Fleischer and Johnston (1982) are indicative, but alternative explanations based upon pooling of heterogeneous data, gene flow between populations, etc., can be proposed.

Despite these reservations, it does seem likely that there are survival differences between sparrows of differing size through periods of inclement weather. These can be explained plausibly in terms of individual vigour associated with position in the social hierarchy, sexual selection and thermoregulatory properties associated with differences in volume and surface area. Whether these differences in survival have any genetic consequences upon the population depends upon the heritability of the attributes involved. Until comparatively recently, estimates of heritability were restricted either to domestic animals, including man (see Falconer 1981), or to organisms that could easily be brought into captivity and reared under laboratory conditions (e.g. Cook 1965, Murray and Clarke 1968). In recent years, field ornithology has advanced sufficiently for data to be obtainable on the breeding performance of birds over a succession of years. Estimates of heritability can be obtained from parent/offspring correlations or sibling analysis (see Boag (1983) and Chapter 2 for several examples). Problems arise over the covariance of some characters, and also the common environment of nestlings, which can artificially raise estimates of similarity and thus the heritability when calculated from sibling resemblance. Many of the studies have been performed using territorial hole-nesting birds, and further problems can arise over territory quality which can combine with limited dispersion to cause the performance of successive generations of descendants to converge in a manner not necessarily associated with genetics.

Nevertheless, these problems are recognized, and efforts are being made either to circumvent them or to control their effects. The results, many of which are little more than preliminary, suggest that most metric attributes are quite highly heritable.

3   DIFFERENTIATION BETWEEN POPULATIONS

Apart from the routine recording of size data, and its use in taxonomy, the first serious study of metric variation in *P. domesticus* was undertaken by Lack (1940). From the analysis of bill and wing lengths of a few samples from North America, he concluded that there was little variation among the New World populations. This result was superseded by a more extensive study by Calhoun (1947), who examined many more populations than Lack, and who measured skeletal as well as plumage dimensions. In contrast to the earlier work, Calhoun found extensive variation in the lengths of wing, humerus and femur between regions of the United States. Although there was some heterogeneity among his samples, he pooled them within climatic zones and found that limb lengths were greater in cold environments. He interpreted this as being an example of Bergmann's rule. It subsequently transpired that Calhoun had chosen characters of the appendicular anatomy, rather than the axial, and the variation of these traits is slightly more complex than his initial conclusions suggest. Nevertheless, they remain a significant step in the understanding of morphological evolution in this species.

The most comprehensive analyses of morphological variation among natural populations of sparrows are those of Johnston (1969 a) and Johnston and Selander (1971, 1973). These three papers examine the relationship between skeletal dimensions, geography and climate in European and North American populations. The most interesting findings concern the results of principal-components analyses of body size and climate. Three components of variation could be distinguished in the skeletal data set, relating to size of body core, limb length relative to body core, and beak size relative to body core, respectively. In North America, body size increases with latitude, but in Europe the reverse holds. However, in both regions, there is a striking correlation between the second component and temperature. Birds from cold climates have relatively shorter limbs than those from warmer places. Such a correlation might be predicted from thermoregulatory considerations, and forms an example of Allen's ecogeographic rule. The third component also shows a negative correlation with temperature in Europe, which is again in agreement with Allen's rule.

The difference between American and European populations in the association between body size and latitude is surprising. The American birds conform to Bergmann's rule that homeotherms are larger in cold climates because the surface area to volume ratio decreases with increasing volume, and so heat loss is reduced. It might be inferred that these differences between the North American populations must have arisen following their arrival from Europe, and this assumption is supported by the analysis reported by Calhoun (1947). His data were somewhat limited since he was compelled to restrict the samples within climatic zones for fear of confounding time and space. The first sample that he could locate had been collected before 1885, within a few years of the species' arrival. These birds were significantly smaller than some from the same area 20 years later, although there is only slight evidence of subsequent divergence. Calhoun (1947) reports that House Sparrows were introduced from Britain and Germany, and comments that the pre-1885 birds were intermediate in size between the smaller British and larger German populations.

Calhoun was careful in the assessment of his measurements and endeavoured to ensure that the differences between means were real rather than artefacts produced by wear, abrasion, moult or shrinkage. It is fairly clear, however, that there is considerable heterogeneity among the samples taken after 1885, so that continued trends cannot be conclusively demonstrated. It is therefore unfortunate that he had only a single sample from the pre-1885 era. While there is no doubt that the dimensions of this sample are statistically different from later birds, it would be more comforting if a few more samples were involved.

Nevertheless, there is evidence here that sparrows increased in size very rapidly in the 20–30 generations following their introduction. Such changes in size have been recorded in other species, and need not necessarily be genetic responses to selection. It was shown by Conterio and Cavalli-Sforza (1957) that the mean stature of Italian conscripts increased by about 1 mm per year, or 30 mm per generation, during the first half of the twentieth century. They suggest that this is probably due to the improvement of living conditions, especially nutrition, hygiene and health, a suggestion that is corroborated by a correlation between stature and socio-economic group. Indeed, it has been shown by Cavalli-Sforza and Bodmer (1971) that mortality differences alone cannot be responsible for the increase in size, which has therefore occurred too rapidly to be due to selection alone. Applying their theoretical analysis to the data in Calhoun (1947), combined with an estimated heritability for wing length of 50% (Boag 1983), shows that this is not the case for North American sparrows: there has been plenty of time for an increase of 1 mm in 30 generations, even with comparatively low selection intensities.

For the variations in body size documented by Calhoun (1947) and Johnston and his colleagues to be genuine adaptations there must be genetic differences at the loci that control size between populations. There is no evidence that this is so amongst sparrows, or in any other wild bird for that matter. In 1973, Johnston wrote, "the tying of genetic to morphologic variation is not trivial for house sparrows; it is precisely such conjunction that needs to be demonstrated if we wish to speak meaningfully of evolution in North American populations of the species". Exactly the same can be said today; not just for the American populations, but even more among the endemic populations in Europe. Its importance has been demonstrated forcibly in a recent paper by James (1983). She transplanted clutches of eggs between the nests of morphologically distinct populations of Red-winged Blackbirds (*Agelaius phoeniceus*). The experiment was limited in size, but the results suggest that the offspring converged in shape towards their foster parents, and away from their natural parents. This suggests that the morphological phenotype is partially, or even largely, controlled by the environment, and less by genetics than had previously been thought. Such a result has been familiar to plant ecological geneticists for some time. Clausen *et al.* (1948) showed many years ago that there was an underlying genetic control of morphology in *Achillea*, but that the local environment could have profound effects within the constraints imposed by genetics. In our own species, Hulse (1968) showed that the children of Swiss immigrants reared in the United States were dramatically bigger than those born and reared in their native cantons in Switzerland.

This could also be having an effect upon Red-winged Blackbirds. Similar genetic/environmental interactions could also be involved in the determination of size and shape in avian populations. If the environmental component of variation was relatively large, the close correlations between morphology and climate that have been reported among species such as House Sparrow could be more easily explained. The direct influence of the ecological and climatological components of the environment upon bodily structure could also explain the apparently rapid differentiation of the North American populations reported by Calhoun (1947). How, or perhaps whether, factors such as differential feeding rates or nutrient quality could have a greater effect upon young birds in a nest than their genetic origins, and thus modify their patterns of growth and subsequent adult size, is a matter of considerable significance. This interaction between environment and genetics can only be conclusively analysed by controlled breeding in a stable environment, for example, by using a wild species that is relatively easy to rear in captivity. Cross-fostering experiments similar to those described by James (1983) controlled against intrapopulation fostering—or even using a third group of birds that are not involved with the transfer—in laboratory conditions would provide suitable data. Indeed, House Sparrow itself might be a suitable target species for such a study, although the one serious drawback to research with House Sparrows is the difficulty of undertaking captive-breeding. However, Mitchell and Hayes (1973) and Washington (1973) have both discussed ways of doing this, so that the research is now not only timely, but possible.

4   BIOCHEMICAL POLYMORPHISMS

The advent of gel electrophoresis to population genetics in the 1960s led to a series of studies of the genetic structure of House Sparrow populations around the world. The first, by Klitz (1973), suffered from a lack of luck, for the loci that he chose to study proved to be relatively invariant. He claimed that sparrows were largely monomorphic, and this result seemed oddly at variance with the rapid morphological evolution that had occurred in the American populations.

A study in Australia by Manwell and Baker (1975) indicated that levels of protein polymorphism might be much higher than Klitz had suggested, and this led Cole and Parkin (1981) to initiate a study of genetic variation amongst British and European populations of the species. They found nine polymorphic loci out of 33 that they were able to visualize, with an observed level of heterozygosity of about 15%. Based upon the evolution of selectively neutral alleles, Ohta and Kimura (1973) have shown that, when a population attains equilibrium, the expected amount of heterozygosity under a system of mutation and random genetic drift is $1 - 1/(1 + 8Nv)^{1/2}$, where N is the population size and v the mutation rate to an electrophoretically detectable allele. This mutation rate has been estimated as 10^{-7} per locus per year from the analysis of amino acid substitutions in protein sequences (Kimura and

Ohta 1971), and the number of sparrows in Britain today is probably about 3·5 to 7·0 million pairs (Sharrock 1976). Substituting these values in the above formula predicts heterozygosities from 61·1 to 71·4%. These are clearly very much higher than the values that Cole and Parkin (1981) obtained. However, it has been shown by Chakraborty and Nei (1977) that, following a bottleneck, it would take $2N/(4Nv + 1)$ generations for a population to regain this equilibrium state. In the case of House Sparrow, this is over three million generations, which is considerably more than the 15 000 years that are estimated to have elapsed since the species emerged from Africa into Europe and Asia (Summers-Smith 1963), and probably longer than the history of the species itself.

The estimate of heterozygosity obtained by Cole and Parkin (1981) is the highest recorded in a series of 30 avian species listed by Barrowclough (1983). The figures are, however, only dubiously comparable, for as pointed out by Barrowclough (1983) and Parkin and Cole (1984, 1985), their values depend very much upon the loci that are screened. The two most variable loci examined by Parkin and Cole were adenosine deaminase and sorbitol dehydrogenase, with per locus heterozygosities of 50 and 45%, respectively. These two enzymes are not regularly examined in other laboratories, and their inclusion will enhance the overall heterozygosities dramatically. Clearly, comparisons between species, or even between populations of the same species, are only meaningful if precisely the same loci are examined in every case.

These initial studies of polymorphism and heterozygosity in sparrows were followed by investigations into the genetic structure of series of populations of sparrows from both sides of the Atlantic. Fleischer (1983) and Parkin and Cole (1984) analysed two sets of adjacent populations, in Kansas and eastern England, respectively, using data from enzyme electrophoresis to estimate genetic similarities. Fleischer's study involved four polymorphic loci over five farm populations, while Parkin and Cole's was more extensive, including 14 variable loci and 15 populations. The two areas were clearly different in their ecology, for the Kansas birds were aggregated around farmsteads, whereas the English ones were effectively continuous across the area of study. The former were consequently more akin to the island or "stepping-stone" model of Kimura and Weiss (1964), while the latter were an example of "isolation by distance" (Wright 1951). Both studies measured the standardized amount of genetic differentiation among sub-populations, F_{ST}, which is effectively the probability that two homologous genes, randomly chosen from a sub-population, are descended from the same gene in that population. Fleischer's values of F_{ST} gave an average of 0·007 6 (SD = 0·002 2), compared with Parkin and Cole's mean of 0·003 45 (SD = 0·003 79). These estimates can also be compared with those listed by Barrowclough (1983), again with caution since some of Barrowclough's are based on very few loci and populations. Considering only those estimates of F_{ST} based upon five loci and five samples, the values obtained by Fleischer (1983) and Parkin and Cole (1985) were consistently lower ($p = 0.05$; Mann–Whitney U-test). Low values of F_{ST} indicate high levels of panmixis, so this result suggests that House Sparrow populations are rather less differentiated than the species listed by Barrowclough.

The attraction of F_{ST} as an estimator of population differentiation is that it is predictable from theory if enough is known about the ecological structure of the populations involved. Thus, both Fleischer (1983) and Parkin and Cole (1984) were able to incorporate survival estimates, population sizes, migration rates, sex ratios, etc., into theoretical models of population genetics to predict values of F_{ST} for their populations: the former's estimate was 0·013 6; the latter's 0·004 84. It is interesting to note that both the observed and predicted values for the North American study are higher than those for England. A value of 0·004 84 implies that, of the total genetic variance, 99·5% is due to variation within the populations, i.e. due to polymorphism, and only 0·5% to interpopulation differentiation. Although the values are small, it does seem that the more discontinuous nature of the Kansas populations is reflected in a greater amount of genetic differentiation.

The similarity of these populations, and their lack of differentiation, contrasts markedly with the situation in western Norway. Here, the populations are very isolated, and show much greater genetic divergence than anywhere else so far examined (Bjordal et al., in preparation). The average value of the coefficient of genetic differentiation (G_{ST}; Nei 1975) is 0·021 5 (SD = 0·007 8), compared with 0·010 8 (SD = 0·005 7) for the east midlands of England. There are several instances where allele frequencies differ significantly among the populations, many of which seem to be totally isolated. Their relationship with populations from elsewhere can be visualized using cluster analysis based upon the similarity between the samples.

There are several different ways of assessing the similarity of pairs of samples from allele frequency data, of which that derived by Nei (1972) is the most widely used. This involves a statistic, D, that is effectively the probability of an allele chosen at random from one population being identical with one chosen at random from another, relative to the probability of identity of two alleles chosen randomly from the same population. Thus,

$$D = J_{XY}/(J_{XX}J_{YY})^{1/2}$$

where J_{XX} and J_{XY} are the probabilities of choosing identical alleles from the same and different populations, respectively. It should be noted that "identical" here means "indistinguishable", and not identical by descent. In fact, an allele is a band on an electrophoretic or isofocusing gel.

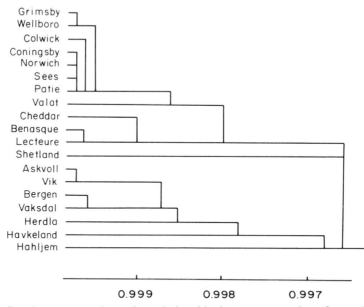

Fig. 2. Dendrogram to show the relationship between a series of samples of *Passer domesticus* taken from western Europe, based upon Nei's coefficient of genetic distance computed for a series of polymorphic enzyme loci. The top 12 samples are from Britain, France and Spain; the lower 7 are from Norway. (After Bjordal *et al.*, in preparation.)

A series of genetic identities from some west European samples was derived by Bjordal *et al.* (in preparation), and these have been subjected to cluster analysis in Fig. 2. It is apparent that the Norwegian birds are very different from those in the south-west part of Europe, including the British Isles. It is believed that the evolution of avian populations in Europe has been strikingly influenced by glaciation events over the last one hundred thousand years (Lack 1971, Parkin 1979). It is possible that the Norwegian populations were founded from eastern Europe following the last glaciation, and that the remainder shown in Fig. 2 emanate from north Africa round the western end of the Mediterranean Sea. If this is the case, the two groups of populations might have been separated for over ten thousand years (see below).

Parkin and his colleagues have extended their analysis of House Sparrow populations to other endemic subspecies from Asia, and the introduced birds from Australia and New Zealand. They have screened the same loci in all samples, and so can directly compare the results from each population. Burke and his colleagues (Burke 1984; and Burke *et al.*, in preparation) have examined two samples from each of four subspecies: the nominate *domesticus*

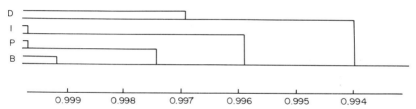

Fig. 3. Dendrogram to show the relationship between four subspecies of *Passer domesticus*, based upon Nei's coefficient of genetic distance using the same loci as Fig. 2: (D) *domesticus*; (I) *indicus*; (P) *parkini*; (B) *biblicus*.

from Britain, *biblicus* from Israel, *indicus* from north India, and *parkini* from Kashmir. The former two of these are from the *domesticus* subspecies group and the latter from *indicus* (see Fig. 1; Vaurie 1956).

Genetic identities were computed between all of the samples, and the dendrogram resulting from cluster analysis of these is shown in Fig. 3. It is clear that populations of the same subspecies are more similar to one another than to other subspecies. Furthermore, *indicus* and *parkini* cluster closer together than to the others. This is not very surprising since they are geographically closer, and also in the same morphological subspecies group. More unexpected is the closer alignment of *biblicus* with these two than with *domesticus*.

An attraction of Nei's estimate of genetic identity is that it is easily converted to a measure of genetic distance:

$$D = -\ln(I)$$

This genetic distance between two populations has been shown by Nei (1975) to increase steadily over time as follows:

$$D_t = D_0 + 2\alpha t$$

where D_0 and D_t are the genetic distances over a period of t years, and α is the rate of substitution of electrophoretically detectable alleles per locus per year. It is thus possible to use genetic distances in order to estimate the rate of evolution when the time-scale is known, or the time of separation when the evolutionary rate has been established.

Parkin and Cole (1985) were able to determine this rate of molecular evolution from the comparison of British and European stocks. It is believed (Summers-Smith (1963) and personal communication) that House Sparrow colonized Britain about 2000 years ago. It seems probable that colonization was by the general spread of flocks of birds rather than the chance arrival of vagrant individuals, and that these birds established themselves around the villages and settlements along the south coast. This was followed by a spread northwards, and sparrows were certainly established on Tyneside, in the north of England, by the seventh century, since they were familiar to the Venerable Bede. Parkin and Cole (1985) estimated the genetic distance between British and European samples, and found the average inter-regional distance to be 0·002 572 (SD = 0·000 147). They took this to be the value of D_t in Nei's formula, and estimated D_0 by assuming that the amount of differentiation between the birds that colonized Britain and the parent stocks at the time of arrival was the same as the differentiation between random continental populations at the present day. It seems likely that these populations will be in some sort of equilibrium, and that any increase in genetic divergence will be counterbalanced by migration and gene flow. The mean genetic distance between seven samples from south-west Europe was 0·001 868 so that

$$0·002\,572 = 0·001\,868 + 2\alpha \times 2000$$

from which $\alpha = 1·76 \times 10^{-7}$.

This result is close to that obtained by Kimura and Ohta (1971) and Nei (1972) from the analysis of amino acid substitutions in a series of proteins. It is also close to the estimated mutation rate for electrophoretically detectable alleles. This, then, was an estimate of the rate of evolution, and could be used to assess the time of separation of the various subspecies studied by Burke *et al.* (in preparation). Summers-Smith (1963) suggested that House Sparrow evolved in Africa, and spread into Europe and Asia through the Rift Valley. Sparrows thus arrived in the Nile Delta, and those populations destined to become the nominate *domesticus* moved westwards across north Africa, and then north into Iberia. The *indicus* birds spread eastwards across Arabia and into the Indian subcontinent. Thus, the populations available to Burke *et al.* that were geographically closest to the ancestral sparrows of the Nile Delta were the *biblicus* samples from Israel.

The genetic distance between the original populations could be estimated as 0·001 2 from the mean intra-subspecies distance, and that between *biblicus* and *domesticus* as 0·005 9. Substituting these in Nei's rate of evolution equation with $\alpha = 1·76 \times 10^{-7}$ gives $t = 13\,350$. The populations of the *indicus* subspecies group could be examined in the same way, and gave $t = 7950$. These results agree reasonably well with the Summers-Smith time-scale, which is based upon historical and zoogeographic considerations. He believes (Summers-Smith 1963; and personal communication) that House Sparrow arrived in the Nile Delta between 10 and 15 thousand years ago, which encompasses the molecular estimate of 13 thousand years for the separation of *biblicus* and *domesticus*. It would clearly be very interesting to examine some of the other subspecies, especially those from the Nile Valley itself.

House Sparrow was introduced into Australia and New Zealand independently, chiefly from the British Isles. Its Australasian populations were established during the period 1860–1872 (Long 1981), largely through the efforts of well-meaning enthusiasts. Organizations such as the Zoological and Acclimatization Society of Victoria strove to encourage an appreciation of the living world in the British colonies, at least partially by making the environments of human settlements in these regions more attractive through the introduction of familiar animals and plants. While such activities would be frowned upon today, they do mean that we have a certain amount of documentary evidence relating to the dates, origins and numbers of the introductions. This can be used in the analysis and interpretation of contemporary population structure.

Parkin and Cole (1985) found that populations from both Australia and New Zealand lacked some of the alleles that are found among contemporary British birds. Such a result would be expected from the founder effect (Mayr 1963) for two reasons. Firstly, small samples taken from a large population are likely to be genetically depauperate, since rare alleles may be omitted owing to sampling effects. Secondly, and equally significant in the longer term, during the early generations following introduction, the populations will still be relatively limited in number, and so susceptible to both inbreeding and random genetic drift. The effects of these will be to reduce genetic variation even more among the introduced populations. In the absence of further introductions, additional alleles can only arise by mutation or introgression following hybridization with related reproductively compatible species.

The genetic distances have also been determined for a series of samples from these two regions and some endemic British populations, based upon precisely the same loci as before (Parkin and Cole 1985). From a theoretical analysis of the founder effect (Mayr 1963), Nei (1978) and Templeton (1980 a,b) derived formulae describing the consequences of a sharp bottleneck upon the genetic distance between a small population and its ancestral stock. Templeton (1980 a) suggested that the distance at the moment of founding would be

$$D_0 = f(1 - G)/(2G)$$

where G is the homozygosity of the base population and f is the coefficient of inbreeding in the founding population. There were several introductions into Australia, and Parkin and Cole calculated that the harmonic mean of the number of founders in any one colony was 86·1. The heterozygosity in the British populations was 14·6% from the 29 loci examined, so that $D_0 = 0·000\,474$. Hence, over 112 years

$$0·003\,224 = 0·000\,474 + 2\alpha \times 112$$

so $\alpha = 1·23 \times 10^{-5}$. This seems an improbably high rate of evolution, being 100 times greater than that between British and European populations. However, Nei and Templeton's calculations relate to a single founding event. It is very likely that the new populations remained quite small for several generations, during which inbreeding and random genetic drift could play a significant role in enhancing the differentiation from the ancestral stocks. Parkin and Cole (1985) showed that the increase in the genetic distance could be accounted for with the earlier, more realistic, rate of evolution if the populations began with an effective size of about 40, and increased by about 50% per generation.

5 DISCUSSION AND CONCLUSIONS

These studies of population and evolutionary genetics have told us a great deal about House Sparrow in both its native and introduced habitats. The morphological variation appears to be under the control of natural selection, since there is a series of correlations between the local climate (macro and micro) and both absolute size and relative proportions of the birds in many populations. There is evidence that sparrows generally are larger in cold places, and that the mortality of the smallest males is higher under conditions of low ambient temperature. This is in agreement with the widely quoted ecogeographic rule of Bergmann, which suggests that animals are larger in cold places. Proponents of this view claim that the size of a homeotherm is regulated by the costs and benefits of energy metabolism. Under the same conditions of temperature, insulation, etc., large animals require more food to keep themselves alive. Heat loss is a significant problem in low external temperatures, and is proportional to the temperature differential across the skin, and also to the surface area that is exposed to the environment. More heat will be lost across a larger body surface, and so in a cold place more energy has to be expended in order to keep the animal at its vital temperature. Advocates of Bergmann's rule claim that, provided a large animal can obtain sufficient food to keep itself alive at all, then it will be at an advantage over a small one in a cold place, because less heat is lost across the body surface per gram of body weight than from a smaller one. McNab (1971) challenged this view on two grounds. Firstly, he claimed that the physics was wrong: the classic exposition of Bergmann's rule depended upon heat loss being related to a weight-specific rate, whereas the animal in fact lives as an intact individual so that the absolute rate of heat loss is the significant parameter. Secondly, the correlations between size and ambient temperature were by no means universal among homeotherms (e.g. Scholander 1955), whereas the size of some poikilotherms correlated positively with latitude and negatively with temperature (e.g. Lindsey 1966). McNab (1971) suggested that the larger size of granivores, such as House Sparrow, in northern latitudes was due to a reduction in competition, and therefore a widening of the range of available food resources. Whether this is true for House Sparrow itself is unresolved, but it is clearly an interesting avenue for speculation and experimentation.

The correlations between reduced extremities and low temperature seem to be less disputed. These are known as Allen's Rule, and again are related to thermoregulation. Relatively little heat is generated in peripheral appendages such as wings and legs, so they act as an area of net heat loss. Johnston and Selander's (1971) analyses showed that the appendicular/axial ratio declined in colder latitudes, and the results of the re-analysis of Bumpus' data (Johnston *et al.* 1972) and the more recent data of Rising (1970) and Fleischer and Johnston (1982) suggest that long-limbed sparrows survive the winter cold less well.

On the other hand, the biochemical data suggest that (some) gene frequencies are less rigorously controlled by selection. The differentiation between geographically close populations in both North America (Fleischer 1983) and England (Parkin and Cole 1984) is relatively slight, and could easily be due to inbreeding and drift within populations that are relatively small and somewhat isolated. The greater divergence between some Scandinavian populations (Bjordal *et al.*, in preparation) may also prove to be due to isolation and inbreeding.

However, there is evidence that selection might be acting at some loci in some populations. Cole and Parkin (1986) have evidence of consistently different allele frequencies at the adenosine deaminase locus between rural and urban populations. While this difference is slight, it relates to an enzyme that plays a significant part in the preliminary metabolism of food in the digestive tract. Associations between such so-called "external" or "non-regulatory" enzymes (Johnson 1974) and population ecology and fitness have been recorded in other species. For example, Baker and Fox (1978) produced evidence of an association between social status and heterozygosity at a peptidase locus in Dark-eyed Junco (*Junco hyemalis*). Evans (1980; chapter 4) found indications of associations between growth rate and genotype at a similar locus in Eurasian Starling (*Sturnus vulgaris*). So it seems possible that some selective effects might be involved in the control of allele frequencies and heterozygosity, but it is true to say that in no bird has a rigorous case been made showing the causal links between the enzymic or genotypic function and the selective agents involved. It is evident that such a case can be made for other vertebrate and invertebrate groups (Koehn *et al.* 1983), and no doubt will eventually be established for avian species too.

In an attempt to link morphological and enzymic variation, Johnston and Klitz (1977) and Fleischer *et al.* (1983) studied the relationship between variance in skeletal characters of House Sparrow and the genotype at a series of protein loci. They found evidence of a lowered morphological variance among individuals that were more heterozygous than the average. These results were contradictory to those of Handford (1980) working with Rufous-collared Sparrow (*Zonotrichia capensis*), although the latter's study involved fewer birds. They confirm the predictions made many years ago by Lerner (1954) that increased heterozygosity should result in greater homeostasis, and therefore less intrapopulation variability in metric traits.

Certain problems still remain unresolved, some of which are particular to House Sparrow, while others are of a more general nature. At a local level, the studies of Parkin and his colleagues have shown that there is a slight but significant differentiation at enzymic loci between the various subspecies of *P. domesticus*. A study of the zone of introgression between *domesticus* and *italiae* in the Swiss Alps (Fothergill *et al.*, in preparation) suggests that there might be some steep gradients in allele frequency across the area of contact that can be related to the amount and direction of cross-boundary movement. It would be informative to examine similar boundaries between other subspecies. Of particular interest is the situation in southern Egypt where the *domesticus* and *indicus* subspecies groups meet. This is almost certainly a zone of secondary contact, formed following the northward spread of *P. d. indicus* from the horn of Africa (Vaurie 1956). Relatively little is known of the genetics of avian speciation, and the structure of hybrid zones is still a matter of great interest (cf. chapters 10 and 15).

This leads on to the general question of the relationship between genic heterozygosity and population fitness in general. It is clear that there are interactions between enzyme heterozygosity and morphological variation, and also between size variation and fitness. There are remarkably few data in this species (or any other for that matter) relating to the genetic fine structure of avian populations, despite the fact that for genetical/demographic studies birds are almost the ideal target. They are relatively easy to trap and mark, their external morphology is comparatively simple to quantify, and blood samples allow the determination of enzyme and protein genotypes. Nests can be located, and from monitoring the contents, the fertility, fecundity, nestling growth rates and survival can all be established. It is thus possible to analyse population structure through time and space more easily than for any other group. A study has been done by Burke (1984) that will show some of the problems and possibilities of this kind of research, undertaken with House Sparrow but applicable to a wide range of species.

The morphological analysis of homeotherm populations is currently a matter for some debate. McNab (1971) has challenged the universality of Bergmann's Rule, and James (1983) has suggested that not all morphological differentiation between populations is genetic in origin. Both of these fields are wide open for rigorous scientific analysis, and House Sparrow is an attractive potential target for further research. The physiology and thermodynamics of this species has been studied for over 40 years (Barnett 1970, Blem 1973, Hudson and Kimzey 1966, Kendeigh 1944, 1973, 1976, Kendeigh and Blem 1974), and the methodology of experimentation is now well understood. It is possible to design experiments to examine the thermodynamics of birds of various sizes and to compare the effects of body size upon thermoregulation and energy dynamics both within and between populations. Similarly, the phenomenon uncovered by James with Red-winged Blackbirds can be resolved by the careful application of quantitative genetics to controlled breeding experiments, again within and between populations, to establish the genetic and non-genetic contributions to the size and shape of a bird's body. Such a study could be undertaken with House Sparrow, using either endemic or New World populations.

Finally, the studies so far undertaken on the rate of evolution of endemic and introduced populations suggest that this is relatively constant, and at a level that is close to the mutation rate. Such a finding is in accord with the theory of neutral evolution (e.g. Kimura 1983). However, the analyses suffer from being based upon the electrophoresis of enzymes. It is well known that this does not disclose all of the variation present in nature. Allozymes exist whose electrophoretic mobility is identical despite profound differences in their physico-chemical properties (e.g. Singh *et al*. 1975). It is thus effectively an analysis several steps removed from the genetic material itself. Techniques are now available for the identification of variation in the base sequence of the DNA itself, and allowing the rapid screening of samples from individuals or populations. It is thus possible to re-work this study at a DNA level, and thereby gain some insight into the true rate of molecular evolution in native and non-native populations. The comparisons of these results with mutation rates and the function of the DNA on the one hand, and the evolution of morphology and enzymes on the other, will be interesting indeed.

ACKNOWLEDGMENTS

Much of my research into House Sparrow population genetics has been jointly undertaken with Stephen R. Cole, who has now returned to his native Australia. I am grateful to him for five years of collaborative research, and to his company, both practical and intellectual. My work has been based at Nottingham, where Professor Bryan Clarke has provided an ideal environment for the study of population genetics and evolution. Laboratory and field assistance have been given by Andrew Bird, Chris Fothergill, Jonathan Lewis, Kevin O'Dell, John Stephen and David Walters. The manuscript has been read and criticized by Drs Terry Burke, Fred Cooke, Peter Evans and Jim Rising, and by Toby Bennett and Jonathan Wetton. To all of them I express my gratitude. Finally, I should like to thank Denis Summers-Smith, who first introduced me to the scientific study of House Sparrows when I was a

402

D. T. Parkin

schoolboy in Newcastle upon Tyne over 30 years ago. The seed that he planted was a long time germinating!

REFERENCES

Anderson, T. R. (1977). Reproductive responses of sparrows to a superabundant food supply. *Condor* **79**, 205–208.

Anderson, T. R. (1978). Population studies of European sparrows in North America. *Occ. Papers Mus. Nat. Hist. Univ. Kansas* **70**, 1–58.

Anderson, T. R. (1979). Experimental synchronization of sparrow reproduction. *Wilson Bull.* **91**, 317–319.

Baker, M. C. and Fox, S. F. (1978). Dominance, survival and enzyme polymorphism in Dark-eyed Juncos, *Junco hyemalis. Evolution* **32**, 697–711.

Barnard, C. J. (1980 a). Flock feeding and time budgets in the house sparrow (*Passer domesticus*). *Anim. Behav.* **28**, 295–309.

Barnard, C. J. (1980 b). Equilibrium flock size and factors affecting arrival and departure in feeding house sparrows. *Anim. Behav.* **28**, 503–511.

Barnard, C. J. (1980 c). Factors affecting flock size mean and variance in a winter population of house sparrows (*Passer domesticus*). *Behaviour* **74**, 114–127.

Barnard, C. J. and Sibly, R. M. (1981). Producers and scroungers: a general model and its application to feeding flocks of house sparrows. *Anim. Behav.* **29**, 543–550.

Barnett, L. B. (1970). Seasonal changes in temperature acclimatization in the House Sparrow, *Passer domesticus. Comp. Biochem. Physiol. A* **33**, 559–578.

Barrowclough, G. B. (1983). Biochemical studies of evolutionary processes. In "Perspectives in Ornithology" (eds A. H. Brush and G. A. Clark), pp. 223–261. Cambridge University Press.

Bjordal, H., Cole, S. R. and Parkin, D. T. Genetic variation in some Norwegian populations of the House Sparrow (*Passer domesticus*), as revealed by enzyme electrophoresis. (In preparation.)

Blem, C. R. (1973). Geographic variation in the bioenergetics of the House Sparrow, *Passer domesticus. Ornithol. Monogr.* **14**, 96–121.

Boag, P. T. (1983). The heritability of external morphology in Darwin's ground finches (*Geospiza*) on Isla Daphne Major, Galapagos. *Evolution* **37**, 877–894.

Boag, P. T. and Grant, P. R. (1981). Intense natural selection in a population of Darwin's Finch (Geospizinae) in the Galapagos. *Science* **214**, 82–85.

Broun, M. (1972). Apparent migratory behaviour in the House Sparrow. *Auk* **98**, 189–191.

Bulatova, N. S., Radjabu, S. I. and Panov, E. N. (1972). Karyological description of three species of the genus *Passer. Experientia* **28**, 1369–1371.

Bumpus, H. C. (1899). The elimination of the unfit as illustrated by the introduced sparrow, *Passer domesticus. Biol. Lect. Marine Biol. Lab., Woods Hole*, pp. 209–226.

Burke, T. A. (1984). The ecological genetics of two populations of the house sparrow, *Passer domesticus.* Ph.D. Thesis, University of Nottingham, UK.

Burke, T. A., Cole, S. R., O'Dell, K. M. C. and Parkin, D. T. Genetic differentiation between sub-species of the House Sparrow, *Passer domesticus.* (In preparation.)

Calhoun, J. B. (1947). The role of temperature and natural selection in relation to the variations in the size of the English Sparrow in the United States. *Am. Natur.* **81**, 203–228.

Castrowiejo, J., Christian, L. C. and Gropp, A. (1969). Karyotypes of four species of birds of the families Ploceidae and Paridae. *J. Hered.* **60**, 134–136.

Cavalli-Sforza, L. L. and Bodmer, W. F. (1971). "The Genetics of Human Populations". Freeman, San Francisco.

Chakraborty, R. and Nei, M. (1977). Bottleneck effects on average heterozygosity and genetic distance with the stepwise mutation model. *Evolution* **31**, 347–356.

Cheke, A. S. (1972). Movements and dispersal among house sparrows, *Passer domesticus*, at Oxford, England, *In* "Productivity, Population Dynamics and Systematics of Granivorous Birds" (eds S. C. Kendeigh and J. Pinowski). Polish Scientific Publishers, Warsaw.

Clausen, J., Keck, D. D. and Hiesey, W. M. (1948). Experimental studies on the nature of species. III. Environmental responses of climatic races of *Achillea*. *Carnegie Inst. Washington Publ.* **581**, 1–129.

Cole, S. R. and Parkin, D. T. (1981). Enzyme polymorphism in the House Sparrow, *Passer domesticus*. *Biol. J. Linn. Soc.* **15**, 13–22.

Cole, S. R. and Parkin, D. T. (1986). Adenosine deaminase polymorphism in the house sparrow, *Passer domesticus*. *Anim. Blood Groups Biochem. Genet.* **17**, 77–88.

Conterio, F. and Cavalli-Sforza, L. L. (1957). Evolution of the human constitutional phenotype: an analysis of mortality effects. *Convegno Genet.*, pp. 3–14.

Cook, L. M. (1965). Inheritance of shell size in the snail, *Arianta arbustorum*. *Evolution* **19**, 86–94.

Cornelius, L. W. (1969). Field notes on *Salmonella* infection in greenfinches and house sparrows. *Bull. Wildlife Dis. Ass.* **5**, 142.

Dawson, D. G. (1970). Estimation of grain loss due to sparrows (*Passer domesticus*) in New Zealand. *New Zealand J. Agric. Res.* **13**, 681–688.

Dawson, D. G. and Bull, P. C. (1970). A questionnaire survey of bird damage to fruit. *New Zealand J. Agric. Res.* **13**, 326–371.

Evans, P. G. H. (1980). Population genetics of the European Starling (*Sturnus vulgaris*). D.Phil. Thesis, Oxford University.

Falconer, D. S. (1982). "Introduction to Quantitative Genetics", 2nd edn. Longman, London.

Fleischer, R. C. (1983). A comparison of theoretical and electrophoretic assessment of genetic structure in populations of the House Sparrow (*Passer domesticus*). *Evolution* **37**, 1001–1009.

Fleischer, R. C. and Johnston, R. F. (1982). Natural selection of body size and proportions in house sparrows. *Nature* **298**, 747–749.

Fleischer, R. C., Johnston, R. F. and Klitz, W. J. (1983). Allozymic heterozygosity and morphological variation in house sparrows. *Nature* **304**, 628–630.

Fothergill, C. J. and Parkin, D. T. Genetic variation in the house sparrow though the boundary between two subspecies in the Swiss Alps. (In preparation.)

Grant, P. R. (1972). Centripetal selection and the House Sparrow. *Syst. Zool.* **21**, 23–30.

Gustafson, D. P. and Moses, H. E. (1953). The English sparrow as a natural carrier of Newcastle disease virus. *Am. J. Vet. Res.* **14**, 581–585.

Handford, P. (1980). Heterozygosity at enzyme loci and morphological variation. *Nature* **286**, 261–262.

Harris, J. A. (1911). A neglected paper on natural selection in the English sparrow. *Am. Natur.* **45**, 314–318.

Hubalek, Z. (1977). Spread of fungi and other micro-organisms by sparrows: a review. *Intl Stud. Sparrows* **10**, 7–25.

Hudson, J. W. and Kimzey, S. W. (1966). Temperature regulation and metabolic rhythms in populations of the House Sparrow, *Passer domesticus. Comp. Biochem. Physiol. A* **17**, 203–217.

Hulse, F. S. (1968). The breakdown of isolates and hybrid vigour among the Italian Swiss. *Proc. XII Int. Congr. Genet.* **2**, 177.

James, F. C. (1983). Environmental components of morphological differentiation in birds. *Science* **221**, 184–186.

Johnson, G. B. (1974). Enzyme polymorphism and metabolism. *Science* **184**, 28–37.

Johnston, R. F. (1969 a). Character variation and adaptation in European sparrows. *Syst. Zool.* **18**, 206–231.

Johnston, R. F. (1969 b). Aggressive foraging behavior in House Sparrows. *Auk* **86**, 558–559.

Johnston, R. F. and Klitz, W. J. (1977). Variation and evolution in a granivorous bird: the house sparrow. *In* "Granivorous Birds in Ecosystems" (eds J. Pinowski and S. C. Kendeigh). Cambridge University Press.

Johnston, R. F., Niles, D. M. and Rohwer, S. A. (1972). Hermon Bumpus and natural selection in the House Sparrow, *Passer domesticus. Evolution* **26**, 20–31.

Johnston, R. F. and Selander, R. K. (1971). Evolution in the House Sparrow. II. Adaptive differentiation in North America. *Evolution* **25**, 1–28.

Johnston, R. F. and Selander, R. K. (1973). Evolution in the House Sparrow. III. Variation in size and sexual dimorphism in Europe and North and South America. *Am. Natur.* **107**, 373–390.

Kalmbach, E. R. (1940). Economic status of the English sparrow in the United States. *U.S. Dept Agric. Tech. Bull.* **711**, 1–66.

Kendeigh, S. C. (1944). Effect of air temperature on the rate of energy metabolism in the English Sparrow. *J. Exp. Zool.* **96**, 1–16.

Kendeigh, S. C. (1973). Monthly variations in the energy budget of the House Sparrow throughout the year. *In* "Productivity, Population Dynamics and Systematics of Granivorous Birds" (eds S. C. Kendeigh and J. Pinowski). Institute of Ecology, Dziekanow, Poland.

Kendeigh, S. C. (1976). Latitudinal trends in the metabolic adjustments of the House Sparrow. *Ecology* **57**, 509–519.

Kendeigh, S. C. and Blem, C. R. (1974). Metabolic adaptation to local climate in birds. *Comp. Biochem. Physiol. A* **48**, 175–187.

Kimura, M. (1983). "The Neutral Theory of Molecular Evolution". Cambridge University Press.

Kimura, M. and Ohta, T. (1971). "Theoretical Aspects of Population Genetics". Princeton University Press.

Kimura, M. and Weiss, G. H. (1964). The stepping stone model of population structure and the decrease of genetic correlation with distance. *Genetics* **49**, 561–576.

Klitz, W. J. (1973). Empirical population genetics of the North American House Sparrow. *Ornithol. Monogr.* **14**, 39–48.

Koehn, R. K., Zera, A. J. and Hall, J. G. (1983). Enzyme polymorphism and natural selection. *In* "Evolution of Genes and Proteins" (eds M. Nei and R. K. Koehn). Sinauer, Massachusetts.

Lack, D. (1940). Variation in the introduced English Sparrow. *Condor* **42**, 239–241.

Lack, D. (1971). "Ecological Isolation in Birds". Blackwell, Oxford.

Lande, R. and Arnold, S. J. (1983). The measurement of selection on correlated characters. *Evolution* **37**, 1210–1226.

Lerner, I. M. (1954). "Genetic Homeostasis". John Wiley, New York.

Lindsey, C. D. (1966). Body size of poikilotherm vertebrates at different latitudes. *Evolution* **20**, 456–465.

Long, J. L. (1981). "Introduced Birds of the World". David & Charles, London.

Lowther, P. E. (1979 a). The nesting biology of House Sparrows in Kansas. *Kansas Ornithol. Soc. Bull.* **30**, 23–28.

Lowther, P. E. (1979 b). Growth and dispersal of nestling House Sparrows: sexual differences. *Inland Bird Banding* **51**, 23–29.

Lowther, P. E. (1979 c). Overlap of House Sparrow broods in the same nest. *Bird Banding* **50**, 160–162.

Manwell, C. and Baker, C. M. A. (1975). Molecular genetics of avian proteins. XIII. Protein polymorphism in three species of Australian Passerines. *Aust. J. Biol. Sci.* **28**, 545–557.

Markus, M. B. (1964). Premaxillae of the fossil *Passer predomesticus* Tchernov and the extant South African Passerinae. *Ostrich* **35**, 245–246.

Mayr, E. (1963). "Animal Species and Evolution". Belknap Press, Harvard.

McGillivray, W. B. (1980). Nest grouping and productivity in the House Sparrow. *Auk* **97**, 396–399.

McGillivray, W. B. (1983). Intraseasonal reproductive costs for the House Sparrow, *Passer domesticus*. *Auk* **100**, 25–32.

McNab, B. K. (1971). On the ecological significance of Bergmann's rule. *Ecology* **52**, 845–854.

Meise, W. (1936). Zur Systematik und Verbreitungsgeschichte der Haus- und Weiden Sperlinge, *Passer domesticus* und *hispaniolensis*. *J. Ornithol.* **99**, 431–437.

Mitchell, C. J. and Hayes, R. O. (1973). Breeding House Sparrows, *Passer domesticus*, in captivity. *Ornithol. Monogr.* **14**, 39–48.

Murphy, E. C. (1978 a). Breeding ecology of House Sparrows: spatial variation. *Condor* **80**, 180–193.

Murphy, E. C. (1978 b). Seasonal variation in reproductive output of house sparrows: the determination of clutch size. *Ecology* **59**, 1189–1199.

Murray, J. J. and Clarke, B. C. (1968). Inheritance of shell size in *Partula*. *Heredity* **23**, 189–198.

Naik, R. M. and Mistry, L. (1970). Breeding season and reproductive rate of *Passer domesticus* in Baroda, India. *Intl Stud. Sparrows* **4**, 15–16.

Nei, M. (1972). Genetic distance between populations. *Am. Natur.* **106**, 283–292.

Nei, M. (1975). "Molecular Population Genetics and Evolution". North-Holland, Amsterdam.

Nei, M. (1978). Estimation of average heterozygosity and genetic distance from a small number of individuals. *Genetics* **89**, 583–590.

O'Donald, P. (1973). A further analysis of Bumpus' data: the intensity of natural selection. *Evolution* **27**, 398–404.

Ohta, T. and Kimura, M. (1973). A model of mutation appropriate to estimate the number of electrophoretically detectable alleles in a finite population. *Genet. Res.* **22**, 201–204.

Parkin, D. T. (1979). "An Introduction to Evolutionary Genetics". Edward Arnold, London.

Parkin, D. T. and Cole, S. R. (1984). Genetic variation in the House Sparrow (*Passer domesticus*) in the east midlands of England. *Biol. J. Linn. Soc.* **23**, 287–301.

Parkin, D. T. and Cole, S. R. (1985). Genetic differentiation and rates of evolution in some populations of the House Sparrow (*Passer domesticus*) in Australia and New Zealand. *Heredity* **54**, 15–23.

Pinowski, J. and Myrcha, A. (1977). Biomass and production rates. *In* "Granivorous
    Birds in Ecosystems" (eds J. Pinowski and S. C. Kendeigh). Cambridge University
    Press.
Rising, J. D. (1970). Age and seasonal variation in dimensions of the House Sparrow,
    Passer domesticus (L.) from a single population in Kansas. *In* "Productivity,
    Population Dynamics and Systematics of Granivorous Birds" (eds S. C. Kendeigh
    and J. Pinowski). Institute of Ecology, Dziekanow, Poland.
Schifferli, L. (1978). Experimental modification of brood size among House Sparrows,
    Passer domesticus. Ibis **120**, 365–369.
Scholander, P. F. (1955). Evolution of climatic adaptation in homeotherms. *Evolution* **9**,
    15–26.
Singh, R. S., Hubby, J. L. and Throckmorton, L. H. (1975). The study of genetic
    variation by electrophoresis and heat denaturation techniques at the octonal
    dehydrogenase locus in the *Drosophila virilis* group. *Genetics* **80**, 637–650.
Seel, D. C. (1960). The behaviour of a pair of House Sparrows while rearing young. *Br.
    Birds* **53**, 303–310.
Seel, D. C. (1966). Further observations on a pair of House Sparrows rearing young.
    Bird Study **13**, 207–209.
Seel, D. C. (1968 a). Breeding seasons of the House Sparrow and Tree Sparrow, *Passer*
    spp., at Oxford. *Ibis* **110**, 129–144.
Seel, D. C. (1968 b). Clutch size, incubation and hatching success in the House Sparrow
    and Tree Sparrow, *Passer* spp., at Oxford. *Ibis* **110**, 270–282.
Sharrock, J. T. R. (1976). "The Atlas of Breeding Birds in Britain and Ireland". BTO,
    Tring, Herts.
Summers-Smith, D. (1963). "The House Sparrow". Collins, London.
Summers-Smith, D. (1985). The systematic position of the sparrows (*Passer*). *In* "The
    Dictionary of Birds" (eds B. Campbell and E. Lack). Poyser, Berkhamsted.
Tchernov, E. (1962). Paleolithic avifauna in Palestine. *Bull. Res. Council Israel* **11**,
    95–131.
Templeton, A. R. (1980 a). Modes of speciation and inferences based upon genetic
    distances. *Evolution* **34**, 719–723.
Templeton, A. R. (1980 b). The theory of speciation via the founder principle. *Genetics*
    94, 1011–1038.
Vaurie, C. (1956). Systematic notes on Palearctic birds. No. 24 Ploceidae: the genera
    Passer, Petronia, and *Montifringilla. Am. Mus. Novitates,* No. 1814.
Washington, D. (1973). Breeding the house sparrow. *Avicult. Mag.* **79**, 109–115.
Wright, S. (1951). The genetical structure of populations. *Ann. Eugen.* **15**, 323–354.
Yom-Tov, Y. (1980). Intra-specific nest parasitism in birds. *Biol. Rev.* **55**, 93–108.

Note Added in Proof
Since writing the section on the evolution of house sparrow subspecies, I have acquired
additional samples of *P.d. italiae* and *P. hispaniolensis.* Discussion of the results of
the electrophoresis of these with Denis Summers Smith has caused me to alter my views
on the history of the species as revealed by the enzymes. An outline of these will be
found in the *Proceedings of the International Ornithological Congress, Ottawa,* to be
published during 1987, and in more detail in the *Biological Journal of the Linnean
Society* during 1988.

13

Lesser Snow Goose: A Long-term Population Study

Fred Cooke

Biology Department, Queen's University, Kingston, Ontario, Canada K7L 3N6

1 INTRODUCTION

Colonial birds provide some unusual advantages for students of avian population genetics. Colonies often provide large numbers of birds in close proximity to one another and many individuals can be obtained for genotype analysis and fitness measures. Additionally, when different segments of the species are isolated in separate colonies, effective population sizes (N_e) and gene flow among these segments can be examined.

Snow Goose is an example of such a colonial bird, often nesting in extremely large colonies ($> 100\,000$ pairs) mostly in the Canadian Arctic. The smaller race, Lesser Snow Goose (*Anser caerulescens caerulescens*), provides an additional advantage for geneticists and evolutionary biologists in that it

AVIAN GENETICS
ISBN 0-12-187570-9

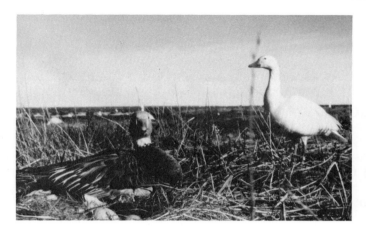

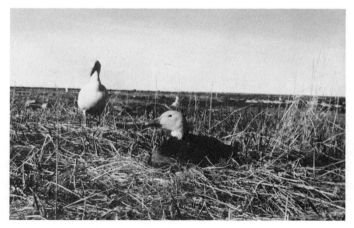

Fig. 1. The two colour phases of Lesser Snow Goose: white and blue (photo-
graph: Pierre Mineau).

occurs in two colour phases, the white and the blue (see Fig. 1). Historical
evidence (Graham 1768, Barnston 1860) indicates that the two phases were
formerly allopatric and merged only in the early twentieth century.
Nevertheless this polymorphism has proved valuable for investigating
selection, drift and gene flow in a similar way to the classical invertebrate
studies such as those carried out on snails and moths.

Of the two races of Snow Geese, the Greater Snow Goose (*A. c. atlantica*) is
monomorphic and nests in the islands of the high Eastern Canadian Arctic. It
has not been studied from a genetical viewpoint and plays no further part in

our story. The Lesser Snow Goose breeds throughout the Arctic, from Baffin Island in Eastern Canada to Wrangel Island in the Soviet Union. The southernmost colony occurs at latitude 55°N on the Hudson Bay coast at Cape Henrietta Maria. Snow Geese participate in large impressive migrations and individuals winter in widely separated areas, depending on breeding location. For example, while most of the Hudson Bay and Baffin Island subpopulations winter along the Texas and Louisiana coasts, the subpopulations from the Western Canadian Arctic and the Soviet Union winter in the Central Valley of California. Smaller wintering populations occur in Maryland, New Mexico, Central Mexico and British Columbia. Much of the data on Lesser Snow Geese has been collected from the Hudson Bay/Foxe Basin subpopulations, estimated at 530 000 breeding pairs in 1973 by Kerbes (1975) and scattered among 16 colonies ranging in size from 200 pairs to 163 000 pairs. There is extensive intermingling of birds from these colonies during migration and on the wintering grounds (where pair-formation occurs), so the possibility of gene exchange among the colonies within this population is considerable. In this chapter I consider types of genetic variation present in this population and the various factors that mould this variation. To conclude, I discuss the present and past distribution of the geese in terms of these various factors.

2 METHODS OF DATA COLLECTION

The bulk of the genetic analysis described herein is based on data collected at the La Perouse Bay Snow Goose colony in northern Manitoba, on the west coast of Hudson Bay. This colony has been under intensive investigation since 1968 and, during this time, has grown from 2000 to over 7000 pairs. Approximately 2000 nests are now monitored each year. Approximately 40% of the adult females and 20% of the adult males in the colony are marked with alphanumeric coloured plastic leg bands, allowing for individual recognition. Family relationships can be determined by the letters and colour of the leg bands. Hatching goslings are marked with a numbered monel metal web tag which identifies each gosling individually and indicates its natal nest and hatch date. The goslings grow rapidly after hatch, feeding in the nearby salt marshes where they remain with their parents in family groups. During this time, the adults undergo a complete moult of the flight feathers. Towards the end of this period, adults and goslings are rounded up and captured; 4000–8000 geese are captured each year and, at this time, they are weighed, measured, aged, sexed and their plumage type recorded.

A US Fish and Wildlife band and a coloured band are applied. If an individual is already banded, the band codes are recorded. Since female Snow

Geese are highly philopatric, they may be caught in several successive years. Female goslings banded during their hatching year frequently return as adults; however, male goslings are rarely seen again since they pair away from the breeding grounds and follow the females back to their natal colonies. A consequence of this dispersal pattern from the geneticist's point of view is that family relationships can be studied best through the female line. For characters which are visible during the first six weeks of life (e.g. basic plumage colour), family data can be obtained, but for those characters that appear only at reproductive maturity (e.g. clutch size, adult plumage), the sample sizes are much lower and are restricted to those goslings which are web-tagged at hatch and subsequently sighted or captured as breeding adults in the colony, two or more years later.

Measures of fitness can be divided into two categories: those concerned with fecundity and those related to viability (Prout 1971). Fecundity is assessed by monitoring as many nests as possible each breeding season. Approximately 600 nests are found at the one egg stage, staked, and visited regularly until hatch. Nest initiation usually occurs in late May and eggs are usually laid at one day intervals, with incubation commencing after the laying of the penultimate or the last egg. Clutch sizes of 2–6 prevail, with an average of 4 to 5. Incubation lasts approximately 23 days and, during this time, an additional 1000–2000 nests are found in order to increase sample sizes. These, and the original nests, are mapped onto large-scale aerial photographs. All nests are visited until the eggs hatch and the goslings leave the nest. Fledging success can be measured among those web-tagged families which are captured during the banding period. Recruitment into the breeding colony can be used as yet another measure of fitness.

Viability of pre-reproductive and of adult birds is assessed using recovery information from banded birds and from birds recaptured or resighted at the breeding colony in subsequent years. Of particular value in these analyses are the large numbers of birds of known age which return to breed at the colony.

3   TYPES OF GENETIC VARIABILITY

3.1   Plumage

The two colour phases of Lesser Snow Goose are quite distinct in adult, yearling and gosling plumages. Until recently (Lemieux and Heyland 1967), the two were considered distinct species, but now most ornithologists concur with the opinion of Cooch (1961) that they should be considered as phases of the same species. There is plumage variation within the phases, particularly among the blue birds, which vary in the amount of white on neck, breast, belly and rump. There is a continuum ranging from birds that are totally dark in these areas to those which are completely white. Goslings of the two phases are quite different, even at hatch. Blue-phase goslings have black legs and dark-coloured down; white-phase goslings have grey legs and yellowish down, at least on the forehead.

Genetic analyses have been carried out on two populations: the Boas River colony on Southampton Island in the Northwest Territories, Canada (Cooke and Cooch 1968), and the La Perouse Bay colony (Cooke and Mirsky 1972, Rattray and Cooke 1984). Genetic analyses of wild populations in the field are fraught with difficulties and there are two which complicate interpretation of the Snow Goose data. First, Snow Geese mate assortatively for plumage colour (Cooch and Beardmore 1959, Cooke *et al.* 1976). This means that techniques of estimating gene frequency based on the use of Hardy–Weinberg equilibrium cannot be used. Secondly, females occasionally lay their eggs in nests other than their own. Such intraspecific nest parasitism results in 5–10% of offspring being unrelated to the birds attending the nests, thus making pedigree analysis difficult. Despite these difficulties there are several lines of evidence pointing to the polymorphism being largely determined by a single major gene with two alleles: B (blue), incompletely dominant to the recessive b (white). These are as follows:

(1) Lack of intermediate plumages in both adults and goslings. The plumages, although variable within each phase, contain few if any birds that cannot be obviously classified as blue or white phase. This eliminates simple polygenic inheritance, but not polygenic inheritance with associated threshold effects.

(2) Blue × blue matings produce 90% blue goslings and 10% white goslings; mixed matings give a slight excess of blue goslings, and white × white matings produce all white goslings, with a few exceptions which are attributable to intraspecific nest parasitism (Table 1).

(3) Using data from individual families, Cooke and Mirsky (1972) investigated the genetics of the dichromatism using a method suggested initially by Hogben (1931), which generates expected segregation ratios from a truncated binomial distribution. If the blue allele (B) is dominant to white (b) then there will be some blue × white crosses where the blue parent is homozygous (BB) and all offspring will be heterozygous blue. In other cases, the blue parent is heterozygous (Bb), such that blue and white offspring are produced with equal frequency. With small family sizes, the proportion of families of size 4 (say) which have 0, 1, 2, 3 or 4 white offspring is generated from the binomial distribution. Since Bb × bb crosses with all blue offspring are indistinguishable from BB × bb crosses with all blue offspring, only those families where at least one white gosling occurs can be tested, hence the term

Table 1. Phase ratios of goslings from different parental nests.

Year		WW No. (%)		Mixed No. (%)		BB No. (%)	
1973	W	2 157 (98·5)		233 (39·0)		52 (7·8)	
	B	32 (1·5)		365 (61·0)		618 (92·2)	
1974	W	2 216 (97·1)		217 (36·3)		73 (10·1)	
	B	65 (2·9)		381 (63·7)		648 (89·9)	
1975	W	2 446 (98·2)		279 (40·7)		79 (9·9)	
	B	45 (1·8)		406 (59·3)		717 (90·1)	
1976	W	2 879 (98·1)		312 (40·1)		80 (9·6)	
	B	55 (1·9)		466 (59·9)		752 (90·4)	
1977	W	2 477 (96·5)		292 (41·2)		93 (11·8)	
	B	91 (3·5)		416 (58·7)		694 (88·2)	
1978	W	2 166 (97·2)		247 (40·1)		75 (10·6)	
	B	63 (2·8)		369 (59·9)		634 (89·4)	
1979	W	3 080 (98·4)		338 (42·6)		79 (8·7)	
	B	50 (1·6)		456 (57·4)		830 (91·3)	
1980	W	3 424 (97·9)		389 (42·5)		81 (8·6)	
	B	75 (1·1)		526 (57·5)		866 (91·4)	
1981	W	3 339 (97·4)		335 (39·6)		93 (10·2)	
	B	91 (2·7)		510 (60·4)		815 (89·8)	
1982	W	3 334 (98·3)		360 (40·2)		132 (12·8)	
	B	59 (1·7)		535 (59·8)		899 (87·2)	
1983	W	3 378 (97·5)		392 (40·3)		104 (9·4)	
	B	86 (2·5)		580 (59·7)		1 006 (90·6)	
1984	W	4 208 (97·8)		479 (41·3)		123 (9·1)	
	B	97 (2·3)		681 (58·7)		1 228 (90·9)	
Total	W	35 104 (97·7)		3 873 (40·5)		1 064 (9·9)	
	B	809 (2·3)		5 691 (59·5)		9 707 (90·1)	

"truncated binomial distribution". If the relative frequency of white and blue goslings conforms to the truncated binomial distribution, then one has strong circumstantial evidence for a single major gene segregating. Table 2 gives observed and expected frequencies of such families from the La Perouse Bay colony. In all cases the binomial model can be fitted to the data. Using similar logic, blue × blue crosses with one or more white offspring can also be analysed using the truncated binomial approach. In these crosses too, observed values conformed to predictions based on the hypothesis of a pair of segregating alleles with blue dominant to white.

(4) There is no evidence of sex linkage. Remembering that females are the heterogametic sex in birds, and assuming sex-linkage, a number of combinations of parental and gosling colours would not be expected. From blue × blue crosses, no white males would be expected. From white male × blue female crosses, all male progeny would be blue and all female

Table 2. Truncated binomial distribution of segregating Snow Goose families from blue × white crosses.

Family size		Number of White offspring				Total
		1	2	3	4	
2	Observed	16	9			25
	Expected	16·7	8·3			
3	Observed	10	13	9		32
	Expected	13·7	13·7	4·6		
4	Observed	20	24	17	4	65
	Expected	16·3	24·4	16·3	4·1	

progeny would be white. Neither prediction is confirmed. As such, the locus appears to be autosomal.

I mentioned earlier that the blue allele was incompletely dominant over the white allele. Thus, heterozygotes are often recognizably different in phenotype from homozygous blues. All white-bellied blues appear to be heterozygotes, but not all dark-bellied blues are homozygous. Thus, the genotype cannot in all cases be deduced from the phenotype. The finding that heterozygotes show considerable variability in their phenotype suggests this variability arises not from the major gene itself but rather from modifier genes or environmental variation. Recent work by Rattray (1981) suggests that environmental variation is the more important insofar as no correlation was detected between the degree of whiteness in the belly among blue adults and their blue offspring (as adults). From 13 light-bellied blue × white crosses, 5 blue offspring were light-bellied and 8 dark-bellied. From 21 dark-bellied blue × white crosses, 9 blue offspring were light-bellied and 12 dark-bellied. Since it is not possible to classify heterozygotes reliably, we have lumped BB and Bb genotypes together in the various analyses of selection and gene flow. This, unfortunately, may obscure effects of heterosis.

3.2 Biochemical

Parkin (unpublished data) has examined 28 enzymes from samples of liver of 25 Snow Geese from La Perouse Bay. He found variation in 13 of these and postulated that they reflected genetic variation. From their variation, he obtained an estimated 14% polymorphism and 5% heterozygosity in the population. From 630 blood samples and an analysis of 5 polymorphic loci he found that blue and white phases differed marginally but significantly from one another. This difference may reflect the different histories of the two phases (see later). Mitochondrial and genomic DNA variation in Snow Geese is covered by Quinn and white in chapter 5; and so is omitted here.

3.3 Quantitative

Although data are available to assess the environmental and genetic components of variation on various morphological measures in Snow Geese, studies at La Perouse Bay have concentrated on estimating the contribution of additive genetic variation to ecologically important traits such as clutch size (Findlay and Cooke 1983, 1987) and hatch date (Findlay and Cooke 1982 a). Since there is a negative correlation between clutch size and relative hatch date within a season (Finney and Cooke 1978), any underlying genetic variability may affect both characters simultaneously.

Clutch-size variation has both environmental and genetic components. Mean clutch sizes at La Perouse Bay vary considerably between seasons (Davies and Cooke 1983) and within seasons. Ankney and MacInnes (1978) showed a positive correlation between nutrient reserves and clutch size, suggesting that birds with the ability or opportunity to store nutrients more effectively before nesting were able to lay more eggs. Age has also been shown to affect clutch size up to at least the age of four years (Rockwell *et al.* 1983). In order to test whether some of the variation in clutch size could be attributed to additive genetic effects, we carried out repeatability and heritability studies as described earlier in this volume by Boag and van Noordwijk (chapter 2).

We limited our analysis to those females for which clutch size was known in at least four seasons ($N = 479$) and obtained a repeatability value (r) of 0·29. Since female Snow Geese are philopatric, often nesting within 50 metres of their nest of the previous year, this similarity within females and difference between females could arise either from genetic differences or permanent environmental effects. If the former, one would expect daugheters to resemble their mothers. To test this, 132 mother–daughter pairs were compared. Since a temporally fluctuating environment may introduce an environmental covariance if mothers and daughters are measured in the same years, only mother–daughter pairs who were measured in different years were included. From these pairs a heritability of 0·21 was calculated, as estimated by a weighted regression of daughter's mean clutch size on mother's clutch size (Fig. 2). Although these values are relatively low, they are significantly higher than zero and suggest that some of the between-individual variation in clutch size arises from additive genetic effects.

Similar repeatability and heritability values were obtained for hatch date (measured as a deviation from the mean hatch date of the colony in a given season). The repeatability value for this character based on a sample of 136

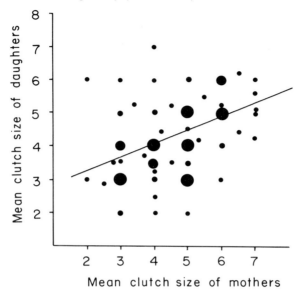

Fig. 2. Weighted regression of daughter's mean clutch size on mother's mean clutch size. Points indicate single observations, larger circles, multiple observations.

females was 0.49 ± 0.14. Since age is known to affect laying date, a second analysis attempted to distinguish phenotypic variation due to age difference between individuals by recalculating individual relative hatch dates as deviations from the mean hatch date of a particular age cohort in a given season. For this sample of 70 birds, repeatability increased to $r = 0.59 \pm 0.11$. An estimate of the heritability of the trait (in this case uncorrected for age) calculated by regression of 136 mother/daughter pairs yielded at $h^2 = 0.44 \pm 0.16$. Again, the similarity between the h^2 and uncorrected r-values suggests that some of the individual variation arises from additive genetic effects.

There are, of course, non-genetic causes of correlations between mothers and daughters. Maternal effects and correlated environments can both introduce a significant source of covariance contributing to the resemblance between relatives. For example, Prevett and MacInnes (1980) demonstrated that families usually remain together throughout the first year of life and thus traditions of migration routes and favoured feeding areas can be transmitted from mothers to daughters. Recall that female philopatry prevails in waterfowl. Since the quality of feeding locations prior to nesting could have a considerable influence upon both clutch size (Ryder 1970) and laying date (and therefore hatch date), the cultural transmission of feeding locales could

Table 3. Phase ratios of major Snow Goose colonies 1955–1963 and recent estimates.

Colony	Early			Recent		
	% blue phase	Year	Reference	% blue phase	Year	Reference
Bowman Bay, Baffin Island	97	1955	Cooch 1963	81	1973	Kerbes
				85–90	1981	Cooch (pers. comm.)
Cape Dominion, Baffin Island	80	1955	Cooch 1963	61	1973	Kerbes 1975
				80	1981	Cooch (pers. comm.)
Koukdjuak, Baffin Island	53	1961	Cooch 1963	41	1981	Kerbes 1975
Cape Henrietta Maria, Ont.	67	1957	Hanson et al. 1972	71	1979	Ross (pers. comm.)
East Bay, Southampton Island	35	1955	Cooch 1963	45	1979	Dupuis-Reed (pers. comm.)
				36	1979–80	Ankney and Abraham (pers. comm.)
Boas River, Southampton Island	33	1961	Cooch 1963	23	1979	Dupuis-Reed (pers. comm.)
				36	1979	Ankney and Abraham (pers. comm.)
La Perouse Bay, Man.	24	1963	Hanson et al. 1972	26–29	1972–84	Cooke
McConnell, R., N.W.T.	17	1961	Cooch 1963	24	1977	Brace (pers. comm.)
	24	1961	Hanson et al. 1972	28	1978	Brace (pers. comm.)
Central Arctic	5	1960	Cooch 1963	15	1976	Kerbes et al. 1983

contribute to the observed correlation between mothers and daughters. Nevertheless, in most cases h^2 was calculated from birds nesting in different years, and Davies and Cooke (1983) provide evidence suggesting considerable year to year variability in the quality of the pre-nesting feeding areas. As such, it appears that some of the variation among females in these two traits can be ascribed to genetic difference.

4 FACTORS AFFECTING THE DISTRIBUTION OF GENES FOR PLUMAGE COLOUR

Having documented the types of genetic variability that have been discovered in Snow Geese, I now examine in greater detail the factors which influence the present-day distribution of one of these, namely, the conspicuous plumage dichromatism, which provides an easy genetic marker for such an investigation. The distribution of the B and b alleles varies in both space and time.

Although blue-phase birds are occasionally seen in all breeding colonies, the vast majority occur among the colonies whose members winter along the Texas and Louisiana coast, and I will concentrate on these colonies in subsequent discussion. In general, blue birds decrease in frequency from east to west and north from a centre of concentration in Southern Baffin Island. Table 3 gives the most recent estimates of the frequency of blue-phase birds in the major Eastern and Central Arctic nesting colonies.

Phase ratios have also varied with time. Changes in phase ratio at the La

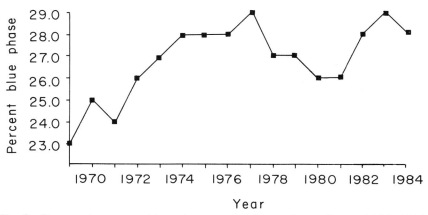

Fig. 3. Changes in per cent blue-phase nesting Lesser Snow Geese, 1969–1984, at La Perouse Bay, Manitoba.

Perouse Bay colony between 1969 and 1984 are shown in Fig. 3. They show a consistent and significant increase in the frequency of the blue phase until 1977, after which the frequency appears to stabilize. Although evidence is lacking of phase ratios at the breeding colonies in earlier centuries (the blue phase was not discovered nesting until 1929 (Soper 1930)), evidence from sightings of migrating geese in the eighteenth, nineteenth and early twentieth centuries shows that the two colour phases were formerly almost allopatric. Graham (1768) reports only 20–30 blue geese among the more than 10 000 white geese shot at the westerly Hudson Bay company settlements of forts Prince of Wales (now Churchill), York and Severn while, at the more easterly forts, the ratios were reversed. Barnston (1860) similarly reports flocks of white birds migrating from the west coast and blue phase from the east coast of Hudson Bay in the fall and Saunders (1917) likewise noted that white birds predominated on the west side of James Bay, while those of the east side were almost exclusively blue.

Within the Gulf Coast wintering areas, the distribution of the colour phases also varies in space and time. In general, blue phase birds predominate in the eastern parts (Louisiana) and white in the west (Texas). There is no continuous clinal variation in phase ratio, but a rather sudden change in frequency at the Texas–Louisiana border. There is evidence that this step cline was more pronounced in former times. McIlhenny (1932) reports that, in the major wintering concentration of blue-phase birds in the Mississippi delta, one might find one white-phase bird to every 65–70 blue phase, while across the Texas border in Galveston, one blue phase to every 75 whites. This indicates much less mixing of the colour phases than at present. A manuscript cited in Oberholser (1974) reports only four records of blue-phase birds in Texas in the nineteenth century.

It might be imagined that the wintering-ground cline corresponded to the breeding-ground cline, with the eastern breeding colonies wintering in the east and the westerly colonies wintering further west. However, the data indicate a more complex pattern, as illustrated from banding data from six Arctic colonies in Table 4. Two important points emerge from this table. First, birds from all the major Hudson Bay colonies can be found throughout the Gulf Coast wintering grounds, suggesting considerable mixing of birds from different colonies. Secondly, even for a particular breeding colony, blue birds tend to have a more easterly wintering distribution than white-phase birds. This probably reflects the maintenance of wintering ground traditions from a time when the two colour phases were more segregated than they are now.

From this admittedly sketchy summary of spatio-temporal variation in the frequency of the two colour phases of Snow Goose, one can readily see that the data provide fertile ground for the population geneticist interested in understanding the factors affecting changes in gene frequencies in natural

Table 4. Direct recoveries and blue phase frequency on the Gulf Coast wintering grounds (25°00′–30°59′N and 85°00′–99°00′W). Parentheses indicate a sample size <10

Colony		Recovery location (degrees longitude)							
		West				East			
		99–97	96	95	94	93	92	91–85	Total
Baffin Island	Number	—	3	8	2	13	18	5	49
	Percentage Blue	—	(33·3)	(62·5)	(50·0)	92·3	94·4	(100)	83·7
Cape Henrietta Maria	Number	1	20	28	21	27	48	14	159
	Percentage Blue	(0)	50·0	42·9	71·4	77·8	89·6	85·7	71·1
East Bay, Southampton Island	Number	8	36	28	47	29	10	6	164
	Percentage Blue	(25·0)	19·4	32·1	38·3	48·3	80·0	(100)	39·0
Boas R. Southampton Island	Number	67	152	169	390	80	33	21	912
	Percentage Blue	16·4	19·7	17·8	28·5	42·5	84·8	52·4	27·9
McConnell River	Number	33	284	259	300	142	68	17	1 103
	Percentage Blue	24·2	18·3	19·7	31·3	36·6	60·3	76·5	28·2
La Perouse Bay	Number	—	37	40	42	14	22	2	157
	Percentage Blue	—	21·6	30·0	31·0	57·1	45·5	(0)	32·5
Grand total	Number	109	532	532	802	305	199	65	2 544
	Percentage Blue	19·3	20·3	22·4	31·4	46·2	73·9	72·3	32·8

populations. This is particularly true since the genetic basis for the plumage dimorphism is well understood.

One possible explanation for the non-random distribution is that the selection pressures operating on the two phases also vary in space and time.

4.1   Selection

Graham Cooch was the first to attempt an explanation for the gene-frequency changes. He noted (Cooch 1961) that, in most colonies, blue-phase birds were increasing within these populations at a rate of 1·2% per annum. At one of these colonies (Boas River, Southampton Island, North-western Territories), he attempted to monitor nest success and survival (based on hunter kill) of the two colour phases. Although rigorous statistical approaches were often lacking, he provided evidence that (1) there were no detectable differences in initial clutch sizes of the two phases; (2) white-phase birds tended to nest earlier than blues in two of the three seasons for which data were collected; (3) in those seasons, blue goslings suffered higher predation rates than their counterparts, and (4) white-phase birds were more likely to exhibit an interrupted migration (i.e. to spend some time in the northern United States) and therefore be more accessible to hunters. Direct evidence that these differences could account for the observed increases in blue frequency were lacking. On the basis of these possible differences and temporal changes in the phase ratios at a number of Arctic breeding colonies, Cooch (1963) predicted that by 1980 most of the Lesser Snow Geese nesting in the Hudson Bay–Foxe Basin colonies would be blue phase. This prediction has not in general been realized, and indeed it is by no means certain that there has been an overall change in the global phase ratio since 1963.

A much more comprehensive investigation of potential differences in both fecundity and viability between the colour phases has recently been carried out by Findlay, Rockwell, Smith and Cooke at the La Perouse Bay colony (Cooke *et al.* 1985, Rockwell *et al.* 1985). They subdivided the life cycle into several different stages and investigated potential differences among components of fitness between females of both phases. They used data collected from 1969 to 1982. Since large sample sizes were available, even small differences in selection pressure between the phases could have been detected. The following components of fitness were compared: total clutch size, final clutch size, number of goslings leaving nest, brood size at fledging, recruitment into the breeding population, partial clutch loss, total clutch loss, partial brood loss, total brood loss, age structure, prereproductive survival, adult survival, age of first breeding and breeding propensity. No differences were found between the two phases for any of these measures in any season, except for pre-reproductive survival in 1976, when significantly fewer immature blue geese were shot. The authors concluded that overall selective differences between the colour phases are inadequate to explain the observed increase in blue-phase birds at La Perouse Bay between 1969 and 1977. It therefore appears that we must look elsewhere for an explanation for these local changes.

The inability to detect selective differences despite large sample sizes and several seasons of data does not necessarily mean that no selection is occurring (or has occurred). Natural selection is a very subtle factor in moulding gene frequencies, and differences between any genotypes might be expected to be small or detectable only at certain times. Moreover, it is conceivable that selective differences may not be detectable at the relatively benign southern breeding colonies, but only under the harsher conditions of the high Arctic. Therefore, we must not conclude from the work at La Perouse Bay that selection is unimportant in affecting gene-frequency changes at the global level, but alternative explanations need to be examined carefully. One potential explanation, suggested by Cooke (1978), is gene flow.

4.2 Gene flow

Gene flow in Snow Geese is manifested by birds hatching in one breeding colony and subsequently nesting successfully in another. While this is most readily documented through bird ringing, the relatively low sampling effect at various colonies makes it difficult to assess these immigration rates. Cooch (1961) recognized that some birds exchanged colonies but underestimated the importance of the phenomenon. Seiger and Dixon (1970) allowed for the existence of 4% annual gene flow between colonies when constructing a computer-simulation model of the role of imprinting (see later) in determining the distribution of the colour phases of Snow Geese. This, too, was an underestimate. Cooke *et al.* (1975) were the first to show that gene flow was much more widespread than previously thought; indeed, immigration rates at the La Perouse Bay colony were estimated at approximately 50% per generation. High exchange rates between colonies reflects two important aspects of Snow Goose life history. First, mate selection occurs during spring migration or on the wintering ground when birds from several colonies are intermixed; secondly, when two birds which mate are from two different colonies, the pair will generally return to the natal colony of the female. This means that whereas almost all females which breed do so in their natal colony, males return to their natal colony only if they happen to choose a female from the same colony. This is unlikely if the male comes from a small colony, but more probable in the larger colonies. Cooke *et al.* (1975) reported that, of 223 goslings from La Perouse Bay which subsequently returned to breed in their natal colony, only eight were males. Since survival is similar in the two sexes, this implies that the vast majority of surviving males were nesting elsewhere. Although most gene flow occurs via the males, females do occasionally change breeding colonies. Of 55 birds banded as goslings at one colony and recovered at another, 4 were females. Geramita and Cooke (1982) also provided evidence of female Snow Geese nesting in a non-natal colony in certain seasons.

Given the high gene flow between colonies, it is surprising that there should remain large differences in the frequency of blue-phase birds at different colonies. Cooke (1978) pointed out that, if gene flow is as large as seems to be the case, phase ratios should tend to equilibrate among colonies. Clearly something else is influencing the distribution of genes for plumage colour at the global level. This brings us to the third major factor influencing gene distribution: non-random mating.

4.3 Non-random mating

Positive assortative mating with respect to plumage colour in Snow Geese was first documented by Cooch and Beardmore (1959) who showed that mixed pairs were considerably less frequent than expected under the assumption of random mating. Moreover, among the two types of mixed matings, matings between a blue male and a white female outnumbered those between a white male and blue female. Cooke and Cooch (1968) showed that positive assortment also occurred within the subdivisions of the blue-phase birds and that heterozygous birds were more likely to be mated with white birds than were homozygous blues. This latter finding led to the hypothesis that mate selection in Snow Geese reflects the imprinting of goslings on the parental phenotype (i.e. birds select a mate of a similar plumage colour to one of their parents). This hypothesis was substantiated by a series of experiments and field observations (Cooke *et al.* 1972, Cooke and McNally 1975, Cooke *et al.* 1976, Cooke 1978) with one modification; namely, sibling colour (as well as parental colour) influences mate choice. Birds from homochromatic families (i.e. all members of the family of the same colour phase) would generally choose a mate of the family colour, whereas birds from a mixed family (both colours represented in the family, either parents or offspring) choose mates of either colour. Under these conditions, we expect a gradual reduction in the frequency of mixed pairs and ultimately complete isolation of the two colour phases, as predicted by Seiger (1967). That this has not happened during the 15-year period of study at La Perouse Bay is illustrated in Table 5 where the frequency of mixed pairs is seen to vary little (14–19%). This constancy of mixed matings led Geramita *et al.* (1982) to suggest that some offspring from pure families chose mates of the opposite colour. In contrast to expectations

Table 5. Pair-bond frequencies and phase ratio of blue and white Lesser Snow Geese, La Perouse Bay, 1969–1984. (Updated from Cooke 1978)

Year	W × W		B × W		W × B		B × B		% blue phase
	No.	%	No.	%	No.	%	No.	%	
1969	439	70	36	6	55	9	98	16	23
1970	619	67	55	6	92	10	162	17	25
1971	411	68	28	5	63	10	102	17	24
1972	850	66	80	7	125	10	231	18	26
1973	929	65	91	6	144	10	272	19	27
1974	900	64	85	6	137	10	279	20	28
1975	947	64	99	7	146	9	286	20	28
1976	893	63	113	8	134	10	271	19	28
1977	984	62	129	8	165	10	310	20	29
1978	1 039	64	133	8	150	9	292	18	27
1979	950	65	113	9	143	10	261	18	27
1980	1 089	65	143	9	150	9	290	17	26
1981	985	66	113	8	126	9	265	18	26
1982	1 166	64	146	8	160	8	360	20	28
1983	1 207	63	149	8	167	9	396	21	29
1984	1 387	64	164	8	205	9	415	19	28

under the imprinting hypothesis advanced above, Table 6 shows that 9·7% of goslings from white parents obtained blue mates, and 21·8% of offspring from blue parents obtained white mates. Thus, it appears that imprinting is not complete, and that some individuals "err" (with respect to the imprinting scenario) when selecting a mate. Cooke (1978) has suggested the mistake rate at 10–15% would be sufficient to account for the observed level of mixed matings and this is close to the observed value.

It appears that, at the proximate level, non-random mating arises from colour preferences which individuals develop as a result of their pre-pairing experience.

In an attempt to determine whether or not there is any selective advantage to mating by positive assortment, Findlay *et al.* (1985) compared pure and mixed pairs with respect to several components of reproductive success, including clutch size, brood size at hatch, brood size at fledging, recruitment into the breeding colony, nest failure, brood loss, and immature and adult mortality of offspring from mixed and pure parentage. For most of these measures, no differences were found among the various pair types but, surprisingly, in some measures higher success was associated with mixed pairs. For example, in 2 of 7 cohorts, significantly higher recruitment rates were found among offspring of mixed parentage relative to pure pairs. Furthermore, nest failure was consistently lower among mixed pairs. These

Table 6. Mate choice of geese of known parentage, 1972–1984

Year	Offspring choice	White	Mixed	Blue	Total
1972	White	2	0	0	2
	Blue	1	0	2	3
1973	White	23	5	2	30
	Blue	4	1	4	9
1974	White	29	8	2	39
	Blue	2	6	11	19
1975	White	43	4	1	48
	Blue	8	8	9	25
1976	White	36	8	0	44
	Blue	3	5	12	20
1977	White	58	12	4	74
	Blue	4	7	19	30
1978	White	40	7	1	48
	Blue	3	6	10	19
1979	White	49	4	3	56
	Blue	4	4	10	18
1980	White	39	13	2	54
	Blue	5	5	11	21
1981	White	47	12	1	60
	Blue	7	5	13	25
1982	White	53	12	8	73
	Blue	4	3	8	15
1983	White	51	9	4	64
	Blue	5	3	12	20
1984	White	79	6	11	96
	Blue	9	7	19	35
Total*	White	549 (90·3%)	100 (62·5%)	39 (21·8%)	688 (72·7%)
	Blue	59 (9·7%)	60 (37·5%)	140 (78·2%)	259 (27·3%)

* It is not strictly valid to total these values since the same pair may be observed in more than one year.

differences, though slight, do suggest that although mixed matings are relatively rare, there may in fact be some reproductive advantage accrued to mixed pairs. These findings are somewhat paradoxical insofar as if there is a selective advantage (albeit slight) to obtaining a mate phenotypically dissimilar to oneself, then why is the population characterized by positive assortment? One possible explanation is suggested by the historical evidence, which indicates that the two phases were allopatric until recently, and became sympatric only in the early part of the twentieth century. As such, species recognition cues developed in the past may still be a potent proximate mechanism for mate choice despite the slight reproductive advantage associated with choosing a mate of opposite colour. If this is correct, one might predict an eventual increase in the frequency of mixed mating and possibly even negative assortment in the population. However, in general, the positive assortative mating tends to maintain phase-ratio differences among colonies. Moreover, because females generally choose a mate of the same colour as themselves, though often from a different colony, intercolony gene flow for the plumage colour gene (and presumably genes tightly linked to it) is reduced.

5 DISCUSSION

5.1 Modelling changes in plumage colour genes

The spatio-temporal distribution of the gene for plumage colour is influenced by gene flow and non-random mating but not, as far as we know, by selection. Clearly, we would like to know the relative importance of each factor (and their interactions) in determining gene distributions. This has been attempted by means of a simplified model by Geramita *et al.* (1982). In the model, they assumed (1) that the lack of fitness differences between the phases found at La Perouse Bay was typical of the other colonies; (2) that the patterns of non-random mating are determined by the colour composition of the family in which a bird was raised, but that the mate choice even for birds from pure families was not always according to the imprinting roles (empirical values for this level of mistake making were assumed); (3) that there was a clinal distribution of colour phases on the Gulf Coast wintering grounds where pair-formation occurred; (4) that females returned to breed at natal colonies and the frequency of gene flow was inversely related to colony size; (5) that all gene flow was by male immigration; and (6) that a certain amount of non-genetical family mixing due to nest parasitism and fostering occurred. With these simplifying assumptions, they predicted slow changes in the phase ratios within individual colonies. In particular, the model suggested a slow increase in blue birds at the predominantly white colonies and a slow increase in white birds at the predominantly blue-phase colonies. In general, these predictions fit the data observed on phase ratio changes at the colonies. According to the model, most of the changes in phase ratio can be explained by gene flow mediated through assortative mating, rather than selection.

There are two corollaries to this explanation of gene-frequency change. First, the model predicts that the frequency of mixed matings is a function of the level of "mistake making" of pure colour. If the pattern of gene frequency distribution in the Hudson Bay–Foxe Basin population primarily reflects gene flow, then one would predict that a slow equilibration of gene frequencies is occurring. A corollary of this is that the phases were formerly more isolated from one another and this is in keeping with the historical evidence that suggests that the two populations were allopatric even at the beginning of the twentieth century. The present and past distributions suggest a white-phase population that bred in the western part of the breeding range and wintered in Texas, and a blue-phase population that bred in Southern Baffin Island and wintered in Louisiana. The present-day distributions still reflect this historical pattern despite the re-establishment of sympatry.

Of course, we do not know for certain whether the two morphs were at one time completely allopatric but, whatever the evolutionary history of their species, it seems plausible that at one or more stages, some of the Arctic populations were dichromatic. If one assumes that the ancestral goose was coloured (most *Anser* geese are grey- or brown-plumaged), then we surmise that, in one or more populations, a white recessive mutation must have become firmly established either through selection or drift. While we can only speculate on most of the past history of the population, the Snow Goose example clearly illustrates the principle that, when examining genetic variability in natural populations, it is necessary to assess the relative importance of several different factors (selection, gene flow, etc.) in moulding that variation.

5.2 Quantitative variation and selection

The accumulation of a considerable amount of family data from La Perouse Bay has allowed us to ask a number of questions relating to selection of quantitative traits. To illustrate what has been achieved in this area, I will summarize the work of Findlay and Cooke (1982 a,b, 1983), Cooke and Findlay (1982) and Cooke *et al.* (1984), who investigated the question of the timing of reproductive events.

Nesting is highly synchronized in Snow Geese, with the vast majority initiating within a two-week period in any one season. Hatching is even more synchronized than laying, due to the negative correlation between initiation date and clutch size (Findlay and Cooke 1982 a). Enhanced synchronization, early nesting, and a short incubation period have been interpreted as adaptations to the short Arctic summer (Cooch 1958), suggesting that there may be strong directional and/or stabilizing selection for the timing of the nesting events. Although laying and hatching are highly synchronized, there is nevertheless considerable interindividual variability within a season, some of which arises from genetic differences among individuals (Findlay and Cooke 1982 a).

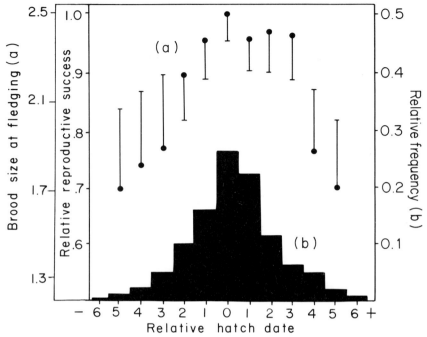

Fig. 4. The relation between reproductive success and relative hatch date.
(From *American Naturalist*, 1982, **120**, 543–547.)

Given intraseasonal variability in the time of hatching, is there any evidence of a selective advantage associated with any particular hatching time relative to the population mean? Findlay and Cooke (1982 b) used fledging success as a measure of reproductive fitness and calculated an effective brood size for each hatch date relative to the population mean. These values were from a pooled sample of females from different seasons but similar data were obtained when individual seasons were examined. Effective brood size was calculated from two values: the brood size at fledging of successful families (i.e. those in which at least one gosling fledged), and the probability of total brood loss. They found that the effective brood size was highest among those birds hatching at the intermediate and most synchronized hatch period (Fig. 4). The early hatching birds were susceptible to total brood loss, though when successful, early families had the highest mean brood size at fledging. The late hatching birds had the lowest brood sites among the successful families. Intermediate hatching birds had slightly lower brood sizes but much lower total brood loss than the early hatching birds. In addition, these authors found greatest nest loss prior to hatch among the early and late laying birds. Both the pre-hatch and post-hatch data therefore suggested stabilizing selection, with highest success accruing to those birds which hatched in the middle period. These are also the most synchronized birds. It was suggested that the reduced success of early and late nesting birds could be attributed to greater predation pressure from Herring Gulls (*Larus argentatus*) and Arctic Foxes (*Alopex lagopus*). During the synchronous nesting period, predator-swamping probably occurs. This appears to provide strong evidence for stabilizing selection for a character in which considerable additive genetic variance has been demonstrated.

The existence of a large additive component of variance for a trait under stabilizing selection presents the theoretical population geneticist with the problem of how such variation is maintained. Several thoretical models have been proposed to explain the persistence of adaptive genetic variation, including mutation (Kimura 1965), frequency-dependent selection (Slatkin 1979), selection in heterogeneous environments (Levene 1953) and migration (Bulmer 1971). Cooke and Findlay (1982) used a migration model to explain the data. They argued that there may be some colonies, perhaps those in the high Arctic, where earlier nesting birds may be more strongly favoured. Selection for different optima may occur in different parts of the breeding range and, given the large amounts of gene flow, the genetic variance could be maintained.

Of course, other explanations are possible. We have seen earlier that the present-day population is probably a mixture of two populations (one blue, one white) which, until relatively recently, were allopatric. If these two populations had different sets of genes controlling the timing of reproduction, the present additive genetic variance may be in transition and, under the present selective regime, may be slowly diminishing.

When investigating the timing of nesting of a synchronized population under stabilizing section it is difficult to know whether synchrony itself is favoured or whether there is simply an advantage to nesting in the middle time-period. Without experimental manipulation we have trouble dissociating the two influences. There is an additional complication. Although the evidence above showed that geese that hatch in the middle time-period produced more fledged goslings, Cooke *et al.* (1984) have recently shown that, if recruitment of females into the breeding populations rather than fledging success is used as the measure of reproductive success, then in general it is the earliest hatching goslings which are recruited into the breeding population at the highest frequency. In three out of seven seasons there was a significantly higher recruitment of goslings from the earliest-hatching nests. These seasons were those when nesting in the colony as a whole was delayed owing to the late disappearance of snow. So it appears that, even at La Perouse Bay (one of the more southerly colonies), there may be directional selection for early nesting, despite a higher fledging success among birds which hatch during the middle period. Perhaps the larger size which can be achieved earlier in early-hatching goslings provides those goslings with greater reserves for the hazardous migration which they undergo.

To recapitulate, in this section I have indicated the advantages of studying natural selection acting on a quantitative character related to reproductive success. Despite strong directional or stabilizing selection, there appears to be considerable additive genetic variation for the character. It seems to be important to look at as many measures of reproductive fitness as possible. If fledging success is taken as the measure, the population appears to be under stabilizing selection. If recruitment of females into the breeding population is the measure, there is evidence of directional selection for early breeding, relative to the population mean.

6 SUMMARY

In this chapter I have shown the various ways in which the genetics of Snow Geese can be studied. Major genes, allozymes, genes affecting quantitative variation, and mitochondrial and nuclear DNA variation have all been examined and used to investigate the genetic structure of the Snow Goose population.

Two examples of the ways in which genetics can be used were presented. In the first the plumage colour in this dimorphic species was shown to be determined by a single gene with the allele for dark plumage incompletely dominant over the allele for white plumage. The temporal and spatial variation in the distribution of the alleles led to the conclusion that the present-day pattern could be explained by gene flow and non-random mating rather than differential selection. Historical evidence suggested that the two colour phases were allopatric as recently as the early years of the twentieth century, and that the present pattern was due to the recent re-establishment of sympatry plus a gene flow pattern modified by non-random mating. In the second example, the timing of hatching was shown to vary genetically among geese and that stabilizing selection was occurring during the fledging stage.

There is still much work to be done on the ecological genetics of Snow Geese. The analysis of genes at the DNA or the protein level has barely started and comparisons of genetic differences between colonies are only just beginning. Nevertheless, the studies of Snow Geese, particularly those at La Perouse Bay, have already shown the value of long-term studies in the elucidation of many important biological findings. They also show the value of integrated studies which consider not only genetical, but also behavioural and ecological approaches to the investigations.

REFERENCES

Ankney, C. D. and MacInnes, C. D. (1978). Nutrient reserves and reproductive performance of female Lesser Snow Geese. *Auk* **95**, 459–471.

Barnston, G. (1860). Recollection of the swans and geese of Hudson Bay. *Ibis* **2**, 253–259.

Bulmer, M. G. (1971). The effect of selection on genetic variability. *Am. Natur.* **105**, 201–221.

Cooch, F. G. (1958). The breeding biology and management of the Blue Goose. Ph.D. Thesis, Cornell University, Ithaca, New York.

Cooch. F. G. (1961). Ecological aspects of the Blue-Snow goose complex. *Auk* **78**, 72–89.

Cooch, F. G. (1963). Recent changes in distribution of color phases of *Chen c. caerulescens*. *Proc. 13th Int. Ornithol. Congr.*, pp. 1182–1194. Ithaca, N.Y.

Cooch, F. G. and Beardmore, J. A. (1959). Assortative mating and reciprocal difference in the blue-snow complex. *Nature* **183**, 1833–1834.

Cooke, F. (1978). Early learning and its effect on population structure. Studies of a wild population of snow geese. *Z. Tierpsych.* **46**, 344–358.

Cooke, F. and Cooch, F. G. (1968). The genetics of polymorphism in the snow goose *Anser caerulescens*. *Evolution* **22**, 289–300.

Cooke, F. and Findlay, C. S. (1982). Polygenic variation and stabilizing selection in a wild population of lesser snow geese (*Anser caerulescens caerulescens*). *Am. Natur.* **120**, 543–547.

Cooke, F., Findlay, C. S. and Rockwell, R. F. (1984). Recruitment and the timing of reproduction in Lesser Snow Geese (*Chen caerulescens caerulescens*). *Auk* **101**, 451–458.

Cooke, F., Finney, G. H. and Rockwell, R. F. (1976). Assortative mating in lesser snow geese (*Anser caerulescens*). *Behav. Genet.* **6**, 127–140.

Cooke, F., Findlay, C. S., Rockwell, R. F. and Smith, J. A. (1985). Life history studies of the lesser snow goose (*Anser caerulescens caerulescens*). III. The selective value of plumage polymorphism: net fecundity. *Evolution* **39**, 165–177.

Cooke, F., MacInnes, C. D. and Prevett, J. P. (1975). Gene flow between breeding populations of Lesser Snow Geese. *Auk* **92**, 493–510.

Cooke, F. and McNally, C. M. (1975). Mate selection and colour preferences in lesser snow geese. *Behaviour* **53**, 151–170.

Cooke, F. and Mirsky, P. J. (1972). A genetic analysis of Lesser Snow Goose families. *Auk* **89**, 863–871.

Cooke, F., Mirsky, P. J. and Seiger, M. B. (1972). Colour preferences in the Lesser Snow Goose and their possible role in mate selection. *Can. J. Zool.* **50**, 529–536.

Davies, J. C. and Cooke, F. (1983). Annual nesting productivity in Snow Geese: Prairie droughts and arctic springs. *J. Wildl. Managem.* **47**, 291–296.

Finney, G. H. and Cooke, F. (1978). Reproductive habits in the Snow Goose: the influence of female age. *Condor* **80**, 147–158.

Findlay, C. S. and Cooke, F. (1982 a). Breeding synchrony in the lesser snow goose (*Anser caerulescens caerulescens*). I. Genetic and environmental components of hatch date variability and their effects on hatch synchrony. *Evolution* **36**, 342–351.

Findlay, C. S. and Cooke, F. (1982 b). Synchrony in the lesser snow goose (*Anser caerulescens caerulescens*). II. The adaptive value of reproductive synchrony. *Evolution* **36**, 786–799.

Findlay, C. S. and Cooke, F. (1983). Genetic and environmental components of clutch size variance in a wild population of the Lesser Snow Goose (*Anser caerulescens caerulescens*). *Evolution* **37**, 724–734.

Findlay, C. S. and Cooke, F. (1987). Repeatability and heritability of clutch size— Lesser Snow Geese. *Evolution* **41**, 452.

Findlay, C. S., Rockwell, R. F., Smith, J. A. and Cooke, F. (1985). Life history studies of the Lesser Snow Goose (*Anser caerulescens caerulescens*). VI. Plumage polymorphism, assortative mating and fitness. *Evolution* **39**, 904–914.

Geramita, J. M. and Cooke, F. (1982). Evidence that fidelity to natal breeding colony is not absolute in female snow geese. *Can. J. Zool.* **60**, 2051–2056.

Geramita, J. M., Cooke, F. and Rockwell, R. F. (1982). Assortative mating and gene flow in the lesser snow goose: A modelling approach. *Theor. Pop. Biol.* **22**, 177–203.

Graham, A. (1768). Diary written between 1768 and 1769. "Observations on Hudson's Bay, Book 2." Hudson's Bay Archives, Winnipeg, Man.

Hanson, H. C., Lumsden, H. C., Lynch, J. J. and Norton, H. W. (1972). Population characteristics of three mainland colonies of the Blue and Lesser Snow Geese nesting in the Southern Hudson Bay region. *Res. Rept* (*Wildl.*) No. 93. Ontario Ministry of Natural Resources.

Hogben, L. (1931). The genetical analysis of familial traits. I. Single gene substitutions. *J. Genet.* **25**, 97–112.

Kerbes, R. H. (1975). Surveys of Lesser Snow Geese with vertical aerial photography. *Can. Wildl. Serv. Report Series 35*, Ottawa, Canada.

Kerbes, R. H., McLandress, M. R., Smith, G. E. J., Beyersbergen, G. and Godwin, B. (1983). Ross' Goose and Lesser Snow Goose colonies in the Central Canadian Arctic. *Can. J. Zool.* **61**, 168–173.

Kimura, M. (1965). A stochastic model concerning the maintenance of genetical variability in quantitative characters. *Proc. Natl. Acad. Sci. USA* **54**, 731–736.

Lemieux, L. and Heyland, J. (1967). Fall migration of Blue Geese and Lesser Snow Geese from the Koukdjuak River, Baffin Island, Northwest Territories. *Natur. Can.* **94**, 677–694.

Levene, L. (1953). Genetic equilibrium when more than one ecological niche is available. *Am. Natur.* **87**, 331–333.

McIlhenny, E. A. (1932). The Blue Goose in its winter home. *Auk* **49**, 279–306.

Oberholser, H. C. (1974). "The Bird Life of Texas". University of Texas Press, Austin. (Manuscript cited is on microfilm at Texas A&M University.)

Prevett, J. P. and MacInnes, C. D. (1980). Family and other social groups in snow geese. *Wild. Monogr.* **71**, 46 pp.

Prout, T. (1971). The relationship between fitness components and population prediction in *Drosophila* I. The estimation of fitness components. *Genetics* **68**, 127–149.

Rattray, A. B. (1981). Genetics of the colour polymorphism of the Lesser Snow Goose: revisited. B.Sc. Thesis, Queen's University, Kingston, Ontario.

Rattray, A. B. and Cooke, F. (1984). Genetic modelling: an analysis of a colour polymorphism in the Snow Goose (*Anser caerulescens*). *Zool. J. Linn. Soc.* **80**, 437–445.

Rockwell, R. F., Findlay, C. S. and Cooke, F. (1983). Life history studies of the Lesser Snow Goose (*Anser caerulescens caerulescens*). I. The influence of age and time on fecundity. *Oecologia* **56**, 318–322.

Rockwell, R. F., Findlay, C. S., Cooke, F. and Smith, J. A. (1985). Life history studies of the lesser snow goose (*Anser caerulescens caerulescens*). IV. The selective value of plumage polymorphism: Net viability, the timing of maturation and breeding propensity. *Evolution* **39**, 178–188.

Ryder, J. P. (1970). A possible factor in the evolution of clutch size in Ross' Goose. *Wils. Bull.* **82**, 5–13.

Saunders, W. E. (1917). Wild geese at Moose Factory. *Auk* **34**, 334–335.

Seiger, M. B. (1967). A computer simulation study of the influence of imprinting on population structure. *Am. Natur.* **101**, 47–57.

Seiger, M. B. and Dixon, R. D. (1970). A computer simulation study of the effects of two behavioural traits on the genetic structure of semi-isolated populations. *Evolution* **24**, 90–97.

Slatkin, M. (1979). Frequency and density-dependent selection on a quantitative character. *Genetics* **93**, 755–771.

Soper, J. D. (1930). "The Blue Goose. An Account of its Breeding Ground, Migration, Nests and General habits." Canadian Department of the Interior, Ottawa, Canada.

14

Polymorphism and Sexual Selection in the Arctic Skua

Peter O'Donald

Emmanuel College, University of Cambridge, Cambridge CB2 3AP, UK

1 INTRODUCTION

The skuas (Stercorariidae: Charadriiformes) consist of about seven species of colonially breeding seabirds related to gulls and terns. They breed in the Arctic and Antarctic, spending the rest of the year at sea. They feed as kleptoparasites and predators. The three smaller species (known as jaegers in North America) breed in the Arctic and typically occur in three morphs ranging from uniformly dark brown morphs to pale morphs which have white neck and belly feathers; intermediates occur regularly. One of these species, the Arctic Skua (*Stercorarius parasiticus*; Parasitic Jaeger in North America), was the subject of my long-term population genetic studies on islands off the northern coast of Scotland. The results of this study are summarized in *The Arctic Skua* (O'Donald 1983). This chapter both updates the conclusions reached in that book and answers some pertinent criticisms offered by certain reviewers.

433

AVIAN GENETICS
ISBN 0-12-187570-9

2   THE GENETICS OF ARCTIC SKUA PHENOTYPES

Three phenotypes, similar in males and females, can be recognized in the Arctic Skua. Some birds are pale with a white or nearly white breast and belly; they may have a dark band across the breast. Other birds are uniformly dark-brown all over. The rest are intermediate: dark with a variable amount of lighter plumage around the cheeks, collar and breast; the bases of the breast and belly feathers are white. Those intermediates with a very broad white base to their belly feathers show a distinctly lighter belly compared to the dark birds, who have no white base to their belly feathers. But the darkest intermediate birds cannot always be distinguished from the dark birds, except by examination of the belly feathers; even then, dark-intermediates merge into darks in a continuous sequence (see O'Donald (1983) for full descriptions of the phenotypes).

These plumage differences appear to be controlled by a single gene, with dark showing incomplete dominance over pale. The intermediates are mostly heterozygous; but the data of individuals from known parents suggest that dark-intermediates may often be homozygous, while some darks may be heterozygous. Plumage changes between the dark-intermediate and dark categories occur from one breeding season to the next, showing that the variable expression is at least partly developmental in origin.

On Fair Isle about 20% of the population is pale. Since pale birds are all homozygous we may estimate the gene frequency of pale by $q^2 = 0.2$; $q = 0.45$ and hence the frequency of dark $q = 0.55$. In view of the assortative mating known to occur in this species, these estimates are only rough approximations.

3   MODELS FOR MAINTAINING POLYMORPHISMS

Many birds are polymorphic for plumage characters (chapter 1). These polymorphisms are usually stable for the frequency of the different plumage phenotypes. Several different modes of selection have been advanced to explain this stability, but as Buckley notes in chapter 1, virtually none has been *proven* to operate in the wild. Some of these mechanisms are as follows.

(1) *Apostasis*, or selection for different phenotypes that hinder predator or prey recognition. Predators may form a "search-image" of their prey (Tinbergen 1960). If a prey species is polymorphic, predators with a search-image of a particular phenotype will take a much higher proportion of this phenotype than its proportion in the population, thus giving rise to selection. Since predators will more often form search-images of the commoner prey, this will produce frequency-dependent or "apostatic" selection (Clarke 1962). The same might apply to predator recognition: prey would more readily recognize common predator phenotypes. This form of selection has been

postulated to explain polymorphism in diurnal birds of prey (Payne 1967, Paulson 1973) and in the Arctic Skua (Arnason 1978).

(2) *Heterozygous advantage.* This will always maintain a polymorphism (Fisher 1922). Hall *et al.* (1966) suggested that heterozygous advantage might explain the polymorphism in *Malaconotus*, Bush Shrikes, which Owen (1967) attributed (also without evidence) to apostasis.

(3) *Diffusion clines.* Diffusion can balance selection for different phenotypes in different areas: a phenotype disadvantageous in a particular area of the species' range is continually replaced by migration from areas where the phenotype is advantageous. In each area there is an equilibrium between diffusion and selection, giving rise to a cline or gradient in frequency from areas where a phenotype is common and advantageous to areas where it is rare and disadvantageous. Theoretically, the point or region in the cline where two phenotypes have equal frequencies should be the neutral point where neither has any selective advantage. The cline in the melanic and pale phenotypes of the Arctic Skua has been the subject of many surveys (e.g Southern 1943, O'Donald 1983). Clines have been studied in many birds. Huxley's survey of the cline of bridled Common Guillemots (*Uria aalge*; Huxley 1938, 1939) was the occasion on which the term was coined. Stable clines are always interesting because they imply the action of selection. But it does not follow that selection is acting on the obvious plumage differences: it may be acting on a pleiotropic effect of alleles of which the plumage polymorphism is merely an incidental manifestation, or it may be acting on alleles closely linked to those for the plumage polymorphism.

(4) *Sexual selection.* O'Donald (1973, 1974, 1977, 1980) has shown that in many different models, sexual selection can maintain a stable polymorphism, either by itself or when balanced by natural selection. This follows because sexual selection is almost always frequency-dependent. In particular, female preference gives rise to a mating advantage of rare males, or "rare male effect": the preferred males mate more often when they are rare, simply because then a relatively greater proportion of females prefer them. If more than one male phenotype is the object of female preference, a globally stable polymorphism will be produced. A polymorphism can also occur if the preferred males suffer a disadvantage in natural selection: as the preferred males become more common, so their sexual selective advantage diminishes until it exactly balances their natural selective disadvantage.

4 MAINTENANCE OF THE ARCTIC SKUA POLYMORPHISM

Arnason (1978) suggested that apostatic selection might maintain the polymorphism of melanic and pale Arctic Skuas: their prey might learn to recognize and avoid the commoner phenotype. He compared the proportion

Table 1. Selection of Arctic Skua phenotypes. The selective coefficients measure the relative selective disadvantages of the phenotypes. Relative fitness is measured by $w = 1 - s$. The phenotype with selective coefficient $s = 0$ has the highest relative fitness $w = 1$

Phenotype	Selective coefficients (s)		
	Males	Females	Both sexes combined
Pale	0·109	0	0·040
Intermediate	0·145	0·012	0·071
Dark	0	0·048	0

of successful pursuits by pale and melanic Arctic Skuas on the south coast of Iceland, where pales occur at a frequency of about 11%. But Arnason's data give scant support to his hypothesis: in one of his comparisons, the rarer pale phenotype was more successful, but this was of doubtful statistical significance. For all comparisons, a combined test showed no significance. Other observations have not supported Arnason's hypothesis (O'Donald 1983).

Extensive demographic data of Arctic Skuas on Fair Isle in Shetland have provided good estimates of the selection acting on the melanic and pale phenotypes (O'Donald 1976, 1983). These calculations (Table 1) show that on Fair Isle, in the south of the Arctic Skua's range where about 80% of the population is melanic, the heterozygotes suffer an overall selective disadvantage. This is a consequence of selection acting differently on males and females and produces a point of unstable equilibrium where the frequency of the pale allele is $q = 0.70$. Since the actual frequency of pale is $q = 0.45$, which is well below its unstable equilibrium, pale should rapidly be eliminated from the population. But roughly stable frequencies have been maintained on Fair Isle and Shetland generally for many generations.

We know that about 45% of breeding birds are immigrants from other populations, so this migration will produce a diffusion of genes from northern populations where pale birds are common (100% are pale above 75°N) and must inevitably balance the loss of the pale genes by selection. Thus, the polymorphism of the Arctic Skua in populations across its latitudinal range is a diffusion cline.

5 SEXUAL SELECTION OF ARCTIC SKUA PHENOTYPES

In the Arctic Skua, melanics have a general reproductive advantage over pales which is partly offset by the pales' slightly younger average age at maturity

(O'Donald 1976, 1977, 1983). Sexual selection is one of the components of the melanics' reproductive advantage. This has been estimated demograpically, but provides no evidence about the behaviour that gives rise to the sexual selection. Do females prefer to mate with melanic males, or do melanic males compete more successfully for mates? In *The Arctic Skua* (O'Donald 1983), I discussed three lines of evidence in favour of the hypothesis of female choice, while rejecting one line of evidence in favour of male competition. On one of these lines of evidence, provided by assortative mating, new data have been obtained since the book's publication. And in view of some reviewers' criticisms of the hypothesis of female preference for melanic males, I will concentrate in the rest of this chapter on the problem of the mechanism of sexual selection in the Arctic Skua.

Arctic Skuas are monogamous. Unless many males are left unmated to provide a pool from which the females can choose their mates or within which the males compete with each other for mates, there can be little variation in the males' chances of finding a mate. But as Darwin originally suggested (Darwin 1871), sexual selection may still take place if some males consistently mate with more fertile or more successful females, while other males mate with less fertile or less successful females. Darwin put forward a subtle theory, based on a premise of the breeding ecology of birds, to explain how different male phenotypes might vary in their mean reproductive success. In Darwin's words, the theory is as follows:

> Let us take any species, a bird for instance, and divide the females inhabiting a district into two equal bodies, the one consisting of the more vigorous and better-nourished individuals, and the other of the less vigorous and healthy. The former, there can be little doubt, would be ready to breed in the spring before the others. . . . There can also be no doubt that the most vigorous, best-nourished and earliest breeders would on an average succeed in rearing the largest number of fine offspring. The males, as we have seen, are generally ready to breed before the females; the strongest, and with some species the best armed of the males, drive away the weaker; and the former would then unite with the more vigorous and better nourished females, because they are the first to breed. Such vigorous pairs would surely rear a larger number of offspring than the retarded females, which would be compelled to unite with the conquered and less powerful males, supposing the sexes to be numerically equal; and this is all that is wanted to add, in the course of successive generations, to the size, strength and courage of the males, or to improve their weapons.

Darwin also explained that the advantage of early breeding would produce sexual selection by female preference; for

> . . . the more vigorous females, which are the first to breed, will have the choice of many males . . . they will select those which are vigorous and well armed, and in other respects most attractive. Both sexes, therefore, of such early pairs would, as above explained, have an advantage over others in rearing offspring; and this has

apparently sufficed during a long course of generations to add not only to the strength and fighting powers of the males, but likewise to their various ornaments and other attractions.

The correlation of earlier breeding date with increased reproductive success that Darwin postulated has now been established for many birds. In the Arctic Skua, which usually lays only two eggs, the average number of chicks fledged by a pair varies from 1·6 chicks for the earliest pairs to 0·6 for the latest pairs breeding about five weeks later in the season. The fledging success declines from the beginning to the end of the breeding season (see O'Donald (1983) for details).

Sexual selection takes place when pairs are formed. The mean breeding dates of Arctic Skua morphs in new pairs are noted in Table 2. These are the mean dates of the hatching of the first egg in number of days after 1st June. Hatching date is easily determined and has been used to measure breeding date; laying date would have been a better measure but is much more difficult to determine. Incubation period varies between 25, 26 and 27 days (median 26 days), showing no phenotypic variation. Hence, hatching date is virtually equivalent to laying date as a measure of breeding date. In mating with new females, pale males are very significantly later in breeding date than intermediate and dark melanic males. Female phenotypes show no significant variation in breeding date, nor do males show any variation between phenotypes in older, established pairs: the variation is solely between the males in new pairs. Pairs that have been together for two years breed an average of 22 days after 1st June. These differences between new and older pairs are shown both by males breeding for the first time as well as by experienced males finding a new mate. The average breeding date for both first-time and experienced males is 30 days in new pairs and 22 days in older pairs. An old pair invariably comes back to its territory of the previous year, and mating soon takes place. A single bird has to set up a territory and attract a mate. This process apparently takes an extra eight days on average. So we can say that to attract a mate, a dark melanic male takes $28·3 - 22·0 = 6·3$ days on average; an intermediate melanic male takes $29·8 - 22·0 = 7·8$ days on average; and a pale non-melanic male takes $33·4 - 22·0 = 11·4$ days on average.

Table 2. Mean number of days after 1st June for hatching of first eggs in new pairs

Sex	Dark	Colour phase Intermediate	Pale
Males	28·3	29·8	33·4
Females	31·1	29·3	31·5

Since earlier breeding is advantageous, as Darwin suggested, melanic males are sexually selected. Given their relative success through the breeding season, the relative selective disadvantage (or selective coefficient) of intermediate and pale males compared to darks can be calculated as $s_I = 0.039$ for intermediates and $s_P = 0.162$ for pales. These values apply only to new pairs. As a measure of sexual selection in the population as a whole, these selective coefficients become $s_I = 0.013$ and $s_P = 0.058$. For the demographic basis of these calculations, the reader should refer to *The Arctic Skua* (O'Donald 1983).

6 PREFERENTIAL MATING

It is often possible to measure natural selection acting on particular phenotypes without knowing what environmental factors give rise to it: Haldane (1924) estimated the selection for melanic moths of the species *Biston betularia* without knowing that melanics and non-melanics were differentially predated by birds on tree trunks where lichens had been killed by sulphur dioxide pollution. Similarly, we can estimate the sexual selection of melanic Arctic Skuas, as we did in the previous section, without knowing how it arises from the mating behaviour. Originally, it seemed likely that competition for territories produced selection for melanic males. Davis and O'Donald (1976 b) found that pale males had the smallest territories and pairs with smaller territories bred later on average during the breeding season, thus fledging a smaller average number of chicks. Hence pale males were at a sexual disadvantage compared to melanic males. Since territory size must partly be determined by the intensity of male competition, which in turn probably depends on androgen levels, the males with larger territories would also be the more active in courting the females, for courtship probably depends on androgen levels. Thus, as we have seen, melanic males would breed earlier than pale males and gain the sexual selective advantage we calculated in the previous section.

Davis and O'Donald's original sample consisted of new males and experienced males who had changed their mates. Only when experienced males changed their mates has a significant difference been observed between the territory sizes of pale and melanic males, and this difference is only barely significant. Data on territory size collected in later years contradicted the earlier data: melanics were then found to have smaller territories, but not significantly so. For all the data collected, territory size showed very little difference between the phenotypes, nor, surprisingly, was any significant heterogeneity found between the different sets of data. However, the earlier breeding of males with larger territories remained highly significant and consistent. Sexual selection of territory size certainly occurs, but this does not lead to sexual selection for melanic phenotypes. The sexual selection of the melanics must depend on behavioural mechanisms other than competition for territory.

Females may prefer to mate with melanic males. Female preference will certainly produce the sexual selection we have observed. The preferred males will have set up their territories alongside the others. As the females arrive to choose their mates, those that prefer the melanics will mate according to their preference. Other females will choose at random. Since melanics are preferentially mated, later females will eventually be left with only the pales to choose from. Exactly as Darwin suggested, the melanics will, on average, have mated before the pales and thus gained a selective advantage from their earlier breeding. I set up computer models to simulate this Darwinian sexual selection in a monogamous bird (O'Donald (1976, 1983); full details can be found in O'Donald (1983)). The models depend on the distribution of breeding dates, the phenotypes that are the objects of female preference, and the sequence of preferential and random matings.

In the simplest version, *Model 1*, a proportion of the females, β, prefers to mate with either dark or intermediate males without discriminating between them: they simply prefer melanics, either dark or intermediate. In this model, as in all the others, the females that have no preferences always mate at random among the different phenotypes of those males that remain unmated on their territories. In *Model 2*, females mate preferentially with dark males first, then with intermediate males if no darks are left unmated. Other females mate at random. In *Model 3*, there are two kinds of female preference. A proportion, α, of the females prefer to mate only with dark males while another proportion, β, prefers either dark or intermediate males indiscrimi- nately. The remainder, $1 - \alpha - \beta$ mate at random. Thus, when $\alpha = 0$, Model 3 becomes the same as Model 1; in terms of mating preference, the allele for dark is then completely dominant. When $\beta = 0$, the dark allele is completely recessive. In general, therefore, Model 3 allows for any degree of dominance of the dark and pale alleles. Finally, in *Model 4*, dark and intermediate melanics are preferred by separate groups of females: α of the females prefer dark males; β prefer intermediate males; $1 - \alpha - \beta$ mate at random. Model 4 is a special case of the more general model in which there is a separate preference for each phenotype. Model 4 produces a stable polymorphism with the dark allele at an equilibrium frequency $p = (\alpha + \frac{1}{2}\beta)/(\alpha + \beta)$. This equilibrium is reached in models of preferential mating with either polygynous or monogamous matings (O'Donald 1980, 1983).

Within each of these four models of mating preference, preferential mating may take place either before random mating (P-models), simultaneously with random mating (S-models), or after random mating (R-models). In the P-models, the females with preferences choose their mates before the females that mate at random. This would correspond to preferential mating, in which females with preferences have a lowered threshold of response towards the males they prefer. If it is advantageous to mate with melanic males, females will be selected that mate more readily with the advantageous males. The females that thus mate preferentially gain the advantage of producing sons that possess the advantageous character of their fathers. Since these sons also tend to carry the genes for female preference, these genes are selected through the advantage gained by the sons of the females that mated preferentially: the preference selects itself, as Fisher originally suggested (Fisher 1930). Mathematical models of this selection show that the preference genes become associated in linkage disequilibrium with the genes for the preferred character (for example, the genes for melanism). A male with the preferred character is likely also to carry the genes for the preference, so selection of the preferred males selects the preference (O'Donald 1962, 1967, 1980, Kirkpatrick 1982). As a gene for the preferred character spreads through a population, a gene for the preference may be expected to undergo a four- to sixfold increase in frequency (O'Donald 1980). It is plausible that a preference may thus evolve by the selection of a gene that lowers a female's response towards an advantageous male phenotype. The P-models would describe this evolutionary outcome. In terms of the four models of the preferences for Arctic Skua phenotypes, we have Models 1P, 2P, 3P and 4P.

In the R-models, random matings precede preferential matings. These models are perhaps less biologically plausible than the P-models. They imply that the females with the preferences have a higher threshold of response than the others, especially against the non-preferred males. In terms of the different preferences, we then have Models 1R, 2R, 3R and 4R.

In the S-models, the simultaneous preferential and random mating implies that each female arrives in succession to choose a mate, making her choice and removing one male from the pool of unmated males. The P- and R-models imply that in an interval or period of the breeding season, a group of females have become ready to breed; the preferential and random matings then occur within the group. The breeding season is thus divided into a succession of intervals, the females in each interval mating as a group. As the intervals become smaller, the P- and R-models converge on the S-models. In the limit, as the intervals become so fine that only one female mates in each interval, the P-, R- and S-models are identical.

The models have been fitted to the actual data of the breeding dates of male Arctic Skuas in new pairs. Table 3 shows the numbers of males breeding in successive weeks of the breeding season. The actual values when each male bred give the mean breeding dates of the phenotypes shown in the previous section. The total number of males in each interval also represents the number of females that reached breeding condition in that interval. The females in

Table 3. Breeding dates of melanic and non-melanic male Arctic Skuas in new pairs

Breeding dates in weekly intervals	Number of males breeding			
	Dark	Intermediate	Pale	Total
10–16 June	2	4	1	7
17–23 June	15	45	4	64
24–30 June	30	67	16	113
1–7 July	17	48	16	81
8–14 July	5	25	15	45
15–21 July	3	10	5	18
Total number	72	199	57	328

each of these intervals express their preferences in accordance with the specific models. The models were fitted to the data by finding the values of the preferences that maximized the log-likelihood of the model (for details of the procedure of fitting the models, see O'Donald (1983)). This procedure finds the maximum likelihood (ML) estimates of the parameters of the model—the proportions of females expressing preferences. In the P- and R-models, weekly intervals give the maximum likelihood.

The results of fitting the models are shown in Table 4. The P-models all give higher likelihoods at their respective maxima than the R-models. As we should expect, the likelihoods and estimates of the S-models are intermediate between the P- and R-models. Also shown in the table is the relative "support" for each model. ("Support" is the difference in the log-likelihoods of the most likely model and the model in question.) It is the increase in log-likelihood produced by the most likely model (see Edwards 1972). Model 3P has the highest likelihood, followed closely by Model 4P and Model 1P. The differences in their log-likelihoods is less than 1·0, which is by no means significant. The R-models, however, are about two units of log-likelihood below the P-models: this represents the support for the P-models. Since two units of log-likelihood correspond roughly to the 5% level of significance, the R-models may be rejected in favour of the P-models. The table also shows that Model 2 is completely ruled out.

Table 4 shows that Model 3P is the best of the models: it fits the data significantly better than Model 2 and the R-models. However, this evidence is not sufficient to show that the model does fit the data adequately: it must also be shown that after fitting no significant residual variation is left to be explained. Given the ML estimates of the parameters of the model ($a = 0·039$, $b = 0·344$), the theoretical distributions of the breeding dates of the phenotypes can be computed. Then from the numbers breeding, as given in Table 3, χ^2 can

Table 4. Maximum likelihood (ML) estimates of female preferences when the models of preferential mating are fitted to the data of Table 1. In Models 2, 3 and 4, α is the proportion of females preferring darks. In Models 1 and 3, β is the proportion preferring dark or intermediate males indiscriminately or, in Model 4, the proportion preferring only intermediate males.

Model	ML estimates of female preferences		Log-likelihood (to base e)	Support for Model 3P
	$\hat{\alpha}$	$\hat{\beta}$		
1P	—	0·382	−501·466	0·471
1R	—	0·194	−503·292	2·297
1S	—	0·286	−502·285	1·290
2P	0·063	—	−505·277	4·282
2R	0·026	—	−505·724	4·729
3P	0·039	0·344	−500·995	0
3R	0·022	0·172	−502·842	1·847
3S	0·026	0·260	−501·836	0·841
4P	0·114	0·262	−501·120	0·125
4R	0·057	0·132	−503.066	2·071
4S	0·085	0·195	−501·997	1·002

be calculated to test the goodness of fit of the model. This test shows that no significant heterogeneity is left in the data after the model has been fitted: the model is a very good fit (see O'Donald (1983) for details).

Since melanism does appear to be a semi-dominant character, it is most satisfactory that a model of semi-dominant preference (Model 3P) best fits the data. But goodness of fit does not prove that preferential mating actually takes place: in the logic of inference, it is almost a truism that goodness of fit does not prove the validity of a model, for other models, which have not been tested, may fit as well or better. Independent corroboration is required.

7 ASSORTATIVE MATING

The fit of Model 3P to the data of breeding dates is one line of evidence in favour of the hypothesis of female preference. Assortative mating provides a second line of evidence, which independently corroborates the hypothesis. Matings are assortative whenever they occur non-randomly with respect to certain phenotypes: one phenotype tends to assort with another. For example, in positive assortative mating (or simply "assortative mating"), phenotypes that are alike assort together; in negative assortative mating (or "disassortative mating"), unlike phenotypes assort together. Data on assortative mating

Table 5. Calculation of expected mating frequencies of different morph-pairs

Mating	Observed number	Hypothetical frequency of matings
Melanic × melanic	a	$\alpha u + \dfrac{u^2(1-\alpha)^2}{1-\alpha u}$
Melanic × pale	b	$\dfrac{2uv(1-\alpha)}{1-\alpha u}$
Pale × pale	c	$\dfrac{v^2}{1-\alpha u}$

are easily obtained by counting the numbers of matings between the various phenotypes. Since the writing of the Arctic Skua book, additional data of mating frequencies have been collected by a very detailed survey of the breeding pairs of Arctic Skuas on the islands of the Orkney archipelago (Meek et al. 1985). Coverage of Arctic Skua populations was virtually complete. These data can be added to those of Fair Isle and Shetland and analysed together. Since the melanics have not been classified into intermediate and dark forms in every set of data, darks and intermediates have all been included in a single class of melanics.

In order to analyse the data, a model of assortative mating must be fitted and parameters estimated. Models of assortative mating have been described by Davis and O'Donald (1976 a) and O'Donald (1983). Suppose that a proportion α of the females mate assortatively with melanic males: the females' preference for the melanic males is expressed only if the females themselves also possess the melanic phenotype. The remaining females mate at random. To conform to the P-model of preferential mating of the previous section, I assume that the assortative matings occur before the random matings. If melanic birds occur in the population at frequency u and non-melanics at frequency $v = 1 - u$, then we should have the hypothetical frequencies of matings corresponding to a sample of observed matings shown in Table 5. Maximum likelihood estimates of the parameters are given by $\hat{u} = (a + \frac{1}{2}b)/(a + b + c)$ and $\hat{\alpha} = (ac - \frac{1}{4}b)/c(a + \frac{1}{2}b)$. A full account of the analysis of the assortative mating is given in Appendix C of *The Arctic Skua* (O'Donald 1983).

Table 6 gives the data on assortative mating, including the new data from the survey on Orkney carried out in 1982 (Meek et al. 1985). The data from Fair Isle, Foula and the rest of Shetland were analysed by O'Donald (1983), who gave details of the statistical methods of analysis. The χ^2 values test the significance of deviations from random mating: they are significant for Foula

Table 6. Numbers of matings between different phenotypes of Arctic Skuas on Orkney and Shetland. Here r is the correlation coefficient of phenotypes of mated pairs. z is Fisher's transformation

$$z = \tanh^{-1}(r)$$

which has an approximately normal distribution with variance

$$\mathrm{var}\,(z) = 1/(n-3)$$

$\bar{z}$ is the weighted mean of the values of z for each area. A χ^2 test of the significance of the variation in z between samples is then given by

$$\chi^2 = \sum (z - \bar{z})^2/\mathrm{var}\,(z) = 5{\cdot}394\,7$$
$$P = 0{\cdot}145 \quad \text{(not significant)}$$

	Areas sampled				
	Orkney	Fair Isle[a]	Foula[b]	Shetland[c]	Total
Melanic × melanic	501	254	144	218	1 117
Melanic × pale	299	119	86	120	624
Pale × pale	58	19	26	38	141
Total	858	392	256	376	1 882
Estimates					
$\hat{x}$	0·177 8	0·215 9	0·389 8	0·443 4	0·298 5
$\hat{u}$	0·758 2	0·799 7	0·730 5	0·739 4	0·759 3
Value of χ^2	2·118 9	1·070 0	5·521 8	11·114 2	19·824 9
Correlation, r	0·049 69	0·052 25	0·146 9	0·171 9	
Transformation, z	0·049 74	0·052 29	0·147 9	0·173 7	$\bar{z} = 0{\cdot}088\,28$

[a] Data from O'Donald (1983).
[b] Data from Davis and O'Donald (1976 a).
[c] Data from O'Donald (1960).

and Shetland, not significant for Orkney and Fair Isle. However, the test of variation in assortative mating (the χ^2 test of variation in z) is not significant: the different χ^2 values for each area are not evidence of variation in the assortative mating. In fact, the non-significant values of χ^2 for Orkney and Fair Isle can be seen to correspond to quite appreciable estimates of assortative mating preference (22% for Fair Isle). Much larger samples would have to be collected in order to obtain a significant result when the mating preference is only about 20%. This insensitivity of the χ^2 test is mainly caused by the high frequency of melanics in these populations. A large proportion of purely random matings will be of the type melanic × melanic. The additional assortative matings do not add much to the numbers of these matings. The χ^2 test will not detect the relatively small deviations from random mating unless the sample is very large indeed. Over all the areas of Orkney and Shetland, the assortative mating is highly significant, and it is not heterogeneous between areas. This can also be demonstrated by an analysis of χ^2. The matings from

Table 7. χ^2 analysis of assortative mating of Arctic Skuas on Orkney and Shetland. The degrees of freedom are found as follows. There are 12 classes. In order to calculate the numbers of matings to be expected in each class on the hypothesis of random mating ($\alpha = 0$), the four sample totals are required, removing four degrees of freedom; the estimate $\hat{u} = 0.7593$ removes one more degree of freedom, leaving seven as shown. After fitting the model of assortative mating, the estimate $\hat{\alpha} = 0.2985$ removes a further degree of freedom, leaving six: three for the variation in frequency and three for the variation in assortative mating. This analysis produces a value of χ^2 for the test of variation in α that is somewhat different from the test using Fisher's z transformation. The difference arises because different models of assortative mating are being tested. Neither test shows significance.

Component of variation	Value of χ^2	Df	Value of P
Assortative mating	19·1249	1	1.22×10^{-5}
Variation in melanic frequency	10·9936	3	0·0118
Variation in assortative mating	3·6187	3	0·306
Total variation	33·7372	7	1.93×10^{-5}

the four areas form a 3×4 contingency table. Assuming that the samples have all been drawn from the same random mating population, each sample supplies two degrees of freedom for χ^2, giving a total of eight degrees of freedom, less one for the estimation of the overall frequency of melanics. Fitting the additional parameters for the assortative mating of melanics removes one further degree of freedom. The six residual degrees of freedom can then be analysed into the variation between areas in phenotypic frequency (three degrees of freedom) and variation in assortative mating (three degrees of freedom). Thus we obtain an analysis of χ^2 given in Table 7. The variation in frequency reflects the northward cline of increasing numbers of pale birds, though the change in frequency is very slight at this extreme southerly part of the Arctic Skua's range. Assortative mating is seen to be highly significant and shows no significant variation in Orkney and Shetland.

There is no evidence in the Arctic Skua that the assortative mating is caused by imprinting, which, as Cooke has shown (1978; and chapter 13), is the cause of assortative mating in the Snow Goose. Imprinting would be a plausible mechanism by which the females acquired their preferences. Alternatively, the preferences may be genetic, having evolved in linkage disequilibrium with the gene preferred. This process necessarily gives rise to assortment in the expression of preference: the linkage disequilibrium between the preference genes and the genes for the preferred character means that females with the preference are also likely to have the genes for the preferred character. O'Donald (1980) showed by computer simulation that in the course of the evolution of preferential mating the linkage disequilibrium would produce up to 20% or more assortative mating among the preferred phenotypes. The assortative mating we have observed thus strongly supports the hypothesis of sexual selection by preferential mating. If females have evolved preferences for melanic males, the assortment we have found in the matings is about what we should expect to find theoretically. This independently corroborates the evidence of the goodness of fit of models of preferential mating. Quite apart from satisfying the predictions of the theory of the evolution of mating preference, assortative mating is by itself sound evidence for the occurrence of some form of female choice. Males are so often undiscriminating in their choice of mates that it is most unlikely they would compete only, or more strongly, for females with the same phenotypes as themselves. As a cause of assortative mating, male competition seems implausible.

The assortative mating of the Arctic Skua thus provides a second and strong line of evidence in favour of the hypothesis of female preference.

8 SEXUAL SELECTION AND MALE EXPERIENCE

Males who have bred in previous seasons should have acquired a competitive advantage over young males breeding for the first time. If sexual selection results from male competition, experienced males should be more successful in finding mates. There is no evidence for this in the Arctic Skua. The times taken to find a new mate are very much the same for both experienced and new males; average breeding dates (measured, as before, in days from 1st June) are in Table 8 (O'Donald 1983).

New and experienced males do not differ significantly in the breeding dates of the phenotypes, but the phenotypes are significantly different. On average, experienced males in new pairs breed as late as new males: they take as long to find a new mate as the new males. This observation appears to refute the hypothesis put forward by Andersson in his review of *The Arctic Skua* (Andersson 1984). As an alternative to the hypothesis of female preference, he suggested that the different breeding dates of the phenotypes were a consequence of the timing of their return to the colony. In Black-legged Kittiwakes (*Rissa tridactyla*), birds seem to return to the colony about ten days

Table 8. Mean number of days after 1st June for hatching of first eggs in new pairs

	Colour phase		
	Dark	Intermediate	Pale
New males	29·71	32·52	32·88
Experienced males	28·05	27·59	33·21

earlier in each successive year of life. Since pale Arctic Skuas are younger when they first breed (4 years old on average, compared to melanics that are 4·5 years old), Andersson suggests that pale males might breed later simply because they are younger and take up territories later: all birds would breed earlier in successive years but with the pales always later than the others. According to Andersson's statement, his theory applies only to first-time breeders, not to experienced males taking a new mate. Yet, as we have seen, experienced pale males are just as late as new pale males. Moreover, if it were true that pale males breed four days later than the others because they are one-half year younger on average, the experienced males, which are more than a year older than new males, would have to breed more than eight days earlier than the new males in order to account for melanics in new pairs being four days earlier than the younger pale males in new pairs. However, experienced males with a new mate are almost as late as males breeding for the first time. A pair that has bred together in previous years is indeed eight days earlier than a new pair; but, when having to find new mates, experienced and new males are at just the same disadvantage and breed just as late as each other, regardless of the age of the male and the number of years he bred in the past. Andersson's interesting suggestion cannot stand.

Cooke (1984), in his review of the book, made a suggestion similar to Andersson's. According to Cooke, melanics may be more successful in reproduction, not because the females prefer them but simply because they are older. Cooke seems to have mistakenly assumed that, in my interpretation, all the variation in reproductive success is caused by sexual selection. This has never been my view. On the contrary, I showed that sexual selection contributes to only a small part of the variation between phenotypes in reproductive success. The detailed tables of breeding date and reproductive success given in Appendix A of *The Arctic Skua* show that females vary as much as males in overall reproductive success but do not vary in breeding date. The evidence for sexual selection is to be seen not in the variation in reproductive success but in the variation in breeding date of males in new pairs. This, as we have seen, does not depend on age.

9 CONCLUSIONS

In this chapter I have reviewed the evidence for sexual selection by female choice in the Arctic Skua. The evidence for sexual selection is clear-cut: melanics take less time to find a mate than pales; melanic males thus breed earlier in the breeding season than pales; and they gain a selective advantage from the general correlation between earlier breeding and increased reproductive success.

The evidence for female choice as the mechanism of sexual selection is indirect. The mating advantage of having a larger territory cannot explain the sexual selection for melanics, because territory size does not vary among the male phenotypes.

Three independent lines of evidence support the hypothesis that females prefer to mate with melanic males. First, the data on breeding dates of the males give an excellent fit to models with female preferences for dark and intermediate males. The models that fit best are those in which the preferential matings precede random matings. These models accord with the hypothesis that female preference evolved by the selection of a gene that lowers the females' threshold of response to mating with melanic males. It can be shown theoretically that this evolution must produce linkage disequilibrium between the gene for the melanism and the gene for the preference. As a result, females with the preference will tend to be melanic; this preference of melanic females for melanic males will produce assortative mating. The assortative mating of melanics thus provides a second line of corroborative evidence for female preference: it accords with the theoretical prediction. In addition, assortative mating is most unlikely to result from male competition: to produce assortment, a male would have to compete more strongly for females with the same phenotype as his own. This seems most implausible.

Male experience seems to have no effect on the time taken to find a mate. Experienced males who have bred in previous years take almost as long to find a mate as new males breeding for the first time. This third line of evidence suggests that male sexual activities have little or no effect on the chances of mating, which must therefore be determined by the females. The suggestion that pale males take longer to find a mate because they are younger is refuted by this evidence, for new pale males take no longer than older pale males with several years' breeding experience behind them.

I therefore conclude that female preference provides much the most likely explanation of the sexual selection of Arctic Skua phenotypes. All the alternative explanations that have so far been put forward have now been excluded.

REFERENCES

Andersson, M. (1984). Review of *The Arctic Skua. Quart. Rev. Biol.* **59**, 322–323.

Arnason, E. (1978). Apostatic selection and kleptoparasitism in the Parasitic Jaeger. *Auk* **95**, 377–381.

Clarke, B. (1962). Natural selection in mixed populations of two polymorphic snails. *Heredity* **17**, 319–345.

Cooke, F. (1978). Early learning and its effect on population structure. Studies of a wild population of Snow Geese. *Z. Tierpsych.* **46**, 344–358.

Cooke, F. (1984). Avian population biology (review of *The Arctic Skua*). *Science* **224**, 277–278.

Darwin, C. R. (1871). "The Descent of Man and Selection in Relation to Sex". John Murray, London.

Davis, J. W. F. and O'Donald, P. (1976 a). Estimation of assortative mating preferences in the Arctic Skua. *Heredity* **36**, 235–244.

Davis, J. W. F. and O'Donald, P. (1976 b). Territory size, breeding time and mating preference in the Arctic Skua. *Nature* **260**, 774–775.

Edwards, A. W. F. (1972). "Likelihood". Cambridge University Press.

Fisher, R. A. (1922). On the dominance ratio. *Proc. Roy. Soc. Edinb.* **42**, 321–341.

Fisher, R. A. (1930). "The Genetical Theory of Natural Selection". Clarendon Press, Oxford.

Haldane, J. B. S. (1924). A mathematical theory of natural and artificial selection. *Trans. Camb. Phil. Soc.* **23**, 19–40.

Hall, B. P., Moreau, R. E. and Galbraith, I. C. J. (1966). Polymorphism and parallelism in the African bush-shrikes of the genus *Malaconotus* (including *Chlorophoneus*). *Ibis* **108**, 161–181.

Huxley, J. S. (1938). Clines: an auxiliary taxonomic principle. *Nature* **1421**, 219.

Huxley, J. S. (1939). Notes on the percentage of bridled Guillemots. *Br. Birds* **33**, 174–183.

Kirkpatrick, M. (1982). Sexual selection and the evolution of female choice. *Evolution* **36**, 1–12.

Meek, E. R., Booth, J. C., Reynold, P. and Ribbans, B. (1985). Breeding skuas in Orkney. *Seabird* **8**, 29–33.

O'Donald, P. (1960). Inbreeding as a result of imprinting. *Heredity* **15**, 79–85.

O'Donald, P. (1962). The theory of sexual selection. *Heredity* **17**, 541–552.

O'Donald, P. (1967). A general theory of sexual and natural selection. *Heredity* **22**, 499–518.

O'Donald, P. (1973). Models of sexual and natural selection in polygynous species. *Heredity* **31**, 145–156.

O'Donald, P. (1974). Polymorphisms maintained by sexual selection in monogamous species of birds. *Heredity* **32**, 1–10.

O'Donald, P. (1976). Mating preferences and their genetic effects in models of sexual selection for colour phases of the Arctic Skua. *In* "Population Genetics and Ecology" (eds S. Karlin and E. Nevo), pp. 411–430. Academic Press, New York.

O'Donald, P. (1977). Theoretical aspects of sexual selection. *Theor. Pop. Biol.* **12**, 298–334.

O'Donald, P. (1980). "Genetic Models of Sexual Selection". Cambridge University Press.

O'Donald, P. (1983). "The Arctic Skua. A Study of the Ecology and Evolution of a Seabird". Cambridge University Press.

Owen, D. F. (1967). The interpretation of polymorphism in the African bush-shrikes. *Ibis* **109**, 278–279.

Paulson, D. R. (1973). Predator polymorphism and apostatic selection. *Evolution* **27**, 269–277.

Payne, R. B. (1967). Interspecific communication signals in parasitic birds. *Am. Natur.* **101**, 363–375.

Southern, H. N. (1943). The two phases of *Stercorarius parasiticus*. *Ibis* **85**, 443–485.

Tinbergen, L. (1960). The natural control of insects in pinewoods. I. Factors influencing the intensity of predation by song-birds. *Arch. Neer. Zool.* **13**, 265–336.

Part IV

Coda

15

Epilogue and Prologue: Past and Future Research in Avian Genetics

P. A. Buckley

Ecology Graduate Faculty and Center for Coastal and Environmental Studies, Doolittle Hall, Rutgers University, New Brunswick, New Jersey 08903, USA

1 INTRODUCTION

The previous four chapters, comprising Part III, represent four quite different, idiosyncratic, yet complementary approaches to performing avian genetic analyses of natural populations of wild birds. Two involved assaying conspicuous well-known plumage polymorphisms and the factors possibly responsible for their maintenance; one looked at the quantitative genetics of fitness in a common Eurasian passerine; and the fourth took a global approach to the evolution and systematics of *Passer domesticus*, a bird with a worldwide distribution and complex evolutionary history. Employing various techniques discussed in earlier chapters, these four chapters give a splendid picture of the opportunities available for using genetics to answer questions of evolutionary, population or ecological importance.

As subjects for genetic studies, birds offer certain advantages. They are very well studied taxonomically; by and large they are diurnal and highly visible,

AVIAN GENETICS
ISBN 0-12-187570-9

behaviourally and ecologically; they are often easy to count, to age and to sex externally by inspection; they are frequently colonial, widely distributed with regular ecological and taxonomic replacements around the world; and range from solitary to colonial in habits; some are extraordinarily sedentary, others globally migratory; and their growth rates are deterministic. Many of them, from waterfowl to various finches, are easily bred in captivity; many others' nests and young are easily locatable in the wild, and individual marking in various ways has long been used successfully with wild birds.

On the debit side, much remains unknown about the genetics of wild birds. Indeed, the very existence of avian Z and W sex chromosomes was shown only in the 1960s, and the fact that the mechanism involves genic balance (as in *Drosophila*) rather than Y-dominance (as in mammals) has only just been demonstrated (Sittmann 1984). As Shields points out (chapter 3), very little is known about the comparative karyotypy of wild birds, to the extent that true variation in diploid number is unknown for any wild bird. Moreover, essentially all avian chromosome work to date has involved the large macrochromosomes; the number, homologies and functional/evolutionary/ecological (?) importance of the unique avian microchromosomes remains a technically intractable enigma. In chapter 1, Buckley demonstrated that even the most basic kinds of information on Mendelian inheritance of, for example, plumage patterns, are known in detail for only one species, Gouldian Finch (*Poephila gouldiae*)—and then only for head and bill colour. Various external plumage polymorphisms have been described for wild birds, but only occasionally are their genetics known, and in only two cases—Lesser Snow Goose (*Anser c. caerulescens*) (chapter 13) and Arctic Skua (*Stercorarius parasiticus*) (chapter 14)—do we have reasonably good ideas why the polymorphism is maintained.

Against this gloomy background there has been set, notwithstanding, a surprising amount of research in avian genetics, described in the preceding chapters. Owing to the vast gaps in our knowledge, this work has ranged from demonstration of basic karyotypy and simple Mendelian inheritance of plumage, to work at the frontiers of population and evolutionary biology (e.g. Corbin 1983) and molecular biology and systematics (e.g. Sibley and Ahlquist 1983). Still, there is no "avian *Drosophila melanogaster*," although Snow Goose bids fair for that spot; its closest competitors are probably Arctic Skua (O'Donald 1983; chapter 14) and in quantitative, ecological genetics, the various Galápagos geospizines being studied by Grant and colleagues.

Birds differ from other vertebrates in a number of ways bearing importantly on their genetics, ecology and evolution, for example in their chromosomes, and in their vagility: volant species have spread far and wide across all the earth's continents, and dispersal of young birds frequently involves intercontinental distance and destinations. This is particularly true for seabirds, but our phenomenological knowledge of the effect is still inadequate, let alone its quantitative description. At the other end of the dispersal spectrum are the often-postulated but all too infrequently quantified sedentary low-dispersal small-population characteristics of tropical oscines and suboscines. Indeed, one of the major problems confronting avian population genetic analyses today is the virtual absence of hard data on effective breeding population (N_e) sizes as well as rates of dispersal of young, and normal cruising ranges ("neighbourhoods") of any breeding adults, critical values for certain calculation of expected gene frequencies. On the other hand, in many birds, clutch sizes are sufficient to enable rapid accumulation of progeny data from parents of known or inferred genotypes; this is augmented in those species, usually passerines, that raise multiple (serial or simultaneous) broods each breeding season. Differences in mobility of birds have been advanced, for example, as the likely reason avian biochemical genetic diversity (heterozygosity) is more uniform and appreciably lower than that of other vertebrates (amphibians, for example, score 10–20 times higher than birds; see discussion below). These differences offer unique opportunities, when coupled with other aspects of avian biology, for conspicuously more work in avian genetics than has been attempted to date. We hope this book will pique the curiosity of (especially) field-oriented ornithologists, overcome a distressingly widespread apprehension of modern genetics, and possibly galvanize them into applying some of the techniques described here to problems of their own, optimally in novel fashion. Meantime, treatment of certain topics—some discussed in previous chapters, some not—is in order.

2   THE NEUTRALITY–SELECTION CONTROVERSY

Both chapters 4 and 10 discussed at some length the methods of allozyme (or isozyme or electromorph) analysis that, beginning in the mid-1960s, have given biologists for the first time reasonable estimates of actual genetic diversity in natural populations. While these approaches took a while to be used with birds, there is now a considerable body of such data reported on by Evans and Corbin. There is, however, additional information that readers should be aware of in properly evaluating biochemical techniques in avian genetics.

Soon after the first allozyme data appeared, certain aspects of their frequency and distributions seemed at variance with traditional notions of the selective value of alleles in natural populations, leading Kimura (1968 a,b) and King and Jukes (1969) to propose the then radical notion that alleles at the various allozymic loci were, as far as natural selection was concerned, equivalent or neutral. Soon thereafter a long series of studies appeared reporting the selective importance of even slight chemical variants (e.g. Ayala and Gilpin 1973, Hedrick *et al*. 1976, Nevo 1978) continuing to the present (e.g. Mueller *et al*. 1985). At the same time an impressive array of theoretical and applied papers appeared in support of the neutral hypothesis (e.g. Maruyama and Kimura 1974, Li 1978, Fuerst *et al*. 1977, Nei and Grauer 1984), summarized in a lucidly written book by Kimura (1983).

Considerable misunderstanding has persisted about exactly what is implied by the neutral theory, which many prefer to call the "neutral mutation–random drift theory". As recently expressed by Kimura (1983), it

> claims that the great majority of evolutionary mutant substitutions are not caused by positive Darwinian selection but by random fixation of selectively neutral or nearly neutral mutants. The theory also asserts that much of the intraspecific genetic variability at the molecular level, such as is manifested in the form of protein polymorphism, is selectively neutral or nearly so, and maintained in the species by the balance between mutational input and random extinction or fixation of alleles. From the standpoint of the neutral theory, evolutionary mutant substitutions and molecular polymorphisms are not two independent phenomena, but simply two aspects of a single phenomenon. In other words, protein polymorphism merely represents a transient phase of molecular evolution (*The Neutral Theory of Molecular Evolution*, pp. 306–307).

> [The theory] does not deny the role of natural selection in determining the course of adaptive evolution, but it assumes that only a minute fraction of DNA changes in evolution are adaptive in nature, while the great majority of phenotypically silent molecular substitutions exert no significant influence on survival and reproduction and drift randomly through the species (p. xi, *op. cit.*).

Moreover, Kimura (1983, pp. 270–271) explicitly recognizes that even though some alleles may be selectively neutral at say, the present time, they could at other times or under other conditions cease to be neutral, and has termed this the "Hartl–Dykhuizen effect" in honour of those first reporting it (Hartl and Dykhuizen 1981). As he notes, even the most hardened selectionist would have little difficulty accepting such a concept.

The utility of the neutral theory lies in its general ability to provide simple and logical falsifiable null hypotheses. It has also generated an extraordinary amount of research in both theoretical and applied population genetics, now having implications for the genetics of wild birds. Increasingly, ornithologists are coming to grips with the impressive amount of data supporting the neutral theory, and are recognizing that the all too often *ad hoc*, *a posteriori* selectionist arguments cannot withstand careful critical testing. Again, this is not to say that some biochemical polymorphisms have not been selected for and/or maintained by selection, but only that they now appear to be in a clear minority.

At the same time that experimental efforts were underway to establish that allozyme polymorphisms are adaptive, theoretical work was mushrooming on both sides of the controversy. In particular, selectionists developed models invoking overdominance, directional selection, habitat selection, frequency-dependent selection, and many others. They are discussed at some length in Kimura (1983) and Nei and Graur (1984) and typically are narrowly focused, with unrealistically limited or biologically remote requirements. Maynard Smith and Hoekstra (1980), by way of example, dissect several models involving heterogeneous environments, eliminating essentially all as unrealistic. Few models have survived rigorous analysis or experimental verification; of those, virtually all are so specific as to have little heuristic or predictive applicability.

R. C. Lewontin—long identified with the selectionist camp and author of one of the most balanced analyses of both views, albeit one now out of date (Lewontin 1974)—has in two recent papers (Lewontin 1985 a,b) acknowledged that there appear to be two major kinds of allozyme polymorphisms—selectively neutral and selectively advantageous—and that, moreover, allozyme loci seem to fall into the following categories: (1) monomorphic or virtually so; (2) "classically polymorphic" with two or three alleles in intermediate frequency; (3) polymorphic with one very common and many very rare alleles; and (4) "clasically polymorphic" plus very many rare alleles. These he arrays on two "axes": one major; one minor. Classical polymorphisms occupy the major axis, and he suggests these "may well be selectively balanced". Those along the minor axis (the remainder, far and away the majority of observed cases), "tolerate amino acid substitutions, which are then essentially neutral to selection". Furthermore, he predicts, logically and quite in keeping with Kimura's (1983) formulation, that minor-axis variation will be uniform across species lines, while major-axis variation should occur among species and among environments.

3 INTERPRETATION OF ALLOZYME ANALYSES

While this approach, coupled with the Dykhuizen–Hartl suggestion, all but weds the neutralists and selectionists, Lewontin (1985 a) raises another interesting question as a straw man: has total (true) heterozygosity been overestimated because of undue emphasis on allozymes? (This in itself is an interesting reflection by one of the pioneers of allozyme analysis, one whose early papers (Lewontin and Hubby 1966, Hubby and Lewontin 1966) revolutionized our ideas about the levels of genetic diversity in natural populations.) He concluded that perhaps we have overestimated heterozygosity, but then dismisses the question by observing that we should abandon gel electrophoresis of proteins and get right down to the business of DNA sequencing, and that population genetics should "rid itself of its preoccupation with assessing the amount of genic variation in natural populations and with understanding the role of selective and nonselective forces". By imperial rescript thus will all population geneticists become biochemical technicians.

Fortunately, analysis of population gene frequencies, including by allozyme techniques, is not going to cease anymore than research in comparative anatomy ended with the discovery of DNA. There are still many essential questions to be asked, patterns to be detected, processes to be explained. It is clear that the F_{ST} technique and its related functions are exceptionally useful, and as outlined in the Evans, Rockwell and Barrowclough, and Corbin chapters, is being put to increasingly informative uses, both explanatory and predictive. Ignoring the question of neutral versus selectively important alleles, F_{ST} scores have told us that in general, the range of values for avian taxa is less than for other vertebrates, and the per cent heterozygosity is appreciably lower (chapters 7 and 10). In particular, fixation or near-fixation of certain alleles has occurred in Blue Grouse (*Dendragapus obscurus*; Redfield *et al.* 1972), Lesser Prairie Chicken (*Tympanuchus pallidicinctus*; Gutierrez *et al.* 1983) and Great Blue Heron (*Ardea herodias*; Guttman *et al.* 1980). Similar values have been found in Pacific coast pinnipeds (Bonnell and Selander 1974) and have been interpreted as evidence of greatly increased gene flow, an assumed correlate of low *H* values (cf. Barrowclough (1983) for birds). However, this explanation seems most unlikely to apply equally to two species of grouse (notoriously sedentary birds) or a colonially breeding waterbird. Rather, as neutral theories of both Kimura (1983) and Gillespie (1985) predict, very low *H* values or even allelic fixation are to be expected in species whose effective breeding population is small—in their models, less than 1000. This is clearly the more logical explanation: grouse are lekking species with a few males normally fertilizing most females, and colonial birds typically behave as reasonably exclusive breeding units, in Great Blue Herons rarely exceeding a few hundred pairs. Findings are thus in accord with neutrality theory, and it is unnecessary to invoke explanations about high levels of gene flow (here, counter-intuitive) or population bottlenecks (hypothetical), both of which have been adduced to explain other observed low levels of heterozygosity.

In like fashion, there is increasing attention being paid to examining the old question of whether there is more genetic variation in "central" or in "peripheral" populations (cf. Mayr 1963, Lewontin 1974). While I am unaware of any such allozymic studies in birds, the issue has been reviewed recently for *Drosophila* (Brussard 1984), where across several species no biologically meaningful or statistically significant central–peripherhal differences were found; indeed, no trends were even apparent. These findings are of course again consistent with neutrality predictions, as was even the sole exception— the isolated Colombian population of *D. pseudoobscura*. The implications for these findings on classical speciation theory are discussed by Brussard (1984), which is recommended reading.

Other questions have been asked of avian F_{ST} data. For example, is different modal clutch size in two populations of California Gull (*Larus californicus*) at widely separated sites attributable to (other) population genetic differences? Zink and Winkler (1983) found that at the loci they studied, the populations were statistically indistinguishable from any two samples drawn from one panmictic unit. They admit it is highly unlikely the allozymes they compared had any relationship to the character under study (clutch size), but nonetheless concluded that clutch size differences were either recently evolved and determined by loci they did not examine, or that they were environmentally labile. These findings, and those from a few similar studies, should be viewed in the light of Lewontin's (1984) caveat about not really ever expecting to find correlations between phenotypic and allozyme characters.

Two recent studies have addressed the questions, respectively, of allozyme variation in sibling species, both of which happened to be tropical (Capparella and Lanyon 1985), and in tropical versus temperate species (Braun and Parker 1985). Neither study found F_{ST} values that differed from those already in the avian literature, again in conformation with neutrality theory. However, the very real questions of dispersal, effective breeding population size (N_e), philopatry, and inbreeding (cf. chapter 6) in tropical species need serious attention, as those variables materially affect rate of genic evolution even of selectively neutral alleles (Kimura 1983). Lastly, genetic comparisons using allozyme data are now being made to assay the taxonomic status, and to infer the evolutionary history, of allopatric bird populations. A recent example is that of Johnson and Zink (1985) involving several taxa in the genus *Vireo*, with disjunct, so-called "leap-frog", distributions. Johnson and Zink's somewhat surprising taxonomic conclusions turn out to be reinforced by other data on song and wing formula. One hopes that similar kinds of analyses will be applied to other avian taxa, especially where large populations are allopatric or allochronic as in many procellariiform seabirds. For a review of the general area of genic heterozygosity and variation in birds, see Johnson *et al.* (1985).

4 PHYLOGENIES, STATISTICAL CONSTRAINTS AND MOLECULAR CLOCKS

The statistical properties of F_{ST} and its relatives, as well as the various genetic distances, are undergoing rigorous examination at the moment. While few successful assaults have been made on the techniques, *pace* Lewontin (1985 b), some useful admonitions have been advanced. For example, Archie (1985), using simulations, suggested that the frequently used parametric independent-sample t-test may not be valid for making heterozygosity comparisons among populations or species because of skewed or bimodal distributions, only sometimes offset by increasing sample sizes. Further, Simon and Archie (1985) offer a mordant demonstration that choice of loci can appreciably affect heterozygosity estimates, so interspecific or interlaboratory comparisons should be done with utmost care. And because of what they regard as lax use of various F-statistics, Weir and Cockerham (1984) recommend a more rigorous approach, but one unfortunately involving yet another set of genetic heterozygosity/relatedness statistics. Their technique has the appreciable advantages, though, of estimating variances by means of jack-knife procedures, as well as making no assumptions about numbers of populations, sample sizes or heterozygote frequencies. Time will tell if this is useful enough to warrant frequent adoption. Those contemplating genetic analyses using F_{ST} and related statistics are advised to pay close attention to the literature.

The existence of a reasonably uniform "molecular clock" is one of the more useful by-products of the neutral theory. While a recent thorough review can be found in Thorpe (1982), the molecular-clock concept embodies several points that bear on the present discussion:

> (1) for each protein, the rate of evolution in terms of amino acid substitutions is approximately constant per year per site for various lines, as long as the function and tertiary structure of the molecule remain essentially unaltered; (2) functionally less important molecules or parts of molecules evolve (in terms of mutant substitutions) faster than more important ones; (3) those mutant substitutions that are less disruptive to the existing structure and function of a molecule (conservative substitutions) occur more frequently in evolution than more disruptive ones; (4) gene duplication must always precede the emergence of a gene having a new function; (5) selective elimination of definitely deleterious mutants, and random fixation of selectively neutral or very slightly deleterious mutants, occur far more frequently in evolution than positive Darwinian selection of definitely advantageous mutants (Kimura 1983, pp. 98–113).

Various measures of genetic distance (see chapter 10) have been used with the methods of cladistics to derive "phylogenetic trees" with presumed true time-scales (calibrated by alignment with known geological or vicariance events) showing divergence of genetic and evolutionary lines. This method was used, for example, in the *Vireo* analysis mentioned above (Johnson and Zink 1985), as well as in many non-avian analyses. Until recently, though, there was considerable disagreement over the methods used to derive phylogenies, as well as over alternative competing phylogenies. Discussion of various approaches takes up most of at least two international journals, and the topic is beyond our interest here, save to mention that recently Felsenstein

Table 1. A conceptual framework for dealing with the empirical observation of a conservative pattern of protein differentiation among closely related avian species (after Avise 1983).

Fundamental alternative possibilities
- A. Avian congeners are younger than most non-avian vertebrate congeners.
- B. Protein evolution is decelerated in birds.

Possible corollaries and ramifications of A
1. Avian genera have been taxonomically "oversplit" relative to other vertebrate genera.
2. Avian speciations occur rapidly.
3. Rates of morphological (e.g., plumage) and behavioural divergence can be different from rates of protein evolution.
4. Morphological and behavioural differences may represent only rather superficial genetic changes.
5. Should be reflected in small genetic distances for entire avian genome.

Possible corollaries and ramifications of B
1. Uniform electrophoretic clock in vertebrates does not exist.
2. May not be reflected in small genetic distances for entire avian genome.
3. Rate of protein evolution influenced by intrinsic properties of birds
    - a. Ecological (e.g., mating system, generation length)
    - b. Evolutionary (e.g., mode of speciation)
    - c. Genetic (e.g., heterozygosity, mutation rate)
    - d. Physiological (e.g., body temperature)

Possible empirical tests of A versus B
1. Examine other portions of avian genome (e.g., by restriction enzymes, sequencing DNA hybridization).
2. More careful study of fossil/biogeographic evidence of ages of avian speciations.

(1985 a,b,c) has paid attention to putting confidence limits on such phylogenies, as well as to some statistical problems generally associated with the process. Nonetheless, it is one generally accepted, that will likely see future applications to avian genetics problems. Lastly, work is only now beginning on the generation of genetic distances using quantitative traits, sometimes in conjunction with allozyme data (e.g. Camussi *et al.* 1985), although not yet with birds.

Earlier, I alluded to the fact that heterozygosity values for birds were lower, and consistently so, than those of other vertebrates. This raises the question of whether the conservative avian pattern is due to the fact that (*a*) avian species are generally younger than non-avian species, or (*b*) that the rate of avian protein evolution is slower than that of other vertebrates. Avise (1983) offers an interesting discussion of the problem, leading to a series of questions, hypotheses and explanations that could form the basis for much future work in avian genetics (Table 1). Also earlier I referred to Lewontin's (1985 a) suggestion that allozyme work be abandoned in favour of dealing directly with DNA. For almost the last ten years, Sibley and Ahlquist have been doing so, attacking the entirety of avian phylogeny and higher-order taxonomy, in a series of impressive papers beginning with "primitive insect eaters" (Sibley and Ahlquist 1980) and continuing, at present, through the suboscines (Sibley and Ahlquist 1985). They have used the techniques of DNA–DNA hybridization against known standards, rather than actual base-pair sequence analysis; the process, theoretical framework and interpretation of results are clearly described in Sibley and Ahlquist (1983), recommended reading for anyone wanting an approachable introduction to a technically daunting procedure.

We are delighted to report in this book that ornithologists are now well on the road to actual DNA-sequence analyses, and we hope this makes Lewontin very happy. Quinn and White (chapter 5) have been analysing both nuclear and mitochondrial DNA and, while they looked at polymorphisms in restriction-fragment lengths not actual base-pair sequences, that technique is the next step. Their excellent summary of this exciting new work in avian genetics is the first available. The mtDNA in particular, owing to its unique maternal inheritance pattern (recently extended to eight generations in *Mus musculus* and *M. spretus* with 99·9% fidelity (Gyllensten *et al.* 1985)), provides an extraordinary, and so far unique, opportunity for avian geneticists, ecologists and evolutionists to answer questions about genetic identity by descent rather than by state, in turn shedding light on an array of vexing topics ranging from paternity to inbreeding, to site tenacity and group adherence, to the still uninvestigated question of gentes in female *Cuculus* cuckoos—long suggested as being maternally inherited without a shred of evidence. mtDNA sequence analysis is an adjunct to other biochemical techniques suggested for lineage tracing, already described in chapters 4 and 6, and is a field being actively worked in at the moment (e.g. Michod and Hamilton 1980, Schwartz and Armitage 1983, Wilkinson and McCracken 1985). Another logical extension of DNA sequencing is its use in generating linkage maps. This would be especially important in avian genetics where complex karyotypy has all but precluded linkage mapping except in a few domestic species (see chapter 3). Botstein *et al.* (1980) outlined a schema for use of human restriction fragment length polymorphisms (RFLPs; see pages 177 and 193) to prepare linkage maps, although the technique is new and has to my knowledge not yet been applied to any birds.

5   GENE FLOW

Rockwell and Barrowclough (chapter 7) offer a particularly lucid example of how the tools of modern population genetics, especially using allozyme frequencies, can be used to estimate gene flow in wild-bird populations. Their analysis should be read in conjunction with a recent review of gene flow by Slatkin (1985), who notes that despite much work examining heterozygosity, genetic distance and gene flow, as yet there exists no theory for estimating gene-flow components from genetic distance. He also discusses at length various direct and indirect approaches to measuring gene flow, offering the sobering observation that while direct measures of gene flow might intuitively be thought better than indirect ones, the former suffer from being only valid when taken, they do not indicate time- or region-averaged gene flow, and probably would miss the exceptional, unique events that might be the most important genetically.

So, despite Lewontin's (1985 b) theoretical/philosophical jeremiad inveighing against the utter futility of indirect measures of gene flow, Slatkin (1985) opts strongly for indirect measures. (His approach to categorization as direct or indirect differs somewhat from that of Rockwell and Barrowclough, but that is minor.) Slatkin discusses as direct methods: dispersal of marked individuals, dispersal of marker alleles, and population extinction and re-colonization histories, noting that while island biogeography theory (cf. MacArthur and Wilson 1967, Diamond and May 1981) is extensive, there has been little development of parallel genetic models (e.g., Slatkin 1977, Maruyama and Kimura 1980). The indirect measures that Slatkin discusses include allelism of lethals; calculation of F_{ST} values; private polymorphisms; using population subsamples; estimating rates of approach to genetic equilibrium conditions; and using a recent tool in population biology known as spatial autocorrelation. In particular, the extinction and recolonization rate approach might be fruitful with birds once theory is in place, but particular caution is needed: very many species of birds nesting colonially extinguish and recolonize sites with some or all of the same individuals, compounding the non-independence statistical problem so often encountered in such studies. Perhaps, further down the road when we know the fine structure of colonial birds from mtDNA or other identity-by-descent techniques (see above), truly cohesive analyses involving these kinds of data can be attempted.

A point raised by many authors is that while genetic theory seems to imply that gene flow induces a conservative effect by retarding evolution, there are instances where evolution persists in spite of significant gene flow. Evans (chapter 4) cites an example of Mute Swans (*Cygnus olor*) maintaining allozyme frequencies in the face of apparently high gene flow. Another problem of long standing involves the holarctic groups of "reddish" crossbills (*Loxia* cf. *curvirostra*). *Curvirostra* is particularly subject to massive irruptions from boreal coniferous forests, with birds breeding hundreds or thousands of kilometres out of their "normal" range. The "species" has thus often been cited as a good example of a passerine approximation to true panmixia (Mayr 1963). If that be the case, then how does one explain that in North America, "*curvirostra*" is highly polytypic (probably eight races: American Ornithologists' Union 1957) and in Eurasia has been split into at least nine subspecies (Vaurie 1959), plus two other taxa variously treated conspecifically or specifically (*scotica*; *pytyopsittacus*)? Population-genetic thinking coupled with life-history information should lead one to question such a taxonomy. Recently, such an analysis in Europe (Knox 1976) confirmed that at least *scoticus* behaves as a good biological species, where it had been previously ascertained that *curvirostra* and *pytyopsittacus* were both ecologically and reproductively segregated. In North America, during a recent "Red" Crossbill invasion, several clearly recognized subspecies were apparently breeding side-by-side in the Adirondack Mountains of New York, with attendant conifer-cone food source segregation (Peterson, J. M. C., *Kingbird* **35**, 139 (1985))! Clearly, either present taxonomy needs revision, or population genetics and speciation theory are way off base. This is certainly a prime opportunity for the application of biochemical techniques, among others.

Population biologists not working with birds (e.g. Ehrlich and Raven 1969, Endler 1977) have questioned the premise that gene flow has a diluting effect by noting the dispersals they had studied were far less than those reported by ornithologists (e.g. Mayr 1963), and that, moreover, selection could offset the levels of gene flow they encountered. It may well be that both approaches are correct: birds (many, at least) do indeed have very great dispersal distances and this can result in demonstrably high levels of gene flow. One has only to consider the example of Snow Goose described by Rockwell and Cooke (1977). Other birds, possibly most tropical land-birds, might well have dispersal distances that approximate those found in plants (i.e. in metres rather than kilometres), such that gene flow may play a radically different role in those animals. This is an area ripe for study.

6   LIFE HISTORY VARIATION

Another important consideration is the genetic consequences of life history variation. It is here that birds should have a conspicuous edge over most other organisms, for birds have been long and well studied ecologically and in other ways pertinent to their life history traits. Indeed, in this regard we are considerably better off than *Drosophila* geneticists: witness Slatkin's lament (1985) that "only the cactophilous and Hawaiian species seem to have a life outside collecting traps". Relatively few birds, however, have had their genetics examined from a life history point of view. Snow Goose (chapter 13) is one, involving a plumage polymorphism, and the various studies on Darwin's Finches (Geospizinae) by P. R. Grant and associates represent another (updated in, among others, Price and Grant (1985), Grant *et al.* (1985), and

Grant (1985)), here involving several species and paying especial attention to quantitative traits. The Darwin's Finch work is also discussed at length in chapters 2 and 8, which provide not only an especially clear assessment of both theoretical and field techniques with quantitative traits, but the first summary of this area's progress with wild birds. Two recent reviews by Istock (1984) and Dingle (1984) provide additional broad and complementary overviews relating genetics, life history and ecology. Accurate measurement of selection under natural conditions in wild birds at varying stages in their life cycle bids fair to become one of the most important ecological genetics techniques usable by ornithologists in the future, and while it will probably not change the outcome of the neutrality–selection argument, will shed considerable light on the mechanics of avian adaptation.

7   POLYMORPHISMS AND THEIR MAINTENANCE

Chapters 1 and 4 discussed, respectively, the two major kinds of avian polymorphisms, external (plumage) and internal (biochemical), reporting in both cases mechanisms alleged to maintain them. Earlier in this summary chapter I discussed the notion now accepted by the majority of population geneticists and a growing number of ornithologists, that most allozymic alleles are selectively neutral. What of plumage polymorphisms?

The observation made in chapter 1, that none of the myriad of postulated mechanisms maintaining plumage polymorphisms has been conclusively proven, stands. There exist very good data that the light- and dark-phase Arctic Skuas on Fair Isle, Scotland, studied so extensively by O'Donald (1983; chapter 14) are maintained by sexual selection favouring darks and natural selection favouring lights, but the blue/white plumage polymorphism in Lesser Snow Geese has been attributed not to any genic balance mechanisms but merely to gene flow (chapter 13). These two cases aside, all the rest—and avian plumage polymorphisms are not rare—are open questions. In view of the findings on allozyme polymorphisms, and the frequency of fully interfertile hybrids between many disparate-appearing bird taxon-pairs, I suggest as a working null hypothesis that henceforth all avian plumage polymorphisms be considered selectively neutral, and that tests be designed solely to falsify that null hypothesis. If such falsification were demonstrated, then and only then, on a case-by-case basis, would it be reasonable to attempt falsification of carefully crafted alternative hypotheses.

This view is not to be considered anti-selection; rather it is likely that some presently unknown portion of avian morphs will prove to be maintained by selection. Their taxonomic distribution hints at some non-random patterns: raptorial and predatory birds in particular show high levels of plumage polymorphism (chapter 1), suggesting the possibility of ecological correlates, perhaps related in some way to reversed sexual-size dimorphism. But it should prove most illuminating to subject some of these systems to neutral-allele analyses in much the way that Price and Boag (chapter 8) calculated selection coefficients for bridling in Common Murres (Guillemots) (*Uria aalge*). The time has clearly come for such an approach.

8 THE GENETICS OF SPECIATION

While the bulk of this book has concerned intraspecific genetic variation, inevitably that leads to the question of when variation crosses the line between intra- and interspecific, assuming acceptance of a biological species definition, which virtually all contemporary ornithologists do. Very much early speciation theory was derived using avian models (Mayr 1942, 1963) augmented by *Drosophila* population genetics (Dobzhansky 1937, 1951). For some time, while population genetics theory expanded, speciation theory languished, reviving episodically in the 1960s and 1970s when papers for and against sympatric speciation proliferated (cf. Futuyama and Mayer (1980) for a discussion). A few books appeared in the late 1970s and early 1980s (Endler 1977,White 1978; Barigozzi *et al.* 1982), but in the 1980s interest in speciation from a population genetics point of view became heightened (e.g. Templeton 1980 a,b, 1981, Lande 1980, 1981, Nei *et al.* 1983). This led to the first integrations of population genetics and quantitative variation that actually made predictions about likely kinds of speciation events given different population structures and kinds of isolating events (as well as their absence)—thus meeting one of Lewontin's (1985 a) dicta about the "proper role" of population genetics. This is not the place for analysis of these papers, but the reader is referred to a few studies that have used these techniques on birds (*Coereba*, Wunderle 1981; *Dendroica*, Barrowclough 1980; *Colaptes*, Moore and Buchanan 1985).

The reproductive-isolation criterion familiar to most of us is an ideal not always met, for a variety of reasons. As such, it has not usually been considered absolute by ornithologists. Yet in a recent analysis of hybrid zones from a narrow but rigorous, modern population genetic point of view, Barton and Hewitt (1985) held to it absolutely: hybridization resulting in gene flow even of neutral alleles, was, by their definition, proof of conspecificity. They argued that the great majority of hybrid zones are maintained in a stable balance between dispersal and selection, however weak, and would thus not likely be on their way to complete reproductive isolation. Notwithstanding this conclusion, narrow but reasonably long-term hybrid zones occur in birds (*Corvus corone* and *cornix*; *Vermivora pinus* and *chrysoptera*; *Sphyrapicus ruber*, *nuchalis* and *varius*, etc.), and recently Grant and Price (1981) demonstrated episodic interspecific hybridization among geospizines. It has also been suggested that transposable elements (see page 469) and mtDNA (see chapter 5) effect regular transfer and likely incorporation of hereditary material among species. It seems worthwhile to investigate in birds whether our species definition should be formally modified to allow even routine passage of demonstrably neutral (or possibly even selectively non-neutral) alleles or genes between otherwise good, biological species. Theory is only beginning to address some of these questions.

Several genetic approaches to identifying species (*contra* subspecies) have been used recently. The first merely compares calculated values of genetic distance (by Nei's D, for example) between subject taxa against values for known species–species and subspecies–subspecies pairs (e.g. Barrowclough 1980). The second uses measures of genetic distance to generate phenograms and phylogenetic trees (e.g. Johnson and Zink 1985). The third is more controversial, that developed by Corbin (1983; chapter 10), where standard genetic distances (Nei's D) are regressed onto F_{ST} values, leading to what Corbin describes as two data arrays each best described by separate rectilinear regression equations, and each with high r^2 values (Fig. 8, page 348). Corbin's interpretation is that differences in the two lines are biologically as well as statistically real, the change in slope indicating speciation events via founder-effect genetic revolutions (*sensu* Mayr 1954). The technique has been dismissed by Barrowclough (1984) as invalid because (*a*) the combined datasets should be treated as one curvilinear array, not two rectilinear arrays; (*b*) D and F_{ST} are related in such a way that a curvilinear relationship is inescapable; and (*c*) in any event a genetic revolution is not indicated by such an analysis. I am aware of no detailed assessment of Corbin's technique, but such an innovative approach to a vexing problem deserves better than summary judgment. As to curvilinearity, the arrays he presents are, on inspection, much more bilinear than curvilinear, and forcing a quadratic function on them seems unwarranted.

Two recent back-to-back review papers addressed the topic of genetic revolutions and founders. Carson and Templeton (1984) concluded that founder-induced speciation via either genetic transilience or founder-flush mechanisms (but not genetic revolution) does occur, although rarely, and can be important in some organisms or situations. Barton and Charlesworth (1984) determined that rapid evolutionary divergence rarely takes place in extremely small populations, that under founder-effect speciation the probability of a genetic revolution leading to reproductive isolation is low, and that if these events have occurred, they would have been under very limiting conditions, such as in the Hawaiian *Drosophila* that Carson has so long studied. Both papers would seem to regard genetic revolutions as the exception, and not the rule, in animal speciation. The importance of gene flow, isolation, and genetic diversity thus loom large in current and future research on the speciation aspects of research in avian genetics, complementing their importance in the study of intrapopulation genetics. Basic population data as well as new theory are needed.

9   GENETICS AND CONSERVATION

While this book has not discussed the application of genetics to the conservation or protection of bird populations, some observations are relevant. First, extremely low levels of genetic diversity do not necessarily mean a population is imperilled. For one thing, small population sizes and/or certain mating patterns inevitably lead to low diversity, or even fixation of the selectively neutral alleles detected by allozyme analysis, without catastrophic results. Second, careful planning and genetical modelling can systematically increase heterozygosity, and reduce inbreeding and its consequences, or accommodate to it, in captive birds. Such as programme was designed for, and worked well with, Speke's Gazelle (*Gazella spekei*), which, from an initial captive herd in the US of only one male and three females had grown to some 29 individuals about 15 years later (Templeton and Read 1983). Inbreeding was impossible to avoid, and new genetic stock was unavailable, so Templeton and Read chose animals that already had had high breeding success under inbreeding conditions. This was augmented by equalizing the average genetic contributions of the four ancestral animals and by allowing the herd's size to increase during selection—in order to optimize conditions for genetic variability. Most if not all inbreeding depression in this small captive population was thereby eliminated.

Cade (1983) reviews the general question of gene exchange among birds as it relates to conservation. He reports on a situation that has had a grim outcome subsequent to his writing that paper. Dusky Seaside Sparrow (*Ammospiza maritima nigrescens*), an endangered taxon formerly restricted to certain marshes in eastern Florida, was sadly reduced to only five captive males. A plan was devised for essentially total reconstitution of the form's genome (subject to the very real founder effect of only five males) by hybridizing these males with females of a closely related race, *A. m. peninsulae*, according to a genetic protocol similar to that used with Speke's Gazelle. Because it was determined that this procedure would violate provisions of the Endangered Species Act forbidding hybrids [*sic*], the experiment was cancelled. As of late 1985, all but two of the original males, plus several backcrosses, remain alive and *nigrescens* as an evolutionary and genetic entity seems doomed. One hopes this kind of anti-scientific blunder will be a singularity, and that efforts to captively breed species such as California Condor (*Gyps californicus*) will follow the gazelle model instead.

Another topic on which there are no studies to my knowledge, at least involving birds, are the inter-relations of gene flow, patch size, genetic diversity, and the geometry and spacing of nature reserves. As rain forest in Amazonia and South-east Asia disappears daily, along with many species of birds, pressure increases for refuge establishment. While there has been much ecological theory addressing the question, its connection with genetic theory, and subsequent application, remains elusive. Nonetheless, especially useful starting places, are Soulé and Wilcox (1980), Frankel and Soulé (1981), and Schoenwald-Cox *et al.* (1983); the journal *Biological Conservation* consistently provides most useful contributions on these essential matters.

Although he did not address genetic questions *per se*, Reed (1980, 1983, 1985) has recently raised important empirical objections to the blanket application of biogeography theory (e.g. MacArthur and Wilson 1967, Diamond and May 1981) and specifically the use of only one variable, area, in the design of nature reserves. He argues forcefully and compellingly for incorporation of additional data such as habitat variability, proximity to colonizing sources, and turnover patterns, and developing the useful notion of "turnover triangles" (Reed 1980). Expansion of his ideas, and eventual incorporation of population genetic data, offers a prime opportunity for avian genetics and applied ecology to interact fruitfully.

10 A LAST WORD

Despite the thoroughness of coverage in this first book on the genetics of wild birds, because it is the first summary of a new field of endeavour, it is appropriate to call attention to additional topics needing more attention or clarification, or which have never been looked at in wild birds. Most of them are familiar to ornithologists with ecology or population biology interests; some pertinent references should serve as entry points. Included are the following:

(*a*) the occurrence and population genetics of transposable genetic elements, also known as TEs or transponsons, and the general question of gene flow between good species via hybridization (cf. Grant and Price 1981, Barton and Hewitt 1985), and by mtDNA, etc. (Rose and Doolittle 1983, Takahata and Slatkin 1983, Temin and Engels 1984, Syvanen 1984, Clegg and Epperson 1985);

(*b*) the evolution of sexual selection, the definition and demonstration of true female-choice mechanisms, and its role *vis-à-vis* natural selection (O'Donald 1980, 1983, Bateson 1983, Maynard-Smith 1985);

(*c*) the interaction between cultural and genetic evolution, especially with predictive, testable models (Cavalli-Sforza and Feldman 1981, Maynard-Smith and Warren 1982);

(d) assessment of the real adaptive significance of traits by direct observation of selection in action (Lande and Arnold 1983, Grant 1985);

(e) reaction-norms, developmental constraints and threshold polygenes: what limits and shapes the expression of genotypes, and the interface between qualitative and quantitative characters (Waddington 1957, Falconer 1981, Maynard Smith 1983, Cheverud 1984, Via and Lande 1985, Alberch 1985).

In this chapter I have taken a clearly non-random walk through avian genetics. While topics I have discussed or mentioned have been those that interest me, and either were not mentioned by other authors or needed additional treatment, their common thread was that I believe each should occupy a prominent place in future studies of the genetics of wild birds.

ACKNOWLEDGMENTS

Ideas, topics and approaches for inclusion in this chapter came, of course, from each of the books' constituent chapters. In addition, particularly useful suggestions and insight, with remarkable overlap, came from Francine G. Buckley, Fred Cooke, Peter Evans, Bertram G. Murray, Arie van Noordwijk, Trevor Price and Gerald F. Shields. The inspiration was theirs, the errors mine.

REFERENCES

Alberch, P. (1985). Developmental constraints: why St. Bernards often have an extra digit and poodles never do. *Am. Natur.* **126**, 430–433.

American Ornithologists' Union (1957). "Check-list of North American Birds", 5th edn. Baltimore, Maryland.

Archie, J. W. (1985). Statistical analysis of heterozygosity data: independent-sample comparisons. *Evolution* **39**, 623–637.

Avise, J. (1983). Commentary (on Barrowclough's chapter). *In* "Perspectives in Ornithology" (eds A. Brush and G. Clark), pp. 262–270. Cambridge University Press.

Ayala, F. J. and Gilpin, M. E. (1973). Lack of evidence for the neutral hypothesis of protein polymorphism. *J. Hered.* **64**, 297–298.

Barigozzi, C., Montalenti, G. and White, M. J. D. (eds) (1982). "Mechanisms of Speciation". Liss, New York.

Barrowclough, G. (1980). Genetic and phenotypic differentiation in a wood warbler (Genus *Dendroica*) hybrid zone. *Auk* **97**, 655–668.

Barrowclough, G. (1983). Biochemical studies of microevolutionary processes. *In* "Perspectives in Ornithology" (eds A. Brush and G. Clark), pp. 223–261. Cambridge University Press, New York.

Barrowclough, G. (1984). *J. Field Orn.*, **55**, 509 [review of Corbin 1983].

Barton, N. H. and Charlesworth, B. (1984). Genetic revolutions, founder effects, and speciation. *Ann. Rev. Ecol. Syst.* **15**, 133–164.

Barton, N. H. and Hewitt, G. M. (1985). Analysis of hybrid zones. *Ann. Rev. Ecol. Syst.* **16**, 113–148.

Bateson, P. (ed.) (1983). "Mate Choice". Cambridge University Press, Cambridge.

Bonnell, M. and Selander, R. K. (1974). Elephant seals: genetic variation and near-extinction. *Science* **184**, 908–909.

Botstein, D., White, R. L., Skolnick, M. and Davis, R. W. (1980). Construction of a genetic linkage map in man using restriction fragment length polymorphisms. *Am. J. Hum. Genet.* **32**, 314–331.

Braun, M. J. and Parker, T. A. (1985). Molecular, morphological and behavioral evidence concerning the taxonomic relationships of "*Synallaxis*" *gularis* and other synallaxines. *In* "Neotropical Ornithology" (eds P. A. Buckley, M. S. Foster, E. S. Morton, R. S. Ridgely and F. G. Buckley), pp. 333–346. A.O.U. *Ornithological Monographs* No. 36.

Brussard, P. F. (1984). Geographic patterns and environmental gradients: the central-marginal model in *Drosophila* revisited. *Ann. Rev. Ecol. Syst.* **15**, 25–64.

Cade, T. (1983). Hybridization and gene exchange among birds in relation to conservation. *In* "Genetics and Conservation: A Reference for Managing Wild Animal and Plant Populations" (eds C. M. Schoenwald-Cox, S. M. Chambers, B. MacBryde and L. Thomas), Chap. 18, pp. 288–309. Benjamin/Cummings, Menlo Park, California.

Camussi, A., Ottaviano, E., Calinski, T. and Kaczmarek, Z. (1985). Genetic distances based on quantitative traits. *Genetics* **111**, 945–962.

Capparella, A. P. and Lanyon, S. M. (1985). Biochemical and morphometric analyses of the sympatric, neotropical sibling species *Mionectes macconnelli* and *M. oleagineus*. *In* "Neotropical Ornithology" (eds P. A. Buckley, M. S. Foster, E. S. Morton, R. S. Ridgley and F. G. Buckley), pp. 347–359. A.O.U. *Ornithological Monographs* No. 36.

Carson, H. and Templeton, A. R. (1984). Genetic revolutions in relation to speciation phenomena: the founding of new populations. *Ann. Rev. Ecol. Syst.* **15**, 97–131.

Cavalli-Sforza, L. L. and Feldman, M. (1981). "Cultural Transmission and Evolution". Princeton University Press, Princeton.

Cheverud, J. M. (1984). Quantitative genetics and developmental constraints on evolution by selection. *J. Theor. Biol.* **110**, 155–171.

Clegg, M. T. and Epperson, B. K. (1985). Recent developments in population genetics. *Adv. Genet.* **23**, 235–269.

Corbin, K. W. (1983). Genetic structure and avian systematics. *In* "Current Ornithology" (ed. R. F. Johnston), pp. 211–244. Plenum, New York.

Diamond, J. M. and May, R. M. (1981). Island biogeography and the design of nature reserves. *In* "Theoretical Ecology: Principles and Application". 2nd edn (ed. R. May), Chap. 10, pp. 228–252. Sinauer, Sunderland, Massachusetts.

Dingle, H. (1984). Behavior, genes and life histories: complex adaptations in uncertain environments. *In* "A New Ecology: Novel Approaches to Interactive Systems" (eds P. Price, C. Slobodchikoff and W. Gaud), Chap. 6, pp. 169–194. J. Wiley & Sons, New York.

Dobzhansky, Th. (1937). "Genetics and the Origin of Species". Columbia University Press, New York.

Dobzhansky, Th. (1951). "Genetics and the Origin of Species", 3rd edn. Columbia University Press, New York.

Ehrlich, P. and Raven, P. (1969). Differentiation of populations. *Science* **165**, 1228–32.

Endler, J. (1977). "Geographic Variation, Speciation, and Clines". Princeton University Press, Princeton.

Falconer, D. S. (1981). "Introduction to Quantitative Genetics", 2nd edn. Longman, London.

Felsenstein, J. (1985 a). Confidence limits on phylogenies with a molecular clock. *Syst. Zool.* **34**, 152–161.

Felsenstein, J. (1985 b). Phylogenies from gene frequencies: a statistical problem. *Syst. Zool.* **34**, 300–311.

Felsenstein, J. (1985 c). Confidence limits on phylogenies: an approach using the bootstrap. *Evolution* **39**, 783–791.

Frankel, O. H. and Soulé, M. E. (1981). "Conservation and Evolution". Cambridge University Press, New York.

Fuerst, P. A., Chakraborty, R. and Nei, M. (1977). Statistical studies on protein polymorphism in natural populations. I. Distribution of single-locus heterozygosity. *Genetics* **86**, 465–483.

Futuyma, D. J. and Mayer, G. C. (1980). Non-allopatric speciation in animals. *Syst. Zool.* **29**, 254–271.

Grant, B. R. (1985). Selection on bill characters in a population of Darwin's Finches: *Geospiza conirostris* on Isla Genovesa, Galápagos. *Evolution* **39**, 523–532.

Grant, P. R., Abbott, I., Schluter, D., Curry, R. L. and Abbott, L. K. (1985). Variation in the size and shape of Darwin's finches. *Biol. J. Linn. Soc.* **25**, 1–39.

Grant, P. R. and Price, T. D. (1981). Population variation in continuously varying traits as an ecological genetics problem. *Am. Zool.* **21**, 795–811.

Gillespie, J. (1985). The interaction of genetic drift and mutation with selection in a fluctuating environment. *Theor. Pop. Biol.* **27**, 222–237.

Gutierrez, R. J., Zink, R. M. and Yang, S. Y. (1983). Genic variation, systematics and biogeographical relationships of some galliform birds. *Auk* **100**, 33–47.

Guttman, S. I., Grau, G. A. and Karlin, A. A. (1980). Genetic variation in Lake Erie Great Blue Herons (*Ardea herodias*). *Comp. Biochem. Physiol.* **66B**, 167–169.

Gyllensten, U., Wharton, D. and Wilson, A. C. (1985). Maternal inheritance of mitochondrial DNA during backcrossing of two species of mice. *J. Hered.* **76**, 321–324.

Hartl, D. L. and Dykhuizen, D. E. (1981). Potential for selection among nearly neutral allozymes of 6-phosphogluconate dehydrogenase in *Escherichia coli*. *Proc. Natl Acad. Sci. USA* **78**, 6344–6388.

Hedrick, P. W., Ginevan, M. E. and Ewing, E. P. (1976). Genetic polymorphism in heterogeneous environments. *Ann. Rev. Ecol. Syst.* **7**, 1–32.

Hubby, J. L. and Lewontin, R. C. (1966). A molecular approach to the study of genic heterozygosity in natural populations. I. The number of alleles at different loci in *Drosophila pseudoobscura*. *Genetics* **54**, 577–594.

Istock, C. A. (1984). Boundaries to life history variation and evolution. *In* "A New Ecology: Novel Approaches to Interactive Systems" (eds P. Price, C. Slobodchikoff and W. Gaud), Chap. 5, pp. 143–168. J. Wiley & Sons, New York.

Johnson, N. K., Barrowclough, G. F. and Zink, R. M. (1985). On the nature of genic variation in birds. *In* "Current Ornithology", Vol. 2 (ed. R. Johnston), Chap. 4, pp. 135–154. Plenum, New York.

Johnson, N. K. and Zink, R. M. (1985). Genetic evidence for relationships among the Red-eyed, Yellow-green and Chivi Vireos. *Wilson Bull.* **97**, 421–435.

Kimura, M. (1968 a). Evolutionary rate at the molecular level. *Nature* **217**, 624–626.

Kimura, M. (1968 b). Genetic variability maintained in a finite population due to mutational production of neutral and nearly neutral isoalleles. *Genet. Res.* **11**, 247–269.

Kimura, M. (1983). "The Neutral Theory of Molecular Evolution". Cambridge University Press, Cambridge.

King, J. L. and Jukes, T. H. (1969). Non-Darwinian evolution. *Science* **164**, 788–798.

Knox, A. G. (1976). The taxonomic status of the Scottish Crossbill *Loxia* sp. *Bull. Br. Orn. Club* **96**, 15–19.

Lande, R. (1980). Genetic variation and phenotypic evolution during allopatric speciation. *Am. Natur.* **116**, 464–479.

Lande, R. (1981). Models of speciation by sexual selection on polygenic traits. *Proc. Natl Acad. Sci. USA* **78**, 3721–3725.

Lande, R. and Arnold, S. (1983). The measurement of selection on correlated characters. *Evolution* **37**, 1210–1226.

Lewontin, R. C. (1974). "The Genetic Basis of Evolutionary Change". Columbia University Press, New York.

Lewontin, R. C. (1984). Detecting population differences in quantitative characters as opposed to gene frequencies. *Am. Natur.* **123**, 115–124.

Lewontin, R. C. (1985 a). Population genetics. *In* "Evolution: Essays in Honor of John Maynard-Smith" (eds P. J. Greenwood, P. H. Harvey and M. Slatkin), pp. 3–18. Cambridge University Press, Cambridge.

Lewontin, R. C. (1985 b). Population genetics. *Ann. Rev. Genet.* **19**, 81–102.

Lewontin, R. C. and Hubby, J. L. (1966). A molecular approach to the study of genic heterozygosity in natural populations. II. Amount of variation and degree of heterozygosity in natural populations of *Drosophila pseudoobscura*. *Genetics* **54**, 595–609.

Li, W.-H. (1978). Maintenance of genetic variability under the joint effect of mutation, selection and random drift. *Genetics* **90**, 349–382.

MacArthur, R. H. and Wilson, E. O. (1967). "Theory of Island Biogeography". Princeton University Press.

Maruyama, T. and Kimura, M. (1974). Geographical uniformity of selectively neutral polymorphisms. *Nature* **249**, 30–32.

Maruyama, T. and Kimura, M. (1980). Genetic variability of effective population size when local extinction and recolonization of subpopulations are frequent. *Proc. Natl Acad. Sci. USA* **77**, 6710–6714.

Maynard Smith, J. (1983). The genetics of stasis and punctuation. *Ann. Rev. Genet.* **17**, 11–25.

Maynard Smith, J. (1985). Sexual selection, handicaps and true fitness. *J. Theor. Biol.* **115**, 1–8.

Maynard Smith, J. and Hoekstra, R. (1980). Polymorphism in a varied environment. How robust are the models? *Genet. Res.* **35**, 45–57.

Maynard Smith, J. and Warren, N. (1982). Models of cultural and genetic change. *Evolution* **36**, 620–627.

Mayr, E. (1942). "Systematics and the Origin of Species". Columbia University Press, New York.

Mayr, E. (1954). Change of genetic environment and evolution. *In* "Evolution as a Process" (eds J. Huxley, A. J. Hardy and E. B. Ford), pp. 157–180. Allen & Unwin, London.

Mayr, E. (1963). "Animal Species and Evolution". Bellknap Press of Harvard University, Cambridge, Massachusetts.

Michod, R. E. and Hamilton, W. D. (1980). Coefficients of relatedness in sociobiology. *Nature* **288**, 694–697.

Moore, W. S. and Buchanan, D. B. (1985). Stability of the Northern Flicker hybrid zone in historical times: implications for adaptive speciation theory. *Evolution* **39**, 135–151.

Mueller, L. D., Barr, L. G. and Ayala, F. J. (1985). Natural selection vs. random drift: evidence from temporal variation in allele frequencies in nature. *Genetics* **111**, 517–554.

Nei, M. and Grauer, D. (1984). Extent of protein polymorphism and the neutral mutation theory. *Evol. Biol.* **17**, 73–118.

Nei, M., Maruyama, T. and Wu, C.-I. (1983). Models of evolution of reproductive isolation. *Genetics* **103**, 557–579.

Nevo, E. (1978). Genetic variation in natural populations: pattern and theory. *Theor. Pop. Biol.* **13**, 121–177.

O'Donald, P. (1980). "Genetic Models of Sexual Selection". Cambridge University Press, Cambridge.

O'Donald, P. (1983). "The Arctic Skua: A Study of the Ecology and Evolution of a Seabird". Cambridge University Press, Cambridge.

Price, T. D. and Grant, P. R. (1985). The evolution of ontogeny in Darwin's Finches: a quantitative genetic approach. *Am. Natur.* **125**, 169–188.

Redfield, J. A., Zwickel, F. C., Bendell, J. F. and Bergerud, A. J. (1972). Temporal and spatial patterns of allele and genotype frequencies at the *Ng* locus in Blue Grouse (*Dendragapus obscurus*). *Can. J. Zool.* **50**, 1657–1662.

Reed, T. M. (1980). Turnover frequency in island birds. *J. Biogeog.* **7**, 329–335.

Reed, T. M. (1983). The role of species-area relationships in reserve choice: a British example. *Biol. Cons.* **25**, 263–271.

Reed, T. M. (1985). Island biogeographic theory in bird conservation: an alternative approach. "Conservation of Island Birds" (ed. P. J. Moors), pp. 23–33. ICBP Tech. Publ. No. 3.

Rockwell, R. F. and Cooke, F. (1977). Gene flow and local adaptation in a colonially nesting dimorphic bird: the Lesser Snow Goose. *Am. Natur.* **111**, 91–97.

Rose, M. R. and Doolittle, W. F. (1983). Molecular biological mechanisms of speciation. *Science* **220**, 157–162.

Schoenwald-Cox, C. M., Chambers, S. M., MacBryde, B. and Thomas, L. (eds) (1983). "Genetics and Conservation: A Reference for Managing Wild Animals and Plant Populations". Benjamin/Cummings, Menlo Park, California.

Schwartz, O. A. and Armitage, K. B. (1983). Problems in the use of genetic similarity to show relatedness. *Evolution* **37**, 417–420.

Sibley, C. G. and Ahlquist, J. E. (1980). The relationships of the "primitive insect eaters" (Aves: Passeriformes) as indicated by DNA–DNA hybridization. *Proc. 17th Int. Orn. Congr.*, pp. 1215–1220.

Sibley, C. G. and Ahlquist, J. E. (1983). Phylogeny and classification of birds based on the data of FNA–DNA hybridization. *In* "Current Ornithology", Vol. 1 (ed. R. Johnston), Chap. 9, pp. 245–292. Plenum, New York.

Sibley, C. G. and Ahlquist, J. E. (1985). Phylogeny and classification of New World suboscine passerine birds (Passeriformes:Oligomyodi:Tyrannides). *In* "Neotropical Ornithology" (eds P. A. Buckley, M. S. Foster, E. S. Morton, R. S. Ridgely and F. G. Buckley), pp. 396–428. A.O.U. *Ornithological Monographs* No. 36.

Simon, C. and Archie, J. (1985). An empirical demonstration of the lability of heterozygosity estimates. *Evolution* **39**, 463–467.

Sittmann, K. (1984). Sex determination in birds: progeny of nondisjunction canaries of Durham (1926). *Genet. Res.* **43**, 173–180.

Slatkin, M. (1977). Gene flow and genetic drift in a species subject to frequent local extinctions. *Theor. Pop. Biol.* **12**, 253–262.

Slatkin, M. (1985). Gene flow in natural populations. *Ann. Rev. Ecol. Syst.* **16**, 393–430.

Soulé, M. E. and Wilcox, B. A. (1980). "Conservation Biology; An Evolutionary-Ecological Perspective". Sinauer, Sunderland, Massachussetts.

Syvanen, M. (1984). The evolutionary implications of mobile genetic elements. *Ann. Rev. Genet.* **18**, 271–293.

Takahata, N. and Slatkin, M. (1983). Evolutionary dynamics of extranuclear genes. *Genet. Res.* **42**, 257–265.

Temin, H. M. and Engels, W. E. (1984). Movable genetic elements and evolution. *In* "Evolutionary Theory: Paths into the Future" (ed. J. W. Pollard), Chap. 7. pp. 173–201. J. Wiley & Sons, Chichester, England.

Templeton, A. R. (1980 a). The theory of speciation via the founder principle. *Genetics* **94**, 101,1–1038.

Templeton, A. R. (1980 b). Modes of speciation and inferences based on genetic distances. *Evolution* **34**, 719–729.

Templeton, A. R. (1981). Mechanisms of speciation—a population genetic approach. *Ann. Rev. Ecol. Syst.* **12**, 23–48.

Templeton, A. and Read. B. (1983). The elimination of inbreeding depression in a captive herd of Speke's Gazelle. *In* "Genetics and Conservation: A Reference for Managing Wild Animals and Plant Populations" (eds C. M. Schoenwald-Cox, S. M. Chambers, B. MacBryde and L. Thomas), Chap. 15, pp. 241–261.

Thorpe, J. P. (1982). The molecular clock hypothesis: biochemical evolution, genetic differentiation, and systematics. *Ann. Rev. Ecol. Syst.* **13**, 139–168.

Vaurie, C. (1959). "The Birds of the Palaearctic Fauna". Vol. 1 "Passeriformes". Witherby, London.

Via, S. and Lande, R. (1985). Genotype–environment interactions and the evolution of phenotypic plasticity. *Evolution* **39**, 505–522.

Waddington, C. (1957). "The Strategy of the Genes". Allen & Unwin, London.

Weir, B. S. and Cockerham, C. C. (1984). Estimating *F*-statistics for the analysis of population structure. *Evolution* **38**, 1358–1370.

White, M. J. D. (1978). "Modes of Speciation". Freeman & Co., San Francisco.

Wilkinson, G. S. and McCracken, G. F. (1985). On estimating relatedness using genetic markers. *Evolution* **39**, 1169–1174.

Wunderle, J. (1981). An analysis of a morph-ratio cline in the Bananaquit (*Coereba flaveola*) on Grenada, West Indies. *Evolution* **35**, 333–344.

Zink, R. M. and Winkler, D. W. (1983). Genetic and morphological similarity of two California Gull populations with different life history traits. *Biochem. Syst. Ecol.* **11**, 397–403.

Index

МИНОХИМ